Register Now for Online Access to Your Book!

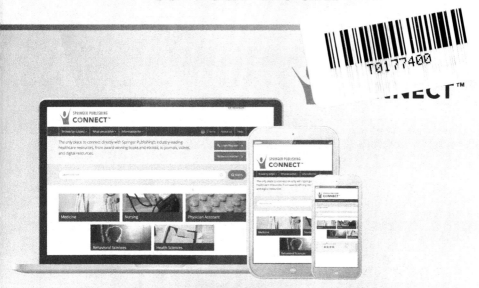

Your print purchase of *Laboratory Screening and Diagnostic Evaluation: An Evidence-Based Approach,* **includes online access to the contents of your book**—increasing accessibility, portability, and searchability!

Access today at:

http://connect.springerpub.com/content/reference-book/978-0-8261-8843-4
or scan the QR code at the right with your smartphone. Log in or register, then click "Redeem a voucher" and use the code below.

5M6G9DWV

Scan here for quick access.

Having trouble redeeming a voucher code?
Go to https://connect.springerpub.com/redeeming-voucher-code

If you are experiencing problems accessing the digital component of this product, please contact our customer service department at cs@ springerpub.com

The online access with your print purchase is available at the publisher's discretion and may be removed at any time without notice.

Publisher's Note: New and used products purchased from third-party sellers are not guaranteed for quality, authenticity, or access to any included digital components.

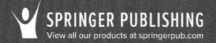

SPRINGER PUBLISHING
View all our products at springerpub.com

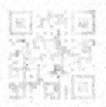

LABORATORY SCREENING AND DIAGNOSTIC EVALUATION

Kelly Small Casler, DNP, APRN-CNP, CHSE, is an assistant professor of clinical nursing at The Ohio State University College of Nursing where she teaches in the Family Nurse Practitioner program. She also teaches in the Doctor of Nursing Practice program and is a doctoral project advisor. Dr. Casler launched her nursing career at the University of Missouri-Columbia where she earned her bachelor of science in nursing (2001) and master of science (2006) degrees. She earned her doctor of nursing practice (2018) from the University of Kansas School of Nursing where her doctoral work focused on primary care of nonalcoholic fatty liver disease. She is a certified healthcare simulation educator (CHSE) and holds a certificate of added qualification in evidence-based practice from the Fuld Institute for Evidence-Based Practice in Nursing and HealthCare. A former ICU and trauma/burn nurse, she now works as a family nurse practitioner at The HealthCare Connection, a federally qualified health clinic in Northern Cincinnati, where you are likely to see an NP student by her side. She resides in Bellbrook, Ohio, with her husband, David, a lieutenant colonel in the United States Air Force, and her sons, Zach and Caleb.

Kate Sustersic Gawlik, DNP, APRN-CNP, FAANP, FNAP, graduated with her doctorate of nursing practice from The Ohio State University and is certified by the American Nurses Credentialing Center as a family nurse practitioner. She also serves as the director of undergraduate health and wellness academic programming, the co-director of Bachelor of Science in Health and Wellness program, and the project manager for the Million Hearts initiatives at The Ohio State University College of Nursing. She has experience in family practice, college health, urgent care, and reproductive care with clinical interests in evidence-based practice, population health, preventive medicine, clinician well-being, education of health professionals, wellness, parental burnout, and cardiovascular disease prevention. Dr. Gawlik is an associate professor of clinical nursing at The Ohio State University. She has taught a variety of undergraduate and graduate nursing courses and serves as a clinical preceptor for advanced practice nursing students. Dr. Gawlik was awarded the Outstanding Faculty Award in 2013 and the Outstanding Leadership Award in 2017. In 2018, she received the American Association of Nurse Practitioners State Award for Excellence for Ohio and was inducted as a Fellow of the American Association of Nurse Practitioners. She is a fellow of the National Academies of Practice. She is co-editor and author of *Evidence-Based Physical Examination: Best Practices for Health and Well-Being Assessment, Evidence-Based Physical Examination Handbook,* and *Assessment and Diagnosis Review for APRN Certification Exams.* She resides in Bexley, Ohio.

LABORATORY SCREENING AND DIAGNOSTIC EVALUATION

AN EVIDENCE-BASED APPROACH

Kelly Small Casler, DNP, APRN-CNP, CHSE
Kate Sustersic Gawlik, DNP, APRN-CNP, FAANP, FNAP

Editors

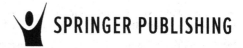

SPRINGER PUBLISHING

Springer Publishing Company, LLC
11 West 42nd Street, New York, NY 10036
www.springerpub.com
connect.springerpub.com/

Executive Acquisitions Editor: Joseph Morita
Director, Content Development: Taylor Ball
Compositor: Amnet

ISBN: 978-0-8261-4087-6
ebook ISBN: 978-0-8261-4093-7
DOI: 10.1891/9780826140937

24 25 / 5 4

Medicine is an ever-changing science. Research and clinical experience are continually expanding
our knowledge, in particular our understanding of proper treatment and drug therapy. The authors, editors, and publisher have made every effort to ensure that all information in this book is in
accordance with the state of knowledge at the time of production of the book. Nevertheless, the authors, editors, and publisher are not responsible for any errors or omissions or for any consequence
from application of the information in this book and make no warranty, expressed or implied, with
respect to the content of this publication. Every reader should examine carefully the package inserts
accompanying each drug and should carefully check whether the dosage schedules therein or the
contraindications stated by the manufacturer differ from the statements made in this book. Such
examination is particularly important with drugs that are either rarely used or have been newly
released on the market.

Library of Congress Cataloging-in-Publication Data:

Names: Casler, Kelly Small, editor. | Gawlik, Kate, editor.
Title: Laboratory screening and diagnostic evaluation : an evidence-based
    approach / Kelly Small Casler, Kate Gawlik.
Description: New York : Springer Publishing Company, 2022. | Includes
    bibliographical references and index.
Identifiers: LCCN 2021058389 (print) | LCCN 2021058390 (ebook) | ISBN
    9780826140876 (paperback) | ISBN 9780826140937 (ebook)
Subjects: LCSH: Medical laboratory technology—Congresses. | Medical
    laboratory technology—Congresses.
Classification: LCC RB37 (print) | LCC RB37 (ebook) | DDC
    616.07/5—dc23/eng/20220204
LC record available at https://lccn.loc.gov/2021058389
LC ebook record available at https://lccn.loc.gov/2021058390

Printed in the United States of America by Gasch Printing.

To my husband, David, who is my rock
and who believes in and unconditionally supports me;
To my nieces, Leah and Cora, who taught me how to be a mom;
To my sons, Zach and Caleb, who remind me of the importance
of play and who even in their young ages understood
my passion for this project (but were excited when
"mommy's book" was finally done); To my parents,
Jim & Debbie, who launched my career by assisting me with
my undergraduate education; To my sisters, Katie and Kim,
who let me practice my "leadership" skills on them growing up;
To my early nursing career mentors in Missouri who taught me
what it truly meant to be a nurse and nurse practitioner;
To The Ohio State University College of Nursing for giving
me a place to grow my passion for nursing excellence and
for supporting this work; To my co-editor, Kate, and our multiple
contributors—this book would not have been possible without
your expertise and dedication to collaboration.

—Kelly Small Casler

I dedicate this book to the wonderful friends, mentors,
and colleagues that I have been so fortunate to have in my life.

I dedicate this book to the best friends anyone could ever ask for—to Jenny,
Roberta, and Chesáre. You never have friends like you do when you were young.
They know where you have been and where you are capable of going.
Most people never have what we have together, an eternal bond that
will withstand the test of time. You are truly remarkable women and
I am so lucky to have you in my life. From the airplane to the nursing home…

To Bernadette Melnyk, the best mentor anyone could ever ask to have.
The support and guidance you have given me over the last 10 years
goes beyond words. To Alice, I couldn't do it without you.
To Kelly, I was the lucky one that you asked me to be part of this project.
Your passion and drive are evident in all that you do.

To all of the readers, clinicians, and students who use this text,
may you always surround yourself with people who inspire you to do more,
see more, and be more.

—Kate Sustersic Gawlik

CONTENTS

III. Evidence-Based Use of Individual Laboratory Tests

RELEVANT TESTS BY BODY SYSTEM

Evidence-Based Use of Laboratory Tests for Cardiovascular Conditions

Evidence-Based Use of Laboratory Tests for Dermatologic Conditions

Evidence-Based Use of Laboratory Tests for Endocrine and Metabolic Conditions

Evidence-Based Use of Laboratory Tests for Gastrointestinal Conditions

Evidence-Based Use of Laboratory Tests for Genitourinary Conditions

Evidence-Based Use of Laboratory Tests for Hematologic and Oncologic Conditions

Evidence-Based Use of Laboratory Tests for Rheumatologic, Immunologic, and Infectious Conditions

Evidence-Based Use of Laboratory Tests for Psychiatric and Neurologic Conditions

Evidence-Based Use of Laboratory Tests for Eye, Ear, Nose, Throat, and Respiratory Conditions

CONTRIBUTORS

Annie Abraham, DNP, APRN, FNP-BC

Clinical Assistant Professor
Louise Herrington School of Nursing
Baylor University
Dallas, Texas

Janyce Cagan Agruss, PhD, APRN, FNP-BC

Associate Professor
Department of Community, Systems and Mental Health Nursing
College of Nursing
Rush University Medical Center
Chicago, Illinois

Olga Amusina, DNP, APRN, ACNP

University of Illinois at Chicago College of Nursing
Chicago, Illinois
NorthShore University HealthSystem
Evanston, Illinois

Anthony M. Angelow, PhD, APN, ACNPC, AGACNP-BC, FAEN, FAANP

Chair, Advanced Practice Nursing
Assistant Clinical Professor
College of Nursing and Health Professions
Drexel University
Philadelphia, Pennsylvania

M. Danielle Atchley, DNP, FNP-C, CPN

Clinical Assistant Professor FNP/MSN Program
Dr. Susan L. Davis, RN & Richard J. Henley College of Nursing
Sacred Heart University
Fairfield, Connecticut;
Family Nurse Practitioner
The Family Clinic
Starkville, Mississippi

LouAnn B. Bailey, DNP, APRN, ACNP-BC, FAANP

Hospitalist Nurse Practitioner
Metro Health Medical Center
Richfield, Ohio

Heidi Bobek, DNP, APRN, FNP-BC

Assistant Professor of Clinical Practice
Family Nurse Practitioner
The Ohio State University College of Nursing
Columbus, Ohio

Melissa Bogle, DNP, FNP-BC, ACNP-BC

Instructor, Southern Illinois University Edwardsville
Family Nurse Practitioner / Acute Care Nurse Practitioner
BJC Alton Memorial Convenient Care
Edwardsville, Illinois

Leah Burt, PhD, APRN, ANP-BC

Clinical Assistant Professor
Director, Adult-Gerontology Primary Care Nurse Practitioner Program
University of Illinois at Chicago
College of Nursing
Chicago, Illinois

Meleana Burt, DNP, APRN-CNP

Adult Nurse Practitioner
The Ohio State University Wexner Medical Center
Columbus, Ohio

Cara A. Busenhart, PhD, APRN, CNM, FACNM

Program Director, Advanced Practice | Program Director, Nurse-Midwifery
Clinical Associate Professor
University of Kansas School of Nursing
Certified Nurse-Midwife
The University of Kansas Health System
Kansas City, Kansas

Jill S. Buterbaugh, DNP, CRNP, FNP-BC, CNE

Assistant Professor of Nursing
Frostburg State University
Frostburg, Maryland

Taylor Butler, PharmD, BCOP, BCPS

Oncology Clinical Pharmacy Specialist
Vanderbilt-Ingram Cancer Center
Nashville, Tennessee

Penelope Callaway, DNP, APRN, FNP-C

Assistant Professor of Nursing
Division of Doctoral Nursing
Family Nurse Practitioner
Indiana Wesleyan University
Marion, Indiana

Carol D. Campbell, DNP, APRN, PMHCNS-BC, PMHNP-BC, FNP-C

Clinical Assistant Professor
College of Nursing
University of Arkansas for Medical Sciences
Little Rock, Arkansas

Kelly Small Casler, DNP, APRN-CNP, CHSE

Assistant Professor of Clinical Nursing
The Ohio State University College of Nursing
Columbus, Ohio;
Family Nurse Practitioner
The HealthCare Connection
Lincoln Heights, Ohio

Amanda Chaney, DNP, APRN, FAANP, AF-AASLD

Nurse Practitioner, Department of Transplant
Chair, Advance Practice Provider Subcommittee
Assistant Professor of Medicine, College of Medicine & Science
Associate in Transplant Medicine
Mayo Clinic
Jacksonville, Florida

Beth Ann Clayton, DNP, CRNA, FAAN

Professor of Clinical Nursing
Director, Nurse Anesthesia Major
University of Cincinnati
Cincinnati, Ohio

Christine Colella, DNP, APRN-CNP, FAANP

Professor and Executive Director of Graduate Programs
Adult Nurse Practitioner
College of Nursing
University of Cincinnati
Cincinnati, Ohio

Susan Corbridge, PhD, APRN, FAANP, FCCP, FAAN

Clinical Professor Emerita of Behavioral Nursing Science
University of Illinois at Chicago College of Nursing
Chicago, Illinois

Kathryn Deshotels, MSN, APRN, FNP-BC

Clinical Assistant Professor
School of Nursing
Sam Houston State University
Huntsville, Texas

Rachel M. Donner, MS, MLS (ASCP)CM

Clinical Laboratory Scientist
Life Sciences Testing Center
Northeastern University
Burlington, Massachusetts

Stephanie C. Evans, PhD, APRN, CPNP-PC, CLC

Assistant Professor
Pediatric Nurse Practitioner
Texas Woman's University
College of Nursing
Dallas, Texas;
Kid Care Pediatrics
Keller, Texas

Beth Faiman, PhD, MSN, APRN-BC, AOCN, FAAN

Department of Hematology and Medical Oncology
Cleveland Clinic Taussig Cancer Institute
Cleveland, Ohio

Sarah Fitz, DNP, APRN, ACNP-BC

Clinical Assistant Professor
Department of Biobehavioral Nursing Science
University of Illinois at Chicago
College of Nursing
Chicago, Illinois

Kate Sustersic Gawlik, DNP, APRN-CNP, FAANP, FNAP

Associate Professor of Clinical Nursing
Family Nurse Practitioner
The Ohio State University
Columbus, Ohio

Retha D. Gentry, DNP, FNP-C

Associate Professor, Graduate Programs
College of Nursing
East Tennessee State University
Johnson City, Tennessee

Darla Gowan, DNP, FNP-BC

Associate Dean of Nurse Practitioner Programs
School of Nursing
IWU-National & Global
Indiana Wesleyan University
Marion, Indiana

Matthew Granger, MS, APRN-CNP

Family Nurse Practitioner
Wexner Medical Center Ross Heart Hospital
The Ohio State University
Columbus, Ohio

Christopher G. Green, PharmD, MSN, APRN-CNP

Family Nurse Practitioner
Community Health & Wellness Partners of Logan County
West Liberty, Ohio

Debra Hain, PhD, APRN, AGPCNP-BC, FAAN, FAANP, FNKF

Professor (tenured), Graduate Coordinator, AGNP Concentration
Florida Atlantic University
Christine E. Lynn College of Nursing
Boca Raton, Florida

Karen Hande, DNP, ANP-BC, CNE, FAANP

Associate Professor
Nurse Practitioner, Supportive Oncology Care
Vanderbilt University School of Nursing
Nashville, Tennessee

Audra Hanners, DNP, APRN-CNP, EBP-C

Assistant Professor of Clinical Practice
The Ohio State University College of Nursing
Family Nurse Practitioner
Columbus, Ohio

Joelle D. Hargraves, DNP, APRN, CCRN-K, CCNS

Associate Professor of Instruction, Undergraduate Program Director
Department of Nursing
College of Public Health
Temple University
Philadelphia, Pennsylvania

Cara Harris, DNP, APRN-CNP, CDCES

Certified Diabetes Care and Education Specialist
Wexner Medical Center East Hospital
The Ohio State University
Columbus, Ohio

Heidi He, DNP, FNP-C

Associate Professor
California State University–Bakersfield
Family Nurse Practitioner
Comprehensive Pulmonary and Critical Care Associates
Bakersfield, California

Danielle Hebert, DNP, MBA, MSN, ANP-BC

Professor of Practice, Nursing
Froelich School of Nursing
Assumption University
Adult Nurse Practitioner
UMass Community Healthlink
Worcester, Massachusetts

Kelli M. Hiller, EdD, MLS (ASCP)CM

Bristol Community College
Fall River, Massachusetts;
Massasoit Community College
Canton, Massachusetts;
Labouré College of Healthcare
Milton, Massachusetts

Deanna Hunt, MS, APRN-CNP

Assistant Professor of Clinical Nursing
Mount Carmel College of Nursing
Columbus, Ohio

Rebecca Hunt, RN, AGNP-BC, MSN

Nurse Practitioner
Stanford HealthCare
Stanford, California

Lynne M. Hutchison, DNP, FNP-BC

Assistant Professor
Chair, Department of Nursing and Health Professions
University of South Carolina Beaufort
Bluffton, South Carolina

Dayna Jaynstein, MSPAS, PA-C, EM-CAQ

Assistant Director, Faculty
Emergency Medicine PA-C
Red Rocks Community College Physician Assistant Program
Denver, Colorado

Lucia M. Jenkusky, DNP, APRN-CNM, C-EFM, FACNM, EBP-C

Assistant Professor of Clinical Practice
Director, Nurse-Midwifery and Women's Health Specialty Tracks
The Ohio State University
Columbus, Ohio

Kimberly R. Joo, DNP, APRN-NP, CNE, EBP-C

Lead Advanced Practice Provider for Urgent Care and Kids Express
Dayton Children's Hospital
Dayton, Ohio;
Assistant Professor
The Ohio State University College of Nursing
Columbus, Ohio

Jane Faith Kapustin, PhD, CRNP, BC-ADM, FAANP, FAAN

Nurse Practitioner
Riverside Medical Associates
Riverdale, Maryland

Pam Kibbe, DNP, APRN-CNP

Associate Clinical Instructor
The Ohio State University College of Nursing
Adult Nurse Practitioner, Hepatology
The Ohio State University Wexner Medical Center
Columbus, Ohio

Elizabeth Kirchner, DNP

Department of Rheumatic and Immunologic Diseases
Cleveland Clinic
Cleveland, Ohio

Nicole Peters Kroll, PhD, APRN, ANP-C, FNP-BC

Clinical Assistant Professor
Dr. Susan L. Davis, RN, & Richard J. Henley College of Nursing
Sacred Heart University
Fairfield, Connecticut

Shannon L. Linder, DNP, APRN-CNP, FNP-BC, PMHNP-BC

Assistant Professor of Clinical Practice
The Ohio State University College of Nursing
Columbus, Ohio

Samara Linnell, MSN, APRN-CNP

Benign Hematology—Family Nurse Practitioner
The Ohio State University Wexner Medical Center and James Cancer Hospital
Columbus, Ohio

Kristopher R. Maday, MS, PA-C, DFAAPA

Program Director, Physician Assistant Program
Associate Professor
University of Tennessee Health Science Center
Memphis, Tennessee

Stephanie L. Marrs, MSN, FNP-BC

Infectious Diseases Nurse Practitioner
Veterans Administration
Oklahoma City, Oklahoma

Randee L. Masciola, DNP, APRN-CNP, WHNP-BC, FAANP

Women's Health Nurse Practitioner
The Ohio State University
Columbus, Ohio

Carolyn McClerking, DNP, APRN-CNP, ACNP-BC

Assistant Professor of Clinical Nursing
Director, Adult Acute Care Nurse Practitioner Program
The Ohio State University College of Nursing
Acute Care Nurse Practitioner
Wexner Medical Center James Cancer Hospital
Columbus, Ohio

Donna Faye McHaney, DNP, MIS, APRN, FNP-C

Clinical Associate Professor
Sacred Heart University
Fairfield, Connecticut

Kymberlee Montgomery, DNP, APRN, WHNP-BC, CNE, FNAP, FAANP, FAAN

Senior Associate Dean of Nursing
Drexel University College of Nursing & Health Professions
Philadelphia, Pennsylvania

Emily Neiman, MS, APRN-CNM, FACNM, C-EFM

Certified Nurse Midwife
The Ohio State University College of Nursing
Columbus, Ohio

Bridget O'Brien, DNP, APRN, FNP-BC, AOCNP

Assistant Professor and Director of Family Nurse Practitioner Program
Rush University College of Nursing
Chicago, Illinois

Kathleen O'Neill, NP

Nurse Practitioner
Dana-Farber Cancer Institute
Boston, Massachusetts

Lisa E. Ousley, DNP, FNP-C

Assistant Professor, Graduate Programs
College of Nursing
East Tennessee State University
Johnson City, Tennessee

Tyler Parisien, EdD, MLS (ASCP)CM

Turtle Mountain Community College
Belcourt, North Dakota

Oralea A. Pittman, DNP, FNP-BC, FAANP

Family Nurse Practitioner
The Ohio State University College of Nursing
Columbus, Ohio

Elyssa Power, FNP-BC

Family Nurse Practitioner
Dana-Farber Cancer Institute
Boston, Massachusetts

John Prickett, MSPAS, PA-C

The James Cancer Hospital, Richard Solove Research Institute
Wexner Medical Center
The Ohio State University
Columbus, Ohio

Danielle A. Quallich, BS

Detroit Medical Center's Children's Hospital of Michigan
General Pediatrics and Adolescent Medicine Clinic
Detroit, Michigan

Susanne A. Quallich, PhD, ANP-BC, NP-C, CUNP, FAANP

Nurse Practitioner, Division of Andrology and Urologic Health
Department of Urology
Michigan Medicine
Ann Arbor, Michigan

Brooke Rengers, MPH, MS, APRN-CNP

Instructor of Clinical Practice
The Ohio State University College of Nursing
Women's Health Nurse Practitioner
The Ohio State University College of Medicine
Columbus, Ohio

Sara Revelle, DNP, APRN-BC, FNP-BC, GNP-BC, NCMP

Family Nurse Practitioner
Boone Health Medical Group;
Adjunct Assistant Professor
University of Missouri Sinclair School of Nursing
Columbia, Missouri

Barbara Rogers, CRNP, MN, AOCN, ANP-BC

Adult Nurse Practitioner
Temple University Fox Chase Cancer Center
Philadelphia, Pennsylvania

Jonathan D. Savant, MHS, PA-C

Physician Assistant
Children's Hospital of Philadelphia
Kidney Transplant Program
Philadelphia, Pennsylvania

Courtney Sexton, MS, CRNP, CPNP-PC

Pediatric Nurse Practitioner
State College, Pennsylvania;
Ideal Pediatric & Adolescent Care
Lewisburg, Pennsylvania

Elizabeth Sharpe, DNP, APRN-CNP, NNP-BC, FAANP, FAAN

Associate Professor of Clinical Nursing
The Ohio State University College of Nursing
Columbus, Ohio

Courtney DuBois Shihabuddin, DNP, APRN-CNP

Assistant Professor of Clinical Nursing
Adult Gerontology Primary Care Nurse Practitioner
The Ohio State University College of Nursing
Columbus, Ohio

Candice Short, DNP, FNP-C, RN

Assistant Professor/Family Nurse Practitioner
East Tennessee State University
Johnson City, Tennessee

Ryan Short, MSN, FNP-BC, RN

Family Nurse Practitioner
Ballad Health Medical Associates, Pulmonology
Kingsport, Tennessee

Rachel Smith-Steinert, DNP, CRNA

Assistant Professor of Clinical Nursing
Assistant Program Director of Nurse Anesthesia Major
University of Cincinnati
Cincinnati, Ohio

Catherine A. Stubin, PhD, RN, CNE, CCRN

Assistant Professor
Rutgers University Camden
Camden, New Jersey

Zachary Stutzman, MS, PA-C, ATC
Physician Assistant
AMITA Orthopedics
Bolingbrook, Illinois

Sean M. Tafuri, BS
Medical Student
California Northstate University College of Medicine
Elk Grove, California

Nancy C. Tkacs, PhD, RN
Associate Professor Emerita
University of Pennsylvania School of Nursing
Philadelphia, Pennsylvania

Tammy L. Tyree, MSN, ACNP-BC, CCRN, CNRN, RNFA
Penn State College of Nursing
University Park, Pennsylvania

Lisa Ward, MS, PA-C
Physician Assistant
Department of Endocrinology/Oncology
The James Cancer Hospital
Columbus, Ohio

Mailey Wilks, DNP, MSN, APRN, NP-C
Nurse Practitioner, Outpatient APRN/PA Coordinator
Department of Hematology and Medical Oncology
Cleveland Clinic Taussig Cancer Institute
Cleveland, Ohio

Lindsay Jamison Wolf, DNP, APRN, CPNP-BC, CNE, CLC
Assistant Professor of Nursing
Director, Graduate Nursing Programs
Keigwin School of Nursing
Brooks Rehabilitation College of Healthcare Sciences
Jacksonville University
Jacksonville, Florida

Elizabeth Wright, MSN, APRN, CNE
Indiana Wesleyan University
Marion, Indiana

Kathleen Wyne, MD, PhD, FACE, FNLA
Division of Endocrinology, Diabetes, & Metabolism
Department of Internal Medicine
Wexner Medical Center
The Ohio State University
Columbus, Ohio

Joan E. Zaccardi, DNP, APN, FNAP-BC, NEA, FAANP
Urogynecology Arts of New Jersey
East Brunswick, New Jersey

Rosie Zeno, DNP, APRN-CNP
Assistant Professor of Clinical Nursing
Pediatric Nurse Practitioner
The Ohio State University College of Nursing
Nationwide Children's Hospital
Columbus, Ohio

REVIEWERS

Anthony Belenchia, PhD
Research/Data Analyst
State of Missouri, Department of Health and Senior Services
Jefferson City, Missouri
Clinical Decision-Making Using Laboratory Tests

Amanda Chaney, DNP, APRN, FAANP, AF-AASLD
Nurse Practitioner, Department of Transplant
Chair, Advance Practice Provider Subcommittee
Assistant Professor of Medicine, College of Medicine & Science
Associate in Transplant Medicine
Mayo Clinic and Hospital
Jacksonville, Florida
Liver Enzymes / Transaminases

Jennifer M. Demma, MSN, APRN-CNM, FACNM
Midwife and Medical Director
Family Tree Clinic
Saint Paul, Minnesota
Testosterone and Sex Hormone Binding Globulin

Kristopher R. Maday, MS, PA-C, DFAAPA
Program Director, Physician Assistant Program
Associate Professor
University of Tennessee Health Science Center
Memphis, Tennessee
BMP-Glucose

Carolyn McClerking, DNP, APRN-CNP, ACNP-BC
Assistant Professor of Clinical Nursing
Director, Adult Acute Care Nurse Practitioner Program
The Ohio State University College of Nursing
Acute Care Nurse Practitioner
Wexner Medical Center James Cancer Hospital
Columbus, Ohio
Troponin

Jennifer Merrill, MD

Endocrinologist
Division of Endocrinology, Diabetes, & Metabolism
Department of Internal Medicine
The Ohio State University Wexner Medical Center
Columbus, Ohio
Autoantibodies in Diabetes/Insulin and C-Peptide

Kelly Skinner, DNP, APRN, FNP

Nurse Practitioner
Midwest Infectious Disease Specialists
Independence, Missouri
Gram Stain, Culture, and Sensitivities

Lisa Ward, MS, PA-C

Physician Assistant
Department of Endocrinology/Oncology
The James Cancer Hospital
Columbus, Ohio
Urine Osmolality

Cindy G. Zellefrow DNP, MSEd, RN, LSN, PHNA-BC, EBP-C

Director; Academic Core Helene Fuld Health Trust National Institute for EBP
   in Nursing and Healthcare at The Ohio State University College of Nursing
Assistant Professor of Clinical Practice
Evidence-Based Practice-CH
Columbus, Ohio
Principles of Evidence-Based Practice for Clinical Decision-Making Regarding Laboratory Tests

FOREWORD

For decades, we have known that evidence-based decision-making and evidence-based practice (EBP) lead to better healthcare quality and safety (i.e., enhanced patient experience) along with improved population health outcomes and reduced costs; this is known as the Triple Aim in healthcare. Yet, these skills are not in the DNA of every practicing clinician, nor are they consistently used as a framework for content in books and curriculum in nursing and health sciences education. As a result, we continue to see approximately 250,000 preventable medical errors across the United States every year, many that result because very well-meaning caring clinicians do not follow the best evidence-based guidelines and make evidence-based decisions. In the year 2000, it was noted that it takes 17 years to translate findings from research to clinical practice to improve healthcare and outcomes. In 2021, findings from a recent study indicated that it takes 15 years. It is hard to believe that it took two decades to decrease the research-practice time gap by 2 years. We absolutely must do better. Stephen R. Covey said, "To know and not to do is really not to know." We know the process of how to make evidence-based decisions and the seven steps of EBP, yet we fall short in this country and all throughout the globe on meeting the EBP competencies and consistently implementing best practices.

Unlike other texts, this book takes an exceptionally strong evidence-based approach to laboratory screening and diagnostic evaluation, incorporating the best and latest evidence into each chapter. My outstanding advanced practice nurse faculty at The Ohio State University College of Nursing, Drs. Kelly Casler and Kate Gawlik, did a masterful job of creating and editing this gold standard book that should be used by all clinicians and incorporated into all nursing and health sciences curriculums. This book is jam-packed with pearls from which both clinicians and patients will greatly benefit. It should be a staple for best laboratory screening and diagnostic evaluation practices.

Bernadette Mazurek Melnyk, PhD, APRN-CNP, FNAP, FAANP, FAAN
Vice President for Health Promotion
University Chief Wellness Officer
Dean and Helene Fuld Health Trust Professor of Evidence-Based Practice,
College of Nursing
Professor of Pediatrics & Psychiatry, College of Medicine
Executive Director, the Helene Fuld Health Trust National Institute for EBP
The Ohio State University
Columbus, Ohio

PREFACE

I (Kelly) have been "tossing around" the premise of this book for almost my entire nurse practitioner (NP) career. I remember being a brand-new clinician and looking for a laboratory reference book to help me in clinical practice. While I found several good options, none quite gave me answers to all my questions or completely fit my needs. Fast forward to the start of my faculty career a decade ago, and I found that many of my students had similar desires for a laboratory reference book. At that time, I started collating tips and pearls in files that I provided as part of my teaching, but I never had as much time as I wanted to really "dive" into the literature. I wanted to see just how much of our laboratory ordering/interpreting practices were due to "tradition" rather than evidence. And then, I completed my doctor of nursing practice and began teaching for The Ohio State University College of Nursing, both of which helped me learn how to be more efficient in evidence review. Moving from Missouri to Ohio also gave me new opportunities for partnerships and collaborations and I realized it might be time to turn my collection of notes into something more. Kate and I began to talk about my idea and she recognized the need for a book of this nature and brought fresh new ideas and perspectives from her experiences in her clinical and faculty practice. And the rest, as they say, is history.

An important aim of this book is to provide a reference and guide in clinical practice and to also spark some ideas for clinical practice improvement, either at the individual patient level or at the system level. Multiple collaborators helped make this book a reality, especially since it was produced during a global pandemic! Being able to bring wisdom together from a variety of professions and specialties is one strength of this book—our contributing authors are from primary care and specialty practices, inpatient and outpatient practices, and are nurse practitioners, physician assistants, physicians, pharmacists, medical lab scientists, clinical nurse specialists, certified nurse–midwives, and certified registered nurse anesthetists. In all, the book summarizes over 3,000 pieces of evidence and incorporates the influence of genetic heritage and gender on the ordering and interpretation of tests. We challenge you to find at least one thing in this book that can change your practice to be more evidence-based. For example, since starting this book, we have changed to performing most of our lipid profiles non-fasting and screening with earlier markers for iron deficiency (i.e., ferritin) rather than hemoglobin.

This book is organized into three sections. Section I (Chapters 1–4) provides foundational information and skills to help the reader appropriately order and interpret laboratory tests. Evidence-based practice is reviewed as are important concepts in laboratory interpretation, such as sensitivity and specificity.

Section II (Chapters 5–10) reviews general circumstances that apply to all laboratory tests; for example, direct-to-consumer genetic testing and preoperative laboratory evaluation. Section III (Chapters 11–168) reviews 150+ individual laboratory tests and is likely where the reader will spend the majority of their time. Each chapter reviews the pathophysiology related to test ordering and interpretation, reviews the available evidence, and provides clinical pearls from practicing clinicians. We have created this section in a way so that the reader can read through several chapters as part of learning activities for a clinical program, or simply flip to the text of interest when a quick reference is needed.

We hope that you find this book useful to clinical practice and enjoy learning pearls from a variety of our contributing authors. We also hope it helps you on your evidence-based practice journey.

Kelly Small Casler and Kate Sustersic Gawlik

ACKNOWLEDGMENTS

Thank you to the authors across professions and disciplines who contributed to or reviewed this text. Your expertise, passion, and desire to move evidence into practice is evident in your contributions. Thank you to our team at Springer Publishing who brought this idea and body of work to fruition, especially Joe Morita and Taylor Ball. Lastly, to all of the clinicians and health sciences' students who use this text, thank you for wanting to be catalysts for change and accelerate evidence-based practice. We will achieve great things together.

ADDITIONAL RESOURCES

Available resources include:

■ **175 Case Studies/Examples**

■ **200 Self-Assessment Questions**

Content can be accessed at http://connect.springerpub.com/content/reference -book/978-0-8261-8843-4

FOUNDATIONAL CONCEPTS FOR EVIDENCE-BASED USE OF LABORATORY TESTS

1. PRINCIPLES OF EVIDENCE-BASED PRACTICE FOR CLINICAL DECISION-MAKING REGARDING LABORATORY TESTS

Kelly Small Casler

EVIDENCE-BASED PRACTICE

Clinicians frequently rely on laboratory tests to augment clinical decision-making. In fact, one study found that nearly all inpatient clinical encounters and nearly one-third of outpatient clinical encounters involved laboratory tests.[1] When they are used in a clinically relevant and cost-effective manner, laboratory tests can improve patient outcomes.[2] Yet, clinicians do not always follow best practice. Some studies estimate that more than half of laboratory test orders may be unnecessary.[3] Patient harm can follow due to, for example, patient anxiety over abnormal results that are really just false positives.[4-6] Unnecessary laboratory test use can also inflate healthcare costs. For example, tests are often done as part of asymptomatic routine health checks, an example of laboratory test overutilization.[3,6,7] One study concluded that the unnecessary use of complete blood count and urinalysis costs the healthcare system 46.1 million dollars.[8] Data also show that underutilization of laboratory tests is a problem, although to a lesser extent.[6]

Evidence-based practice (EBP) is a solution to laboratory test over- and underutilization. Therefore, its role in clinical decisions regarding laboratory tests cannot be understated. EBP is also critical to achieving high value care, defined as providing high-quality care at the lowest cost possible.[9,10] High-value care has been a primary target for healthcare improvement efforts for years and international leaders continue to develop laboratory test best practices to minimize healthcare overspending and improve patient outcomes.[11,12]

EBP is the process of applying internal and external evidence (evidence from research, quality improvement efforts, etc.) to patient care and combining the research findings with clinician expertise and patient preferences and values. All three pillars are equally important to EBP; much like a three-legged stool must have three legs to function correctly, so EBP needs all three EBP pillars to function correctly (Figure 1.1). When one pillar is neglected or broken, EBP does not occur (Figure 1.2).

THE EVIDENCE-BASED PRACTICE PROCESS

Several models of EBP exist to guide the clinician. Some of the most widely used models include the Iowa Model for Evidence Based Practice, the Johns

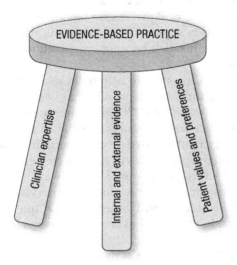

FIGURE 1.1. Evidence-based practice as a three-legged stool, depicting the three pillars of EBP.
Source: Courtesy of the Helene Fuld Health Trust National Institute for Evidence-Based Practice in Nursing and Healthcare; Columbus, Ohio.

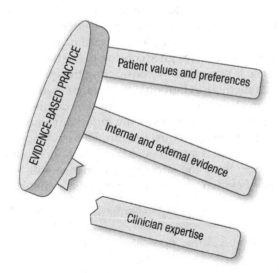

FIGURE 1.2. If even just one of the pillars of evidence-based practice is ignored, EBP does not function as intended, just as if one leg broke off a three-legged stool. *Source:* Courtesy of the Helene Fuld Health Trust National Institute for Evidence-Based Practice in Nursing and Healthcare; Columbus, Ohio.

Hopkins Evidence-Based Nursing Model, and Melnyk and Fineout-Overholt's seven steps of EBP, the model that will be described in the text that follows.[13]

Step Zero Through Three: Finding the Best Practices

In Step Zero, clinicians generally begin the EBP process by having an inquiring spirit and constantly asking "What is best practice?"[13] Clinicians also must champion EBP as a priority for their organization because organizational support is critical to making EBP changes.

In Step One, clinicians design a PICOT question to help them search the literature of the last several years in an effort to understand what best practice is. Structuring questions into a formal method like PICOT assures an efficient and applicable retrieval of relevant studies and literature.[14,15] Table 1.1 provides an example of a PICOT question that might be used when determining best practice regarding laboratory tests and describes each of the five elements that might be part of a PICOT question. All five elements are not always included depending on the focus. The focus can be on meaning (nonintervention), treatment, or diagnosis, for example. Sometimes, in a meaning PICOT question, there is not a comparison (C) element. In the PICOT example (diagnosis focus) in Table 1.1, the time (T) element is not applicable.

In Step Two, each element of the PICOT question is used as a key word for a literature search. Synonyms for the key words may also be used and the key words and synonyms are used with Boolean operators (AND, OR) to search the databases. Common databases, such as the Cumulative Index to Nursing and Allied Health Literature (CINAHL), Scopus, Google Scholar, and Pubmed are used to query the literature.

Step Three is completed after relevant literature is retrieved. In this step, the clinician begins the task of appraising the strength of the evidence, which is determined by evaluating both the *level of evidence* and the *quality of evidence*.[13] The level of evidence is ranked by research design according to the hierarchy listed in Box 1.1. Quality of evidence is evaluated by considering the quality and appropriateness of the research methods. High-quality research assures validity, reliability, and applicability to clinical practice and is further clarified in Table 1.2. Both quality of evidence and level of evidence are important since a higher level of evidence does not automatically equate to stronger evidence. For example, a randomized controlled trial is level II evidence, but if poorly designed the quality is considered weak; thus, the strength of evidence will be weak. Conversely, some low levels of evidence such as case reports or cohort studies

TABLE 1.1: EXAMPLE PICOT QUESTION REGARDING LABORATORY TESTING

Question: In patients with epigastric pain, how does amylase compared to lipase perform for diagnosis of pancreatitis?

PICOT ELEMENT	MATCHING CONCEPT FROM PICOT QUESTION ABOVE
Population (P)	Patients with epigastric pain
Intervention or Issue of Interest (I)	Amylase
Comparison (C)	Lipase
Outcome (O)	Pancreatitis diagnosis
Time (T)	(element not used in this question)

Box 1.1: Factors Used to Determine Quality of a Study

- Clear description of study methods
- Clear description of sampling
- Appropriate sampling method (with an a priori power analysis if a quantitative study)
- Reported effect size
- Reported statistical significance
- Findings and design applicable to practice
- Designed to minimize bias

will have strong quality of methodology, and if they are numerous enough in quantity, the studies, collectively, may be strong enough to initiate EBP change. For example, multiple case reports and cohort studies in the 1950s and 1960s established the strong correlation of smoking to lung cancer, which resulted in substantial public health efforts.[13,14] Additionally, the focus of some PICOT questions may be better answered by lower rather than higher levels of evidence. For example, diagnosis-focused PICOT questions (a main focus for this book) are answered well by cohort studies (level IV) and not just randomized control trials (level II). As the clinician reviews the retrieved evidence for quality, they should expect laboratory test research reports to follow the Standards for Reporting Diagnostic Accuracy Studies (STARD) 2015. The 30 standards of STARD 2015 require reporting of the usual quality of research methods such as sampling, statistical measures, and applicability to real-life practice, but do so in a standardized way that allows easy comparison of multiple studies.[16]

Clinicians should also be aware of the Quality Assessment of Diagnostic Accuracy-2 (QUADAS-2)[17] tool, an evaluation tool used to assess laboratory test research quality. Although designed for authors completing systematic reviews of multiple studies, the QUADAS-2 can also be used to judge the quality of research on new laboratory tests.[16] The tool guides readers through a meticulous evaluation of the study quality including their sampling methods, bias potential, and applicability.[17] Using QUADAS-2 can help evaluate research for any potential bias. There are several types of bias that can threaten the quality and validity of laboratory test research (Table 1.3).

TABLE 1.2: MELNYK AND FINEOUT-OVERHOLT LEVELS OF EVIDENCE (HIGHEST TO LOWEST)
I. Systematic reviews and metanalyses
II. Randomized controlled trials
III. Nonrandomized controlled trials
IV. Controlled cohort studies
V. Uncontrolled cohort studies
VI. Qualitative studies; case studies; descriptive studies
VII. Expert opinion

Source: Melnyk BM. *Evidence-Based Practice in Nursing & Healthcare: A Guide to Best Practice.* 4th ed. Wolters Kluwer Health; 2019.

TABLE 1.3: BIAS IN LABORATORY TEST RESEARCH	
Verification bias	Verification bias can make a diagnostic test performance look better than it is. When new laboratory tests are studied, their performance should be compared against a gold standard or reference test. Sometimes researchers may use a comparison test that is not the current gold standard or they may use multiple comparison tests.[18,19] Both choices can lead to verification bias.
Review bias	Review bias occurs when researchers are not blinded to the performance of the laboratory test and gold standard tests that are being studied. Ideally, the researchers collecting and reporting results should do so while blinded to the information.[18]
Spectrum bias	Spectrum bias occurs when the participant sample does not reflect that of the population the laboratory test will be used for. Ideally, participants in the study should have a wide range of symptom severity for the condition of interest, including not having the disease.[20]

Clinical practice guidelines (CPGs) may also be encountered during the literature search and can be used to guide best practice. A quality CPG strives to consolidate findings from several research studies and expert opinions to guide clinical practice recommendations. However, CPGs are not perfect and need quality appraisal. Clinicians can reference the Appraisal of Guidelines for Research & Evaluation (AGREE) II instrument to evaluate the quality of CPGs.[21]

Two organizations are known for providing high-quality CPGs regarding laboratory tests. Choosing Wisely (www.choosingwisely.org/) provides EBP recommendations for clinical care guidance. Eighteen percent of the recommendations regard the use of laboratory data.[3] Choosing Wisely strives to provide guidance toward using laboratory tests that are truly necessary, avoid harm, and provide high-value care. The United States Preventive Services Task Force (USPSTF) (www.uspreventiveservicestaskforce.org/uspstf/) makes EBP recommendations regarding laboratory test use that aredirected toward screening and prevention.[22] The USPSTF is an interdisciplinary task force comprised of 16 experts in evidence-based disease prevention.

Step Four: Translating Evidence Into Practice

In Step Four, after appraising the collected evidence, clinicians will synthesize the collected literature to understand the answers the literature provides. Then, clinicians combine these synthesis findings with their clinical expertise and the preferences and values of the patient. These steps translate the literature into clinical practice to make meaningful impacts on health outcomes and care value. Clinical expertise regarding laboratory tests involves knowing the limitations of laboratory tests and how to determine accuracy of laboratory tests. These concepts are discussed further in the next chapter.

Patient preference and values have a significant impact on decisions regarding laboratory testing. For example, patients may prefer not to have to fast for a test that screens for diabetes mellitus. Therefore, a hemoglobin A1C or random plasma glucose may be used over a fasting plasma glucose. Perhaps, most importantly, is the concept of patient healthcare cost. In one survey, at least one-fourth of U.S. citizens were concerned about the high costs of healthcare.[23] This emphasizes the importance of bringing the patient view into clinical decisions and only recommending laboratory tests that are consistent with high value care. However, although patients have concern over healthcare costs, sometimes patient desires can drive the overuse of laboratory tests. Interestingly, patients do not seem to negatively view laboratory overtesting in the same manner as pharmaceutical over-treatment.[24,25] This can make it challenging for clinicians to provide high value care and likely signals a need on the part of clinicians to improve patient health literacy on the ramifications of inappropriate laboratory test use. It may help for patients to know that although they express the desire to confirm negative results to calm their fears of disease, this practice does not always reduce patient anxiety.[26]

Step Five and Six: Demonstrating Evidence-Based Practice Impact

Step Five of the EBP process involves collecting data regarding the effect of EBP change. As the clinician identifies and implements EBP practice changes, it is important to illustrate the impact of the change through data. This data will illustrate for other clinicians how to replicate the practice changes and achieve the same impact in their organizations. For example, even if you as the sole clinician eliminate performing complete blood counts (CBCs) as part of your routine physical laboratory work for patients (because of what you learned in this book), it would be important to track how much money that saved your patients.

Step Six involves disseminating the results of EBP change and sustaining EBP changes. In an era of evidence-based laboratory utilization and high value care, knowing how to order and use laboratory tests in an EBP way is only one small piece of the EBP puzzle.[5] Clinicians should openly disseminate findings and collaborate with colleagues to expand EBP change. Likewise, teaming with others to develop interventions that could improve evidence-based laboratory practices is important and needed for a larger impact. Laboratory utilization committees, electronic health record (EHR) order entry alerts, EHR clinical decision support, and improved EHR interoperability are all examples of collaborative approaches that advance and sustain EBP and reduce laboratory care costs.[2–4,27–30]

REFERENCES

Full list of references can be accessed through Springer Publishing Company Connect™ at the following link: http://connect.springerpub.com/content/reference-book/978-0-8261 -8843-4/part/part01/toc-part/ch001

2. CLINICAL DECISION-MAKING USING LABORATORY TESTS: THINKING LIKE A CLINICAL EXPERT

Kelly Small Casler

THINKING LIKE A CLINICAL EXPERT

The ability to correctly apply laboratory tests to a clinical situation involves clinical expertise. The clinical expert understands the limitations of laboratory tests as well as key concepts surrounding their use. This chapter and the chapters that follow seek to outline important pearls and foundational knowledge regarding laboratory testing. You will find similar pearls regarding individual laboratory tests written throughout this text.

When using laboratory tests as part of clinical decision-making it is important to understand:

- No test is 100% perfect at predicting the presence or absence of a condition. Patients should be educated on this fact and clinicians should recognize the limitations of laboratory test accuracy when using results to make clinical practice decisions.
- Laboratory tests do not replace a good history and physical examination and must always be interpreted within the clinical context and condition of the patient.[1]
- Laboratory tests range in prices. The clinician should always keep in mind the costs of laboratory tests to the patient and healthcare system.
- Most often, trends in laboratory findings are more important than one single abnormal reading. Laboratory tests should be compared to a patient's previous results.
- If there is more than one abnormal laboratory test, the clinician should prioritize differential diagnoses that account for all the abnormal tests. Additionally, clinicians should look for differential diagnoses that account for not only the laboratory abnormalities but also the history and physical examination findings. Further, if imaging or other diagnostic tests have been completed, these also need to be considered in context with laboratory results and history/physical examination findings.
- Laboratory tests are not without harm and should not be ordered without strong clinical rationale because false positives can lead to significant patient anxiety and excess follow-up testing. The usefulness of a test depends on when and how it is used; diagnostic tests are, therefore, best used when there is a high pretest probability of a condition.
- Laboratory tests should not be ordered unless they will change the management plan.[2]

■ Clinicians should use internal evidence to guide laboratory interpretation and/or decisions based on laboratory findings. For example, a patient's urinalysis to evaluate for cystitis may test positive for nitrites, causing the clinician to have a high index of suspicion for *Escherichia coli* (*E. coli*) as the pathogen of cause. However, knowing the local antibiotic resistance patterns using the hospital or clinic antibiogram may allow the clinician to predict that the culture sensitivities would show a resistance to trimethoprim/sulfamethoxazole and avoid this antibiotic. Figure 2.1 shows an example of an antibiogram.

DETERMINING TEST ACCURACY

When reviewing the evidence regarding laboratory study quality as described in Chapter 1, clinicians should be familiar with various statistical measures of laboratory test accuracy that will be reported. These accuracy measures are used to determine how valid a new laboratory test is compared to previously used tests (gold standard test) and if it is accurate enough to be used in the real clinical world. Once a new laboratory test enters the clinical world, clinicians can also use accuracy measures reported in the research to guide decisions about whether it would be useful to incorporate the test into clinical decision-making. The common measures of accuracy are described in the text that follows and are calculated using a 2×2 table, or contingency table. A 2×2 contingency table example is shown in Figure 2.2. Table 2.1 summarizes the accuracy measures that will be reviewed in the following sections.

Sensitivity and Specificity

Sensitivity and specificity reflect the performance of a laboratory test in correctly identifying the absence or presence of a condition compared to a gold standard test. Sensitivity and specificity are determined by starting with a sample of people that either have or do not have a condition of interest. This concept is illustrated in Figures 2.3 and 2.4. There is not a general agreed upon ideal value at which a test is considered to have ideal sensitivity or specificity. However, most clinicians look for a sensitivity or specificity of 90% or higher to feel a test is useful to practice.

To determine sensitivity, a sample of people that have the condition are selected to undergo testing and the percentage of patients the test correctly identifies as a positive result is recorded. Sensitivity is also called the true positive rate since it reflects the amount of people with the condition that the test correctly identifies as positive. Therefore, a test with high sensitivity helps to rule out a condition because it has very few false negatives.

To determine specificity, a sample of people that do not have a condition are selected and undergo testing and the percentage of patients that the test correctly identifies as negative is reported. Specificity is also called the true negative rate since it reflects the amount of people without the condition that the test correctly identifies as negative. Therefore, a highly specific test has good ability to rule in a diagnosis because it has very few false positives.

False negative rates and false positive rates are also used to describe laboratory test accuracy. The false positive rate reflects how often people without

Gram (-)	# of patients	Aminoglycosides			B-Lactams			Cephalosporins				Quinolones		Others
		Amikacin	Gentamicin	Tobramycin	Ampicillin	Imipenem	Piperacillin Tazobactam	Cefazolin	Cefoxitin	Ceftriaxone	Ceftazidime	Ciprofloxacin	Nitrofurantoin	TMP/SMX
Echericha coli	4	100	100	100		100	100		100	100	100	75		
Klebsiella sp	13	100	84.6	92.3	38.5	100	92.3	84.6			100	38.5	92.3	38.5
Proteus sp	7	71.4	57.1	71.4		85.7	85.7			57.1	57.1		28.6	71.4
Pseudomonas aeruginosa	13	100	83.3	92.3	91.7		100		81.8	100	100	30.8		69.2

Gram (-)	# of patients	Penicillins				Cephalosporins		Quinolones		Others						
		Penicillin	Ampicillin	Oxacillin	Nafillin	Cephalothin	Ceftriaxone	Ciprofloxacin	Moxifloxacin	Gentamicin	Linezolid	Rifampin	Tetracycline	TMP/SMX	Vancomycin	Nitrofurantoin
Staph aureus (all)	8	0	0	0	0			0	0	87.5	100	100	100	100	100	100
Methicillin resistant (MRSA)	8	0	0	0	0				0	87.5	100	100	100	100	100	100
Methicillin susceptible (MRSA)	0															
Enterococcus sp	4	100	100					50		75	100	100	25	100	100	100

FIGURE 2.1. Example of an antibiogram. Antibiograms use internal data to guide clinical interpretation of laboratory tests. In an antibiogram, the first column lists organisms that were tested for on the sensitivity of a culture. The second column denotes the number of individuals that tested positive for that organism and the following columns denote the percentage of those organisms susceptible to the corresponding antibiotic. The yellow boxes indicate that there is not information available for that combination of bacteria and antibiotic. Clinicians can inquire with clinic or hospital infectious disease or laboratory leadership teams to obtain their local antibiogram.

Source: Figure from Agency for Healthcare Research and Quality. Concise Antibiogram Toolkit Getting Started—Sources of Data 2014. https://www.ahrq.gov/sites/default/files/wysiwyg/professionals/quality-patient-safety/patient-safety-resources/resources/nh-aspguide/module2/toolkit1/cat_sources.pdf.

	Individuals with influenza according to gold standard test	Individuals without influenza according to gold standard test		
Positive influenza rapid test	TP (N = 85)	FP (N = 5)	Total testing positive = 90 (TP+FP)	PPV = 94.4% $\left[\dfrac{TP}{Total\ testing\ positive} \right]$
Negative rapid influenza test	FN (N = 15)	TN (N = 95)	Total testing negative = 110 (FN+TN)	NPV = 86.3% $\left[\dfrac{TN}{Total\ testing\ negative} \right]$
	Total with disease = 100 (TP+FN)	Total without disease = 100 (FP+TN)	N = total number of tests (200)	
	Sensitivity = 85% $\left[\dfrac{TP}{Total\ with\ disease} \right]$	Specificity= 95% $\left[\dfrac{TN}{Total\ without\ disease} \right]$		

FIGURE 2.2. Two by two (contingency) table using an example of a new rapid influenza test. The example consists of testing on 200 patients (100 with influenza according to the gold standard and 100 without influenza according to the gold standard). FN, false negative; FP, false positive; N, number; PPV, positive predictive value; TN, true negative; TP, true positive.

the condition are incorrectly identified as positive on the test and calculated by subtracting the specificity from 1. False negative rates reflect how often people with the condition are incorrectly identified as negative on the test and are calculated by subtracting the sensitivity from 1. Although false positive and false negative rates are impossible to avoid, they have a critical influence on patient care. For example, a test for early detection of cancer with a high false negative rate would be problematic due to the possibility of missing a critical diagnosis that needs early treatment. For this reason, screening tests are usually required to have high sensitivity so they will have a low false negative rate. However, a test with a high false positive rate is also problematic since it can cause overdiagnosis and lead to unnecessary follow-up testing and/or treatment. Prostate-specific antigen is an example of a test with an high false positive rate.[3] Some studies show up to two-thirds of individuals who have a positive result do not really have prostate cancer. However, these patients are subjected to multiple follow-up tests related to the false positive test finding. Due to this, diagnostic tests require a high specificity, resulting in lower false positive rates.

Sometimes the problem with sensitivity and specificity occurs from selecting the wrong cutoff value for which a test result equates to a positive or negative result (for more on this concept see the section on receiver operator curves). Sometimes a cutoff level is set too low. This results in a high sensitivity so that more people with the condition will be identified but could end up sacrificing

TABLE 2.1: KEY STATISTICS USED IN LABORATORY TEST ACCURACY

	DEFINITION	CALCULATED BY	USEFUL FOR
Accuracy	Percentage of tests that were able to correctly identify absence or presence of condition	TP + TN /N	Identifying the overall performance of a test
Sensitivity (true positive rate)	Percentage of those with a condition that test positive	TP / (TP+FN)	If high, ruling out a diagnosis by a negative result
Specificity (true negative rate)	Percentage of people without a condition that test negative	TN / (TN+FP)	If high, ruling in a diagnosis by a positive result
False positive rate	Percentage of those without a condition that test positive	1−specificity	If low, ruling in a diagnosis by a positive result
False negative rate	Percentage of those with a condition that test negative	1−sensitivity	If low, ruling out a diagnosis by a negative result
Positive predictive value	Percentage of people who test positive and actually have the condition	TP / (TP+FP)	Identifying the influence of prevalence on testing
Negative predictive value	Percentage of people who test negative and actually do not have the condition	TN / (TN+FN)	Identifying the influence of prevalence on testing
Positive likelihood ratio (LR+)	How likely a positive test predicts having a condition. Compares true positive rate to false positive rate	Sensitivity / (1−specificity)	Ruling in a diagnosis when the prevalence is unknown
Negative likelihood ratio (LR-)	How likely a negative test predicts not having a condition. Compares true negative rate to false negative rate	(1−sensitivity) / specificity	Ruling out a diagnosis when the prevalence is unknown
Receiver operating curve (ROC)	A plot that helps determine the thresholds for test performance	Graph compares true positive to false positive rate,	Determining cut off values
Area under the ROC (AUROC)	Percentage of space under a ROC	Uses ROC graph to calculate.	Comparing performance of several tests

FN, false negative; FP, false positive; N, number; PPV, positive predictive value; TN, true negative; TP, true positive.

specificity since a positive value will diagnose more people than really have the disease. The opposite is true for raising the cutoff value. Specificity becomes high but the sensitivity becomes so low that too many patients are missed.

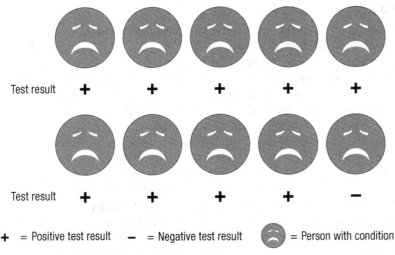

FIGURE 2.3. A simplified depiction of 90% sensitivity.

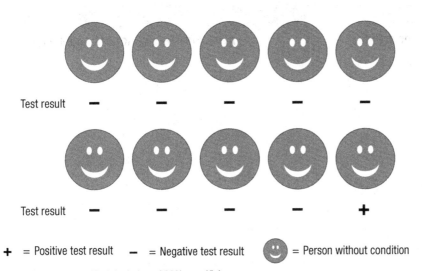

FIGURE 2.4. A simplified depiction of 90% specificity.

Predictive Values

Unlike sensitivity and specificity, predictive values help describe the performance of a test when the presence or absence of a condition is not known ahead of time. Predictive values can also capture the influence of disease prevalence on test accuracy. Positive predictive value (PPV) reflects the probability that a positive test result is a true positive (and not a false positive). PPVs are influenced by test specificity and condition prevalence. When specificity is higher and a condition more prevalent, the PPV will be improved. A negative predictive value (NPV) reflects the probability that a negative result is a true negative (and not a false negative). When a condition has lower prevalence, the NPV is improved.

Likelihood Ratio

Likelihood ratios (LRs) express how well a laboratory result predicts the presence or absence of a condition. A negative likelihood ratio (LR–) predicts how well a negative laboratory result helps to rule out a condition. It is the ratio of false negative rate (something clinicians want to avoid) to specificity (something clinicians find beneficial). Conversely, a positive likelihood ratio (LR+) predicts how well a laboratory result helps to rule in a condition. It is the ratio of sensitivity to the false positive rate. For both positive and negative LRs, the further away from one, the stronger or more predictive the test. LRs are helpful since they help predict probability of disease when it is unknown whether the patient has or does not have the condition—a concept that reflects real life practice. LRs are also helpful since they do not rely on prevalence values like PPV and NPV.

In 2002, McGee[4] expanded on the predictive ability of LRs by proposing an approximate estimation of the percent probability of a disease based on the LR (Table 2.2) Many clinicians use these probability estimations in clinical decision-making today.

TABLE 2.2: LIKELIHOOD RATIOS AND PROBABILITY ESTIMATES	
LIKELIHOOD RATIO	**APPROXIMATE CHANGE IN PROBABILITY (%)**
Values between 0 and 1 decrease the probability of disease.	
0.1	–45
0.2	–30
0.3	–25
0.4	–20
0.5	–15
1	0
Values greater than 1 increase the probability of disease.	
2	+15
3	+20
4	+25
5	+30
6	+35
7	
8	+40
9	
10	+45

Source: McGee S. Simplifying likelihood ratios. J Gen Intern Med. 2002;17(8):646–649. doi:10.1046/j.1525-1497.2002.10750.x

Receiver Operating Curve and Area Under the Receiver Operating Curve

Many laboratory tests are designed as a numerical value along a continuous scale rather than a dichotomous, positive, or negative result. The challenge for researchers then becomes to determine a cut off after which to call a test positive or negative for a condition of interest. Examples of this concept include the level at which glucose is considered diagnostic (or positive) for diabetes or the level at which a troponin is considered diagnostic of myocardial infarction. The receiver operating curve (ROC) is used to guide this process (Figure 2.5).[5] The ROC allows researchers to compare sensitivity to specificity and determine the optimal cutoff points for predicting the presence or absence of a condition.

To plot a ROC, the performance of the test of interest is plotted on an X and Y axis. The X axis is the false positive rate (1–specificity) and the Y axis is the true positive rate (sensitivity). Test accuracy data from multiple participants and/or studies are plotted individually, and a line drawn to connect the plots. As a plot point moves left, specificity improves. As a plot point moves up, sensitivity improves. A test with perfect sensitivity (100%) and perfect specificity (100%) would be plotted in the top left corner of the ROC graph and a perfect ROC would be a straight line that starts in the lower left-hand corner, travels north, and makes a 90-degree right turn at the upper, left-hand corner. Note that a test with perfect sensitivity and specificity is unrealistic in real life, but the plot point(s) closest to the upper left-hand corner are usually chosen as the best cutoff value. A center diagonal line splitting the graph in half shows where

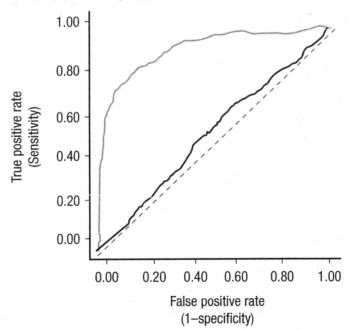

FIGURE 2.5. Receiver Operating Curve (ROC). The gray line represents a test with good to excellent ROC and the black line represents a poor ROC. The dotted line represents a line of no benefit where the test performs no better than a random coin flip.

test accuracy is no better than a random coin flip (sensitivity 50%; specificity 50%). By visualizing the sensitivity and specificity in this manner, researchers can evaluate the performance of a test and where to set a cutoff value for positive and negative tests.[6] This process has been used to develop several cutoff values, for example, what lactate level predicts sepsis mortality.[7]

Sometimes there are several available diagnostic or screening tests for one purpose and researchers need to determine the best performer among the group. Additionally, researchers may want to compare the performance of a new test to others currently being used. For this task, a measure called area under the ROC curve (AUROC) is calculated. AUROC does not compare the cutoff thresholds of the tests, but instead the overall curve from the data for each test. Better performing tests have more "area under the curve", or AUROC, because the ROC is close to the left and top of the graph. Generally, an AUROC of 0.7 or better is considered acceptable. An AUROC above 0.8 is considered excellent.[8] Figure 2.6 illustrates the concept of AUROC.

Odds Ratios and Number Needed to Screen

In diagnostic and screening test research, odds ratios (ORs) and number needed to screen (NNS) are often reported. Both help illustrate the effect that testing can have in a clinical situation. ORs describe the magnitude of association of a positive or negative test with a condition. The greater the OR from 1, the greater the association. The NNS, sometimes also called the number needed to test (NNT), reflects the number of people that will need to be tested over time to prevent one death or one adverse outcome. Both measures help determine the impact of a laboratory test.[9] For example, the fecal immunochemical screening test for

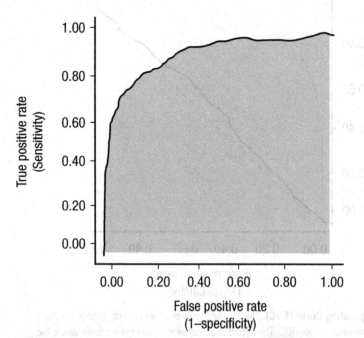

FIGURE 2.6. Area under the receiver operating curve (AUROC). The gray shaded area shows the AUROC.

colon cancer has a NNS of 238. This means that clinicians would need to test 238 patients to detect 1 case of colon cancer.[10]

Bayesian Reasoning

When clinicians use laboratory tests, they are usually most interested in knowing the probability of a patient having or not having a disease based on the test result. This clinical reasoning method is called Bayesian reasoning. Bayesian reasoning uses Bayes theorem, a statistical formula, to determine the probability of an outcome based on a preceding event, such as a patient's family history risk factors or the prevalence of disease in a community. These preceding events help determine the pretest probability, the probability of a condition in a patient prior to testing with a laboratory test. Pretest probabilities can be determined from epidemiologic prevalence studies or they may be estimated by the clinician.[11]

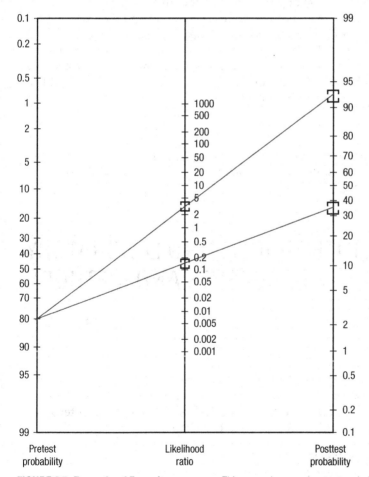

FIGURE 2.7. Example of Fagan's nomogram. This example uses a pretest probability of 80% and two tests: test one (procalcitonin test in our hypothetical example) with a +LR of 3 and test two with a +LR of 0.15 to show the corresponding posttest probabilities if the laboratory test is positive (test one = 94% posttest probability and test two = 35% posttest probability). *Source:* Levin RF, Feldman HR. *Teaching Evidence-Based Practice in Nursing.* 2nd ed. Springer Publishing Company; 2013, Fig. 15.5.

Once the laboratory test result is received, the LR or PPV of the test is combined with the pretest probability to determine the post-test probability of a diagnosis. For example, clinicians can ask themselves, "If a patient has shortness of breath and fever (pretest probability) and then a positive procalcitonin test, what is the probability (posttest probability) that the patient has pneumonia?" Hypothetical data to illustrate this example follows. Suppose a recent cohort study showed that patients with fever, cough, and shortness of breath had an 80% pretest probability of pneumonia. The calculated LR+ of the procalcitonin for pneumonia is 3. In Bayesian reasoning, the question would be, "What would be the posttest probability of the patient having pneumonia?" This type of information proves useful when deciding the management plan for this patient.

In 1975, Terence Fagan[12] developed a nomogram based on Bayes theorem to assist with Bayesian reasoning and determine posttest probability. This nomogram allows visual calculation of probabilities rather than statistical calculation as is done with Bayes theorem. Using Fagan's nomogram and the previous hypothetical pneumonia example, the posttest probability of pneumonia would be 94% (Figure 2.7). Figure 2.7 shows an example of Fagan's nomogram. Despite the usefulness of Fagan's nomogram and Bayes theorem, the LR probability table by McGee (Figure 2.4) is more commonly used due to ease of use and less need for timely calculations or drawing.

REFERENCES

Full list of references can be accessed through Springer Publishing Company Connect™ at the following link: http://connect.springerpub.com/content/reference-book/978-0-8261-8843-4/part/part01/toc-part/ch002

3. INTRODUCTION TO LABORATORY PROCESSES AND METHODS

Kelly Small Casler

To appropriately use laboratory tests in clinical practice, it is important for the clinician to have a good understanding of basic laboratory principles. The principles that have the largest influence on clinical decision-making, interpretation, and quality of care will be reviewed in this chapter.

ROLES OF LABORATORY TESTS

Laboratory tests are used for three primary roles: screening, diagnosis, and monitoring.[1] Often, laboratory tests have multiple roles. For example, hemoglobin can be used as a screening test for pediatric anemia at the 12-month well child visit. It can also be used as a diagnostic test if anemia is suspected in a menstruating woman with fatigue and heavy menstrual cycles. Finally, hemoglobin can be used to monitor the treatment response of a patient with iron deficiency anemia. The three primary roles of laboratory testing are reviewed in further detail in the text that follows.

- **Screening**. A laboratory test is used for universal or targeted screening when it is ordered as part of prevention efforts to detect a condition early before signs or symptoms are present. Universal screening refers to screening patients with no risk factors while targeted screening only screens individuals with certain risk factors for a condition. Appropriate use of laboratory screening tests as a preventative effort is an important component of high value care.[2] Higher sensitivity is usually valued over higher specificity in laboratory screening tests. Thus, false positives are seen more commonly than false negative results.

- **Diagnosis**. A laboratory test is used for diagnostic purposes when it is ordered as part of the clinical decision-making process when a diagnosis is suspected based on signs or symptoms. When designing and evaluating diagnostic laboratory tests, specificity is prioritized over sensitivity. Thus, false negative results are more likely to occur compared to false positive rates.

- **Monitoring**. A laboratory test is used for monitoring of care in several instances. A laboratory test may be used to monitor for effectiveness of a treatment (most commonly, medication) or for side effects or risks from the treatment. Laboratory tests may also be used to determine when treatments should start or conclude or for determination of prognosis for patients with chronic conditions.

PHASES OF THE LABORATORY PROCESS

The laboratory process consists of three distinct phases (Table 3.1).[3] The first phase is the preanalytical phase. This phase includes activities that must happen before a specimen makes it to the laboratory for the test to be conducted. Examples of events in this phase include order entry, phlebotomy, and collection and/or labeling of specimens. The second laboratory phase is the analytical phase, which occurs when the laboratory test is conducted. Finally, the postanalytical phase occurs after the test has concluded and the result is received. Entering, reporting, and interpreting the laboratory result are examples of actions in this phase. Quality improvement in laboratory science usually concentrates on identifying and correcting errors in one of the three phases.

TABLE 3.1: COMMON LABORATORY ERRORS BY STAGE

Preanalytical Stage	Most errors occur in this stage.[4,5]
	Examples of preanalytical errors include ordering of unnecessary or incorrect laboratory tests, incorrect labeling, incorrect specimen collection, and patient misidentification.
Analytical Stage	These types of errors are the least common.
	Examples of errors in this phase include laboratory procedure in-adherence and equipment failure.
Postanalytical Stage	These errors result when results are entered or transcribed incorrectly or when a laboratory test is misinterpreted.[6] An example would include relying on a laboratory test with poor sensitivity to rule out a critical diagnosis.

DETERMINING NORMALITY OF RESULTS

Laboratory data are usually reported as either a dichotomous result (positive or negative) or a numerical value. For those labs reported as a numerical value, a range of values considered to be normal, called a reference interval (RI), accompanies the value. The values at the upper and lower end of the RI are called reference limits. Some laboratory tests are also reported as numerical values but are reported with a decision limit, instead of an RI. A decision limit is a dividing line between numerical values that help to discriminate between patients that have or do not have a condition of interest.[7] Values above a decision limit are usually associated with the condition of interest, while those below the value are not. An example of common laboratory tests that use decision limits include troponin and brain natriuretic peptide. Some laboratory tests may report multiple decision limits such as occurs with glucose testing, where there are different decision limits ("cutoffs") to determine a normal glucose, an elevated glucose level associated with impaired glucose tolerance, and glucose levels consistent with diabetes.[8]

Laboratory tests that use decision limits or dichotomous results tend to have a more rigorous evaluation of performance using ROCs and sensitivity/specificity. In contrast, those laboratory tests reported as numerical values with RIs may have less rigor and standardization in their determination. Because of these imperfections, RIs should be viewed as more of a guide rather than an exact determination of normality.[9] One reason for this suggestion is that extensive variability exists in how RIs are determined. Ultimately, the performing laboratory leadership determines the RI reported with laboratory results. The RI may be chosen from several options such as machine manufacturer kit inserts, published literature, textbooks, or historical data.[10]

Sometimes "in-house" studies are conducted by a laboratory to develop RIs, but only 120 individuals (and sometimes even fewer) are required for RI development sample size.[11] Often, this sample is not reflective of the diverse patient age, sex, ethnicity, race, and health comorbidities that occur within patient populations the laboratory test is intended for. Additionally, when laboratory data is collected from the sample, most RIs are chosen to reflect the middle 95% of values collected. This means that even results received in 5% of the healthy persons used in the study to establish RI will be categorized as abnormal or outside the RI.[8] Therefore, if a patient's laboratory result falls outside a specified RI, disease may not always be present[7] since 5% (2.5% below and 2.5% above the reference limit) of values obtained from the healthy individuals in the RI study also fall outside the RI cutoff.[8] Although additional clinical follow-up may be warranted in some of these cases, it is also possible that the out of range value is of no consequence. This concept emphasizes the importance of using the clinical laboratory tests along with other clinical data acquired from the history and physical.

The laboratory and pathology community continue to work on improving the quality of RI determination. Recent focus has been on harmonization and standardization of RI, since there is much variation between RIs at institutions.[9,11–13] Other areas of future work are focusing on the improvement of RIs. These include examining differences in RIs based on ethnicities and race, differences of RIs based on sex (including the determination of appropriate RIs for transgender individuals), more precise RIs for pediatric age groups, and more precise RIs for those patients in critical care.[7,11] Recent work with pediatric populations has proposed continuous RIs based on growth, similar to the Centers for Disease Control and Prevention (CDC) weight and height growth charts, to reflect the fluid nature of laboratory results as children age.[14] Canada has expanded research on national standardized RIs[15] and Germany has used data mining from electronic health records to improve accuracy of RIs.[16] In the United States, many laboratories participate in the CDC voluntary standardization and quality assurance programs, especially for laboratory tests that are the most vulnerable to variation. Two examples are the Hormone Standardization (HoSt) Program and the Vitamin D Standardization Certification Program (VDSCP). In both programs, third parties assess the precision and bias of results provided by laboratories and provide guidance on process improvement.[17]

Another challenge for clinicians when determining normality of results is variation. Clinicians often order laboratory tests for patient monitoring to determine if a treatment has been effective or to see if a clinical condition has worsened. These instances require clinical decision-making regarding comparison of serial laboratory testing results. To interpret these serial results appropriately, clinicians must recognize the influence that analytic and biologic variation can have on laboratory values. Analytic variation is variation that occurs related to the phases of the laboratory process described previously. There is potential for changes between time points of serial laboratory testing, depending on how frequently (or infrequently) a patient's laboratory test is repeated. Examples of causes for analytic variation include reagent deterioration, human errors, or variation in techniques, such as pipetting.[18] Additionally, if different laboratories or manufacturer products are used for each serial result, there is greater potential for analytic variation. For example, one study found more than a 4-fold variation between parathyroid hormone results when specimens from the same patient were tested on different manufacturer kits.[19] Biologic variation is variation that occurs related to patient physiology or environment. Examples include laboratory tests that are collected during different nutrition states, mood/stress states, or times of day (morning versus evening).[18]

Because of analytical and biologic variation, clinicians are challenged to decide if the differences of serial laboratory results are due to true change in condition/health status or if the change is simply related to the analytic or biologic variation described previously. Reference change values (RCV) refer to a statistical measure used to calculate the potential analytic and biologic variation.[18] RCV is usually reported as a percentage; for a change in a laboratory value to be considered to be from a true health status change, the percent change in the laboratory value would need to be greater than the RCV percent. However, the process of determining accurate RCVs and using them to help clinicians interpret serial laboratory data is imperfect and continues to evolve.[20] Currently, there are no efficient resources that list RCVs for clinicians. However, Canadian experts recently made great strides in this endeavor by providing clinicians with an online, interactive tool (www.bmj.com/content/368/bmj.m149/related) to determine RCV. Unfortunately, clinicians in the United States may not find this tool useful as it is based on the International System of Units (abbreviation: SI) (i.e., mmol/L), whereas the United States uses conventional/traditional units (sometimes called US Standard units) (i.e., mg/dL). Although conversion factors are available to switch between SI and conventional/traditional units,[21] the time required for conversion of the US conventional/traditional units is unlikely to make this tool an efficient resource for US clinicians. However, some laboratory results have conversions that are one to one (i.e., mEq/L to mmol/L for sodium or potassium).[22] Also helpful is that conversion factors between SI and traditional/conventional units are easily accessible and a calculator for conversion can be found at https://www.amamanualofstyle.com/page/91.

TYPES OF LABORATORY TESTING

There are a wide variety of techniques used to collect and test specimens for laboratory analysis. This section will review some of the most common techniques.

Blood, Plasma, and Serum Testing

Laboratory tests that test blood can be performed on venous, arterial, or capillary samples. Capillary blood samples are usually used for point of care testing. Venous and arterial blood samples can be combined in laboratory tubes with anticoagulants or other additives. Some additives hasten clotting to allow for quicker analysis while others allow for separation of whole blood into components, such as serum or plasma. Serum separation tubes allow whole blood samples to clot inside the tube, and the serum separation additives allow the serum to dislodge from the clot and move into the upper part of the tube. The serum can then be extracted for testing. This serum separating process is commonly used for chemistry panels (Figure 3.1). Tubes with plasma-separating additives (EDTA) allow the blood to separate into plasma, a buffy coat that contains white blood cells and platelets, and red blood cells, which settle at the bottom of a tube (Figure 3.2). This plasma-separating process is commonly used when assessing a complete blood count and/or peripheral smear. After collection, samples can be assessed for the analytes of interest. Photometry involves

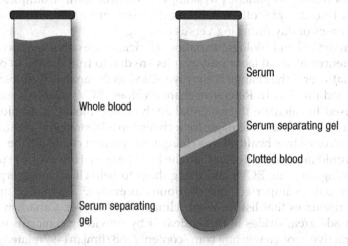

Whole blood

Serum separating gel

Serum separating tube—before centrifuge

Serum

Serum separating gel

Clotted blood

Serum separating tube—after centrifuge

FIGURE 3.1. Serum separating tube before and after centrifugation.

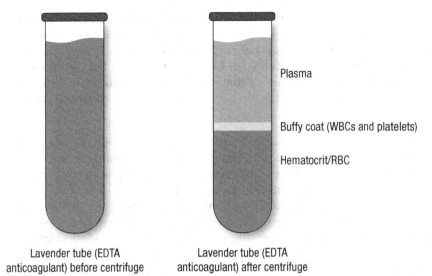

Lavender tube (EDTA anticoagulant) before centrifuge

Lavender tube (EDTA anticoagulant) after centrifuge

FIGURE 3.2. Anticoagulant-treated tube before and after centrifugation. EDTA, ethylenediaminetetraacetic acid; RBC, red blood cell; WBC, white blood cell.

mixing a sample with reagent to produce a color reaction. The strength of the color reaction is measured by the photometer and translated into a number value reflecting concentration of the analyte in the specimen. Flow cytometry uses a laser to measure the amount of cells present in a liquid.[3] Electrochemical measurements are also commonly used in chemistry measurements. Ion selective electrodes measure the flow of current through a membrane specific to the ion of interest. Sodium, potassium, and chloride are often measured in this way.

Microbiology: Gram Stain, Culture, and Sensitivity
Microbiology techniques are used to identify infectious microbes. Samples from a variety of sites can be used in microbiologic testing: sputum, blood, mucous membranes, wound exudates, urine, and others can all be tested for suspected infection. One of the oldest techniques used in microbiology is gram stain microscopy. This technique was developed in 1884 and is still used today as a preliminary way to identify bacteria and divide them into two groups. After the specimen of interest is applied to a slide, violet dye is applied. The slide is washed and then prepared with a counterstain of red dye. Gram positive bacteria retain the violet dye while gram-negative bacteria take up the red dye from the counterstain.[23]

Cultures are also used to identify infection. A culture can be used to identify aerobic and anaerobic bacteria as well as virus and fungi. The suspected type of infection will influence what culture medium is used. For example, viruses require host cells to replicate and will need a culture medium impregnated with host cells. Blood cultures are often mixed in a liquid culture medium, referred to as broth. Other samples may be applied to agar plates and additives may be added to encourage the suspected bacteria to grow. A drawback to the use of cultures is the long turnaround time which can include several days. Additionally, some bacteria will not grow in traditional culture mediums. Along with cultures, antibiotic sensitivities are often performed.

Sensitivities determine the antibiotic susceptibility of the microbes grown during culture. Testing is completed to determine the minimum inhibitory concentration, which is the lowest concentration of an antimicrobial that inhibits growth. If there is only limited inhibition of growth, the antibiotic is listed as resistant. Those antibiotics that have complete effect are listed as susceptible and those with an effect in between are listed as indeterminate.[24]

Immunoassay

Immunoassays (IAs) are a type of test that look for the binding between antibodies (immunoglobulins) and antigens. An IA can be designed to test for either the presence of the antigen or the antibody in a sample, usually blood. Examples of commonly used tests that look for the presence of antibodies are tests for West Nile virus, hepatitis B, or rheumatoid factor. Examples of commonly used IA that test for antigens include thyroid-stimulating hormone and Prostate Specific Antigen. There are different ways to perform IAs, which are described in the text that follows.

Enzyme-linked immunosorbent assay (ELISA) can provide quantitative or qualitative results and looks for the presence of antibodies in a patient's blood. In ELISA, an enzyme reacts with a specific substrate and a color change appears. The process begins by coating wells of a testing plate with an antigen of interest. Patient serum is then added to the wells. If there are antibodies in the patient serum specific to the antigen, they will bind to the antigen in the wells of the testing plate. Any unbound substances are flushed out of the wells and then the wells are filled with animal serum that contains antibodies. These antibodies attach to the human antibodies that are left over from the first process. Finally, a substrate is added to the wells that bind with the animal antibodies to produce a color change. These color changes are either seen by the naked eye or are read by digital imaging.

Western blot assays test for proteins in blood or tissue. Samples from patients are placed in a gel and electrophoresis is used to separate the antigens of interest from the blood. The antigens are then transferred onto a holding membrane where they are exposed to antibodies. Then the sample is tested using either digital imaging (chemiluminescence) or color imaging (fluorescence).

Lateral flow IAs are the simplest type of immunoassay available and often used in point of care testing. For a lateral flow immunoassay, a sample of blood or urine is placed on the sample pad that is housed in a testing cassette or strip. As the sample migrates across the cassette or strip, the antigens and antibodies in the sample will combine with their complementary area on the pad. The combined antigen-antibody complex allows a color change visible to the naked eye. This process usually takes 10 to 15 minutes.[25]

Molecular Diagnostics

An area of rapid expansion in laboratory testing is molecular diagnostics. These tests specifically look for genetic material regarding the condition of interest.

Fluorescence in situ hybridization (FISH) is a microscopic technique developed in the 1980s. FISH looks for specific DNA sequences by applying a fluorescently tagged probe whose job it is to seek out a unique sequence of DNA on a microbe. To begin the test, the sample is heated, which separates the microbe's

DNA strands. Then the fluorescent tagged probe is added to the sample. If the DNA sequence of interest exists, the tagged DNA sequence will adhere (hybridize) and the fluorescence can be seen under microscope. FISH has a quicker result time than cultures. FISH is useful to identify bacteria that do not easily grow in culture medium and is also used in cancer diagnosis such as leukemia.[26]

Nucleic acid amplification tests (NAATs) define a large group of test methods that amplify genetic material of specimens to look for microbes of interest. They can be performed on ribonucleic acid or DNA. The most common NAATs are polymerase chain reactions (PCR) and reverse transcriptase PCRs. Regardless of method used, the overall premise of NAAT is to amplify or make extra copies of the DNA/RNA so that enough material exists to allow identification. The amplification process is completed during a process called thermal cycling which heats and then cools the specimen during repeated cycles. Once enough copies have been made, the specimen DNA/RNA copies are placed next to the DNA/RNA of a pathogenic organism of interest. Both samples are placed in a gel and then electrical current is applied in a process called electrophoresis. When the sample results match, the result is a positive test. The benefits of NAAT include that it is less labor intensive compared to culture or microscopy and there is a quicker turnaround. A major drawback is the cost. For example, NAAT for tuberculosis testing is 4x more expensive than sputum smear microscopy and this can be cost-prohibitive for low or middle income countries.[27]

REFERENCES

Full list of references can be accessed through Springer Publishing Company Connect™ at the following link: http://connect.springerpub.com/content/reference-book/978-0-8261 -8843-4/part/part01/toc-part/ch003

4. LABORATORY POLICY AND REGULATIONS

Kelly Small Casler

Like medical devices and pharmaceuticals, laboratory tests are subject to oversight and policies to assure safety and efficacy. Appropriate use of laboratory methods requires an understanding of the basic regulatory methods regarding laboratory testing.

CLINICAL LABORATORY IMPROVEMENT AMENDMENTS

The Centers for Medicare and Medicaid Services began regulation of laboratory testing in 1988 through the Clinical Laboratory Improvement Amendments (CLIA). Some laboratories, such as Veterans Affairs hospital laboratories, are not subject to CLIA regulations, however. The purpose of CLIA is to ensure high-quality laboratory results and testing practices. Laboratories must follow CLIA regulations to achieve certification and accreditation. Laboratories are certified by state regulating bodies (usually health departments) and can be accredited by one of several national accrediting organizations such as the Commission on Office Laboratory Accreditation, College of American Pathologists, and The Joint Commission.[1]

FEDERAL DRUG ADMINISTRATION

Laboratory tests are considered medical devices. As such, the Food and Drug Administration (FDA) is responsible for their oversight. The FDA assures quality test performance prior to any marketing of commercial laboratory tests. When new laboratory tests are developed, manufacturers must submit through one of three pathways for approval as a new test for commercialization. The first two approval pathways, de novo and premarket approval, are used when there is no comparable laboratory test on the market. The specific pathway chosen will depend on the complexity of the test. If a comparable laboratory test currently exists in the market, manufacturers can submit equivalency data, much like the generic pharmaceutical approval practice. This pathway is referred to as 510K.[2]

Manufacturers must also achieve FDA approval for new diagnostic indications or for new collection processes of prior approved tests. A recent example is the resubmission of a nucleic acid amplification test (NAAT) for chlamydia and gonorrhea to add extragenital sites (pharyngeal and rectal) as an approved collection site.[3]

Some laboratories will design and manufacture tests without the intent for commercialization and for only use within their own laboratory. These tests are referred to as laboratory developed tests (LDTs).[4,5] These tests are not subject to FDA regulatory oversight, which is one of the reasons for their popularity. LDTs were extensively used during the SARS-CoV-2 pandemic.

In times of domestic, military, or public health emergencies, the FDA may issue emergency use authorization (EUA) to certain diagnostic tests, allowing them to forgo approval through the pathways described earlier. The benefits of the test must outweigh any known or potential risk according to scientific evidence available at the time the EUA is initiated.[6] Once the EUA is rescinded, the tests must be submitted for approval in the usual manner. EUA also allows for new, previously unapproved uses of already established tests, such as a new collection procedure or sites as described earlier with NAAT testing. Several diagnostic tests came to the market under EUA during the SARS-CoV-2 pandemic.

COMPLEXITY ASSESSMENT AND CERTIFICATIONS

Oversight of laboratory tests through the regulatory roles of the FDA and CLIA are complementary. The FDA regulates the quality of laboratory tests, whereas CLIA regulates the quality of the laboratories conducting the tests. When manufacturers initially submit laboratory tests for FDA approval, the FDA will review submitted data to categorize the test into one of three complexity categories defined by CLIA[1]: waived, moderate, and high complexity.

Box 4.1: Criteria Used to Rank Complexity of Laboratory Tests

- Calibration, quality control, and proficiency testing measures
- Characteristics of operational steps
- Interpretation and judgment
- Knowledge
- Reagents and materials preparation
- Training and expertise
- Troubleshooting and equipment maintenance

Source: Federal Drug Administration. CLIA categorizations. https://www.fda.gov/medical-devices/ivd-regulatory-assistance/clia-categorizations.

The FDA uses seven criteria (Box 4.1) to categorize the test into the appropriate complexity category. Tests that are in the waived category are tests that have low complexity and can be completed outside of a traditional laboratory, often as a point of care test (POCT). Moderate and high complexity tests must be completed in a laboratory. However, some moderately complex tests may be approved to be performed outside the laboratory and near the point of care by properly trained clinicians using a microscope. These exceptions are made because performing the test at the point of care will improve the timeliness of care, allowing the clinician to have the result sooner to assist with clinical decision- making. Examples of these provider-performed microscopy tests are described in Box 4.2.

CLIA regulates laboratory practices through the provision of CLIA certificates. The type of CLIA certificate that is applied for depends on the goals of the site and complexity of the tests it needs to perform (Table 4.1).

POINT OF CARE TESTING AND DIRECT-TO-CONSUMER TESTS

POCT refers to laboratory tests completed outside of the laboratory, near where patient care is occurring.[7] Examples of laboratory tests that can be completed as POCTs include glucose, urinalysis, lipid testing, international normalized ratio, heterophile antibody tests, hemoglobin, urine human chorionic gonadotropin, influenza, and rapid strep antigen tests.[8] Moving testing outside of the

Box 4.2: Provider-Performed Microscopy

- Fecal leukocyte examination
- Fern test
- Nasal smears for granulocytes
- Potassium hydroxide mounts (skin or vaginal elements)
- Qualitative semen analysis
- Stool examination for pinworms
- Urine sediment microscopy
- Wet mount/hanging drop

Source: Data from Centers for Disease Control and Prevention. *Provider-Performed Microscopy (PPM) Procedures.* 2019. https://www.cdc.gov/labquality/ppm.html.

TABLE 4.1: SUMMARY OF CLINICAL LABORATORY IMPROVEMENT AMENDMENTS CERTIFICATES

Certificate of Waiver	Site is approved to perform waived tests (low complexity) such as POCTs
Certificate of Provider-Performed Microscopy	Site is approved to conduct provider-performed microscopy procedures.
Certificate of Registration	Site is approved to perform moderate or high complexity testing while awaiting a compliance visit by the state department of health.
Certificate of Compliance	Issued to site after survey visit if the laboratory is determined to be in compliance with regulations
Certificate of Accreditation	Issued to laboratory by an accrediting organization

Source: Data from Centers for Disease Control. *Test Complexities.* 2018. https://www.cdc.gov/clia/test-complexities.html; Federal Drug Administration. *CLIA Categorizations.* https://www.fda.gov/medical-devices/ivd-regulatory-assistance/clia-categorizations.

laboratory and nearer to the patient can improve clinical care outcomes and cost effectiveness through better turnaround times, decreased need for laboratory personnel, and fewer errors in specimen collection/handling. However, POCTs can have drawbacks. Not all insurance carriers reimburse for every POCT, and POCTs may result in more overhead costs due to employee time needed to run quality controls and keep accurate records.[8] Additionally, sometimes conducting the test at the point of care may be more costly than sending the sample to the clinical laboratory.[8] However, when overall costs are considered, such as length of stay, re-admission rates, and efficiency, POCTs actually present cost savings.[9-12] POCTs can also improve patient satisfaction.[13]

Some POCTs are FDA approved for direct-to-consumer marketing for at home use (Box 4.3). One of the most common examples is urine pregnancy tests. To be approved for direct-to-consumer marketing, companies must demonstrate that the tests perform in the at-home setting similar to the clinical setting.[14]

Box 4.3: Current Food and Drug Administration-Approved Direct-to-Consumer Point of Care Testing for Home Use

- Follicle-stimulating hormone (to assess menopause and ovulation)
- Hepatitis C
- Human immunodeficiency virus
- Prothrombin time
- Urine pregnancy tests (human chorionic gonadotropin)
- Vaginal PH

Source: Data from U.S. Food and Drug Administration. *Home Use Tests.* 2019. https://www.fda.gov/medical-devices/vitro-diagnostics/home-use-tests

REFERENCES

Full list of references can be accessed through Springer Publishing Company Connect™ at the following link: http://connect.springerpub.com/content/reference-book/978-0-8261-8843-4/part/part01/toc-part/ch004

EVIDENCE-BASED USE OF LABORATORY TESTS RELATING TO GENETICS AND SPECIAL CIRCUMSTANCES

5. DIRECT-TO-CONSUMER GENETIC TESTING

Deanna Hunt and Kelly Small Casler

BACKGROUND AND OVERVIEW

In 2003, the completion of the Human Genome Project allowed new, genetic opportunities for health problem diagnosis and screening.[1] Traditionally, genetic testing has been ordered by healthcare clinicians after determining which genetic tests are needed based on family or personal history. The patient would then return to review the results with the clinician.[2] More recently, however, patients have started using commercial, direct-to-consumer (DTC) genetic testing. With DTC genetic testing, the consumer can purchase a genetic test through different online vendors or companies or even at a local pharmacy. These tests are not covered by health insurance and do not involve the patient's healthcare team. Initially, DTC genetic tests were cost-prohibitive, but a significant drop in price in the last decade has led to increased popularity of these tests.[3]

The focus of DTC genetic testing differs according to the company's emphasis or foci.[4] Once a consumer orders a DTC test, they obtain samples from either saliva or cells within the mouth.[5] Using the DNA collected, the company produces results through an internal program and ultimately sends a report to the consumer. DTC genetic tests may test for relatively general concepts like hair pattern or ancestral information.[5] Others may offer testing for chronic disease (Box 5.1). Pharmacogenetic tests are also available through DTC testing, which informs the consumer of how they might respond to a drug or if they are more likely to have an adverse drug reaction.[6] Newer DTC genetic tests offer testing for athletic performance prediction.[7] Regardless of testing foci, DTC genetic tests only examine a small fraction of the more than 20,000 genes within the human body, and many times they are not individualized to the purchasing consumer. Currently, there are dozens of companies that offer the testing and the number is growing, as is the capability of these tests.[2]

One drawback with DTC genetic testing is the lack of regulation and oversight.[8] DTC genetic testing initially came to market without oversight from the Food and Drug Administration (FDA). However, in 2010, the FDA began requiring approval of these tests just as for other laboratory tests.[9] Further, DTC genetic tests have varying levels of evidence that support each of their claims, with some companies offering high levels of scientific evidence and data to support, and others offering minimal data.[10] Other limitations of DTC testing include the lack of genetic privacy, invalid or inaccurate results, limited health counseling included with test results, and the risk that the results would lead to an inability to obtain life, disability, or long-term healthcare insurance (genetic

Box 5.1: List of Chronic Disease Genetic Risk Testing Offered by a DTC Test*

- Alpha-1 antitrypsin deficiency
- Celiac disease
- Early onset primary dystonia
- Parkinson disease
- Factor XI deficiency
- Gaucher disease type 1
- Glucose 6 phosphate dehydrogenase deficiency
- Hereditary hemochromatosis
- Hereditary thrombophilia
- Late-onset Alzheimer's disease

*Remember that DTC tests may not include all variants that can lead to chronic disease, and therefore can provide false reassurance to the patient.

DTC, direct to consumer.

Source: Data from Food and Drug Administration. FDA allows marketing of first direct-to-consumer tests that provide genetic risk information for certain conditions. Published April 6, 2017. https://www.fda.gov/news-events/press-announcements/fda-allows-marketing-first-direct-consumer-tests-provide-genetic-risk-information-certain-conditions.

discrimination).[11] The concern for genetic discrimination is a complex issue since protection at the state level varies. At the federal level, the Genetic Information Nondiscrimination Act (GINA) provides some protection. However, GINA does not generally protect against discrimination if a patient is already having symptoms of a genetic disease; it only limits insurers from refusing to cover asymptomatic patients with a positive genetic test for a chronic disease.[12]

The role of DTC genetic testing in patient care is controversial and unclear. A recent systematic review of European position statements and guidelines found more risks than benefit.[13] Yet, one study found that DTC negative genetic tests reduced patient anxiety although this may simply be false reassurance.[8,14] While some experts argue that the results could help motivate patients to change unhealthy lifestyles, one study refuted this argument.[15,16] The varying data and controversies can place a significant strain on clinicians. Further, clinicians may not be prepared to counsel patients about tests due to lack of training, lack of testing validity, and lack of time.[4] Although there have been recent efforts to move genetic testing to primary care instead of directly to the consumer,[17] this is challenging since primary care providers feel undereducated to recommend and interpret genetic testing.[18,19] Clinicians wishing to educate themselves on genetic testing can find education modules from the Jaxson Laboratory at https://learn.education.jax.org/browse/hpe/

EXPERT RECOMMENDATIONS

Several organizations have made position statements regarding DTC genetic testing:

- The American Medical Association and the National Society of Genetic Counselors encourages patients to seek care and guidance of a physician, healthcare provider, or genetic counselor when using DTC genetic testing.[20,21]

- The American College of Obstetricians and Gynecologists (ACOG) recommended against DTC genetic testing, stating the tests have the potential to cause harm as a result of misinterpretation and the potential for inaccurate results.[2]
- The Association for Molecular Pathology supports DTC genomic testing under specific conditions and opposes DTC genetic testing when the tests provide information that is not clinically valid.[22]
- The U.S. FDA published a warning letter to consumers to emphasize that DTC are not a substitution for traditional healthcare evaluations and care.[10]
- Choosing Wisely Canada recommends a thorough understanding of risks and limitations of DTC testing when using it to make health-related decisions.[23]

INDICATIONS

Screening

- A patient requiring targeted genetic testing due to family or personal medical history should not use DTC genetic tests and instead seek care from a clinician including a genetic counselor, physician, physician assistant, or advanced practice registered nurse.

Diagnosis and Evaluation

- Not indicated

Monitoring

- Not used

INTERPRETATION

- DTC genetic testing results are sent to the consumer along with an interpretation report; however, results are often misinterpreted in this approach.[3] Further complicating interpretation is that each company has its own (and often different) reference values, using the pool of results from prior customers or public DNA sequencing reports.[24]
- DTC genetic testing does not always provide conclusive results.[5,8] One evaluation showed that for twins, the concordance rate between three different companies was only 52.7% to 84.1%.[24]
- Results can cause false reassurances.[8]
- There is a high risk of false positives. One evaluation showed up to a 40% false positive rate.[4,25]

FOLLOW-UP

- There is no clear consensus on how to follow-up a patient's DTC genetic report.
- There is a concern for potential unnecessary and inappropriate follow-up testing and utilization of healthcare resources as a result of DTC genetic testing.[4]

PEARLS & PITFALLS

- Ideally, DTC genetic testing should be paired with a genetic counseling visit since patients don't always follow up on important findings reported on DTC tests.[26]
- DTC genetic testing usually lacks comprehensiveness. Although companies advertise that they are testing for genetic conditions, they may in fact not be completely testing for all genetic variants that can cause a particular disease.[25]
- There are privacy concerns related to DTC genetic testing and who will have access to the genetic material.[4] It is important that the consumer be aware that genetic data from their sample can be used for research purposes.[5]
- One study found that public advertising videos available to the public about DTC testing lacked accuracy.[27]

PATIENT EDUCATION

- https://www.genome.gov/Pages/PolicyEthics/GeneticTesting/DTC_handout.pdf
- https://ghr.nlm.nih.gov/primer/dtcgenetictesting/directtoconsumer
- http://www.mayoclinicproceedings.org/article/S0025-6196(17)30772-3/fulltext
- https://www.choosingwisely.org/patient-resources/making-smart-decisions-about-genetic-testing/

RELATED DIAGNOSES AND ICD-10 CODES

Encounter with genetic testing	Z76.89
Encounter with genetic counseling	Z71.83
Counseling for genetic conditions	Z71.9

REFERENCES

Full list of references can be accessed through Springer Publishing Company Connect™ at the following link: http://connect.springerpub.com/content/reference-book/978-0-8261-8843-4/part/part02/toc-part/ch005

6. CANCER GENETIC TESTING FOR BREAST AND GYNECOLOGIC CANCER SCREENING

Deanna Hunt

PATHOPHYSIOLOGY REVIEW

Breast cancer is the most common cancer affecting women with an average lifetime risk reported to be about 12%.[1] Breast cancer most commonly forms within the lobules, the mechanism in which the breast creates milk, and the ducts, the mechanism in which milk is transported through the breast and the lobules, of the breast. Cancer of the breast develops in the duct 80% of the time and the lobules totaling about 10% of annual breast cancer diagnoses.[1] Breast cancer develops as a result of environmental and genetic factors. The cancer is classified by location and pathologic markers, which are determined by estrogen, progesterone, and human epidermal growth factor receptor 2 (HER-2/neu) proteins on the outside of the cancer cell. Cancer therapies are often targeted at these proteins. Common genetic variants associated with breast cancer are variants within the *BRCA1* and *BRCA2* genes. The risk of developing breast cancer in a woman with a *BRCA1* mutation is 57% in her lifetime and 49% with a *BRCA2* mutation.[1] While the *BRCA1* and *BRCA2* gene mutations are widely known, there are other genes associated with ovarian cancer (Table 6.1).

Gynecologic cancer originates within a woman's reproductive organs. Types of gynecologic cancer include cervical, ovarian, uterine (endometrial), vaginal, or vulvar cancer. Each of these cancers is unique and has different risk factors, including hereditary or genetic. Approximately 20% of ovarian cancer cases are caused by germline or genetic mutations. Of the germline ovarian cancer cases, between 65% and 85% of these mutations are within the *BRCA1* and *BRCA2* gene.[2] Mutations within the *BRCA* genes impair DNA repair, which allows for damaged mutations to stay in the DNA. These mutations persist, accumulate, grow, and divide without a controlled way to stop them as a result of the mutation within the tumor suppression genes, *BRCA1* and *BRCA2*. While the *BRCA1*

TABLE 6.1: CANCER-SUSCEPTIBLE GENES	
CANCER	**CANCER-SUSCEPTIBILITY GENES**
Breast cancer	*BRCA1, BRCA2, CDH1, PALB2, PTEN, STK11, TP53, ATM, BRIP1, CHEK2, FANCD2, RAD51C*
Ovarian cancer	*BRCA1, BRCA2, ATM, BRIP1, EPCAM, MLH1, MSH2, MSH6, RAD51C*
Endometrial cancer	*EPCAM, MLH1, MSH2, MSH6, PMS2, PTEN*

and *BRCA2* gene mutations are widely known, there are other genes associated with ovarian cancer (Table 6.1).[2]

Endometrial or uterine cancer may also be caused by a germline or genetic mutation. Approximately 2% to 5% of endometrial cancer cases are a result of these mutations, most commonly Lynch syndrome.[3,4] Lynch syndrome is an autosomal dominant syndrome caused by germline mutation in a mismatch repair (MMR) gene. The mismatch repair is a process that corrects mistakes made when DNA is copied. The MMR genes (*MLHL, MSH2, MSH6, PMS2,* and *EPCAM*) are normally cancer protective and work to prevent a person from getting cancer.[5] Those with Lynch syndrome have a 40% to 60% lifetime risk of endometrial cancer, as well as a 6% to 8% risk of ovarian cancer.[4,6] Other gynecologic cancers including cervical, vaginal, and vulvar cancer are typically not caused by genetic mutations and instead are caused by the HPV virus.[7]

OVERVIEW OF LABORATORY TESTS

Genetic testing in the United States continues to change and evolve. As a result of the 2013 Supreme Court of the United States ruling stating that human genes cannot be patented, genetic testing is now much more available and accessible.[8] There are several clinical laboratories that offer multigene, or panel, genetic testing, made much easier through next-generation sequencing methods. Next-generation sequencing is used to determine a section of the nucleotide sequencing of a person's genome. This is done through technologies that have the capability to process multiple DNA sequences in parallel.[9] Multigene panel tests have the ability to use next-generation sequencing to test for multiple genes at once.[10,11] Multigene testing has the ability to test for more than 50 genes at once, oftentimes at the same price as single-gene testing. The benefit of multigene testing is not only the cost, but that these panels can be specific to the cancer type including ovarian or endometrial. It is important that these tests be ordered by a cancer genetic professional in order to determine the most appropriate panel for the patient.[10,12] There can be problems with multigene testing. Genes recognized by the multigene panel can be associated with a questionable cancer risk or may even have a variant with uncertain significance.[12] Prior to testing, it is important to review possible result outcomes.

When thinking about genetic testing, it is important to consider the costs of these tests. Most health insurance plans cover the cost of genetic testing in the setting of cancer and when recommended by a physician, but it is important to first check with the insurance plan. Currently, Medicare covers the cost of genetic counseling and testing in patients with a personal history of cancer. Additionally, Medicare will cover *BRCA1* and *BRCA2* testing under certain conditions. Medicaid programs offer coverage for *BRCA* testing as well; however, coverage varies by state. With the passage of the Affordable Care Act (ACA) in 2010, health insurance plans can now no longer refuse coverage or charge more for coverage due to a person's preexisting health condition, an important legislative win for genetic testing protection in cancer patients.[13]

INDICATIONS

Screening—Universal

- Genetic testing for gynecologic oncology:
  - The U.S. Preventative Services Task Force (USPSTF) recommends against routine screening for ovarian cancer in asymptomatic women without a known high-risk hereditary cancer syndrome. Grade: D recommendation.[14]
  - The USPSTF does not recommend routine screening for ovarian cancer using any method.[14]
  - There are no recommendations for endometrial cancer screening in the general population.[6]
- Genetic testing for breast oncology:
  - The USPSTF has found adequate evidence that genetic counseling and testing are moderate in women with a family history associated with an increased risk of harmful mutations within the *BRCA1* and *BRCA2* genes.[15]
  - The USPSTF has found adequate evidence that the benefits of genetic counseling and testing are small to none in women without a family history associated with an increased risk of harmful mutations within the *BRCA1* and *BRCA2* genes.[15]

Screening—Targeted

- Clinicians are responsible for managing cancer screening and surveillance based on a personalized approach. They often use recommendations from health organizations, outlined in the text that follows, and work in conjunction with genetic counselors when appropriate. Genetic counselors are experts in educating and providing risk management for patients with an inherited disease. While they do not order specific genetic tests, they provide recommendations for the clinician to order. Genetic counselors are also responsible for interpreting results and counseling patients.[16]
- Several organizations including the National Comprehensive Cancer Network (NCCN), the American Society of Human Genetics, the American College of Medical Genetics and Genomics, USPSTF, and Society of Gynecologic Oncology (SGO) have all developed criteria to help providers in deciding who should undergo genetic testing (Table 6.2).
- The SGO recommends that all women diagnosed with epithelial ovarian, fallopian tube, and peritoneal cancers receive genetic counseling and be offered genetic testing.[17]
- The SGO recommends that all women diagnosed with endometrial cancer be assessed for Lynch syndrome.[17]
- Breast cancer targeted screening is reviewed in Table 6.2.

INTERPRETATION

- Must be interpreted by multidisciplinary healthcare team (including genetic counselor) and in context of patient history

TABLE 6.2: INDICATIONS FOR GENETIC TESTING IN BREAST CANCER

Indication to test: Personal history	Female with breast cancer diagnosed age *younger than 45* or male diagnosed at any age[18]	Breast cancer diagnosed age *46–50* with any of the following: • Unknown family history • Second breast cancer diagnosis at any age • More than one blood relative with breast, ovarian, prostate, or pancreatic cancer[18]	Triple negative breast cancer at age *younger than 60*[8]	Diagnosis of multiple primary breast cancers first diagnosed between the ages of 50 and 60[18]	Any new diagnosis of epithelial ovarian, tubal, and peritoneal cancers at ANY age[18]
Indication to test: No personal history of breast cancer and positive family history	Person who is directly related to a female with breast cancer diagnosed age *younger than 45* or male diagnosed at any age[18]	Person who is directly related to a woman with breast cancer diagnosed age *46–50* with unknown family hx, second breast cancer diagnosis at any age, or more than one blood relative with breast, ovarian, prostate, or pancreatic cancer[18]	Person who is directly related to a woman diagnosed with triple negative breast cancer at age *younger than 60*[8]	Person who is directly related to a woman diagnosed with multiple primary breast cancers first diagnosed between the ages of 50 and 60[18]	Person who has a probability of 2.5%–5% BRCA ½ pathogenic variant based on prior probability models (e.g., greater than 10% Tryer-Cuzick, greater than 70% BRCAPro, 5% CanRisk)[18]
Indication to test: No personal or family history of cancer	Person with a blood relative with known pathogenic variant[18]	Person of Ashkenazi Jewish descent[18]			

FOLLOW-UP

■ Consider referral to genetic counselor for repeat genetic testing if family history changes.

PEARLS & PITFALLS

■ Informed consent is required.
■ Prior to testing:
  ● Review implications for family members (Table 6.3).[12]
  ● Review the risks, benefits, and limitations (Table 6.3).[12]
  ● Review possible outcomes including variants of uncertain significance.[12]

TABLE 6.3: CONSIDERATIONS, LIMITATIONS, AND RISKS OF GENETIC TESTING

Considerations of testing	If more than one family member is affected with a highly inherited cancer (breast, ovarian), consider testing the family member who was youngest at diagnosis or had other classic features of the disease.[18]	In children 18 years and younger, testing is *not* recommended when results would not impact the medical management of the patient.[18]	If there is a recommendation to complete testing when no affected family member is available, an unaffected family member should be considered.[18]	Consider multigene testing when a person tests negative for a single syndrome, but their history is suggestive of an inherited susceptibility. This is especially important if a person completed genetic testing many years ago prior to the technology advancements with multigene testing.[18]	Commercial tests may differ in specific genes analyzed with varying forms of RNA analysis. Consider only using companies certified by CAP (College of American Pathologists).[18]
Risks for testing	Finding a variant of unknown significance, which is a genetic alteration that might actually represent a benign finding leading to unclear clinical decision-making.[18]	Risk of false positives resulting in overscreening and overtreating[18]	Multigene panel testing increases the risk of finding a variant of unknown significance without clear clinical significance, leading to anxiety in the carrier.[18]	Genetic testing may not be approved by all insurance companies, leading to worsening health disparities for those of lower socioeconomic status.[19]	Expected long-term financial consequences of predictive genetic testing due to overscreening and overtreating[19]
Limitations of testing	Use in caution in patients who have received allogenic bone marrow transplant might have donor contamination in results[18]	Probability of variant detection is poorly affected when there is little known about family history (adopted family members)[18]	Significant limitations in result analysis when testing an unaffected family member[18]	When a person is found to have a variant of unknown significance there is no clinical recommendations for testing or management of family members[18]	Error rate for commercial companies and direct-to-consumer tests providing *ancestry* and sometimes health information is substantial and should not be used for clinical decision making[18]

- Consider psychologic issues and problems associated with genetic counseling and genetic testing[12]
- Psychologic issues may affect:
  - Declining genetic counseling and testing[12]
  - Uptake of genetic counseling and testing[12]
  - Impact of risk perception[12]
  - Impact of health beliefs[12]
  - Consider personality characteristics.[12]

PATIENT EDUCATION

- https://www.NCCN.org (Free access and log in)
- https://www.sgo.org/

RELATED DIAGNOSES AND ICD-10 CODES

Ovarian cancer	C56.9
Uterine cancer (endometrium)	C54.1
Breast cancer	Z85.3

REFERENCES

Full list of references can be accessed through Springer Publishing Company Connect™ at the following link: http://connect.springerpub.com/content/reference-book/978-0-8261-8843-4/part/part02/toc-part/ch006

7. GENETIC TESTING FOR PHARMACOTHERAPY

Christopher G. Green

PHARMACOGENOMICS—OVERVIEW

The field of pharmacogenomics developed from the work on the Human Genome Project.[1] How a patient's unique DNA, enzymes, and proteins interact with medications can lead to vastly different outcomes from one patient to the next. The primary areas where genetics and medications interact include pharmacokinetics (drug uptake, transport, and breakdown) and pharmacodynamics (drug receptors and disease-specific targeted drug development).[2,3] Interpatient genetic differences occur when a nucleotide sequence is altered—through insertion, deletion, or switching. This leads to variability among nucleotide sequences and corresponding variability in pharmacokinetic and/or pharmacodynamic responses in patients.[4]

Gene variants, or alleles, are often classified using a star allele nomenclature system.[4] The alleles are named by a star (*) followed by a number that corresponds to an activity level for the enzyme in question. The *1 is usually associated with a lack of any discovered variations and therefore "normal" activity. Alleles notated with a number other than 1 indicate a variation from the norm. When paired together, star alleles can be described by how they confer enzymatic activity.[4,5] Levels of activity are categorized from poor to ultra-rapid metabolizers.[4]

Though a relatively new field in Pharmacology, there are organizations that are dedicated to research and guideline development for actionable prescribing decision-making. The Pharmacogenomics Knowledge Base (PharmGKB) is a database that compiles primary and secondary data for genes and medications. The database includes resources on genotype-based drug dosing, prescribing guidelines, and drug labeling with biomarker information, along with pharmacokinetic and pharmacodynamic drug-centered pathways.[6] The Clinical Pharmacogenomics Implementation Consortium (CPIC) is a shared project between PharmGKB and the Pharmacogenomics Research Network (PGRN).[7] The CPIC is considered the gold standard for pharmacogenomic guidelines.

OVERVIEW OF LABORATORY TEST(S)

In most settings, it is unlikely that clinicians in primary care can order pharmacogenetic testing to be performed by their local laboratory or hospital. For clinicians interested in finding a reference laboratory, the National Institutes of Health maintains a searchable Genetic Testing Registry.[8,9] Pharmacogenetic testing is often performed either on a single gene or in concert with multiple genes as part of a broad panel.[8,10] While some tests have assigned CPT codes, not all genetic tests yet have codes assigned.[10,11] Examples of CPT codes for selected genetic tests include[10]:

- Test for variation in CYP2C19: 81225
- Test for variation in CYP2D6: 81226
- Test for variation in VKORC1: 81355

Test samples provided are typically saliva or blood.[11] The type of tests to be performed, interpretation of results, and the format in which results are presented vary from laboratory to laboratory. Costs for testing are variable as is insurance coverage for genetic testing. A recent review of 41 insurers demonstrated that approximately 40% of gene-drug tests were covered.[12]

INDICATIONS
Screening
- At present, universal screening for pharmacogenetic variations is not recommended by the Food and Drug Administration (FDA).[13]
- Choosing Wisely provides additional recommendations against universal screening based on clinical society guidance for the presence of specific genetic conditions.[14]

- Targeted screening may be appropriate based on recommendations from the manufacturer and guidance by the FDA for certain populations.[13,15]
- Additional information and links to guidelines for specific agents are available at the CPIC website.[16]
- Sections within the package inserts where genetic testing recommendations are referenced are provided by the FDA on a drug-per-drug basis.[15]

Diagnosis and Evaluation

Testing for pharmacogenetic variability may be most valuable in the following scenarios:

- To determine the best option within a class of medications with varying pathways for metabolism.[4,13–17]
- After treatment failure with more than one medication within a class.[4,13–17]
- Prediction of possible side effects due to use of a medication where variants in genetic makeup could lead to more severe negative outcomes.[4,13–17]

Monitoring

- There is no generally recognized monitoring for pharmacogenomic testing outside of any monitoring specific to the patient's condition or medications they are taking.
- Choosing Wisely provides recommendations regarding repeat testing:
  - "Don't order a duplicate genetic test for an inherited condition unless there is uncertainty about the validity of the existing test result."[17]

INTERPRETATION

Pharmacokinetic-based testing focused on drug metabolism and breakdown looks at two mechanisms—phase I and phase II reactions. Phase I reactions involve oxidation, reduction, and hydroxylation, and the focus is primarily on Cytochrome P450 (CYP450) polymorphisms. Phase II reactions involve conjugation that leads to an increase in hydrophilicity to aid in excretion.[18]

When looking at CYP450, there are four isoenzymes that impact the most commonly prescribed medications: 2C9, 2C19, 2D6, and 3A4.[4] Depending on the variation seen, patients can be categorized as to how effectively they can metabolize a medication impacted by the relevant isoenzyme(s) as shown in Table 7.1.[3,4,18–20]

An allele-by-allele polymorphism or enzyme-by-enzyme description is not practical for the purposes of this text. However, a list compiled by the FDA is available at: www.fda.gov/medical-devices/precision-medicine/table-pharmacogenetic-associations. This list provides tables of drugs, genes, and affected polymorphisms that include descriptions of the gene-drug interaction.[13]

Phase II specific testing impacts the second part of drug metabolism. The two most common gene-drug variants seen in clinical practice involve thiopurine S-methyltransferase (TPMT) and nucleoside diphosphate-linked moiety X (NUDT15).[3] Medications impacted by TPMT and NUDT15 metabolism include 6-mercaptopurine, azathioprine, and thioguanine. Similar to phase I changes in alleles, loss of function prevalence can lead to poor metabolism and toxicity of the medications and their metabolites. The CPIC has a guideline for thiopurine

TABLE 7.1: CYP450 ENZYME PHENOTYPE

PHENOTYPE	DESCRIPTION OF GENETIC MECHANISM	PHARMACOKINETIC IMPACT
Ultra-rapid	Carries two increased function alleles	Reduced half-lives, increased metabolic breakdown, increased rate of therapeutic failure Prodrugs activated by the enzyme: increased concentrations, increased toxicity
Rapid	Carries one normal function and one increased function allele	Similar effects as seen with ultra-rapid metabolizers, but to a lesser extent
Normal	Carries two normal function alleles	Patient should have a normal or expected risk/benefit profile consistent with results seen in clinical studies
Intermediate	Carries one normal function and one no function allele OR one no function and one increased function allele	Similar effects as seen with poor metabolizers, but to a lesser extent
Poor	Carries two no function alleles	Longer half-lives, decreased metabolic breakdown, increased rate of side effects and toxicity. Prodrugs activated by the enzyme: decreased concentrations, increased rate of therapeutic failure

Sources: Data from Anker JVD, Reed MD, Allegaert K, Kearns GL. Developmental changes in pharmacokinetics and pharmacodynamics. *J Clin Pharmacol.* 2018;58:S10–S25. doi:10.1002/jcph.1284; Black EL, Hocum BT, Black KJ. The future: pharmacogenetics in primary care. *Prim Care Rep.* 2014;20(10):113–128; Caudle KE, Dunnenberger HM, Freimuth RR, et al. Standardizing terms for clinical pharmacogenetic test results: consensus terms from the Clinical Pharmacogenetics Implementation Consortium (CPIC). *Genet Med.* 2016;19(2):215–223. doi:10.1038/gim.2016.87; Roden D, McLeod H, Relling M, et al. Pharmacogenomics. *Lancet.* 2019;394:521–532. doi:10.1016/ S0140-6736(19)31276-0; Wake D, Ilbawi N, Dunnenberger H, Hulick P. Pharmacogenomics: prescribing precisely. *Med Clin North Am.* 2019;103(6):977–990. doi:10.1016/j.mcna.2019.07.002.

dosing based on TPMT and NUDT15 variations.[21] A third genetically variable enzyme is Dihydropyrimidine dehydrogenase (DPYD), which metabolizes pyrimidine-based oncology agents such as 5-fluorouracil and capecitabine. Loss of function alleles with DPYD similarly confer an increased risk of toxicity with use of these agents.[22]

Drug transport and uptake are the other portion of pharmacokinetics where genetic differences can impact patient outcomes. The solute carrier organic anion transporter (SLCO1B1) gene provides encoding for organic anion transporting polypeptide (OATP1B1), a drug transporter that carries medications into cells.[19] Impacts on medications are classified as increased, normal, decreased, or poor function as outlined in Table 7.2.[20] Depending on the pharmacologic action and the toxicity mechanism of the medications impacted, transport differences could lead to greater or lesser action along with greater or lesser risk of toxicity. Examples of medications impacted by SLCO-mediated polymorphisms include methotrexate, simvastatin (and statins in general), and montelukast.[23–25]

TABLE 7.2: DRUG TRANSPORTER PHENOTYPE

PHENOTYPE (FUNCTION)	DESCRIPTION OF GENETIC MECHANISM	PHARMACOKINETIC IMPACT
Increased	One or more increased function alleles	Increased function of transporter—more drug taken into the cells
Normal	Normal and/or decreased function alleles in various combinations	Normal function expectations
Decreased	Normal, decreased, and/or no function alleles in various combinations	Decreased drug transport—clinical impact is between normal and poor
Poor	No function and/or decreased function alleles in various combinations	Minimal and possibly no transporter function—minimal to no drug taken into the cells

Sources: Data from Black EL, Hocum BT, Black KJ. The future: pharmacogenetics in primary care. *Prim Care Rep.* 2014;20(10):113–128; Caudle KE, Dunnenberger HM, Freimuth RR, et al. Standardizing terms for clinical pharmacogenetic test results: consensus terms from the Clinical Pharmacogenetics Implementation Consortium (CPIC). *Genet Med.* 2016;19(2):215–223. doi:10.1038/gim.2016.87.

Another drug transport-related gene of interest is the adenosine triphosphate binding cassette (ABC) family. The *ABCB1* gene encodes for the p-glycoprotein transporter (Pgp).[19] While OATP carries medications into cells, Pgp is an efflux transporter that moves drugs out of cells. Polymorphisms in the *ABCB1* gene can lead to alterations in the expression of Pgp and influence how much drug is expelled for clearance.[19,26,27] P-glycoprotein can be further influenced by medications that can directly inhibit or induce the Pgp, which continues to be a growing area in pharmacogenomics.[27]

Pharmacokinetic interactions apply to those enzymatic differences that impact how a drug moves through the body, whereas pharmacodynamic interactions look more at the body's response to the drug. This often occurs at the receptor site and is impacted by genetic variations that address drug affinity to receptors, or genetic differences that allow for a drug to target specific mutations in a receptor to modulate its action.[3] Genes of interest from the pharmacodynamic perspective include: vitamin K epoxide reductase subunit 1 (VKORC1), glucose-6-phosphate dehydrogenase (G6PD), human leukocyte antigen (HLA), ryanodine receptor 1 (RYR1), and cystic fibrosis (CF) transmembrane conductance regulator (CFTR).[3] Unlike the graded levels seen with kinetic type polymorphisms, pharmacodynamic variations are often expressed as positive or negative, susceptible or non-susceptible.[16,20]

Patients who are on warfarin can have varying levels of response based on expression of VKORC1 variants that would make them more or less sensitive to warfarin. Warfarin can also be impacted by polymorphic variants in CYP2C9 and CYP4F2.[28] Algorithms for dosing warfarin based on polymorphic variation are available.[29] For individuals with G6PD deficiency, there are numerous drugs that are of concern.[30] To date, CPIC only has a guideline written for patients prescribed rasburicase.[31] The *RYR1* gene has implications for the use of succinylcholine and inhaled anesthetics. Patients who are positive for one of

50 variants of the *RYR1* gene, or a second gene with a similar outcome profile (CACNA1S), have a higher rate of malignant hyperthermia when exposed to these medications.[32]

The *CFTR* gene represents a unique application of combining pharmaco-dynamics with pharmacogenomics. Defects in the *CFTR* gene are the cause of CF. The identification of the G551D-CFTR variant led to the development of a targeted drug therapy (ivacaftor) to modulate the effects CFTR has on mucus, sweat, saliva, and digestive enzymes.[33] Patients diagnosed with CF can undergo testing and, if the specified variant is present, can be considered for treatment.

Application of HLA variants is more complex. Testing results typically indicate whether a person is positive or negative for a high-risk allele.[20] If positive, it is generally not advised to use medications that would be directly impacted by this genetic polymorphism. A commonly cited example is the presence of the HLA-B*15:02 allele and an increased risk of Stevens-Johnson syndrome (SJS) in patients of Asian descent.[3,34,35] For patients with European ancestry, the HLA-A*31:01 allele is associated with an increased risk of SJS and drug–skin reactions.[3,35]

FOLLOW-UP

- Follow-up testing is generally not indicated.[17]
- As this is a growing and evolving field, new genetic polymorphisms may be identified and may be applicable to a patient who was previously tested.
- Decisions to retest patients should include whether this will impact their care.

PEARLS & PITFALLS

- Not all tests will be covered by the patient's insurance plan. It is advisable to discuss this with the patient and consider having them connect with their insurer to see about coverage prior to ordering a test.[12]
- Translation of results from genetic testing to electronic medical records and compatibility with clinical decision support tools is not universal.[4]
- Interpretation of results can be challenging as not all laboratories report their results in a similar fashion.[36]
- The Genetic Information Non-discrimination Act (GINA) protects patients from discrimination for health insurance. It does not protect from discrimination for life, disability, or long-term care insurance.[37] This should be discussed with patients prior to testing.
- Consider a comprehensive panel versus a focused one if the cost is comparable. This may prevent the need for repeat testing.[11,19]
- Pharmacogenetic testing can be helpful in guiding therapy in a patient with a history of treatment failures.[4]
- Testing can aid in reducing the risk of severe adverse drug reactions (ex. Carbamazepine and HLA-B*15:02 conferring risk for SJS).[4]

PATIENT EDUCATION

- https://www.choosingwisely.org/patient-resources/making-smart-decisions-about-genetic-testing/
- https://medlineplus.gov/lab-tests/pharmacogenetic-tests/
- https://www.genome.gov/FAQ/Pharmacogenomics
- https://www.cincinnatichildrens.org/service/g/genetic-pharmacology/education

RELATED DIAGNOSES AND ICD-10 CODES

- ICD-10 coding is matched to the disease being evaluated or the medication being monitored. Examples include:

Warfarin and VKORC1, CYP2C19, CYP4F2 testing:
- Long-term use of anticoagulants   Z79.01

Carbamazepine and HLA-B*15:02 testing:
- Epilepsy, unspecified, intractable, without status epilepticus   G40.919

Panel for psychiatric medication testing due to treatment failure for depression:
- Major depressive disorder, single episode, unspecified   F32.9

Encounter for other screening for genetic and chromosomal abnormalities   Z13.79

REFERENCES

Full list of references can be accessed through Springer Publishing Company Connect™ at the following link: http://connect.springerpub.com/content/reference-book/978-0-8261-8843-4/part/part02/toc-part/ch007

---

8. EVIDENCE-BASED USE OF LABORATORY TESTS IN THE PERIOPERATIVE SETTING

Rachel Smith-Steinert and Beth Ann Clayton

BACKGROUND

According to the Centers for Disease Control and Prevention (CDC), approximately 48.3 million surgeries were performed in the United States in 2010.[1] To improve surgical care, patients seek preoperative screening to optimize medical conditions. When deciding which laboratory tests are necessary in the preoperative preparation phase, one must understand the ramifications and implications of results. Appropriate laboratory values and diagnostic tests are vital to determine a patient's anesthetic and surgical risk and to determine if any other procedures are necessary to minimize risk before surgery.[2]

The disputable issue is which tests are needed for what patient population, surgery, and setting. Preferably, test results would determine the presence of disease; however, literature shows most tests only increase or decrease the probability of disease.[3] Literature has revealed asymptomatic disease has little surgical risk implication. Narr et al. demonstrated in a healthy cohort of patients, who had no preoperative testing, no deaths or major perioperative morbidity occurred. The authors concluded that routine testing was not indicated in this population.[4]

For numerous reasons, the argument for performing routine testing is not recommended and it is debatable whether most ordered laboratory results impact the surgical course. The literature shows routine tests are ordered for a multitude of reasons but often are unrelated to findings based on the specific patient's history and examination.[2] Some of the rationale clinicians report are:

- Following customary practice or institutional mandates
- To further evaluate a known disease state
- To diagnose asymptomatic, unknown disease which is modifiable
- To detect nonmodifiable disease which could affect risk assessment[2]

The 2012 American Society of Anesthesiologists Practice Advisory for Paranesthesia Evaluation states that routine preoperative tests do not make an important contribution to preanesthetic evaluation of an asymptomatic patient.[5] When a plethora of routine preoperative tests are ordered, abnormal test results alter patient care only 0.22% to 0.56% of the time.[6] Golub et al. reviewed the records of 325 patients who had undergone preadmission testing prior to ambulatory surgery. Of these, 272 (84%) had at least one abnormal screening test result, whereas only 28 surgeries were delayed or canceled.[7]

Another rationale against routine laboratory testing is the exorbitant cost of this practice, annually estimated to be billions of U.S. dollars. Literature estimates 10% of the more than $30 billion spent on laboratory testing goes to preparing patients for procedures.[2] In the dynamic field of healthcare costs, there is a powerful push to drive down medical expenditures. Bernstein et al. demonstrated hospitalization and length of stay with delays in surgery were attributed to preoperative testing, with little to no changes in medical management or perioperative course.[8] All medical professionals can practice fiscal responsibility when preparing patients for surgery by only ordering necessary tests.

Lastly, the practice of routine laboratory testing can produce false positives and lead to unnecessary further testing.[2] Risks, benefits, and costs must all be weighed when ordering preoperative testing. Clinical discernment is needed to perform a risk assessment and requires addressing the following fundamental questions when ordering lab work and interpreting results:

- Are the patient's risk factors modifiable?
- Will delaying the procedure to obtain testing add to perioperative risk or patient morbidity?
- What interventions during the preoperative period can be implemented to reduce risk?
- Has the patient been provided enough information to make an informed decision concerning the risks, benefits, and alternatives?[2]

Risks of further testing, such as cardiac catheterization, can yield surgical delays, patient discomfort, or injury. Benefits may produce a safer anesthetic plan or improved medical management. A conclusion of most studies is that *routine* preoperative laboratory and procedure screening is not cost-effective or predictive of postoperative complications and is unnecessary when an extensive history and physical examination do not suggest any patient abnormalities.

Preoperative *specific testing* should occur only after review of the medical record, the patient is interviewed, history and physical is complete, and the type and risk of the planned procedure and anesthesia are understood.[9] It is recommended that surgical facilities develop *testing protocols* with medical staff input to determine indications for laboratory and diagnostic screening. When protocols are followed for ordering preoperative tests, the total number of tests have been reduced 50% to 60%, and the appropriateness of the tests have improved.[10] After careful inspection of the patient's medical history and physical assessment, *specific*, indicated testing can be ordered, suited to each individual. Overall, diagnostic testing results are deemed current within 6 months of the scheduled surgery if the results are normal and if the patient's current health indicates no change has occurred since the test was performed.[2]

The preoperative evaluation of the older adult patient should include assessing physiologic age by reviewing functional status and comorbidities. Barnett reports geriatric syndromes such as frailty, cognitive dysfunction, polypharmacy, and malnutrition should all be reviewed due to their implication in increased perioperative risk.[11] Laboratory testing should be based on underlying disease and not age alone.[11]

TEST SPECIFIC INDICATIONS

Box 8.1 summarizes evidence-based rationales for preoperative laboratory evaluation, which are described in the text that follows.

Box 8.1: Indications for Laboratory Testing

Hemoglobin and Hematocrit

- Age less than 6 months (less than 1 year if born prematurely)
- Hematologic malignancy
- Recent radiation or chemotherapy
- Renal disease
- Anticoagulant therapy
- Procedure with moderate to high blood loss potential
- Coexisting systemic disorders (e.g., cystic fibrosis, prematurity, severe malnutrition, renal failure, liver disease, congenital heart disease)

White Blood Cell Count

- Leukemia and lymphomas
- Recent radiation or chemotherapy
- Suspected infection that would lead to cancellation of surgery
- Aplastic anemia
- Hypersplenism
- Autoimmune collagen vascular disease

Serum Chemistry

- Renal disease
- Adrenal or thyroid disease
- Chemotherapy
- Pituitary or hypothalamic disease
- Body fluid loss or shifts (e.g., dehydration, bowel prep)
- Central nervous system disease

(continued)

Box 8.1: Indications for Laboratory Testing (*continued*)

Potassium

- Digoxin therapy
- Diuretic therapy
- ACE inhibitors or angiotensin receptor blockers

Creatinine and Blood Urea Nitrogen

- Cardiovascular disease (e.g., hypertension)
- Renal disease
- Adrenal disease
- Diabetes mellitus
- Diuretic therapy
- Digoxin therapy
- Body fluid loss or shifts (e.g., dehydration, bowel prep)
- Procedure requiring radiocontrast

Blood Glucose Level

- Diabetes mellitus
- Current corticosteroid use
- History of hypoglycemia
- Adrenal disease
- Cystic fibrosis

Liver Enzyme Tests

- Hepatic disease
- Exposure to hepatitis
- Therapy with hepatotoxic agents

Coagulation Studies

INR, Prothrombin Time, and Partial Thromboplastin Time

- Leukemia
- Hepatic disease
- Bleeding disorder
- Anticoagulant therapy
- Severe malnutrition or malabsorption
- Postoperative anticoagulation to establish a baseline

Platelet Count and Bleeding Time

- Bleeding disorder
- Abnormal hemorrhage, purpura, history of easy bruising

Urinalysis

- Not indicated as a routine screening test

Pregnancy Test

- Possibility of pregnancy

Medication Levels

- Monitor for medications (e.g., theophylline, phenytoin, digoxin, carbamazepine) if patient exhibits signs of ineffective therapy, potential drug side effects, or poor drug compliance or has recently changed medication therapy without documentation of the drug level

ACE, angiotensin-converting enzyme; INR, international normalized ratio (prothrombin time).

Source: Adapted from Nagelhout J, Elisha S. *Nurse Anesthesia.* 6th ed. Elsevier; 2018:342.

Hemoglobin and Hematocrit

Loss of blood is an expected occurrence in the surgical patient population. Blood loss may be more than anticipated; thus, known preoperative hemoglobin (Hgb) and hematocrit (HCT) facilitates planning and preparation. An abnormal result may alter perioperative management. The results of the surgical procedure and surgeon can predict the risk of perioperative transfusion and guide the need for type and screen or crossmatch.[9] Routine preoperative Hgb or HCT testing is not supported by literature; however, comorbidities to consider ordering Hgb and HCT include:

- Age less than 6 months
- Older adult

- Hematologic malignancy
- Recent radiation or chemotherapy
- Renal disease
- Anticoagulant therapy
- Procedure with moderate to high blood loss potential
- Coexisting systemic disorders (e.g., cystic fibrosis, prematurity, severe malnutrition, renal failure, liver disease, congenital heart diseases)[2,5,9]

White Blood Cell Count

Evidence does not exist regarding the possible harm from an elevated white blood cell count (WBC) detected preoperatively. Therefore, obtaining a WBC count in asymptomatic patients does not seem justified.[12] Comorbidities to consider in ordering WBC count include:

- Leukemia and lymphomas
- Recent radiation or chemotherapy
- Suspected infection that would lead to cancellation of surgery
- Aplastic anemia
- Hypersplenism
- Autoimmune collagen vascular disease[2]

Electrolytes and Blood Urea Nitrogen (Bun)/Creatinine

There are numerous guidelines to assist with ordering of serum chemistries. The only conclusive evidence is that routine ordering in asymptomatic adults is not necessary.[3] No trials have documented changes in postoperative outcomes who had electrolyte testing before a procedure.[13] Comorbidities to consider when ordering serum chemistries include:

- Endocrine disorders of the adrenal or thyroid gland
- Hypertension
- Heart failure
- Renal and liver dysfunction
- Diabetes mellitus
- Pituitary or hypothalamic disorders
- Central nervous system disease
- Specific medications
  - Chemotherapeutic agents
  - Diuretics
  - Angiotensin-converting enzyme (ACE) inhibitors
  - Angiotensin receptor blockers
  - Nonsteroidal anti-inflammatory drugs
  - Digoxin
- Perioperative therapies (i.e., bowel preps and/or presence of dehydration)[11]
- High-risk procedures (those with high probabilities of requiring invasive monitoring, blood administration, and postoperative care in a critical care area[3])
  - Major emergency surgery, specifically in the older adult
  - Aortic and other major vascular procedures

- Peripheral vascular surgery
- Prolonged procedures associated with fluid shifts (i.e., large abdominal or bowel surgeries, complicated spine procedures)[14]

A serum potassium level should be obtained within 7 days of surgery for patients receiving diuretics or digitalis.[2] One method of assessing the probability of CO_2 retention postoperatively, which can be important in the management of patients with sleep apnea or pulmonary hypertension, is evaluation of the serum bicarbonate. A normal serum bicarbonate value will virtually exclude the diagnosis of chronic CO_2 retention.[3]

Glucose
A blood glucose result the day of surgery is recommended for patients who have a diagnosis of

- Diabetes mellitus
- A history of hyper- or hypoglycemia
- Cystic fibrosis
- Adrenal dysfunction
- Central nervous system disease
- Corticosteroid or any medication used to control blood sugar.
- High-risk procedures

Wang et al. found in a population of 6,683 patients without known diabetes, preoperative glucose was a marker for postoperative complications.[15] However, it is not routine to test this population.

Liver Transaminases
Liver transaminase testing is not indicated unless acute hepatitis, significant liver dysfunction, or cirrhosis is present. Patients with these disease processes are at an increased risk of perioperative complications and death.[9]

Liver transaminase tests are appropriate in patients with visible ascites and associated infection-related comorbidities. There is no evidence to support an increased incidence of perioperative events in patients with asymptomatic elevations in transaminases, bilirubin, or prothrombin time (PT). Albumin level, an indicator of malnutrition or malabsorption, is utilized in several risk calculators and a predictor of poor outcomes.[9]

Coagulation Studies
Activated partial thromboplastin time (aPTT) and PT are useful diagnostic tests in patients who have a history of bleeding. They have not been shown to have value as screening tests in asymptomatic patients.[9] The PTT and PT were developed to identify clotting factor deficiencies in vitro and are not predictive of clinical bleeding. Coagulation testing in patients with no risk factors for coagulopathy or no history of bleeding does not predict perioperative bleeding.[16] A thorough patient history assessing for bleeding abnormalities is important. Query should include a family history of coagulation concerns, history of increased bleeding with previous surgical procedures or tooth extraction, liver

and renal dysfunction, and intake of anticoagulants.[9] A study of neurosurgery patients compared an assessment of patient history with preoperative coagulation testing and demonstrated that patient history had a higher sensitivity for the detection of bleeding.[17]

Routine coagulation evaluation is not recommended unless the patient history suggests a coagulation disorder, liver disease, malnutrition, or the patient is taking anticoagulants.[9] An aPTT is indicated with a personal or family history of a bleeding disorder, unfractionated heparin (UFH) use, and in patients with an undiagnosed hypercoagulable condition. A PT is indicated in patients with alcohol abuse, personal or family history of bleeding disorder, hepatic disease, malabsorption, malnutrition, and warfarin use. Comorbidities to consider when ordering PT or partial PT include

- Leukemia
- Hepatic disease
- Renal dysfunction
- Bleeding disorder
- Anticoagulation therapy
- Severe malnutrition or malabsorption[2,3,5,9]

Comorbidities to consider when ordering platelet count include:

- Bleeding disorder
- Abnormal hemorrhage, purpura, history of easy bruising[2]

Bleeding time previously was utilized to determine the presence of qualitative platelet defect. However, recently authors suggest that the test is not reliable and should not be obtained.[3]

Pregnancy Testing

Patients may present for surgery with an undetected pregnancy. The detection of pregnancy in a patient scheduled to undergo a nonobstetric surgery may lead to surgery cancellation, change in surgical procedur, or alteration of perioperative management. The American Society of Anesthesiologists Task Force on Preanesthesia Evaluation reports the literature is inadequate to apprise individuals whether anesthesia causes harmful effects in early pregnancy.

Preprocedural pregnancy testing guidelines vary at medical facilities. It is reasonable to consider pregnancy testing in women of childbearing age and for whom the results may alter decision-making and perioperative management.[2,5] Obtaining a menstrual cycle history is recommended as no test has 100% accuracy. Serum human chorionic gonadotropin (beta-hCG) performed within 7 to 10 days of the procedure will reliably predict pregnancy. Most urine pregnancy tests detect B-hCG levels of 25 to 50 mIU/mL. These urine tests have a high rate of false negatives 6 to 7 days post-conception because B-hCG levels are low at that time (10 mIU/mL). Thus, a serum hCG level to detect pregnancy is reasonable less than 6 weeks postconceptual age and a urine test is adequate to detect pregnancy 6 weeks after the last menstrual period.[9]

Medications

Medication levels should be drawn if the patient exhibits or reports signs of inadequate treatment, side effects, or poor drug compliance, or if they have been newly prescribed any of the following drugs:

- Theophylline
- Phenytoin
- Digoxin
- Carbamazepine[2]

SUMMARY

The preoperative assessment provides an invaluable opportunity to complete a thorough history and physical examination and determine whether patients need preprocedural testing. Additional tests should be conducted if the information to be obtained will result in changes in the perioperative management of the patient. There is significant evidence to support no need for laboratory tests in patients of any age undergoing minimally invasive procedures.

REFERENCES

Full list of references can be accessed through Springer Publishing Company Connect™ at the following link: http://connect.springerpub.com/content/reference-book/978-0-8261 -8843-4/part/part02/toc-part/ch008

---

9. THERAPEUTIC DRUG MONITORING: PEAK AND TROUGH

Christopher G. Green

PHARMACOKINETICS REVIEW

Pharmacokinetics describes the way medications move through the body from the time they are taken or given until they have been cleared from the system. There are four main elements that impact this process: absorption, distribution, metabolism, and elimination (ADME).[1] Each of these functions in turn can impact the result of drug level monitoring and the clinician should consider potential effects on test results on an individualized basis.

Absorption of medications is impacted by several variables. Medications may be immediate or delayed release or designed to release at a specific point within the gastrointestinal (GI) tract.[1,2] The pH differences in the stomach and different portions of the small intestine can also impact release, dissolution, and therefore absorption of drugs.[2] Modifications to the gastrointestinal (GI) tract, such as with gastric bypass procedures, can modify transit time and affect absorption.[1,2] Enzymes located in the stomach and intestines can metabolize or partially metabolize medications as can the presence or absence of certain bacteria in the GI system.[1,2] Food (or its absence) can impact some medications with respect to breakdown and dissolution. Drug transport proteins can be a factor in uptake by the GI tract prior to distribution via the bloodstream.[1]

Distribution of medications to the organs, tissues, and target sites depends on factors related to the physical makeup of the location and varying physiologic processes. From a physical standpoint, whether a drug is lipophilic, lipophobic, hydrophilic, or hydrophobic and the characteristics of the target site can affect how well a drug will be distributed.[2] For example, if a drug is highly lipophilic, it would be expected to distribute well into fatty tissue. Physiologic processes, such as the extent of protein binding, also impact distribution of the drug.[1,2] If a medication is highly protein bound, a higher free portion could be expected with a drug level when the protein is deficient or when a new medication has displaced it. Similarly, free drug is active drug, so an increased response would be expected.[1,2] Similar to absorption, the permeability of membranes can impact distribution of drugs.[1] A common example is the central nervous system, where the blood-brain barrier prevents entry of most medications.[1]

Metabolism of medications occurs through a variety of mechanisms. The liver is responsible for most drug metabolism, but other areas of the body also can metabolize some medications to varying degrees.[1,2] Two types of reactions occur, divided into phase I or phase II, to break down drugs. Phase I reactions include oxidation, reduction, and hydroxylation. The Cytochrome P450 enzyme (CYP450) system is one example of an enzymatic process for phase I metabolism.[1] Phase II reactions focus on increasing water solubility through conjugation mechanisms.[1] A metabolite is the outcome of phase I or II mechanisms, and they may have similar, different, or no effect on the body compared to the original drug.[1,2]

Elimination of medications is essentially the removal of the drug and its metabolites from the system.[2] The most common routes of elimination are renally or via the biliary tract.[1,2] For renal elimination, glomerular filtration, tubular excretion, and tubular reabsorption govern how effectively a medication is cleared.[1] Hepatobiliary excretion is more complex. There are fewer effective measures to predict clearance rates for medications that undergo this route of elimination.[2] Damage to liver cells responsible for enzymatic metabolism can impact the drug level. Injury to the biliary tree or illnesses that reduce biliary excretion can reduce elimination of medications.[2]

OVERVIEW OF LABORATORY TEST(S)

The information presented in Table 9.1 includes selected drugs where peak or trough monitoring are useful in guiding therapy. This is not an all-inclusive list of medications that can be tested for therapeutic drug monitoring. Additionally, the focus is on drug monitoring for commonly used or encountered medications in outpatient settings. Medications given intravenously are not included as these are often monitored in an inpatient setting and typically subject to internal protocols for management. Some important concepts to consider prior

TABLE 9.1: MEDICATIONS MONITORED BY TROUGH LEVELS

MEDICATION	TIME TO STEADY STATE*	TIMING OF DRAW	THERAPEUTIC RANGE / TOXIC LEVEL
Carbamazepine[3–5]	2–6 days (chronic) 21–28 days (initial dosing due to auto-induction)	30 minutes before dose	Therapeutic: 4–12 mg/L Toxic: Not defined
Cyclosporine[3,6]	2–6 days	30–60 minutes before fourth dose	Therapeutic: 50–500 mcg/L – varies based on type of transplant Toxic: > upper limit of normal dependent on type of transplant
Digoxin[3,7]	7–10 days	30–60 minutes before dose and at least 6 hours after a dose	Therapeutic: 0.5–2.0 mcg/L -in CHF: 0.5–1.0 mcg/L Toxic: > 2.0 mcg/L
Ethosuximide[3,4,8]	5–15 days	30 minutes before dose	Therapeutic: 40–100 mg/L Toxic: Not defined
Lithium[3,9]	3–7 days	30 minutes before dose and at least 12 hours after a dose	Therapeutic: 0.6–1.2 mEq/L -Older adult: 0.4–0.8 mEq/L -Bipolar disorder: < 1.2 mEq/L Toxic: > 1.5 mEq/L
Phenobarbital[3,4]	2–4 weeks	30 minutes before dose	Therapeutic: 10–40 mg/L Toxic: > 50 mg/L
Phenytoin[3,10]	2–6 days	30 minutes before dose and at least 6–9 hours after an oral dose	Therapeutic: 10–20 mg/L (total) -Free level: 1–2 mg/L Toxic: > 20 mg/L (total), > 2 mg/L (free)
Sirolimus[3,11]	5–7 days	30–60 minutes prior to fourth dose	Therapeutic: 5–20 mcg/L – varies based on type of transplant and concomitant immunosuppressant use Toxic: Not defined
Tacrolimus[3,12]	2–5 days	30 minutes before dose	Therapeutic: 4–20 mcg/L – varies based on type of transplant and concomitant immunosuppressant use Toxic: Not defined
Valproic acid[3,4,13]	3–7 days	30 minutes before dose	Therapeutic: 50–100 mg/L (epilepsy) -Bipolar disorder: 50–125 mg/L Toxic: Poorly defined. Risk when > 150 mg/L

*Time to steady state assumes chronic dosing unless otherwise specified.

to drawing a level include timing of the draw, steady state achievement, and patient-specific factors.[3] Timing relates to whether a peak or trough (pre-dose) level is most appropriate for clinical decision-making. Steady state is when a medication has reached a period where three to four half-lives of the medication have passed. This is the time when a medication should have reached the target, or therapeutic, range.[2,3] Patient-specific factors are important with respect to the medication being tested. Consistent with the ADME concepts previously discussed, changes in any of these processes could impact the timing of a lab draw.[2,3] If a medication is renally eliminated, a draw to check for toxicity as opposed to efficacy might be performed when there is a concern for potential drug accumulation.[3,4] Sampling is often done via blood draw, but saliva has been described as an option for some anti-epileptic medications.[3,4]

Monitoring of peak drug levels is most commonly performed with theophylline in the outpatient setting. Theophylline takes 2 to 3 days to reach steady state. A peak level should be performed 1 to 2 hours after the dose for immediate release products. For delayed and sustained release versions, the peak level is best performed 4 to 8 hours after the dose. The therapeutic range is 5 to 20 mg/L and a toxic level is seen above 20 mg/L.[3,14]

CPT Codes for Listed Tests

Carbamazepine	80156		Phenytoin	80185
			• Free phenytoin	80186
Cyclosporine	80158		Sirolimus	80195
Digoxin	80162			
			Tacrolimus	80197
Ethosuximide	80168		Valproic acid	80164
Lithium	80178			
			Theophylline	80198
Phenobarbital	80184			

INDICATIONS
When and Why to Order

As mentioned, there are several drugs for which a laboratory test exists to report a drug level. For the anti-epileptic medications alone, there are at least 21 and as many as 24 medications on the market that have an available blood test.[3,4] How does a clinician determine which drugs to order a test for? What factors play into this decision? The answer is that a variety of factors help the clinician decide if ordering a drug level will be beneficial. In general, if the clinician feels a drug level will help with dosing of the medication, assessing for toxicity, or monitoring both for clinical benefit and toxicity when used long term, then a drug level should be considered.[15,16]

There are specific factors that should also be weighed by the clinician when ordering a drug level. One factor to consider is whether the drug in question has a narrow therapeutic range.[15,16] Examples of several of these medications are in Table 9.1. Straying outside of a narrow range can lead to toxic effects and being below the range can often lead to a lack of clinical benefit.

In the setting of impaired drug clearance, it may be valuable to establish that the drug level is not approaching a potentially toxic level. When there is variability expected in how a patient's body may handle a drug pharmacokinetically, blood levels can serve as an additional marker to guide decision-making.[15,16] As an example, if a patient has chronic renal failure and the medication being used is highly excreted in the urine, a blood level may help to prevent unintended toxicity and allow for continued benefit by guiding dosing.[15,16] Another example where the pharmacokinetics may be altered is when a new and interacting medication is introduced. If the new medication induces or inhibits metabolism of the reference drug, then the ordering of a level may help to guide short-term therapy changes and avoid toxicity.[15,16]

For monitoring to be useful, there needs to be an established relationship between the drug level and the observed clinical effect.[3,15,16] In the absence of this, a drug level alone has little meaning. For drugs with very wide therapeutic indices, or little correlation with blood level to either toxicity or efficacy, performance of a level in unlikely to impact therapy decisions or the care of the patient.

Lastly, monitoring of blood levels can be of value when there is the potential for known dose-related adverse effects.[15,16] One of the better examples of this is with lithium.[3,9,15,16] As the lithium level rises, there has been correlation shown with which side effects are more likely.[9,17] When a clinician is evaluating a patient who takes lithium and has complaints of nausea, diarrhea, and polyuria, knowing the correlation between level and side effect can prompt the ordering of a drug level.[9,17]

INTERPRETATION

Therapeutic drug monitoring levels can serve as a useful guide to medication management. It is important to consider that the level alone is not and should not be the only criteria used to make a treatment decision. While it may be ideal to have a result in the range, it may not be necessary to make an adjustment in every case when a subtherapeutic result is returned. Consider the patient's clinical state: Are they free of symptoms? Are you seeing the intended response even though the level is a little low? Are you seeing a toxic effect even though the level is in the range? For this last item, consider the drug phenytoin, which is highly protein bound. If the total level is normal, but the patient is experiencing signs of toxicity, is it possible the free portion is elevated for some reason? Check the timing of the draw as well. Even though patients are instructed to have their tests done at a specific time, it does not mean they followed through on this advice nor that the laboratory drew the test within the preferred window. It is crucial to treat the patient, not the level—let the level be supporting evidence, but not the only piece of information that is considered.[15,16]

FOLLOW-UP

Follow-up testing may be indicated for the patient. The clinician should take into account whether the level that comes back is subject to variability in the near and long term. If a new medication was started that interacts with the reference drug, then short-term follow-up testing may be warranted. Similarly, in the absence of signs and symptoms of toxicity and evidence of clear benefit in a stable patient, repeat testing would be of little value. Periodic monitoring may be the better approach in this situation.[15,16]

RELATED DIAGNOSES AND ICD-10 CODES

When possible, use the diagnosis code for the condition the medication is currently treating. For example, with lithium being used for bipolar disorder, current episode, manic without psychotic features, mild, code F31.11 would be utilized.

Encounter for therapeutic drug level monitoring	Z51.81
Adverse effect of iminostilbenes (carbamazepine)	T42.1X5
Adverse effect of cardiac stimulant glycosides and drugs of similar action	T46.0X5
Adverse effect of succinimides and oxazolidinediones (ethosuximide)	T42.2X5
Adverse effect of barbiturates (phenobarbital)	T42.3X5
Adverse effect of hydantoin derivatives (phenytoin)	T42.0X5
Adverse effect of other anti-epileptic and sedative-hypnotic drugs	T42.6X5

REFERENCES

Full list of references can be accessed through Springer Publishing Company Connect™ at the following link: http://connect.springerpub.com/content/reference-book/978-0-8261-8843-4/part/part02/toc-part/ch009

10. GENETIC TESTING FOR PRESCRIBING IN MENTAL HEALTH

Carol D. Campbell

PHYSIOLOGY REVIEW

Psychiatric medications are utilized in the treatment of psychiatric disorders. An individual's response to psychiatric medications can vary. Response to medications depends on numerous factors such as age, sex, body composition, and other medications, as well as an individual's genetic makeup which influences pharmacokinetics and pharmacodynamics.[1] Personalized medicine has emerged in the treatment of psychiatric disorders based on pharmacogenomics and pharmacogenetics. Pharmacogenomics (PGx) refers to the study of DNA and RNA variance related to medication response impacting gene function but can change and/or be influenced by various individual factors such as age, sex, and environment. Pharmacogenetics is the study of DNA structural variations and impact on drug metabolism, efficacy, and tolerability. DNA remains stable and does not change with time or age. Thus, PGx is related to gene function that is influenced by the environment, whereas pharmacogenetics is concerned with single genes and their structure, but both have a part that includes metabolism of medication (Figure 10.1). PGx is based on the cytochrome P450 enzyme system, primarily with the liver, and involves genes coding to produce cytochrome P450 enzymes. Ideally, PGx testing examines individuals' ability to metabolize medications and ultimately their response to medications to increase medication efficacy and minimize the risk of toxicity.

OVERVIEW OF LABORATORY TEST(S)

Laboratory evaluation of PGx testing can be assessed by drug metabolism (CPT code 0029U), pain management for opioid use disorder (CPT code 0078U), psychiatry 14 gene panel (CPT code 0173U), and psychiatry 15 gene panel (CPT code 0175U). Panel testing provides a comprehensive view of multiple genes which may be beneficial when utilizing PGx adverse medication effects, issues with medication response, issues related to polypharmacy, or for preemptive testing, where testing is completed prior to prescribing medications with the intent to guide medication selection.[2] Additionally, PGx testing can be ordered for a specific single gene. In some instances, a single gene test may provide better precision of a specific gene than when that same gene is tested in a panel.

INDICATIONS

Screening
■ There is insufficient evidence for universal PGx screening in the general population.
■ The U.S. Food and Drug Administration (FDA) has advised clinicians and patients against making medication selections and dosages from PGx testing results as there is insufficient evidence to support its utilization for most medications.[3]

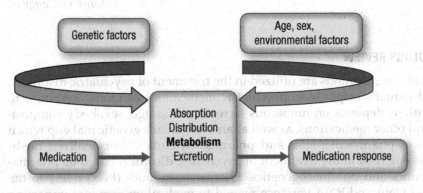

FIGURE 10.1. Factors influencing variation in medication response.

- The FDA recommends genetic prescreening for the HLA-B*15:02 allele before prescribing carbamazepine to patients of Asian descent as those positive for HLA-B*15:02 may be at increased risk for Stevens-Johnson syndrome/toxic epidermal necrolysis (SJS/TEN).[4]
- The FDA does not recommend prescreening for oxcarbazepine. However, there are warnings and precautions to avoid oxcarbazepine in HLA-B*15:02 positive individuals due to the risk of SJS/TEN unless the benefits clearly outweigh the risks.[5]

Diagnosis and Evaluation

- There are over 250 FDA-approved medications with information related to PGx in their labeling (i.e., adverse reactions, medication interactions, use in specific populations, precautions, and warnings) in many areas including psychiatry.[4]
- Guidelines and evidence related to genes and psychiatric medications are expanding. Refer to Table 10.1 for a list of common psychiatric medications, the associated genes, and available evidence-based guidelines on prescribing considerations.

TABLE 10.1: COMMON PSYCHIATRIC MEDICATIONS, GENES, AND PHARMACOGENOMICS GUIDELINES AND EVIDENCE

MEDICATION	GENE(S)	GUIDELINE(S)/EVIDENCE
Amitriptyline	CYP2C19, 2D6	CPIC Guideline for CYP2D6 and CYP2C19 genotypes and dosing of tricyclic antidepressants[6]
Citalopram	CYP2C19, SLC6A4, GRIK4, HTR2A, FKBP5, COMT, TXNRD2	CPIC Guideline for CYP2D6 and CYP2C19 genotypes and dosing of selective serotonin reuptake inhibitors[7] Polymorphisms in GRIK4, HTR2A, and FKBP5 show interactive effects in predicting remission to antidepressant treatment[8]
Clomipramine	CYP2C19, 2D6	CPIC Guideline for CYP2D6 and CYP2C19 genotypes and dosing of selective serotonin reuptake inhibitors[7]
Clozapine	ANKK1, DRD2, MCR4, HTR2C	Genetic variation and the D2 dopamine receptor: implications for the treatment of neuropsychiatric disease[9] The combined effect of CYP2D6 and DRD2 Taq1A polymorphisms on the antipsychotics daily doses and hospital stay duration in schizophrenia inpatients[10] Pharmacogenetic associations of antipsychotic drug-related weight gain: A systematic review and meta-analysis[11]
Desipramine	CYP2D6	CPIC Guideline for CYP2D6 and CYP2C19 genotypes and dosing of tricyclic antidepressants[6]
Doxepin	CYP2C19, 2D6	CPIC Guideline for CYP2D6 and CYP2C19 genotypes and dosing of tricyclic antidepressants[6]

(continued)

TABLE 10.1: COMMON PSYCHIATRIC MEDICATIONS, GENES, AND PHARMACOGENOMICS GUIDELINES AND EVIDENCE (*continued*)

MEDICATION	GENE(S)	GUIDELINE(S)/EVIDENCE
Escitalopram	*CYP2C19, SLC6A4, COMT, TXNRD2*	CPIC Guideline for CYP2D6 and CYP2C19 genotypes and dosing of selective serotonin reuptake inhibitors[7] Interaction between serotonin transporter gene variants and life events predicts response to antidepressants in the GENDEP project[12]
Fluoxetine	*FKBP5, COMT, TXNRD2*	Polymorphisms in GRIK4, HTR2A, and FKBP5 show interactive effects in predicting remission to antidepressant treatment[8]
Fluvoxamine	*CYP2D6, COMT, TXNRD2*	CPIC Guideline for CYP2D6 and CYP2C19 genotypes and dosing of selective serotonin reuptake inhibitors[7]
Imipramine	*CYP2C19, 2D6*	CPIC Guideline for CYP2D6 and CYP2C19 genotypes and dosing of tricyclic antidepressants[6]
Mirtazapine	*CYP2D6, FKBP5*	Multicenter study on the clinical effectiveness, pharmacokinetics, and pharmacogenetics of mirtazapine in depression[13] Polymorphisms in GRIK4, HTR2A, and FKBP5 show interactive effects in predicting remission to antidepressant treatment[8]
Nortriptyline	*CYP2D6*	CPIC Guideline for CYP2D6 and CYP2C19 genotypes and dosing of tricyclic antidepressants[6]
Olanzapine	*ANKK1, DRD2, MCR4, HTR2C*	Genetic variation and the D2 dopamine receptor: implications for the treatment of neuropsychiatric disease[9] Pharmacogenetic associations of antipsychotic drug-related weight gain: A systematic review and meta-analysis[11]
Paroxetine	*CYP2D6, HTR1A, FKBP5, COMT, TXNRD2*	CPIC Guideline for CYP2D6 and CYP2C19 genotypes and dosing of selective serotonin reuptake inhibitors[7] Polymorphisms in GRIK4, HTR2A, and FKBP5 show interactive effects in predicting remission to antidepressant treatment[8] SSRI response and HTR1A[14]
Risperidone	*CYP2D6, ANKK1, DRD2, MCR4, HTR2C*	DPWG Guideline for risperidone and CYP2D6[15] Genetic variation and the D2 dopamine receptor: implications for the treatment of neuropsychiatric disease[9] Pharmacogenetic associations of antipsychotic drug-related weight gain: A systematic review and meta-analysis[11]
Sertraline	*CYP2C19, CYP2D6, COMT, TXNRD2*	CPIC Guideline for CYP2D6 and CYP2C19 genotypes and dosing of selective serotonin reuptake inhibitors[7]
Venlafaxine	*CYP2D6, FKBP5*	Polymorphisms in GRIK4, HTR2A, and FKBP5 show interactive efects in predicting remission to antidepressant treatment[8]

Monitoring

- Low levels of evidence suggest that PGx guided treatment with antidepressants results in improved treatment response when compared to standard care.[16–18]

- PGx testing can potentially be useful in decreasing risks of side effects in specific patient populations. However, broad use of PGx testing is not well supported by the current available evidence.

INTERPRETATION

- PGx panel test results are provided in the form of categorized information generally by genotype (i.e., CYP2C19, CYP2D6) and phenotype (i.e., rapid metabolizer) that correspond with recommendations that are based on an integrated analysis of multiple genetic variants that affect metabolizing enzyme function.[2,6,7]
- Recommendations for medication use are typically reported as: use as normally prescribed, use with caution, or use with extreme caution.[2,6,7]
- Patients are classified as poor/slow, intermediate, normal/extensive, or rapid/ultrarapid/fast phenotype metabolizers.[2,6,7]
- Poor/slower metabolizers are more likely to benefit from lower medication dosages to avoid toxicity.[2,6,7]
- Rapid/ultrarapid/fast metabolizers may require higher medication dosages to achieve therapeutic effects.[2,6,7] Table 10.2 provides a summary of phenotype metabolizers, descriptions, and effects.[2,6,7]

TABLE 10.2: PHENOTYPE METABOLIZERS, DESCRIPTIONS, AND EFFECTS

PHENOTYPE METABOLIZERS	DESCRIPTION	EFFECTS
Poor/slow metabolizer (PM)	An individual with absent or no enzyme activity due to genetic variants for a specific metabolizing enzyme	Medications are broken down extremely slowly by enzymes which create increased risk for toxicity due to slow elimination. Pro-drugs are less effective due to slower activation.
Intermediate metabolizer (IM)	An individual with decreased enzyme activity due to genetic variants for a specific metabolizing enzyme	Medications are broken down slightly slower by enzymes which require a lower dosage to prevent toxicity. Pro-drugs may be less effective due to slower metabolism.
Normal/extensive metabolizer (NM)	An individual with normal enzyme activity	Medications prescribed at FDA approved dosages produce expected outcomes.
Rapid/ultrarapid/fast metabolizer (RM)	An individual with increased enzyme activity due to (multiple) genetic variants or copies of a specific metabolizing enzyme	Medications are broken down and eliminated quickly by enzymes which reduces the effectiveness of medications. Pro-drugs activated quicker causing increased risk for toxicity.

Sources: Data from Hicks JK, Sangkuhl K, Swen J, et al. Clinical Pharmacogenetics Implementation Consortium Guideline (CPIC) for CYP2D6 and CYP2C19 genotypes and dosing of tricyclic antidepressants: 2016 update. *Clin Pharmacol Ther.* 2017;102(1):37–44. doi:10.1002/cpt.597; Hicks JK, Bishop JR, Sangkuhl K, et al. Clinical Pharmacogenetics Implementation Consortium (CPIC) guideline for CYP2D6 and CYP2C19 genotypes and dosing of selective serotonin reuptake inhibitors. *Clin Pharmacol Ther.* 2015;98(2):127–134. doi:10.1002/cpt.147; Nicholson WT, Formea CM, Matey ET, Wright JA, Giri J, Moyer AM. Considerations when applying pharmacogenomics to your practice. *Mayo Clin Proc.* 2021;96(1):218–230. doi:10.1016/j.mayocp.2020.03.011.

FOLLOW-UP

■ Several evidence-based guidelines for PGx testing are available from professional organizations, such as the Clinical Pharmacogenetics Implementation Consortium (CPIC). The CPIC guidelines assist clinicians in guiding medication therapy and dosage based on existing PGx results. However, the guidelines do not provide recommendations regarding when clinicians should utilize PGx testing.[6,7,19]

PEARLS & PITFALLS

■ In general, psychiatric medications should be prescribed to maximize safety and minimize risk of side effects by starting at a low dose and increasing the dose as tolerated. Therapeutic drug monitoring of blood serum levels of medications (i.e., lithium) and adjusting the dosage accordingly may be adequate.[1]
■ Clinicians will likely encounter PGx testing results in practice even if they did not personally order the testing. Thus, it is important to have a working knowledge regarding PGx.[2]
■ Anticipate that as PGx evolves, it will play a role in the future of psychiatric practice.
■ PGx testing has the potential to be a powerful tool but it does not overrule the necessity for clinical assessment and judgment.

PATIENT EDUCATION

■ https://medlineplus.gov/genetics/understanding/genomicresearch/pharmacogenomics/

RELATED DIAGNOSES AND ICD-10 CODES

Major depression disorder	F32.9
• Single episode, unspecified	
Anxiety disorder, unspecified	F41.9
Opioid use disorder	F11.20
Adverse effect of unspecified drugs	T50.905A

Note this is not an exhaustive list of diagnoses and codes.

REFERENCES

Full list of references can be accessed through Springer Publishing Company Connect™ at the following link: http://connect.springerpub.com/content/reference-book/978-0-8261-8843-4/part/part02/toc-part/ch010

SECTION III

EVIDENCE-BASED USE OF INDIVIDUAL LABORATORY TESTS

11. 17 HYDROXYPROGESTERONE

Lisa Ward

PHYSIOLOGY REVIEW

17 Hydroxyprogesterone (17 OHP) is an inactive steroid hormone produced mainly in the adrenal cortex. It is a precursor hormone that is converted into the active hormone cortisol. Several enzymes are needed to complete this conversion to cortisol. If one or more of these enzymes is deficient or dysfunctional, an inadequate amount of cortisol is produced causing 17 OHP and other androgens to be produced in excess (Figure 11.1).[1-4] This excess 17 OHP is seen in an inherited condition called congenital adrenal hyperplasia (CAH). Due to circadian rhythms, 17 OHP levels rapidly decline during the course of the day; therefore, early morning testing is critical for accurate assessment.[5-7]

CAH is a group of inherited disorders caused by gene mutations associated with cortisol-related enzyme deficiencies.[1] The severe form of CAH can cause life-threatening salt wasting crisis in newborn infants and often causes ambiguous genitalia. The milder form of CAH may not present until after adolescence and may result in precocious puberty, hirsutism, and infertility in women.

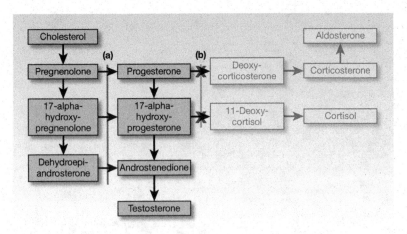

FIGURE 11.1. Congenital adrenal hyperplasia. In congenital adrenal hyperplasia the 21-hydroxylase enzyme is absent and cannot complete the conversion of steroid precursors to aldosterone and cortisol and instead all steroid precursors are focused on adrenal androgen production. *Sources:* Lexicomp Online. *Lab Tests and Diagnostic Procedures.* UpToDate; 2019; Yedinak C, Hurtado CR, Leung AM, et al. Endocrine system. In: Tkacs NC, Hermann LL, Johnson RL, eds. *Advanced Physiology and Pathophysiology: Essentials for Clinical Practice.* Springer Publishing Company; 2020, Figure 17.23.

OVERVIEW OF LABORATORY TEST

The 17 OHP lab testing (CPT code 83498) is used to screen for CAH and for monitoring cortisol replacement therapy in CAH patients. Due to the disrupted hypothalamus-pituitary-adrenal axis, the 17 OHP laboratory test is often done in conjunction with other endocrine laboratory tests: ACTH, renin, and androstenedione.[4]

INDICATIONS

Screening

- The Endocrine Society and European Society for Pediatric Endocrinology recommends all newborn screening programs should incorporate 17 OHP screening to evaluate for CAH and the 17 OHP test is often part of the newborn screening panel in many states in the United States.[4,7,8]
- The UK Society for Endocrinology recommends a 17 OHP be done in all infants with ambiguous genitalia.[9]
- Currently, newborn screening for congenital abnormalities, including CAH, is a mandatory practice in many countries worldwide.[10]
- The Japanese Society of Pediatric Endocrinology recommends universal screening for neonates.[5]

Diagnosis and Evaluation

- A 17 OHP should be ordered in any infant or young child with signs and symptoms of adrenal insufficiency[1,3]:
  - Lethargy
  - Failure to thrive
  - Dehydration
  - Hypotension
- To evaluate any child presenting with precocious puberty
- To evaluate males with infertility
- To evaluate for adrenal causes of adult acne, hirsutism, and irregular menses.[11]
- Evaluation for androgen-secreting adrenal and ovarian neoplasms.[9]

Monitoring

- Used to guide therapy in CAH.[12]
- In patients with 18 months or fewer with CAH, the 17 OHP should be measured every 3 months until age 2 years old.[7,8]
- In adolescent and adult CAH patients, 17 OHP should be measured every 6 to 12 months.[5,8]

INTERPRETATION

- Normal values are dependent upon age and sex (see Table 11.1).
- A 17 OHP level of greater than 10,000 ng/dL establishes the diagnosis of CAH (see Table 11.2).[3,10,13]
- A 17 OHP level of greater than 1,000 ng/dL but less than 10,000 ng/dL typically reflects the milder form of CAH.[8]

TABLE 11.1: 17 OHP (NG/DL) REFERENCE INTERVALS

CHRONOLOGICAL AGE	MALE	FEMALE
Premature infants	≤405	
Term infants (>24 hours old)	<100	
Adolescent	12–190	18–200
Male ≥20 years old	≤220	–
Menstruating females	–	20–430
Postmenopausal	–	≤45
Pregnancy	–	80–575

TABLE 11.2: 17 INTERPRETATION OF OHP (NG/DL) ABNORMAL RESULTS

CHRONOLOGICAL AGE	SWCAH*	NCCAH**
Premature infants	>500–800 ng/dL needs further testing	
Term infants (>24 hours old)	>10,000 ng/dL	>1,000 ng/dL
Children/ Adolescent/ Adults	>5,000 ng/dL	200–1,000 ng/dL needs further testing >1,000 ng/dL

*SWCAH- salt-wasting CAH is the more severe form of CAH.
**NCCAH- Non-classic CAH is the milder form of CAH.

FOLLOW-UP

■ Genotyping may be indicated when 17 OHP results remain equivocal and a CAH diagnosis cannot be made.[7,9]

PEARLS & PITFALLS

■ In newborn infants with significantly elevated 17 OHP levels, it is likely the infant has CAH.[5,13] If 17 OHP is only moderately elevated, the infant may have the milder form of CAH.[1]

■ Baseline 17 OHP must be tested after 48 to 72 hours of life, as levels are physiologically high at birth, before rapidly falling.[3,5,7,13,14,] In infants with CAH, 17 OHP levels will progressively rise over time.

■ A normal 17 OHP result means the patient likely does not have CAH.[1]

■ Female infants have lower 17 OHP levels when compared to male infants.[8,13]

■ Low or decreasing 17 OHP levels in a CAH patient indicate response to treatment. Conversely, high or increasing 17 OHP levels indicate inadequate response to treatment.

■ An early morning laboratory collection done prior to patient taking steroid medication gives the most optimal result.[5,7]

- False positives may occur in premature, sick, or stressed infants.[2,5,7,13,14]
- 17 OHP levels are significantly lower in obese males.[15,16]

PATIENT EDUCATION

- https://patient.info/doctor/congenital-adrenal-hyperplasia-pro
- https://caresfoundation.org/

RELATED DIAGNOSES AND ICD-10 CODES

Congenital adrenal hyperplasia	E25.0
• This applies to CAH, 21-hydroxylase deficiency, SWCAH	
Ambiguous genitalia	Q56.4
Hirsutism	L68.0
Precocious puberty	E30.1

REFERENCES

Full list of references can be accessed through Springer Publishing Company Connect™ at the following link: http://connect.springerpub.com/content/reference-book/978-0-8261 -8843-4/part/part03/toc-part/ch011

12. ADENOVIRUS CONJUNCTIVITIS TEST

Annie Abraham

PHYSIOLOGY REVIEW

Viral conjunctivitis, an infection of the conjunctiva, is the most common form of conjunctivitis. Human adenoviruses (HAdV) are responsible for around 65% to 90% of all cases of viral conjunctivitis.[1-6] HAdV is a non-enveloped double-stranded DNA virus of the genus *Mastadenovirus* and *Adenoviridae* family.[1,7] HAdV causes different types of ocular infections in humans including pharyngoconjunctival fever and epidemic keratoconjunctivitis.[1,7,8] While adenoviral conjunctivitis is highly contagious, it is self-limited, with symptoms lasting for about 2 weeks.[1,2,9]

Transmission of the HAdV virus occurs through direct contact with the infected person and contaminated surfaces such as medical equipment and water in swimming pools.[1,9] Once the virus enters the eye, an immune response is triggered, and proinflammatory cytokines are released into the conjunctiva. Inflammation of the conjunctiva causes dilation of the blood vessels and capillary leakage, resulting in symptoms such as conjunctival hyperemia and edema.[1]

OVERVIEW OF LABORATORY TESTS

The following laboratory tests may be used to confirm the diagnosis of viral conjunctivitis in symptomatic patients:

- The AdenoPlus test is a CLIA waived test (CPT code 87809-QW- RT or LT, "infectious agent antigen detection by immunoassay with direct optical observation; adenovirus").[10] It is a point-of-care test that detects conjunctivitis within 10 minutes. The test is performed by collecting a tear sample from multiple areas of the inferior palpebral conjunctiva. The test is assembled, placed in a buffer solution for 10 minutes, and then interpreted.[1,5] The AdenoPlus test has high specificity (92% to 98%) compared to polymerase chain reaction (PCR) analysis and can be used to diagnose symptomatic patients with adenoviral conjunctivitis.[3,5,11] The sensitivity of the AdenoPlus has shown to range from 33.3% to 93% (see Table 12.1).[3,5,6,11]
- Cell culture with confirmatory immunofluorescence assay (CC-IFA) (CPT code 87252, "viral culture, general") is performed, preferably prior to initiation of antibiotics, on a sample of the conjunctival discharge. The results are typically reported within 1 to 2 weeks.[1,11,12] Sensitivity of CC-IFA is 85% and specificity is 99%.[11]
- A conjunctival specimen is sent to the laboratory for real-time PCR analysis (CPT code 87799, "adenovirus DNA, Quantitative Real-Time PCR") and results are reported within 24 hours.[1,2,11] Sensitivity is 93% and specificity is 97%.[13]

INDICATIONS

Screening

There are no universal or targeted screening recommendations for adenoviral conjunctivitis.[6]

Diagnosis and Evaluation

- Diagnosis of adenoviral conjunctivitis can be made based on the presenting clinical symptoms of conjunctivitis.[6] Symptoms usually begin unilaterally and then spread to the opposite eye in a few days. The patient's history may be significant for current upper respiratory tract infection (URI) or recent exposure to someone with a URI.[6] Other clinical manifestations of acute viral conjunctivitis include watery eyes, edema of the eyelids, presence of conjunctival follicles, enlarged and tender preauricular lymph nodes, and bilateral cervical lymphadenopathy. Other diagnoses to consider

TABLE 12.1: STEPS OF ADENOPLUS TESTING	
Step 1	Collect the tear sample from the conjunctiva.
Step 2	Assemble the test.
Step 3	Place in buffer solution for 10 minutes.
Step 4	Interpret the test.

are bacterial conjunctivitis, herpetic conjunctivitis, acute hemorrhagic conjunctivitis, and COVID-19 conjunctivitis. Patients with matted shut eyes are more likely to have bacterial conjunctivitis.[6] The pharyngoconjunctival fever serotype is common in children who present with acute follicular conjunctivitis along with fever, sore throat, and enlarged periauricular lymph nodes.[1,13] More serious symptoms, such as changes to visual acuity, are seen in conditions such as epidemic keratoconjunctivitis.[6,8,9]

- The American Academy of Ophthalmology suggests using point-of-care adenoviral tests to prevent misdiagnosis, avoid inappropriate use of antibiotics in the setting of viral conjunctivitis, counteract antibiotic resistance, and minimize medical expenditure.[6,9,12]

Monitoring

- Adenoviral conjunctivitis is a self-limiting infection, with no need for routine monitoring.[1,9]

INTERPRETATION

- The AdenoPlus test can be interpreted after 10 minutes of development. A red and a blue line together indicate a positive test, while a blue line alone indicates a negative test.[1,5]
- Both PCR and CC-IFA detect the presence of HAdV in the conjunctival specimen.[1,11]

FOLLOW-UP

- PCR or viral culture should be used to confirm a negative AdenoPlus test.[2,3,12]

PEARLS & PITFALLS

- The rapid test is not widely utilized due to reimbursement challenges.[14]
- The AdenoPlus test has not been approved by the FDA to be used in children.[3]
- It is important to carefully follow the collection instructions to avoid user error and false negative results.

PATIENT EDUCATION

- https://www.cdc.gov/conjunctivitis/about/diagnosis.html
- https://www.choosingwisely.org/patient-resources/antibiotics-for-pink-eye/

RELATED DIAGNOSES AND ICD-10 CODES

Unspecified acute conjunctivitis, bilateral	H10.33
Other mucopurulent conjunctivitis, unspecified eye	H10.029
Unspecified conjunctivitis	H10.029
Conjunctivitis due to adenovirus	B30.1
Viral conjunctivitis, unspecified	B30.9

REFERENCES

Full list of references can be accessed through Springer Publishing Company Connect™ at the following link: http://connect.springerpub.com/content/reference-book/978-0-8261 -8843-4/part/part03/toc-part/ch012

13. ADRENOCORTICOTROPIC HORMONE (ACTH) AND ACTH STIMULATION TEST

Lisa Ward

PHYSIOLOGY REVIEW

Adrenocorticotropic hormone (ACTH) is a hormone produced by the pituitary gland that stimulates the production of cortisol. Cortisol is a steroid hormone produced by the adrenal glands that is important for regulating glucose, protein, and lipid metabolism, suppressing the immune system's response, and helping to maintain blood pressure.[1,2] This process of stimulating ACTH production in the pituitary is done via the hypothalamic-pituitary-adrenal axis (HPA)[1,3] (Figure 13.1). Normally, ACTH levels increase when cortisol is low and decrease when cortisol levels are high. Levels of ACTH vary throughout the day in a diurnal variation with the highest in the morning and lowest at night.[1,4,5] Abnormal levels of ACTH can be caused from dysfunction in the pituitary or adrenal glands or from ectopic secretion.[1] Conditions that interfere with the HPA can result in an excess or deficiency of cortisol. Conditions that specifically affect ACTH and cortisol production include Cushing disease, Addison disease, and hypopituitarism.[6]

OVERVIEW OF LABORATORY TEST

Laboratory evaluation of ACTH can be assessed by ACTH (CPT code 82024). For most accurate results, testing should be done between 6 and 10 a.m.[4] ACTH lab tests require a special refrigerated centrifuge to immediately separate plasma from cells; then, the specimen needs to be immediately frozen.[3,4,6] ACTH concentrations vary considerably depending on physiologic conditions and therefore should always be evaluated simultaneously with cortisol.[3,4] Different assay methods can vary and cannot be used interchangeably.[4,6] ACTH can also be measured as part of the ACTH stimulation test. In this test, the protocol consists of the following[2,4,7]:

- Baseline ACTH and cortisol levels are drawn.
- Patient given injection/infusion of 250 mcg of cosyntropin.
- Cortisol levels are drawn at 30 and 60 minutes post injection.

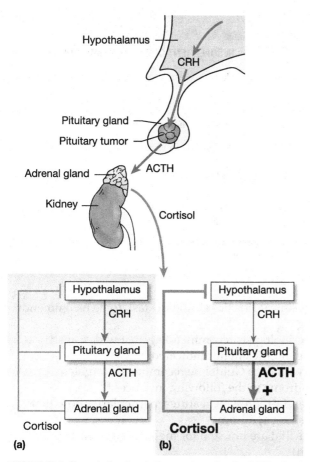

FIGURE 13.1. Hypothalamic-pituitary-adrenal axis. ACTH-stimulated cortisol production: The HPA axis and negative feedback. **(a)** In the normal HPA axis, hypothalamic CRH stimulates pituitary release of ACTH, resulting in stimulation of cortisol synthesis and secretion, and growth promotion of all of the adrenal gland layers. Cortisol also provides negative feedback to the pituitary and hypothalamus, inhibiting excessive ACTH and CRH secretion. **(b)** In Cushing disease, an ACTH-secreting pituitary adenoma continuously secretes supranormal amounts of ACTH, driving adrenal gland hyperplasia and excessive cortisol secretion. Negative feedback via increased cortisol inhibits hypothalamic CRH secretion but is ineffective at reducing ACTH secretion from the autonomously activated tumor cells. ACTH, adrenocorticotropic hormone; CRH, corticotropin-releasing hormone; HPA, hypothalamic-pituitary-adrenal. *Source:* Yedinak C, Hurtado CR, Leung AM, et al. Endocrine system. In: Tkacs NC, Hermann LL, Johnson RL, eds. *Advanced Physiology and Pathophysiology: Essentials for Clinical Practice.* Springer Publishing Company; 2020, Figure 17.13.

INDICATIONS

Screening

- Universal screening of ACTH and cortisol is discouraged due to overlap of symptoms from more common comorbidities (e.g., metabolic syndrome) and high rate of false positives.

TABLE 13.1: SYMPTOMS OF EXCESS AND INSUFFICIENT CORTICOL	
EXCESS CORTISOL SYMPTOMS	**INSUFFICIENT CORTISOL SYMPTOMS**
Truncal obesity	Muscle weakness
Buffalo hump	Unintentional weight loss
Round, red face	Increased skin pigmentation
Fragile, thin skin	Diarrhea, nausea, vomiting
Purple striae	Dizziness
Muscle weakness	Salt cravings
Acnes, hirsutism, recurrent skin infections	Fatigue

Sources: Data from *ACTH, Serum*. Mayo Clinical Laboratories website. https://endocrinology.testcatalog.org/show/ACTH; Labtestsonline.org. *ACTH: at a glance.* 2021. https://labtestsonline.org/tests/ACTH; Lexicomp Online. *Lab Tests and Diagnostic Procedures.* UpToDate; 2019.

- The Endocrine Society Clinical Practice Guideline task force recommends against widespread testing.[8,9]
- As a general rule, endocrinologists recommend against widespread screening because it is neither efficient nor indicated.[10]
- The U.S. Endocrine Society Practice Guideline recommends targeted screening for Cushing syndrome in the following instances.[8,9]
  - Patients with multiple and progressive features, particularly those that are more predictive of Cushing syndrome
  - Patients with symptoms that are unusual for their age (e.g., early osteoporosis, hypertension)
  - Children with diminished growth and increasing weight
  - Patients with adrenal incidentaloma

Diagnosis and Evaluation

- The Endocrine Society recommends acutely ill patients with unexplained symptoms undergo ACTH testing as part of the diagnostic workup to rule out adrenal insufficiency.[11]
- Use ACTH along with cortisol levels to evaluate patients with signs or symptoms suggestive of cortisol alterations (Table 13.1).

Monitoring

- In patients with suspected iatrogenic adrenal insufficiency who fail ACTH stimulation testing, further tapering of iatrogenic steroids should continue. Then at 3-month intervals, repeat ACTH stimulation testing until results are normal or patient is unable to further reduce iatrogenic steroids for fear of unhealthy outcome.[1,5]
- ACTH can be used as a means to monitor therapeutic steroid replacement in adrenal insufficient patients and should be repeated every 3 to 6 months.[2,7,11,12]

TABLE 13.2: INTERPRETATION OF CORTISOL AND ACTH		
DISEASE	CORTISOL	ACTH
Cushing syndrome	↑	↑
Adrenal tumor	↑	↓
Ectopic ACTH	↑	↑
Addison disease	↓	↑
Hypopituitarism	↓	↓

ACTH, adrenocorticotropic hormone.
Sources: Data from Labtestsonline.org. *ACTH: at a glance.* 2021. https://labtestsonline.org/tests/ACTH; Lexicomp Online. *Lab Tests and Diagnostic Procedures.* UpToDate; 2019.

INTERPRETATION

- Adult reference interval for morning ACTH levels: 7–60 ng/L[3,7]
- For a ACTH stimulation test, cortisol levels greater than 18 ng/L 30 to 60 minutes after cosyntropin injection are considered normal. Results below this level exclude suspicion of adrenal insufficiency.[4,7]
- Random ACTH levels are of limited diagnostic use due to diurnal variability, episodic secretion, and the wide reference interval.[3]
- The co-interpreation of ACTH and serum cortisol level will help to clarify the clinical picture. Interpretation of the results can be complex depending upon disease process, but Table 13.2 gives general guidance.[1,3,5,6]

FOLLOW-UP

- Suspicion for adrenal insufficiency (low morning cortisol levels) needs to be evaluated with an ACTH stimulation test[2,6] The ACTH stimulation test is the gold standard confirmatory test to diagnose adrenal insufficiency.[1,13,14]
- Suspicion for excess cortisol needs to be evaluated by tests for hypercortisolism (dexamethasone suppression test, salivary cortisol testing, and 24-hour urinary cortisol testing).[4,8,9,15]

PEARLS & PITFALLS

- In critically ill patients, both ACTH and cortisol rises in response to illness. After the initial phase, cortisol remains high, but ACTH levels may decline.[14]
- Exogenous steroid use can suppress the HPA axis.[12,13,16] Patients should taper and/or stop all exogenous steroids, if able, at least 4 weeks prior to stimulation testing[12,16] for most accurate assessment of HPA axis recovery.
- Stress may increase ACTH secretion,[6] therefore, patients should avoid emotional stress for 12 hours preceding laboratory tests.[3]
- Certain medication (e.g., oral/topical/inhaled steroid, mifepristone, megestrol, estrogen, insulin, lithium) can cause false abnormal results.[3,4,6]

- Falsely elevated ACTH levels can occur in patients who have developed human antimouse antibodies or heterophilic antibodies.[3,4]
- Patients with major depressive disorders, particularly older patients, may have increased ACTH levels.[8,9]
- Baseline morning ACTH levels help to differentiate primary versus secondary adrenal insufficiency.[14]
- Chronic opioid use can cause HPA suppression, thus causing false abnormal results.[13]
- Synthetic ACTH is first-line treatment for infantile spasms.[1]
- Ectopic ACTH production is often associated with small cell carcinoma of the lung, thymic tumors, or neuroendocrine/carcinoid tumors.[7]

PATIENT EDUCATION

- https://www.labcorp.com/resource/acth-stimulation-test

RELATED DIAGNOSES AND ICD-10 CODES

Adrenal insufficiency	E27.40	Cushing disease	E24.9
Addison disease	E27.1	Ectopic ACTH	E24.3
Iatrogenic adrenal insufficiency	E27.3	Iatrogenic Cushing syndrome	E24.2

REFERENCES

Full list of references can be accessed through Springer Publishing Company Connect™ at the following link: http://connect.springerpub.com/content/reference-book/978-0-8261 -8843-4/part/part03/toc-part/ch013

---

14. ALDOSTERONE, RENIN, AND THE ALDOSTERONE-TO-RENIN RATIO

Lisa Ward

PHYSIOLOGY/PATHOPHYSIOLOGY REVIEW

Renin is an enzyme secreted by the kidney in response to low blood pressure and decreased sodium. Secretion of renin initiates the renin-angiotensin-aldosterone system (RAAS) causing the adrenal gland to secrete aldosterone (see Figure 13.1). Aldosterone is a mineralocorticoid that increases blood pressure by vaso-constriction, water and salt retention, and potassium excretion. Excess aldoste-rone can exist from overactivity in the adrenal gland (primary aldosteronism) or excess activity in the RAAS (secondary aldosteronism). Normally, as the aldosterone level rises, the plasma renin activity level (PRA) falls, resulting in a measurable ratio of the two. This mechanism is true of primary aldosteronism, but in secondary aldosteronism, both aldosterone and renin rise in conjunction.

OVERVIEW OF LABORATORY TEST

The aldosterone/renin ratio (aldosterone-to-renin ratio or ARR) is a laboratory test to detect primary aldosteronism (PA) in high-risk, hypertensive patients. Laboratory evaluation of the ARR can be assessed by testing aldosterone (CPT code 82088) and renin (CPT code 84244) and is calculated as the ratio of the serum aldosterone (in ng/dL) divided by renin (in ng/mL/hour). The ARR should be interpreted along with the actual values of renin and aldosterone. In general, an ARR greater than 20 to 25 is indicative of possible PA. The patient's posture should be noted at the time of lab collection as levels may be affected by upright versus supine posture. Morning is the most accurate time for lab collection due to diurnal rhythm of aldosterone and renin secretion.

INDICATIONS

Screening

■ Universal screening for ARR is not recommended. Testing is not indicated in the presence of mild hypertension, or when the diagnosis would not change the management.[1]

■ It is not recommended to screen for ARR in older, normokalemic patients with mild hypertension (i.e., blood pressure controlled on single medication).[2]

■ The Endocrine Society Clinical Guidelines recommend using ARR to screen for PA in patients who meet one of the following criteria[3]:
  ● Sustained blood pressure of greater than 150/90 in three separate measurements taken on different days
  ● People who have hypertension resistant to three conventional antihypertensive drugs
  ● People whose hypertension is controlled but needs four or more medications
  ● People with hypertension and an adrenal mass
  ● People with hypertension and hypokalemia
  ● People with hypertension and sleep apnea
  ● People with hypertension and family history of early-onset hypertension or stroke before age 40
  ● All hypertensive first-degree relatives of patients with confirmed PA

■ The American Heart Association recommends screening with ARR in all patients who fit the definition of resistant hypertension[4]:
  ● Hypertensive patients with blood pressure above goal despite concurrent use of three or more antihypertensive agents
  ● Three or more antihypertensive agents of different classes
  ● Antihypertensive agents are administered at maximally tolerated doses and appropriate dosing frequency

TABLE 14.1: INTERPRETATION OF ALDOSTERONE AND RENIN LEVELS

	ALDOSTERONE	RENIN	ARR	ADDITIONAL INFORMATION
Primary aldosteronism	High	Low	Increased (>30)	Referred to as "Conn syndrome" (hypokalemia is a common finding also, so look for a low potassium)
Secondary aldosteronism	High	High	Decreased (<10)	
Adrenal insufficiency	Low	High	Decreased	Addison's disease
Cushing syndrome	Low	Low	Normal or increased	

ARR, aldosterone renin ratio.

Diagnosis and Evaluation

- Aldosterone, renin, and aldosterone/renin ratio are used to evaluate for PA in the setting of resistant hypertension as previously outlined.[3,5,6]

Monitoring

- Normal ARR should be repeated in patients with high clinical suspicion of PA after appropriate interfering medications have been discontinued.
- If ARR is normal on repeat testing, PA has been ruled out. No further monitoring is needed.

INTERPRETATION

- Table 14.1 assists with interpretation of the aldosterone, renin, and ARR level.
- In general, a renin level lower than 1 ng/L, aldosterone level higher than 10 ng/L, or ARR of greater than 20 is considered suspicious for PA, especially if hypokalemia is also noted.[7]
- Secondary aldosteronism should be suspected when aldosterone and renin level are both elevated.[8]
- If PA is unlikely, differential diagnosis of ARR elevation includes licorice ingestion[9,10]; Cushing syndrome[7,9]; Liddle syndrome[9,11]; congenital adrenal hyperplasia[9,11]; and secondary aldosteronism caused by any condition that decreases blood flow to the kidneys, decreases blood pressure, or lowers sodium levels (e.g., dehydration, congestive heart failure, cirrhosis of the liver, kidney disease, or preeclampsia).[10]

FOLLOW-UP

- Patients with an abnormal ARR should be referred to an endocrinologist for continued follow-up with one of four confirmatory tests.[1,7,11]
  - Oral sodium loading
  - Saline suppression test

TABLE 14.2: FACTORS THAT MAY INFLUENCE THE ACCURACY OF ARR TESTING

FACTOR	INFLUENCE ON ARR	MANAGEMENT
Age older than 50	Increases	Adjustment of cutoff values
Female	Increases	Adjustment of cutoff values
Increased salt intake	Decreases	Minimal effect on ARR; no adjustment
Hypokalemia	Decreases	Potassium should be in normal range and corrected before measurement
Standing	Increases	Patient should be seated upright for 5 to 15 minutes before laboratory collection
Renal impairment	Decreases	No specific recommendations
Oral birth control/ estrogen replacement therapy	May increase or decrease	Stop taking medication 4 weeks prior to test
Pregnancy	May increase or decrease	Postpone test until 4 to 6 weeks post-partum
Stress	Increases	Patient should be seated upright for 5 to 15 minutes before laboratory collection
Aldosterone antagonists/ potassium sparing diuretics	Decreases	Stop taking medication 4 weeks prior to test
ACE-inhibitor/ARBs	Decreases	Stop taking medication 2 weeks prior to test

ARR, aldosterone renin ratio.

- Fludrocortisone suppression test
- Captopril test

PEARLS & PITFALLS

- Hypokalemia should be corrected prior to testing.
- Accuracy of renin and aldosterone testing can be affected by many medications and biologic factors (Table 14.2).[6,10]
- Between 4 to 6 weeks prior to testing, patients should discontinue aldosterone antagonists (e.g., spironolactone, eplerenone) and potassium-sparing diuretics (e.g., triamterene, amiloride) if possible.
- Alpha blockers (e.g., doxazosin), hydralazine, and non-dihydropyridine calcium channel blockers (extended-release verapamil) can be continued.
- Chronic ingestion of licorice can induce a syndrome similar to mineralocorticoid excess.[10,12] Therefore. patients should stop licorice ingestions 4 weeks prior to testing.

PATIENT EDUCATION

- https://www.labcorp.com/help/patient-test-info/aldosterone-and-renin

RELATED DIAGNOSES AND ICD-10

Hyperaldosteronism	E26.0
Hypokalemia	E87.6
Hypertension secondary to endocrine disorder	I15.2

REFERENCES

Full list of references can be accessed through Springer Publishing Company Connect™ at the following link: http://connect.springerpub.com/content/reference-book/978-0-8261-8843-4/part/part03/toc-part/ch014

---

15. ALPHA-1 ANTITRYPSIN DEFICIENCY

Sarah Fitz, Leah Burt, Olga Amusina, and Susan Corbridge

PHYSIOLOGY/PATHOPHYSIOLOGY REVIEW

Alpha-1 antitrypsin (AAT) is an enzyme inhibitor made in the liver. Its primary function is to protect lung tissue from breakdown.[1] Alpha-1 antitrypsin deficiency (AATD) is a genetic condition in which variant alleles lead to decreased serum levels of AAT. This causes decreased enzyme inhibition, which leads to lung tissue destruction and emphysema. In the liver, sequestration of abnormal AAT proteins leads to hepatocyte destruction. Because obstructive lung disease and cirrhosis can often be attributed to other etiologies, AATD is an underrecognized condition. Recognition of AATD is imperative, as it is treatable for some patients who can receive augmentation therapy to increase serum AAT levels.[2] Table 15.1 reviews types of AAT deficiencies.

Lung tissue is exposed to many environmental elements that can cause immune responses. During immune responses, proteases are released and serve to destroy potentially harmful proteins. Proteases also have the potential to damage the lung tissue itself but are usually appropriately inhibited by AAT, as AAT is the protease inhibitor found at the highest concentration in the lungs.[3] Also, AAT likely has some anti-inflammatory effects that are also lung-protective, leaving the lungs more vulnerable when AAT is deficient.[3] In the state of AATD, there is an insufficient level of AAT to inhibit destruction of elastin in lung tissue, which leads to loss of elasticity in the tissue and, thus, obstructive lung disease.[1] As such, severe AATD is a proven genetic risk factor for chronic obstructive pulmonary disease (COPD). Obstructive lung disease caused by AATD is notable for being found in all lobes of the lung and is predominantly found in the lung bases.[1]

The liver is one of the primary sites of AAT production. In homozygous ZZ mutation, the final stage of AAT protein folding is abnormal, and this leads to a large

TABLE 15.1: DEFINITIONS AND EXAMPLES OF GENETIC ABNORMALITIES CAUSING AAT DEFICIENCY

TERM	DEFINITION	PHYSIOLOGY IN ALPHA-1 ANTITRYPSIN DEFICIENCY
Alpha-1 antitrypsin (AAT)	Enzyme inhibitor which inhibits destruction of proteins by protease enzyme[1]	When deficient, the proteases destroy proteins at a higher rate, which can result in lung tissue destruction.
Protease	Enzyme which degrades and destroys proteins	Normally kept in check (at appropriate level) by AAT, but detrimental when AAT is deficient.
Autosomal recessive	Inherited genetic trait for which both parents must be carriers for offspring to inherit trait	If both parents carry the alleles for abnormal AAT sequences, the offspring can be carriers and may also exhibit clinically significant traits of AAT deficiency
Genotype	Genetic blueprint composed of multiple gene alleles	Normal genes are *M*. A person who does NOT have AAT will have two *M* genes (*MM*). A person may have the genotype for abnormal AAT sequences, but may not exhibit phenotypic characteristics consistent with AAT deficiency (see *phenotype* later in this table). Most people with severe AAT deficiency have two *Z* genes (*ZZ*). Another deficient gene combination is *SZ*, although this gene combination is less likely to cause lung or liver problems than *ZZ*. *Z* allele identification on genotype testing is highly associated with increased risk for obstructive pulmonary disease.[2]
Phenotype	Physiologic expression of genotype; observable characteristics	Clinical characteristics of abnormal AAT alleles are highly variable depending on each person's genotype and individual expression of the genotype. The two most common manifestations are obstructive lung disease and hepatic cirrhosis or fibrosis.
Allele	Version of a gene. Humans can have two or more variants (alleles) for a given gene	Two specific alleles (one from each parent) code for more than one hundred genotypic variants of AAT deficiency.
SERPINA1	Gene that encodes the AAT protein	The SERPINA 1 genes in AAT disorders have deviant sequences.

portion inappropriately staying inside hepatocytes.[4] Many of these abnormal proteins are destroyed, but some aggregate and lead to hepatocyte apoptosis. This is the primary cause of liver disease, but it is theorized that environmental and other genetic factors contribute to which individuals develop liver disease. Fewer people exhibit AAT deficiency-related liver disease than pulmonary disease, but it is one of the more common causes of hepatic failure, behind viral hepatitis, alcoholic cirrhosis, and chronic cholangitis.[3] Of note, AATD can also be associated with C-anti-proteinase 3-positive (ANCA)-positive vasculitis (granulomatosis with polyangiitis [GPA]), panniculitis (subcutaneous nodules), or bronchiectasis.[1]

Lung manifestations of AAT deficiency are usually present in early adulthood, but AATD is likely underdiagnosed, with many people being diagnosed with smoking-related COPD or asthma. While this chapter focuses on adult AATD, clinicians should note that neonates with homozygous genotype can develop neonatal hepatitis syndrome,[3] so it is recommended that neonates with unexplained jaundice or hepatitis undergo further evaluation.

OVERVIEW OF LABORATORY TEST

Serum Alpha-1 Antitrypsin Levels (CPT Code 82103)

Serum AAT levels quantify the amount of AAT protein present in blood serum and can be assessed using nephelometry (most common) or latex-enhanced immunoturbidimetric assay (less common).[5] Different genetic variants of AATD produce a unique range of serum levels of AAT proteins. Quantification of AAT serum level alone is insufficient to assess AATD. Not only do AAT levels fluctuate during pregnancy, childhood, and inflammatory states, but some mildly deficient genotypes may have normal serum AAT levels.[6,7] In addition, serum AAT levels do not quantify genetic risk.[8,9] The guideline-recommended, most sensitive, and specific test for inherited airflow deficiency is targeted genotype testing of the S and Z alleles. Sensitivity of AAT levels in identifying patients with genetic variants for AAT vary based on the genotype and existence or lack of inflammatory state in that individual patient. Studies have shown that AAT levels have higher sensitivity for people with homozygous ZZ genotype, while sensitivity is lower for those with heterozygous genotypes.[10,11]

Genotype Variant Testing

Genotype variant testing is most often accomplished through targeted genotyping OR isoelectric focusing (IEF).[5] Before undergoing genotype variant testing, patients should take part in both pre- and post-testing genetic counseling.[5]

Targeted genotyping (CPT code 81332) is a useful test to rapidly identify or exclude most common AAT variants.[5] It detects the normal (M) and most common pathogenic gene mutations seen in AAT deficiency (often, F, I, S, and Z, although varies by individual laboratory).[10] Polymerase chain reaction (PCR) technology rapidly amplifies small amounts of genes to quantifiable amounts that can then be functionally analyzed using primers specific to known sequences.[5] Laboratories must test for specific alleles in order to detect them; therefore, providers should know which alleles are specifically tested for in their laboratory.[5] The COPD Foundation recommends genotyping for the S and Z alleles, at a minimum.[6]

IEF; "protein phenotyping" or "PI typing" (CPT code 82104) identifies specific variant AAT proteins and employs electrophoresis techniques to separate proteins based on their isoelectric points. In other words, this technique distinguishes specific protein types based on how fast the proteins move when given a gentle electrical stimulus. For example, the Z protein migrates the slowest, and the F protein migrates the fastest. It is considered the gold standard for protein identification and should be used secondarily to genotyping.[10] Interpretation is complex and should be undertaken by a geneticist or specialized care provider.[5] In certain less-common cases, targeted genotyping and IEF may be either nondiagnostic or produce results deviating from clinical findings. In these instances, providers should consider genetic origin of blood samples. Does the patient have a parent with a history of a liver transplant? Has the patient undergone a hematopoietic cell transplant themselves? If the answer is "yes" to either of these questions, then laboratory results might be affected. Because AAT proteins have genetic origins in hematopoietic cells but are physically produced by the liver, altering either of these vital systems may skew results.[11]

Gene sequencing ("whole gene sequencing" or "SERPINA1 Gene, Full Gene Analysis") (CPT code 8149) is a molecular analysis and identification of individual AAT gene sequences and able to detect rarer (or unrecognized) AAT variants because gene sequencing does not rely on specific, laboratory-dependent primers.[5,12] The test maps out the DNA composition of individual AAT genes, and is useful if the serum AAT level and genotype do not correspond, if clinical features cannot be explained by reported genotype, or in instances of rare variants or null alleles. Interpretation is complex and should be performed by experienced geneticists or specialized care providers. Depending on the institution and local legislation, this test may require informed consent.[8]

INDICATIONS

Screening

■ Widespread screening of the general population is not recommended.[5] Any person with a diagnosis of COPD should be screened at least once, regardless of age or ethnicity.[6]

Diagnosis and Evaluation

■ AAT concentration and genotyping testing is indicated for patients with clinical features that prompt suspicion for increased likelihood of AAT disorder (summarized in Table 15.2).[5-7]

■ Prioritizing diagnostic testing only to individuals most at risk will help lessen possible psychologic stressors and genetic discrimination that can be associated with screening.[7]

Monitoring

■ Once a diagnosis of AAT deficiency is made, it is not necessary to retest or monitor genotyping or AAT levels.

INTERPRETATION

■ Targeted genotype testing should be interpreted in concert with AAT levels, as outlined in Figure 15.1.

■ AAT concentrations
● Less than 20 micromol/L (100 mg/dL) is defined as potential deficiency if nephelometry is used, although some sources report a low of 80 mg/dL as a low-normal finding.[13] Less than 113 mg/dL (18.4 to 21 µmol/L) is a potential deficiency if latex-enhanced immunoturbidimetric assay is used.[14]

TABLE 15.2: CLINICAL FINDINGS THAT WARRANT CONSIDERATION OF AATD EVALUATION

Family history	*AAT deficiency[2]
	Emphysema
	*COPD[2]
	Liver disease
	Panniculitis
	Bronchiectasis
Lung disease	*Any patient with COPD including early onset <40 years[2,3]
	*Irreversible airflow limitation or obstruction after bronchodilator treatment[1,3]
	Adult-onset asthma
	*Asymptomatic patients with risk factors and persistent, obstructive airflow pattern[1,3]
	Unexplained bronchiectasis[3]
	Emphysema with absence of risk factors OR *prominent basilar hyperlucency[2] OR onset age ≤ 45 years
Liver disease	*Perinatal hepatitis, jaundice, or cirrhosis[2]
	Cirrhosis (children, adults)
	Hepatocellular carcinoma
	Hepatomegaly
	*Unexplained liver disease (neonates, children, adults)[1,3]
Laboratory values	Persistent, mild to moderate elevated ALT, AST
	Low alpha$_1$-globulin or presence of two bands in alpha$_1$ globulin region on SPEP
Skin disease	*Adult necrotizing panniculitis[1,3]
	*Perinatal panniculitis[2,3]
Other conditions	Antiproteinase 3-positive (ANCA) vasculitis
	*Perinatal vasculitis[2]
	*Granulomatosis with polyangiitis[3]

* Priority diagnostic testing recommendation.

[1]American Thoracic Society Grade A Recommendation.

[2]European Respiratory Society Enhanced Suspicion Group.

[3]COPD Foundation Practice Guideline Recommendation.

AAT, alpha-1 antitrypsin; AATD, alpha-1 antitrypsin deficiency; COPD, chronic obstructive pulmonary disease.

Sources: McElvaney NG. Diagnosing α1-antitrypsin deficiency: how to improve the current algorithm. *Eur Respir Rev.* 2015;24(135):52–57; Miravitlles M, Herr C, Ferrarotti I, et al. Laboratory testing of individuals with severe alpha1-antitrypsin deficiency in three European centres. *Eur Respir J.* 2010;35(5):960–968; Sandhaus RA, Turino G, Brantly ML, et al. The diagnosis and management of alpha-1 antitrypsin deficiency in the adult. *Chronic Obstr Pulm Dis.* 2016;3(3):668–682. doi:10.15326/jcopdf.3.3.2015.0182; Teckman JH, Blomenkamp KS. Pathophysiology of alpha-1 antitrypsin deficiency liver disease. In: Borel F, Mueller C., eds. *Alpha-1 Antitrypsin Deficiency. Methods in Molecular Biology,* vol 1639. Humana Press; 2017. doi:10.1007/978-1-4939-7163-3_1

- Clinicians should follow cutoff values at their local laboratory.
- Nephelometry: Less than 20 μmol/L (100 mg/dL) should be evaluated further.
- Latex-enhanced immunoturbidimetric assay: Less than 113 mg/dL (18.4 to 21 μmol/L) should be evaluated further.[14]

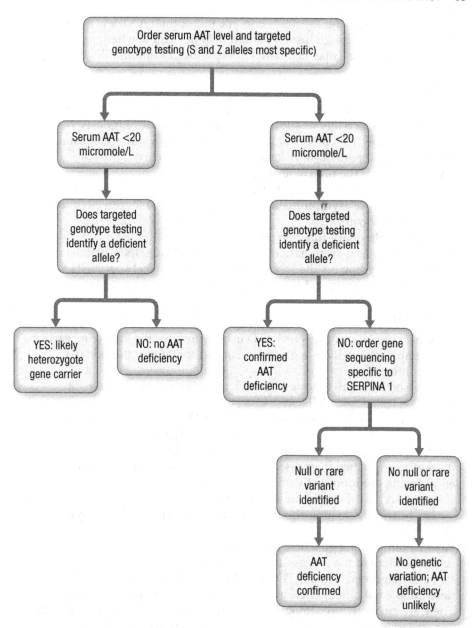

FIGURE 15.1. Algorithm for guideline-based testing and interpretation. AAT, alpha-1 antitrypsin.

- S and Z allele genotyping should be interpreted by an experienced geneticist.[6]
  - Patients with homozygous or heterozygous genotypes consistent with AAT *and* a subtherapeutic AAT serum level are diagnosed with AATD.
  - Patients with a normal genotype and decreased or borderline low AAT levels require more extensive gene sequencing sent to evaluate for less common genotypes.

- Patients with a heterozygous genotype but normal AAT level do not have AATD. A thorough history should help determine whether a patient's liver or lung disease may be related to exposures or modifiable risk factors.

FOLLOW-UP

- Evaluating AAT level alone is not recommended; patients need genotyping performed concurrently or subsequently to confirm the diagnosis. If AAT level is low, concurrent or follow-up genotype testing can ensure identification of patients at risk for clinical disease (even if they are asymptomatic at the time of testing).[6]
- Individuals who have been tested and found to have abnormal AAT genotypes but are asymptomatic should be monitored for development of clinical disease with:
  - Annual pulmonary function testing[6]
  - Annual physical examination, liver function testing, INR, platelet count[6]
- Positive genotyping results should be referred to clinical specialists for expanded genotyping and treatment.[6]

PEARLS & PITFALLS

- Clinical expressions of severe AATD usually involve the lung (e.g., early onset emphysema); liver (e.g., cirrhosis); and sometimes the skin (e.g., panniculitis).
- Any person with a diagnosis of COPD, regardless of race or ethnicity, should be tested for AATD.
- Features more likely to be associated with AATD include emphysema in younger persons (i.e., 45 years old or younger), nonsmokers or with minimal smoking history, a family history of emphysema and/or liver disease, unexplained liver disease, and/or with radiographic features of emphysema predominantly in the lung bases.
- If serum AAT level is low but initial genotype testing does not show variant alleles, further evaluation should be undertaken with a full genotype evaluation.
- Patients undergoing genetic testing need genetic counseling to improve understanding of the process and reduce anxiety.
- Patients diagnosed with AATD should meet with a genetic counselor to determine what other genetically related relatives should seek testing.
- There are currently no demographic characteristics or clinical findings that can effectively rule out AATD,[6] but it is more common among Caucasians from Europe and North America.[3]

PATIENT EDUCATION

- https://www.alpha1.org/newly-diagnosed/learning-about-alpha-1/testing-for-alpha-1/
- https://www.lung.org/lung-health-diseases/lung-disease-lookup/alpha-1-antitrypsin-deficiency/symptoms-diagnosis

RELATED DIAGNOSES AND ICD-10 CODES

Alpha-1-antitrypsin deficiency	E88.01	Hepatic fibrosis	K74.0
Chronic obstructive pulmonary disease	J44.9	Bronchiectasis	J47.0
Cirrhosis	K74.6	Granulomatosis with polyangiitis (GPA)	M31.3

REFERENCES

Full list of references can be accessed through Springer Publishing Company Connect™ at the following link: http://connect.springerpub.com/content/reference-book/978-0-8261 -8843-4/part/part03/toc-part/ch015

16. AMMONIA

Kelly Small Casler and Amanda Chaney

PHYSIOLOGY REVIEW

Ammonia is produced in the small bowel and colon from the breakdown of urea into ammonia and carbon dioxide. The kidneys and muscles also contribute to production of ammonia in smaller amounts.[1] Ammonia is primarily metabolized by the liver and is excreted by the kidney and liver.[2,3] It is a compound that can pass through the blood-brain barrier, causing cerebral irritation and swelling. Excess ammonia accumulation in the brain is felt to be partly responsibility for the neuropsychiatric symptoms seen in hepatic encephalopathy (HE).[3]

OVERVIEW OF LABORATORY TEST

Ammonia can be measured via venous (plasma or serum) or arterial blood. It is generally felt that there is no difference in accuracy between venous or arterial blood as long as specimens are analyzed quickly and placed on ice immediately after collection.[2,4,5] However, in HE caused by acute liver failure (ALF) one source suggests arterial ammonia levels are more accurate.[1]

INDICATIONS

Screening
- Not indicated and especially discouraged by Choosing Wisely.[6]

Diagnosis and Evaluation
- Ammonia levels are indicated in evaluating for urea cycle disorders.[7]
- In evaluation of mental status changes in patients with chronic liver disease (CLD), ammonia levels are not useful for HE evaluation. Diagnosis

and severity classification of HE should be determined using clinical examination and West Haven Criteria.[2,3,5,6,8–10]

■ In evaluation of mental status changes in the presence of ALF, ammonia is helpful for diagnosis and higher levels of ammonia do correlate with severity of HE. This correlation is not seen in patients with CLD.[2,11,12]

Monitoring

■ Do not use to monitor recovery and treatment response in HE from CLD; use clinical examination instead.[2,8]
■ Can be used for monitoring therapy during ALF.[11,12]
■ In one study a level greater than 200 µg/dL predicted cerebral herniation in patients with ALF.[13]
■ In one study, levels greater than 120 µmol/L resulted in increased risk of dying from ALF (7.1 OR).[14]
■ High ammonia levels in patients with acute or chronic liver failure have worse prognosis.[15,16]
■ Elevations in ammonia for more than 3 days in ALF may indicate poorer prognosis.[17]

INTERPRETATION

■ Levels should be less than 50 µmol/L.[18]
■ When interpreting ammonia levels, care must be taken to consider conditions other than HE that can cause elevated ammonia levels (Box 16.1).

FOLLOW-UP

■ Elevated ammonia levels do not rule out the possibility of other differential diagnoses of mental status changes, so care must be taken in the initial diagnosis phase.[8]

Box 16.1: Conditions Other Than HE Associated With Elevated Ammonia Levels

■ Alcohol
■ Gastrointestinal bleeding (increases ammonia production)
■ Hemolytic states (hemolytic disease of newborn)
■ Portosystemic shunting (decrease ammonia excretion)
■ Medications: some chemotherapy, valproic acid, barbiturates, narcotics, diuretics, steroids
■ Renal disease
■ Reyes syndrome
■ Shock
■ Total parenteral nutrition (increases ammonia production)
■ Urea cycle disorders
■ Urinary tract infection caused by organisms that produce urease

HE, hepatic encephalopathy.

Sources: Data from Elgouhari HM, O'Shea R. What is the utility of measuring the serum ammonia level in patients with altered mental status? *Cleve Clin J Med.* 2009;76(4):252–254. doi:10.3949/ccjm.76a.08072; Ge PS, Runyon BA. Serum ammonia level for the evaluation of hepatic encephalopathy. *JAMA.* 2014;312(6):643. doi:10.1001/jama.2014.2398; Petel D, Prasad C, Rupar T, et al. Hyperammonemic encephalopathy as a manifestation of Reye syndrome in a previously-healthy 14-year-old girl: a case report. *Pediatr Med.* 2020;3:16. doi:10.21037/pm-20-51

PEARLS & PITFALLS

- Prolonged tourniquet use can cause false high ammonia levels.[2,8]
- Samples should be placed on ice and evaluated within 15 minutes.[19,20]
- Although guidelines report monitoring ammonia levels in HE "may be appropriate" to follow treatment efficacy[5] a recent study supports ammonia levels are unnecessary during therapy[21] and more recent literature recommends against monitoring ammonia during HE due to poor sensitivity/specificity for HE.[8,22]
- In one study, ammonia levels remained elevated up to 48 hours after HE resolution.[4]
- Use of ammonia to diagnose HE significantly increases costs, but does not improve diagnosis or management.[23]

PATIENT EDUCATION

- https://www.webmd.com/a-to-z-guides/ammonia-test#1

RELATED DIAGNOSES AND ICD-10 CODES

| Hepatic encephalopathy | K72.90 | Chronic liver disease | E72.10 |
| Acute and subacute liver failure | K72.00 | Hyperammonemia | E72.20 |

REFERENCES

Full list of references can be accessed through Springer Publishing Company Connect™ at the following link: http://connect.springerpub.com/content/reference-book/978-0-8261 -8843-4/part/part03/toc-part/ch016

---

17. ANDROSTENEDIONE

Lisa Ward

PHYSIOLOGY REVIEW

Androstenedione (AE) is an inactive steroid hormone precursor to androgen and estrogen sex hormones. Although it is often considered a male sex hormone, AE is also found in females. AE is produced by the ovaries in females, testes in males, and adrenal glands. LH from the pituitary gland stimulates the testes and ovaries to release AE, while the pituitary hormone adrenocorticotropic hormone (ACTH) stimulates the adrenal gland to release AE. The body then converts AE into testosterone and estrogen.[1,2] AE levels peak near birth and then rapidly fall during the first year of life. With the onset of adrenarche, AE gradually rises and accelerates the onset of puberty, and reaches adult levels by 18 to 20 years old.[3] Excessive AE in infants can cause ambiguous genitalia and can cause precocious puberty in adolescents. Elevated AE in adult males typically is asymptomatic,[3] whereas in females, excess may cause virilization. Inadequate levels of AE can cause failure of sexual characteristics development (pubic hair/body hair growth in males and menses in females).

OVERVIEW OF LABORATORY TEST

Laboratory evaluation of AE can be assessed by androstenedione (CPT code 500152). Due to the diurnal pattern of AE, serum levels will vary during the day with the peak at 7 a.m. and the nadir at 4 p.m.[2,4,5]AE levels also vary with women's menstrual cycles, are higher in pregnancy, and will abruptly decline after menopause.[6] Because of its origins, AE can be a useful marker of adrenal gland function, of androgen production, and of ovary and testicle function.[1,3] The AE laboratory test is often done as a confirmatory test when other hormone testing, such as 17 hydroxyprogesterone (OHP), dehydroepiandrosterone sulfate (DHEAs), or testosterone, is abnormal.[2,6]

INDICATIONS

Screening

- The Endocrine Society, American College of Obstetricians and Gynecologists (ACOG), American Society for Reproductive Medicine, European Society of Endocrinology, and the International Menopause Society recommend against universal AE screening because a correlation between symptoms and androgen levels has not been established.[6]
- The Endocrine Society and International Evidence-Based Guidelines recommend evaluating AE levels when screening women with suspected PCOS,[7,8] even if total and free testosterone levels are not elevated.[9,10]

Diagnosis and Evaluation

- The Endocrine Society recommends evaluating androgen levels, including AE, in all women with hirsutism.[7,8]
- ACOG recommends evaluating AE in adolescents with hyperandrogenic symptoms.[5,11]
- AE is used to evaluate the cause of precocious puberty, virilization, and ambiguous genitalia.
- AE is used to diagnose CAH.
- AE is used to evaluate the cause of infertility, amenorrhea, persistent or late-onset acne, and hirsutism in women.[5,11,12]
- AE is used to evaluate the cause for delayed puberty.
- AE is used to evaluate adrenal gland function and to distinguish androgen-secreting tumors in the adrenal glands from those that originate in the ovaries or testicles.[1]
- AE is used to evaluate for PCOS.[11]

Monitoring

- In CAH patients, AE is monitored every 3 to 6 months for assessing disease control.[4,13]

- In hyperandrogenic adolescence, repeat AE every 3 to 6 months to assess response to treatment until condition is stable, then monitor annually.[5]
- If patient is medically treated for androgen deficiency, androgen levels should be done 3 to 6 weeks after initiation of therapy and every 6 months thereafter to assess androgen excess.[6]

INTERPRETATION

- In infants, normal reference intervals are given for premature and full-term infants[3]:
  - Premature infants:
    - 26 to 28 weeks: 92 to 282 ng/dL
    - 31 to 35 weeks: 80 to 446 ng/dL
  - Full-term infants:
    - 1 to 7 days: 20 to 290 ng/dL
    - 1 month to 1 year: less than 69 ng/dL
- Normal levels of AE vary with age and Tanner development and are described in Table 17.1
- An elevated level of AE indicates increased adrenal, ovarian, or testicular production.
- A low level of AE may be due to adrenal gland dysfunction, adrenal insufficiency, or to ovarian or testicular failure.[2] Drugs that induce hepatic enzymes or affect lipid metabolism, as well as other steroid hormones, can also cause low AE levels.[3]
- Small fluctuations of AE levels can be normal; however, a pronounced increased level greater than 500 ng/dL may indicate underlying conditions such as CAH or adrenal cancer.[1–3,10,11]
- Differential diagnosis of elevated AE includes PCOS, CAH,[3] precocious puberty, hirsutism, adrenal gland tumor, anabolic substance use/abuse, and ovarian/testicular tumors.
- Differential diagnosis of decreased AE includes ovarian/testicular failure and delayed puberty.

TABLE 17.1: ANDROSTENEDIONE

		MALE	FEMALE
Tanner stage	Age (years)	Reference interval (ng/dL)	Reference interval (ng/dL)
Stage I (prepubertal)	<9	<51	<51
Stage II	~9–14	31–65	42–100
Stage III	~10–15	50–100	80–190
Stage IV	~11–16	48–140	77–225
Stage V	~12–18	65–210	80–24
Adults	>18	40–150	30–200

Sources: Data from *Androstenedione, Serum.* Mayo Clinical Laboratories website. https://endocrinology.testcatalog.org/show/ANST; Lexicomp Online. *Lab Tests and Diagnostic Procedures.* UpToDate, Inc; 2019.

FOLLOW-UP

■ Drugs that induce hepatic enzymes (e.g., carbamazepine, imipramine, phenytoin) or affect lipid metabolism, as well as other steroid hormones, can also cause low AE levels.[3] These drug-induced changes likely are not significant enough to cause diagnostic confusion. If clinically concerned, the patient should stop all interacting medications for 4 weeks, and testing should be repeated.

■ An elevated AE is not diagnostic of a specific condition; it usually indicates the need for further testing to pinpoint the cause.[1]

■ Most mild-to-moderate elevations in AE do not have a recognizable cause and could be due to AE supplements.[2] If supplement use is suspected, the patient should stop all supplements and repeat AE laboratory testing in 4 to 6 weeks to determine if results normalized.

■ Elevated levels greater than 500 ng/dL may indicate adrenal cancer, adrenal tumor, or CAH; therefore, further diagnostic testing and endocrinology referral is warranted:

   ● In infants with ambiguous genitalia and/or children below age 9 with precocious puberty, continued workup for CAH is needed, including DHEAs, 17 OHP, ACTH, and cortisol laboratory testing.[3]

   ● In symptomatic or asymptomatic adults, abdominal imaging is needed to rule out adrenal gland tumor.

PEARLS & PITFALLS

■ An increased level is not diagnostic of a specific condition; it usually indicates the need for further hormonal testing to determine the cause.[2]

■ When monitoring CAH patients treated on glucocorticoid steroids, normal AE levels indicate effective treatment, whereas elevated AE levels indicate the need for medications adjustment.

■ AE is elevated in 90% of patients with PCOS[9] and are diagnostic for excess ovarian androgens.[14]

■ Simultaneous measurement of AE along with testosterone and DHEA-S leads to more accurate diagnosis of PCOS.[15,16]

■ AE levels increase in pubertal boys for about 2 years prior to significant increases in testosterone. AE testing is not typically used to monitor this process.[2,4]

■ Adrenal AE is the major source of androgens in postmenopausal women.

■ AE levels are decreased in obesity and aging.[17]

■ AE levels are typically significantly increased in adults with persistent acne.[12]

■ Androstenedione has been marketed as a dietary supplement in the United States for its anabolic steroid effects. These supplements can cause increased levels of AE.[3]

■ AE may be measured as part of testing for athletes using performance-enhancing drugs since the NCAA has banned androstenedione supplements.[3]

PATIENT EDUCATION

■ https://www.yourhormones.info/hormones/androstenedione/

RELATED DIAGNOSES AND ICD-10 CODES

Androgen excess	E28.1	Precocious puberty	E30.1
Congenital adrenal hyperplasia	E25.0	Polycystic ovarian syndrome	E28.2
Ambiguous genitalia	Q56.4	Adrenal nodule	E27.9
Hirsutism	L68.0		

REFERENCES

Full list of references can be accessed through Springer Publishing Company Connect™ at the following link: http://connect.springerpub.com/content/reference-book/978-0-8261-8843-4/part/part03/toc-part/ch017

18. ANTIPARIETAL CELL ANTIBODY AND INTRINSIC FACTOR

Lynne M. Hutchison

PHYSIOLOGY REVIEW

The stomach is lined with mucus-secreting epithelial cells which provide a protective barrier for the surface of the stomach. In addition, the stomach mucosa contains parietal cells, which secrete hydrochloric acid and intrinsic factor. Hydrochloric acid is involved in the chemical breakdown of ingested substances. Intrinsic factor is needed in order to absorb vitamin B12.[1] Vitamin B12 is found in foods of animal origin. During digestion, B12 is released from the animal protein and is bound to intrinsic factor. This complex of B12-intrinsic factor protects vitamin B12 from digestion by intestinal enzymes until it can be absorbed in the ileum. This process can be interrupted by the use of proton pump inhibiting drugs, sprue, gastrectomy, or gastric bypass surgery, resulting in a deficiency of intrinsic factor which leads to a deficiency in vitamin B12. This can result in pernicious anemia.[1] In patients with pernicious anemia, nearly 90% are positive for antiparietal cell antibody (APCA) [also called gastric parietal cell antibodies (GPCAB)], and of these patients, nearly 60% also have positive anti-intrinsic factor antibodies. There is research suggesting these antibodies contribute to the destruction of the gastric mucosa. Along with presence of APCAs in patients with atrophic gastritis, gastric ulcers, and gastric cancer, it can also be present in other autoimmune-related diseases including but not limited to thyroiditis, myxedema, type 1 diabetes, Addison disease, and iron-deficiency anemia.[2]

OVERVIEW OF LABORATORY TEST

Laboratory evaluation of parietal cell functioning is often done in conjunction with a workup for pernicious anemia. The functioning of parietal cells can be assessed by evaluating the level of intrinsic factor blocking antibody (CPT code 86340).[3] If present, this antibody impedes the action of intrinsic factor, and indirectly, the absorption of vitamin B12. In addition, parietal cell functioning can be assessed by evaluating the APCA [also referred to as GPCAB levels] (CPT code 83516)[4] or GPCAB with reflex to titer (CPT code 86256)[4] and, when present, is suggestive of pernicious anemia or other related autoimmune diseases. This test has a high degree of sensitivity greater than 90% but a low degree of specificity. This is due to autoantibodies pre-dating symptoms by several years.[5]

INDICATIONS

Screening

■ Universal or targeted screenings are not recommended.

Diagnosis and Evaluation

■ Test for autoantibodies to intrinsic factor and parietal cells in individuals who have biochemical evidence of vitamin B12 deficiency without another obvious cause.[6,7]
■ A combination of testing for both intrinsic factor blocking and gastric parietal cell antibodies, with fasting gastrin levels, is recommended as an adjunct to histologic diagnosis of atrophic gastritis.[7]

Monitoring

■ No routine monitoring is recommended once diagnosis is established.[6,7]

INTERPRETATION

■ See Table 18.1 for test result interpretation.

FOLLOW-UP

■ Abnormal results should be interpreted in combination with available history data, complete blood count, vitamin B12 levels, and histologic findings.[8,9]

TABLE 18.1: INTERPRETATION OF PARIETAL CELL FUNCTIONING		
TEST	**REFERENCE INTERVAL**	**METHODOLOGY**
Intrinsic factor blocking antibody [IF blocking antibody][4]	Reported as positive or negative	Immunoassay
Antiparietal cell antibody*[5]	< or = 20.0 Units: Negative 20.1–24.9 Units: Equivocal > or = 25.0 Units: Positive	ELISA

*Also called gastric parietal cell antibody.

■ There is a pernicious anemia diagnostic panel available which includes IF blocking antibody, methylmalonic acid, and vitamin B12 (CPT codes 82607, 83921, 86340).

PEARLS & PITFALLS

■ Samples for intrinsic factor blocking antibody should not be collected from patients who have received vitamin B12 injection therapy within the last week.[8,9]
■ APCAs are found in more than 90% of patients with pernicious anemia.
■ APCAs can be elevated with atrophic gastritis, Hashimoto thyroiditis, myxedema, Addison disease, and type 1 diabetes in addition to pernicious anemia. No differences in laboratory results have been identified based on age or sex. They are found in 60% of atrophic gastritis and 22% of gastric ulceration diagnoses as these conditions occur before the onset of the anemia. APCAs are also found in 30% to 40% of patients with the following conditions: Addison disease, autoimmune thyroiditis, insulin-dependent diabetes, and ovarian failure.[5]
■ APCAs are not associated with duodenal ulcer or gastritis.

PATIENT EDUCATION

■ https://medlineplus.gov/ency/article/003351.htm
■ https://labtestsonline.org/tests/intrinsic-factor-antibody

RELATED DIAGNOSES AND ICD-10 CODES

Atrophic gastritis	K29.40
Pernicious anemia	D51.0
Vitamin B12 deficiency, unspecified	D53.9

REFERENCES

Full list of references can be accessed through Springer Publishing Company Connect™ at the following link: http://connect.springerpub.com/content/reference-book/978-0-8261 -8843-4/part/part03/toc-part/ch018

19. ANTIBODIES MEASLES, MUMPS, AND RUBELLA

Donna Faye McHaney

PHYSIOLOGY REVIEW

Vaccines such as the measles, mumps, and rubella (MMR), and varicella (MMRV) are recommended around the world and are based on the scientific principle of how they prevent and protect individuals against infection. It has been shown that these vaccines reduce both morbidity and mortality in both high- and low-income countries. MMRV are considered typical childhood infections with a good prognosis. However, they are highly contagious and can lead to serious complications. As individuals age, the risk of complications increases but have proven to be effective overall. Vaccination remains one of the most effective and safest interventions available to the public for primary prevention of infectious disease.[1-3] Immunity, both direct and indirect, is induced in individuals who are vaccinated and can create herd immunity among populations.[1,4]

Immunity is an essential aspect of vaccinations. The ability of the human body to tolerate foreign or indigenous materials is known as immunity, although it is generally specific to single organisms or related organisms. The immune system can identify foreign organisms and eliminate them, providing protection from infectious diseases such as MMRV.[5] The immune response is a defense against antigens that stimulates the immune system. This response involves the production of protein molecules by B-lymphocytes (B cells) and T-lymphocytes or cell-mediated immunity. The two basic mechanisms for acquiring immunity are shown in Table 19.1. The MMR and varicella antibody tests are commonly used to determine vaccination history and immunity in addition to identifying active infections.

OVERVIEW OF LABORATORY TEST

A variety of laboratory tests may be performed depending on the reason for the test and/or the presentation of signs and symptoms of MMRV. Some of the most recommended tests are listed in Table 19.1 along with Current Procedural Terminology (CPT) codes. Sample reports for some of the tests can be found in Table 19.2.

Measles, Mumps, and Rubella Antibodies (IgG) Panel, Immune Profile

The MMR Antibodies IgG Panel, Immune Profile is also known as the MMR antibodies panel (CPT codes 86735, 86765, 86762) and includes measles antibody (IgG), mumps virus antibody (IgG), and rubella antibody (IgG). The CPT codes for these are listed in Table 19.2. Serologic status can be determined to diagnose measles, mumps, and rubella viruses. Exposure to a virus or even previous vaccinations will yield a positive result which is considered adequate.[6] Evidence of immunity to measles, mumps, and rubella is important. Presumptive immunity

TABLE 19.1: PASSIVE AND ACTIVE IMMUNITY	
PASSIVE IMMUNITY	**ACTIVE IMMUNITY**
Able to achieve immunity in a short period of time.	Development of active immunity requires a longer amount of time (e.g., days or even weeks).
Provides rapid, short-term protection.	Immunity is long term; can last a life span.
Does not produce the antibody.	Additional exposure to the same antigen results in a greater response of the antibody.
Acquired when an individual is given the antibodies (through fetal transmission or by receiving immunoglobulin)	Acquired through immunization or infection with the disease.

Sources: Data from Alder R, Fallon LFJ, Hessen MT. *Immunization and vaccination.* Magill's Medical Guide (Online Edition). 2021. Centers for Disease Control and Prevention. The Pink Book: epidemiology and prevention of vaccine-preventable diseases. https://www.cdc.gov/vaccines/pubs/pinkbook/mumps.html.

evidence to measles, mumps, and rubella can be measured by this panel for purposes of routine vaccination, for those students at post-high school level, and for international travelers.[6]

Polymerase Chain Reaction to Detect Mumps, Measles, Rubella, and Varicella Zoster Virus

When testing for measles or mumps with the PCR test, a positive result indicates that there is a current viral infection. Depending on the strain of measles or mumps virus, there may be information that can help determine the source of the infection, such as travel to a specific country or exposure to someone with an active infection. The CDC can use the results of the genetic test to identify outbreak cases and prevent further spread of the virus.[8]

If a negative result is yielded from the test, signs and symptoms may be due to something else. It is important to note that a negative result means a person does not have an active infection. The virus may have been present in too low of numbers to detect. If there is a negative result but an infection is still strongly suspected, then the test should be repeated or a follow-up test repeated.[8]

The PCR laboratory test (CPT code 87798) is recommended to be used to confirm any suspected cases of varicella, confirm if varicella is the cause of outbreaks, confirm varicella in severe or unusual cases, determine susceptibility to varicella, or if adverse events suspected to be related to a vaccine are caused by vaccine-strain varicella zoster virus (VZV).[6]

Fluorescent Antibody Assay

The direct fluorescent antibody assay (DFA) is used to diagnose VZV. Positive results require the morphology of the organism or cells to distinguish them from background fluorescence. PCR assays are more sensitive than DFA and are used instead of traditional testing methods. The PCR assay may be used in combination with the DFA or when information is still needed when the magnitude of the infection is in question.[7,9]

TABLE 19.2: TEST TYPES, ORGANISMS TESTED FOR, TURNAROUND TIME, AND NOTES

TEST	ORGANISMS	LAB TURNAROUND TIME	NOTES
Measles, mumps, rubella (MMR) immunity profile (MMR antibodies panel)	Measles antibody, IgG Mumps antibody, IgG Rubella antibody, IgG	1–2 days[6,7]	This is a serum specimen test. Causes of rejection include hemolysis; lipemia; and gross bacterial contamination.
Polymerase chain reaction (PCR) to detect varicella zoster virus (VZV) (VZV, DNA by real-time PCR)	Chickenpox (Varicella)	4–5 days[6,7]	This test is sensitive when used with skin lesions (vesicles, scabs, maculopapular lesions). The specimen can be obtained from cerebrospinal fluid (CSF), whole blood, or swab.
Varicella-zoster virus antibodies (IgG, IgM) (VZV Ab IgG and IgM,chickenpox IgG and IgM Ab, herpes zoster IgG and IgM Ab)	Chickenpox (Varicella)	1–4 days[7]	Detect IgM antibodies specific for VZV to confirm VZV acute infection. If a patient presents more than 9 days after a rash appears this assay should not be used.
Fluorescent antibody assay (DFA)	Chickenpox (Varicella)	1–3 days[7]	DFA is less sensitive than PCR.
Viral culture	Chickenpox (Varicella)	9–12 days[6,7]	Not recommended since the viral culture takes longer to generate results.
Virus culture, rapid, varicella zoster virus (VZV) (chickenpox culture Culture, varicella zoster virus Shingles culture VZV culture)	Isolation of varicella-zoster	5–6 days[6,7]	Used in the diagnosis of varicella-zoster virus (i.e., chickenpox and shingles).

Sources: Data from LabCorp. *Varicella Zoster Virus (VZV), DNA PCR.* https://www.labcorp.com/tests/138313/varicella-zoster-virus-vzv-dna-pcr; Quest Diagnostics. https://testdirectory.questdiagnostics.com/test/test-detail/5259/mmr-igg-panel-measles-mumps-rubella?cc=MASTER.

Virus Culture, Rapid, Varicella Zoster Virus

The virus culture, rapid, VZV test (CPT code 87254) is used in the diagnosis of varicella-zoster virus (i.e., chickenpox and shingles). Clinical diagnosis must be made in conjunction with the patient's presenting signs and symptoms. This test does not differentiate between an active infection or a past infection. However, if there is a positive result, it indicates the patient has antibodies to VZV. This test may not be sensitive enough to detect any antibodies so if a negative result is obtained, it may not indicate susceptibility to a VZV infection.[6]

INDICATIONS

Screening

■ Universal screening for MMR and varicella antibodies is not recommended.[10]
■ Targeted screenings should be considered in the following populations if immunity is unknown:
  ● Healthcare clinicians[8]
  ● Individuals who are pregnant or looking to become pregnant [8,10]
  ● College students (as required by the individual colleges/universities)[8]
  ● International travelers who will be visiting regions where active infections are prevalent[8]

Diagnosis and Evaluation

■ Individuals who present with signs/symptoms of measles.
  ● Signs and symptoms
    ■ Generalized rash lasting 3 or more days[11,12]
    ■ Temperature of 101 °F or higher (38.3 °C or higher)[11,12]
    ■ Prodrome cough, coryza, and/or conjunctivitis.[11,12]
    ■ Rash or Koplik spots[11,12]
    ■ Fever[11]
    ■ Lymphadenopathy[11]
  ● Common differential diagnoses
    ■ Mucocutaneous lymph node syndrome (Kawasaki disease)[11]
    ■ *Roseola infantum* (*exanthem subitum*)[11]
    ■ *Erythema infectiosum* (fifth disease)[11]
    ■ Enterovirus[11]
■ Individuals who present with signs/symptoms of mumps.
  ● Signs and symptoms
    ■ Prodromal symptoms[8,13]
      ● Low-grade fever
      ● Anorexia
      ● Malaise
      ● Headache
    ■ Pain, tenderness, and swelling in one or both parotid salivary glands.[13]
    ■ Regardless of age or vaccination status and travel history, mumps should be suspected in all patients with parotitis or mumps complications.[13]
  ● Common differential diagnoses[14]
    ■ Influenza A
    ■ Parainfluenza virus types 1 and 3
    ■ Coxsackie A virus
    ■ Cytomegalovirus or Epstein-Barr virus
    ■ HIV
    ■ Acute bacterial suppurative parotitis (*Staphylococcus aureus* and *Streptococcus* spp.)
    ■ Recurrent parotitis
    ■ Drug reactions, allergies, tumors, immunologic diseases

- Individual who presents with signs/symptoms of rubella infection.
  - Signs and symptoms[15]
    - Rash
    - Cough
    - Runny nose
    - Low-grade fever
    - Headache
    - Mild pink eye (redness or swelling of the white of the eye)
    - General discomfort
    - Swollen and enlarged lymph nodes
  - Common differential diagnoses[16,17]
    - *Erythema infectiosum* or "fifth disease"
    - *Roseola infantum* or *exanthem subitem*
    - Infectious mononucleosis (Epstein-Barr virus or cytomegalovirus)
    - HIV infection
    - Scarlet fever
    - Mycoplasma infection
    - Juvenile idiopathic arthritis and adult-onset Still disease
    - Acute cutaneous lupus erythematosus
- Individuals who present with signs and symptoms of varicella infection.
  - Signs and symptoms[18]
    - Rash that turns into itchy, fluid-filled blisters that eventually turn into scabs.
    - Fever
    - Tiredness
    - Loss of appetite
    - Headache
  - Common differential diagnoses[19]
    - Herpes simplex
    - Enteroviral infections
    - Impetigo
    - Rickettsialpox
    - Insect bite

Monitoring
- No monitoring is required once antibodies are determined.

INTERPRETATION
- MMR vaccine antibody testing takes into consideration interpretation of the measles antibody immune status, the mumps antibody immune status, and rubella immune status.[9]
- The PCR test is sensitive when used with skin lesions (vesicles, scabs, maculopapular lesions).[6]
- Both the VZV Ab (IgG) and VZV Ab (IgM) should be considered for varicella.
- See Table 19.3 for a summary of reference intervals.

TABLE 19.3: REFERENCE RANGES FOR MEASLES, MUMPS, RUBELLA, AND VARICELLA ANTIBODY TEST

TEST	REFERENCE INTERVALS	RESULTS
Measles antibody (IgG), immune status[6]	AU/mL Interpretation a) <13.50 b) 13.50–16.49 c) >16.49	a) Not consistent with immunity b) Equivocal c) Consistent with immunity. The presence of measles IgG suggests immunization or past or current infection with measles virus.
Mumps virus antibody (IgG), immune status[6]	AU/mL interpretation a) <9.00 b) 9.00–10.99 c) >10.99	a) Not consistent with immunity b) Equivocal c) Consistent with immunity. The presence of mumps IgG antibody suggests immunization or past or current infection with mumps virus
Rubella antibody (IgG), immune status[6]	Index interpretation a) <0.90 b) 0.90–0.99 c) ≥1.00	a) Not consistent with immunity b) Equivocal c) Consistent with immunity. The presence of rubella IgG antibody suggests immunization or past or current infection with rubella virus.
Polymerase chain reaction (PCR)[9]	a) No pathogen DNA present b) Pathogen DNA present	a) Negative b) Positive
Fluorescent antibody assay (DFA)[9]	a) Unbonded antibodies b) Bonded antibodies	a) Negative b) Positive
VZV Ab (IgG)[6]	a) < 135.00 b) 135.00–164.99 c) ≥ 165.00	a) Negative—Antibody not detected b) Equivocal c) Positive—Antibody detected.
VZV Ab (IgM)[6,7]	a) 0.0–0.90 b) 0.91–1.09 c) ≥ 1.10	a) Negative b) Equivocal c) Positive

Sources: Data from LabCorp. *Varicella Zoster Virus (VZV), DNA PCR.* https://www.labcorp.com/tests/138313/varicella-zoster-virus-vzv-dna-pcr; Minnich LL, Goodenough F, Ray CG. Use of immunofluorescence to identify measles virus infections. *J Clin Microbiol.* 1991;29(6):1148–1150. doi:10.1128/JCM.29.6.1148-1150.1991; Quest Diagnostics. https://testdirectory.questdiagnostics.com/test/test-detail/5259/mmr-igg-panel-measles-mumps-rubella?cc=MASTER.

FOLLOW-UP

- If the PCR test is completed with a negative result and infection is still strongly suspected, then the test should be repeated or a follow-up test repeated.[8]
- Measles and mumps—evaluate for measles or mumps in individuals presenting with clinical signs and symptoms.[20]

PEARLS & PITFALLS

- Antibodies produced by the immune system in response to a measles or mumps infection or vaccine are detected when testing for antibodies.

Antibody tests are used to determine whether you are immune, diagnose an active case, or to track outbreaks.[8,20]

■ A positive PCR test for measles or mumps means a person has a current viral infection and does not confirm immunity.[8]

■ A negative PCR test may indicate a person is not infected and signs and symptoms are due to another cause. However, a negative result does not necessarily rule out an active infection due to low numbers that cannot be detected in the sample. Repeat the test if infection is strongly suspected.[8]

■ Live vaccines including MMR and varicella should not be given to individuals who are immunocompromised, pregnant, have a history of bleeding disorders or tuberculosis, received a recent blood transfusion, have severe, life-threatening allergies, or received other vaccinations within the past month.[21]

PATIENT EDUCATION

■ https://vaccineinformation.org/[12]
■ https://www.cdc.gov/vaccines/hcp/vis/vis-statements/mmr.pdf[12,20]
■ https://www.immunize.org/handouts/measles-mmr-vaccines.asp[12]
■ https://www.cdc.gov/vaccines/hcp/patient-ed/conversations/downloads/vacsafe-mmr-color-office.pdf[22]

RELATED DIAGNOSES AND ICD-10 CODES[23]

Encounter for immunization	Z23	Mumps without complications	B26.9
Delinquent immunization status	Z28.3	Rubella	Z20.4
Lapsed immunization schedule status	Z28.3	Varicella	Z20.820
● Status (post)		Antibody response	Z01.84
■ Delinquent immunization	Z28.3		
■ Lapsed immunization schedule	Z28.3	Immunity status testing	Z01.84
■ Under immunization	Z28.3		
■ Under immunization status	Z28.3	Immunity status	Z01.84
Measles	B05		

REFERENCES

Full list of references can be accessed through Springer Publishing Company Connect™ at the following link: http://connect.springerpub.com/content/reference-book/978-0-8261-8843-4/part/part03/toc-part/ch019

20. ANTIDIURETIC HORMONE

Lisa Ward

PATHOPHYSIOLOGY REVIEW

Antidiuretic hormone (ADH), also known as vasopressin or arginine vasopressin, is made in the hypothalamus and is stored in the posterior pituitary. ADH maintains water homeostasis in the body by binding to receptors in the kidney and initiating water reabsorption.[1] The synthesis and release of ADH is regulated by the hypothalamus in response to changes in fluid osmolality and changes in blood volume via a negative feedback loop (Figure 20.1).[2-5] ADH deficiency is called diabetes insipidus (DI) and central DI is caused when hypothalamic ADH production is decreased or when pituitary release is hindered.[2,3] Nephrogenic DI occurs when production and release of ADH are normal, but the body does not recognize or use it appropriately. Decrease in production or secretion of ADH causes polyuria, increased serum osmolality, and decreased urine osmolality.[4] If the kidney does not respond to ADH, this can cause excessive thirst, frequent urination, dehydration, and hypernatremia.[6] Excess production of ADH is called syndrome of inappropriate ADH (SIADH) which can lead to decreased urine output, decreased serum osmolality, and increased urine osmolality.[4] Patients often will experience nausea, headaches, disorientation, lethargy, and hyponatremia in this situation.[2,6,7]

OVERVIEW OF LABORATORY TEST

The ADH test alone is not diagnostic of a specific condition.[6,8,9] Thus, abnormalities of ADH are usually diagnosed by testing serum osmolality (CPT code 83930), urine osmolality (CPT code 83935), and serum sodium (CPT code 84295).[2] However, serum ADH (CPT code 046557) testing in addition to these laboratory tests is used in the differential diagnosis of SIADH, DI, chronic hyponatremia, and psychogenic water intoxication and is performed as part of water deprivation and water loading tests[4,6,7] (Tables 20.1 and 20.2). If ADH testing is ordered, the laboratory test typically co-tests the serum/urine osmolality and serum sodium; thus, rarely does the clinician need to order separate testing.[4,10] ADH plasma testing requires a frozen specimen.[9]

INDICATIONS

Screening

- Universal screening using ADH is not recommended.

Diagnosis and Evaluation

- European and United States guidelines suggest against using ADH as a means to evaluate hyponatremia because urine osmolality more accurately reflects vasopressin activity and is a more reliable laboratory test.[11]

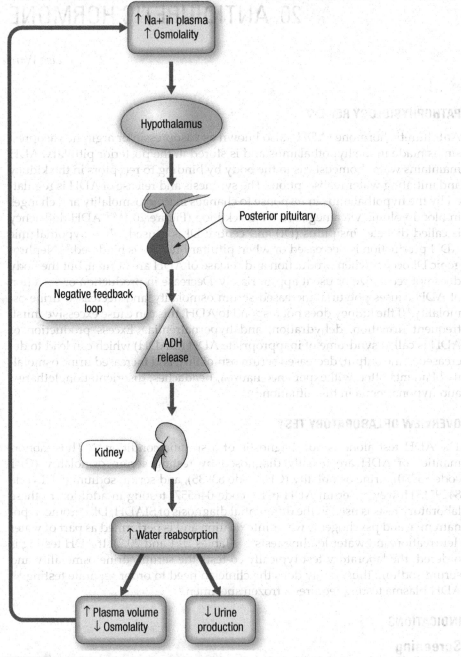

FIGURE 20.1. ADH negative feedback loop. ADH, produced in the hypothalamus and stored in the posterior pituitary, is secreted in response to serum osmolality and blood volume. ADH promotes the kidney to absorb water, causing decreased urine production and decreased blood osmolarity. As blood osmolarity decreases, a negative feedback mechanism causes decrease in ADH secretion. *Sources:* Gounden V, Jialal I. Hypopituitarism. In: *StatPearls*. StatPearls Publishing; 2020; Rotondo F, Butz H, Syro LV, et al. Arginine vasopressin (AVP): a review of its historical perspectives, current research and multifunctional role in the hypothalamo-hypophysial system. *Pituitary*. 2016;19(4):345–355. doi:10.1007/s11102-015-0703-0.

TABLE 20.1: WATER DEPRIVATION ANTIDIURETIC HORMONE STIMULATION TEST

Details	• Used to confirm diagnosis of DI and to distinguish the type of DI • Must be done under medical supervision. No oral intake is allowed until testing is complete. • Baseline serum ADH and blood and urine osmolality test performed; urine volume and urine osmolality are measured hourly. Once urine osmolality is stable (<30 mOsm/kg change for 2 consecutive hours), serum osmolality, serum sodium, and ADH levels are drawn. Then, synthetic ADH is given to patient. Urine osmolality is measured 1 hour later.
Interpretation	• Low serum ADH and increased urine osmolality after synthetic ADH administration = central DI • High serum ADH and no change in urine osmolality = nephrogenic DI

ADH, antidiuretic hormone; DI, diabetes insipidus; SIADH, syndrome of inappropriate diuretic hormone.

Sources: Data from Hoorn EJ, Zietse R. Diagnosis and treatment of hyponatremia: compilation of the guidelines. *J Am Soc Nephrol.* 2017;28(5):1340–1349. doi:10.1681/ASN.2016101139; Hui C, Radbel JM. Diabetes Insipidus. In: *StatPearls.* StatPearls Publishing; 2021. Labtestsonline.org. *ADH: at a glance.* 2021. https://www.testing.com/tests/antidiuretic-hormone-adh/; Sonani B, Naganathan S, Al-Dhahir MA. Hypernatremia. In: *StatPearls.* StatPearls Publishing; 2020.

TABLE 20.2: WATER LOADING ANTIDIURETIC HORMONE SUPPRESSION

Details	• Used to help diagnosis SIADH • Must be done under medical supervision. Must not be done on patients with significant hyponatremia because water load will worsen hyponatremia. • Test is performed 2 hours after patient has light breakfast. Baseline serum and urine osmolality are collected. Patient is then given 20 mlLkg of water to drink over a 15- to-30- minute period. Urine quantity and plasma/urine osmolality and ADH are measured hourly for 4 hours.
Interpretation	• In healthy patients, plasma osmolality will drop by >5 mOsm/kg and urine will become diluted. • In patients with SIADH, urine osmolality will be <100 mOsm/kg, decreased serum sodium, high urine osmolality, elevated ADH = SIADH

ADH, antidiuretic hormone; SIADH, syndrome of inappropriate diuretic hormone.

Sources: Data from Labcorp.com. *Water loading test.* 2021. https://www.labcorp.com/resource/water-loading-test; Lexicomp Online. *Lab Tests and Diagnostic Procedures.* UpToDate, Inc; 2019; Spasovski G, Vanholder R, Allolio B, et al. Clinical practice guideline on diagnosis and treatment of hyponatraemia [published correction appears in Eur J Endocrinol. 2014 Jul;171(1):X1]. *Eur J Endocrinol.* 2014;170(3):G1–G47. doi:10.1530/EJE-13-1020

- The European Society of Intensive Care Medicine, the European Society of Endocrinology, and the European Renal Best Practice Clinical Practice Guidelines do not believe that measurement of ADH contributes to the diagnosis of SIADH.[12]
- This is typically ordered along with urine/serum osmolality and serum sodium.[2]
- It may be ordered for patient with hyponatremia of unidentified cause.
- It may be ordered in patients with polydipsia and polyuria to evaluate for suspected DI.

Monitoring
- ADH is not used in monitoring.

INTERPRETATION
- Reference interval:[9]
  - ADH: 0.0 to 4.7 pg/mL

	PLASMA OSMOLARITY	URINE OSMOLARITY	URINE VOLUME	ADH
TABLE 20.3: OSMOLARITY AND ANTIDIURETIC HORMONE INTERPRETATION				
Defective urine concentrating ability (e.g., CKD)	↑	↔	↑	↑
↓ Water intake	↑	↑	↓	↑
↑ Solute intake	↑	↑	↓	↑
↑ Fluid intake in response to thirst	↑	↑	↓	↑
↑ Spontaneous fluid intake	↓	↓	↑	↓

Source: Data from Kanbay M, Yilmaz S, Dincer N, et al. Antidiuretic hormone and serum osmolarity physiology and related outcomes: what is old, what is new, and what is unknown? *J Clin Endocrinol Metab.* 2019;104(11):5406–5420. doi:10.1210/jc.2019-01049.

- It is typically interpreted in conjunction with osmolarity and serum sodium levels (Table 20.3).
- Table 20.4 provides a general overview of causes of increased or decreased ADH.
- ADH production temporarily increases during stress, exercise, pain, standing position, and during the night.[1,6]
- Interpretation as part of a water deprivation or water loading test is discussed in Tables 20.1 and 20.2.

FOLLOW-UP

- If hyponatremia is also present, tests for causes of hyponatremia are needed (e.g., congestive heart failure, liver/kidney disease, thyroid disease).[2]
- If SIADH is suspected, follow-up testing of abnormal results will be guided by the Schwartz and Bartter Clinical Criterion for diagnosing SIADH (Table 20.5).
- Copeptin may be used in addition to ADH to aid in the evaluation for DI and is more convenient than water deprivation testing. Copeptin measurement is of little diagnostic value in suspected SIADH and is not recommended.[13]

PEARLS & PITFALLS

- Assays are complex to perform and lack sensitivity and specificity. Therefore, it is important to test plasma osmolality concurrently with ADH levels.[4]
- Serum osmolarity of 286 mOsm/L is the threshold for thirst perception and ADH release.[8]
- In general, the ability to concentrate urine typically decreases with age.
- A spot urine osmolality of 100 mOsm/kg or less always indicates maximally dilute urine.[12]

TABLE 20.4: DIFFERENTIAL DIAGNOSIS OF ABNORMAL ANTIDIURETIC HORMONE LEVELS

CAUSES OF ELEVATED ADH	CAUSES OF DECREASED ADH
Dehydration	Drinking large volumes of water
Trauma, pain, exercise	Hypertension
Surgery	Patient lying supine
Lung disorders (cystic fibrosis, emphysema, tuberculosis)	Children, older adult
Nervous system disorders (epilepsy, Guillain Barré syndrome, MS)	Central diabetes insipidus
HIV/AIDS	Hypernatremic states
Adrenal insufficiency	
SIADH	
Hyponatremia, edema, oliguria (congestive heart failure, liver/kidney disease, thyroid disease)	
Hypertension	
Supine position	

ADH, antidiuretic hormone; AIDS, acquired immunodeficiency syndrome; HIV, human immunodeficiency virus; MS, multiple sclerosis; SIADH, syndrome of inappropriate diuretic hormone.

Sources: Data from Cuzzo B, Padala SA, Lappin SL. Physiology, vasopressin. In: *StatPearls.* StatPearls Publishing; 2020; Hoorn EJ, Zietse R. Diagnosis and treatment of hyponatremia: compilation of the guidelines. *J Am Soc Nephrol.* 2017;28(5):1340–1349. doi:10.1681/ASN.2016101139; Hui C, Radbel JM. Diabetes insipidus. In: *StatPearls.* StatPearls Publishing; 2021; Labtestsonline. org. *ADH: at a glance.* 2021. https://www.testing.com/tests/antidiuretic-hormone-adh/; Rotondo F, Butz H, Syro LV, et al. Arginine vasopressin (AVP): a review of its historical perspectives, current research and multifunctional role in the hypothalamo-hypophysial system. *Pituitary.* 2016;19(4):345–355. doi:10.1007/s11102-015-0703-0; Sonani B, Naganathan S, Al-Dhahir MA. Hypernatremia. In: *StatPearls.* StatPearls Publishing; 2020; Sterns R, Emmet M, Forman J. Pathophysiology and etiology of the syndrome of inappropriate antidiuretic hormone secretion (SIADH). In: Post TW, ed. *UpToDate.* UpToDate Inc.; 2021; Yasir M, Mechanic OJ. Syndrome of inappropriate antidiuretic hormone secretion. In: *StatPearls.* StatPearls Publishing; 2020.

- Postoperative DI is the most common complication after pituitary surgery.[14]
- Advanced CKD usually impairs water excretion, thus causing ADH evaluation to not be as reliable.[11]
- Several medications influence ADH levels (Table 20.6).

PATIENT EDUCATION

- https://www.labcorp.com/resource/water-loading-test
- https://www.labcorp.com/resource/water-deprivation-test

RELATED DIAGNOSES AND ICD-10 CODES

Syndrome of inappropriate antidiuretic hormone secretion (SIADH)	E22.2	Hyponatremia	E87.1
		Hypernatremia	E87.0
Diabetes insipidus (DI)	E23.2		

TABLE 20.5: SCHWARTZ AND BARTTER CLINICAL CRITERION FOR DIAGNOSIS OF SYNDROME OF INAPPROPRIATE ANTIDIURETIC HORMONE

ESSENTIAL CRITERIA	AUXILIARY CRITERIA
Serum sodium <135 mEq/L	Serum uric acid <4 mg/dL
Serum osmolality <275 mOsm/kg	Serum urea <21.6 mg/dL
Urine sodium >40 mEq/L	Failure to correct hyponatremia after 0.9% saline administration
Urine osmolality >100 mOsm/kg	Fractional sodium excretion >0.5%
Patient is clinically euvolemic	Fractional uric acid excretion >12%
Absence of other causes of hyponatremia (adrenal insufficiency, hypothyroid, hypopituitary, diuretic use)	

Sources: Data from Mentrasti G, Scortichini L, Torniai M, et al. Syndrome of inappropriate antidiuretic hormone secretion (SIADH): optimal management. *Ther Clin Risk Manag.* 2020;16:663–672. doi:10.2147/TCRM.S206066; Spasovski G, Vanholder R, Allolio B, et al. Clinical practice guideline on diagnosis and treatment of hyponatraemia [published correction appears in Eur J Endocrinol. 2014 Jul;171(1):X1]. *Eur J Endocrinol.* 2014;170(3):G1–G47. doi:10.1530/EJE-13-1020; Yasir M, Mechanic OJ. Syndrome of inappropriate antidiuretic hormone secretion. In: *StatPearls.* StatPearls Publishing; 2020.

TABLE 20.6: MEDICATIONS INFLUENCE ANTIDIURETIC HORMONE

↑ADH PRODUCTION	↓ADH PRODUCTION	↑EFFECT OF ADH ACTION ON KIDNEYS[6]
Amitriptyline	Ethanol	Desmopressin
Barbiturates	Lithium	Metformin
Carbamazepine	Phenytoin	NSAIDs
Chlorpropamide		Oxytocin
Cyclophosphamide		
Desipramine		
Ecstasy		
Morphine		
Nicotine		
SSRIs		

NSAIDs, nonsteroidal anti-inflammatory drugs; SIADH, syndrome of inappropriate antidiuretic hormone.

Sources: Data from Sterns R, Emmet M, Forman J. Pathophysiology and etiology of the syndrome of inappropriate antidiuretic hormone secretion (SIADH). In: Post TW, ed. *UpToDate.* UpToDate Inc.; 2021; Yasir M, Mechanic OJ. Syndrome of inappropriate antidiuretic hormone secretion. In: *StatPearls.* StatPearls Publishing; 2020.

REFERENCES

Full list of references can be accessed through Springer Publishing Company Connect™ at the following link: http://connect.springerpub.com/content/reference-book/978-0-8261-8843-4/part/part03/toc-part/ch020

21. ANTI-MÜLLERIAN HORMONE

Jill S. Buterbaugh

PHYSIOLOGY REVIEW

Anti-Müllerian hormone (AMH) is secreted in granulosa cells of developing follicles in the ovary and is used as a measure of ovarian function, also termed functional ovarian reserve.[1-3] Serum AMH levels correspond to the number of developing follicles that could potentially ovulate in response to follicle-stimulating hormone (FSH) and is primarily used to predict response to FSH dosing protocols in infertility treatments.[3-6] AMH levels are also used as a predictor of natural or disease-related menopause including genetic abnormalities, autoimmune disease, response to chemotherapy/radiation therapy, and infections.[2,3,6] AMH has been confirmed as a tumor marker, in addition to inhibin B, for primary and recurrent granulosa cell tumors of the ovary.[1,3] Women with polycystic ovarian syndrome (PCOS) have been found to have 2- to 3-times higher levels of serum AMH than females with normal ovaries, so levels may assist in the diagnosis of this disorder.[2,3,6-10]

In the prepubescent male, AMH is the most useful marker to determine testicular functioning in the evaluation and treatment of mono- or cryptorchidism, Kleinfelter syndrome, intraabdominal functional testicular tissue, suspicion of central hypogonadism, micropenis, absence of or precocious puberty, prepubertal macro-orchidism, and disorders of sex devlopement.[11,12] AMH is also of benefit for the identification of sex-cord stromal testicular tumors.[12]

OVERVIEW OF LABORATORY TEST(S)

There is currently no international standard for testing AMH levels.[13] There is no gold standard to predict stimulated ovarian response, but AMH levels are beginning to be accepted as a preferred marker.[6] Laboratory testing varies by laboratory and the assay that is used. Some laboratories use anti-Müllerian hormone (CPT code 82350) and require that it be specified as male or female. Other laboratories use anti-Müllerian hormone assay (CPT code 82397: analysis using chemiluminescent technique) also identified as Müllerian-inhibiting substance.

INDICATIONS

Screening

- There are no published recommendations for universal screening with AMH.
- Women at high risk of diminished ovarian reserve who indicate desire for future conception can have targeted screening with AMH.[2,3,5,6,14]
  - Cancer treated with gonadotoxic therapy
  - Pelvic irradiation
  - Advanced reproductive age

- Familial history of premature menopause
- Sex chromosome genetic conditions
- Ovarian injury (endometriosis, injection, ovarian surgery)
- Unilateral oophorectomy
- Smoking[15]

Diagnosis and Evaluation

- Used to evaluate infertility in combination with FSH, estradiol, and inhibin B levels.[1,2]
- Used to evaluate women over 35 years of age who have not conceived after 6 months.[11]
- Used to identify males with symptoms of hypogonadotropic hypogonadism in delayed puberty.[5,12–14]
- Used to differentiate ovarian granulosa cell tumors.[1,3,5,6]

Monitoring

- May be of benefit to monitor testicular function.[5]
- May be of benefit to monitor restoration of ovarian function post-chemotherapy or radiation therapy in certain cancers.[6,13,14]

INTERPRETATION

- Interpretation of levels varies depending on the assay used.[14]
- May be elevated two- to three-fold in the setting of PCOS.[2,3,6,7,9,10]
- Will be reduced in the presence of primary ovarian failure.[2,3,5,6]

FOLLOW-UP

- There are no standard recommendations for follow-up testing. It should be determined on a case-by-case basis and depends largely on the working diagnosis.

PEARLS & PITFALLS

- Stability of the AMH assays are variable and interpretation is not able to be standardized; therefore, there is variability in the sensitivity and specificity of the test results.[13]
- Reproducibility of test results depend on intra/inter-assay differences, laboratory differences, sample stability, and unknown factors.[13]
- AMH should be used in addition to FSH and estradiol levels in functional ovarian reserve screening.[14]
- When tests suggest low functioning ovarian reserve, counseling that there may be a narrow window of opportunity to conceive is suggested.[14]
- AMH levels do not predict failure to conceive.[8,14]
- There are conflicting research findings on how the menstrual cycle influences AMH level. Most evidence suggests levels need to be drawn during the early follicular phase.[6,13,14]
- There are conflicting research findings regarding the impact of hormonal contraception on AMH. Low AMH levels have been identified with oral contraception and hormone secreting intrauterine devices.[6]

- Body mass index may impact AMH levels, possibly due to the effects of leptin.[6]
- Seasonal variations in AMH have been identified, suggesting a potential influence of vitamin D.[6,16,17]
- Research had identified that there is a reduction in AMH levels after bariatric surgery in women without PCOS. Vitamin deficiencies and hormonal imbalances have been suggested, but not confirmed, to be the cause.[18]
- Low AMH has been associated with increased cardiovascular risk including worsening lipid profiles, increased insulin resistance, and C-reactive protein in premenopausal women.[17]
- Ethnicity and age may play a role in AMH levels. In one study, peak AMH levels were higher in women of Chinese genetic heritage compared to women of European heritage at age 25. Over the next two decades, these individuals had faster declines in AMH levels compared to women with Black heritage or Caucasian race.[6]
- AMH levels appear to be lower in those with autoimmune diseases.[3,5]

PATIENT EDUCATION

- https://medlineplus.gov/lab-tests/anti-Müllerian-hormone-test/

RELATED DIAGNOSES AND ICD-10 CODES

Primary ovarian failure	E28.3	Testicular hypofunction	E29.1
Other ovarian dysfunction	E28.8	Delayed puberty	E30.0
Polycystic ovarian syndrome (PCOS)	E28.2		

REFERENCES

Full list of references can be accessed through Springer Publishing Company Connect™ at the following link: http://connect.springerpub.com/content/reference-book/978-0-8261 -8843-4/part/part03/toc-part/ch021

22. ANTINEUTROPHIL CYTOPLASMIC ANTIBODIES

Elizabeth Kirchner

PHYSIOLOGY REVIEW

Antineutrophil cytoplasmic antibodies (ANCAs) are serum tests used to aid in the diagnosis of ANCA-associated vasculitis (AAV). AAV refers to a group of disorders which affect the small blood vessels (capillaries, arterioles, and venules) and are defined by leukocyte migration to blood vessel walls with resultant damage. AAV is a chronic relapsing disease which can affect individuals of any age or race. The incidence of AAV ranges from 0.5 to 14 per million, and the prevalence is estimated to be 46 to 184 per million.[1] ANCAs are a group of autoantibodies directed against enzymes contained in neutrophil and monocytes. The main antigenic targets of ANCAs are proteinase 3 (PR3), a protease, and myeloperoxidase (MPO), a lysosomal enzyme. Damage that occurs in AAV is typically the result of either breach of vessel integrity (bleeding) or narrowing of vessels to the point of restricted blood flow. Either event causes inadequate blood flow to downstream organs and tissues; damage may occur in any organ but the skin, kidneys and lungs are most commonly affected.[2] There are three subtypes of AAV: granulomatosis with polyangiitis (GPA), microscopic polyangiitis (MPA), and eosinophilic granulomatosis with polyangiitis (EGPA).[3] Any of the subtypes of AAV can be life or organ threatening and therefore prompt recognition and diagnosis is of paramount importance.

OVERVIEW OF LABORATORY TEST

There are two ANCA assays widely used in commercial laboratories: indirect immunofluorescence (IA, CPT code 86021) and enzyme-linked immunosorbent (ELISA, CPT code 86256). Both assays are able to detect the two most relevant target antigens in vasculitis as previously described: PR3 and MPO.[4] IA is more sensitive for detecting these antigens, whereas the ELISA is more specific. Therefore, both assays should be performed if AAV is suspected.[5] In order to differentiate between MPO and PR3 patterns, specimens are typically screened by IA on ethanol-fixed neutrophils, formalin-fixed neutrophils, and HEp-2 slides. A positive IA is often automatically reflexed by the laboratory to a follow-up ELISA.

In patients with AAV, which antibody is positive may indicate the manifestations the disease is likely to exhibit. Patients who are PR3-ANCA positive are more likely to have ear, nose, throat, and respiratory tract disease. This test is also referred to as cytoplasmic ANCA (C-ANCA). Patients who are MPO-ANCA positive are more likely to have renal, cutaneous, and pulmonary disease.[6] MPO-ANCA is also referred to as perinuclear ANCA (P-ANCA).

INDICATIONS

■ ANCAs are used in the diagnosis of AAV.

Screening

■ Universal and targeted screenings are not recommended. ANCA has a low positive predictive value for AAV in unselected populations.[7]

Diagnosis and Evaluation

■ ANCA is not diagnostic in itself but supports a diagnosis of AAV and helps distinguish between various types of vasculitis. Specific signs and/or symptoms which may prompt the clinician to order ANCA testing include:
  ● Fever, fatigue, weight loss, arthralgias—these are nonspecific and on their own are not enough to justify testing.
  ● History of eye inflammation (scleritis)
  ● Persistent nasal crusting, epistaxis

- Unexplained hemoptysis
- Glomerulonephritis
- Palpable purpura
- Markedly elevated erythrocyte sedimentation rate (ESR) and/or C-reactive protein (CRP)

Monitoring

- The clinical utility of ANCA as a marker of disease activity in AAV has been long-debated.
  - For patients who have had renal or pulmonary manifestations of AAV, an increase in ANCA values may be predictive of relapse and therefore periodic monitoring of ANCA may be clinically useful.[7]
  - Conversely, ANCA levels have not been found to correlate with relapse in patients with nonrenal/nonpulmonary disease.[7]

INTERPRETATION

- A positive MPO or PR3 ANCA in a patient with clinical symptoms of AAV is highly sensitive for generalized GPA or MPA, but only 60% sensitive for patients with limited disease. Only 40% of patients with EGPA will have a positive ANCA test.[7] Therefore, it is important to interpret the test results in the context of the suspected disease.
- A positive ANCA is not definitively diagnostic for AAV. There are many other causes of a positive ANCA result. Since the treatment for AAV is high dose steroids, it is of utmost importance that infection be ruled out before immunosuppression is initiated. Other conditions that can cause a positive ANCA are included in Table 22.1.

FOLLOW-UP

- If ELISA testing is ordered without IA screening and is positive, there is no need to perform IA testing.[12]
- A positive PR3-ANCA in a patient with nasal/septal disease but no other signs or symptoms of AAV should prompt the clinician to ask the patient about cocaine use (current or prior). If needed, a test specific for cocaine-induced midline destructive disease (HNE-ANCA) may be ordered.[13]
- Any patient diagnosed with AAV (whether by clinical diagnosis or laboratory-confirmed) requires urgent, careful follow-up by a multidisciplinary team and may need a biopsy of the affected site.

PEARLS & PITFALLS

- ANCA is a very poor screening test outside of specific clinical settings. It should only be ordered in patients for whom clinical suspicion for an ANCA-associated disease is high.
- Reliability of ANCA results varies between laboratories. When possible, a referral to a tertiary referral center, vasculitis center, or large teaching hospital is preferable to having an ANCA drawn at a smaller laboratory.
- There are many diseases associated with a positive ANCA. PR3-ANCA is also highly specific to ulcerative colitis and can be used to support accurate

TABLE 22.1: CONDITIONS ASSOCIATED WITH A POSITIVE ANCA

Drug-induced vasculitis (usually MPO-ANCA with a high titer)[8]

- Exposure to anti-thyroid drugs
- Hydralazine
- Minocycline
- Allopurinol
- Penicillamine
- Procainamide
- Thiamazole
- Clozapine
- Phenytoin
- Rifampicin
- Cefotaxime
- Isoniazid
- Indomethacin
- Dual positivity (PR3 and MPO) may indicate exposure to levamisole, usually in the context of cocaine use.

Autoimmune gastrointestinal disorders[10]:

- Ulcerative colitis
- Primary sclerosing cholangitis
- Crohn's disease
- Autoimmune hepatitis

Other rheumatic conditions (usually MPO-ANCA with a positive IA but negative ELISA)[9]

- Rheumatoid arthritis
- Systemic lupus erythematosus
- Sjögren's syndrome
- Inflammatory myopathies
- Juvenile idiopathic arthritis
- Reactive arthritis
- Relapsing polychondritis
- Systemic sclerosis
- Antiphospholipid syndrome

Other[11]

- Cystic fibrosis
- Bacteremia
- Subacute bacterial endocarditis
- Tuberculosis
- Leprosy
- Buerger's disease
- Malaria
- Preeclampsia
- Eclampsia
- Diffuse alveolar hemorrhage
- Chronic graft-versus-host disease
- Acute parvovirus B19 infection
- Acute mononucleosis

classification of inflammatory bowel disease. ANCA can also be used along with anti-*Saccharomyces cerevisiae* antibodies (ASCA) to differentiate ulcerative colitis from Crohn disease.[14]

PATIENT EDUCATION

- https://www.rheumatology.org
- https://www.eular.org
- https://www.vasculitisfoundation.org

RELATED DIAGNOSES AND ICD-10 CODES

Granulomatosus with polyangiitis (formerly known as Wegener's granulomatosis)	M31.3
Eosinophilic granulomatosis with polyangiitis (formerly known as Churg Strauss syndrome)	M30.1
Microscopic polyangiitis	M31.7

REFERENCES

Full list of references can be accessed through Springer Publishing Company Connect™ at the following link: http://connect.springerpub.com/content/reference-book/978-0-8261-8843-4/part/part03/toc-part/ch022

23. ANTINUCLEAR ANTIBODIES

Elizabeth Kirchner

PHYSIOLOGY REVIEW

Autoimmune disease arises when the body loses immunologic tolerance and attacks self-molecules.[1] For this to occur, the immune system must not only mistake "self" for "non-self" but must also identify self-molecules as a danger or threat.[2] When it does so, the immune system may create antibodies (in this case, autoantibodies) to attack the "threat."

Many diseases fall under the umbrella of autoimmunity, from type 1 diabetes to multiple sclerosis to Hashimoto thyroiditis to rheumatoid arthritis, as well as dozens of others. Some diseases have associated autoantibodies, which not only provide insight into the pathophysiology of the disease but also provide a convenient diagnostic tool. One laboratory abnormality that several autoimmune diseases have in common is antinuclear antibodies (ANAs).[3] ANAs are antibodies directed against any of a number of proteins found in the cell nucleus. A positive ANA can be found in several rheumatic diseases as well as autoimmune thyroid disease, inflammatory bowel disease, and certain liver diseases, lung diseases, cancers, and infections.[4] The clinical utility of ANA testing varies widely between autoimmune diseases; this should be carefully considered before ordering an ANA.

There are typical ages of onset for most autoimmune diseases, but overall autoimmunity is a phenomenon that affects all age groups. On the other hand, there is a clear difference in incidence between genders, as women account for over 75% of those affected by autoimmune disease.[5]

OVERVIEW OF LABORATORY TEST

ANA testing was developed in the 1950s and grew out of the first test specifically for SLE, the detection of the "LE cell." The realization that LE cell testing was neither sensitive nor specific enough to be clinically useful led to the development of immunofluorescence assay (IFA) techniques.[6] Binary IFA testing (that is, strictly positive or negative) had high sensitivity but low specificity, so laboratories started reporting titers and staining patterns in an effort to increase specificity. Over time, the sensitivity of ANA testing was improved even more by the adoption of the use of HEp-2 substrate instead of rodent tissue.[6]

IFA (CPT code 86038) is considered the gold standard for ANA testing by the American College of Rheumatology.[7] An alternative testing method for ANA is via an enzyme immunoassay (EIA) (CPT code 86038). The antinuclear antigen is coated on to a microtiter plate and incubated with the patient's serum. An enzyme-labeled antibody is added, and the optical density of the substrate reaction is graded against a cutoff to give a positive/negative result. EIA testing for ANA has a high negative predictive value but a low positive predictive value[8]; therefore, confirmatory testing with IFA is needed for positive EIA results.

INDICATIONS

Screening

- Universal and targeted screenings are not recommended.

Diagnosis and Evaluation

- ANA is not diagnostic by itself but is often used in the diagnostic decision-making process when patients present with symptoms consistent with a possible autoimmune disease that has a high incidence of positive ANA. Each autoimmune condition presents slightly differently and the diagnostic workup often includes multiple components. Refer to Table 23.1 for a list of common conditions that are associated with an elevated ANA.

TABLE 23.1: AUTOIMMUNE DISEASES ASSOCIATED WITH A POSITIVE ANTI-NUCLEAR ANTIBODY	
DISEASE	**SENSITIVITY (%)**
Mixed connective tissue disease	100
Systemic lupus erythematosus	90–100
Systemic sclerosis	95
Drug-induced lupus	80–95
Autoimmune hepatitis	70
Primary biliary cholangitis	50–70
Sjögren's syndrome	60
Graves'/Hashimoto's	50
Rheumatoid arthritis	45
Juvenile idiopathic arthritis	15–40
Raynaud's syndrome	40
Idiopathic pulmonary hypertension	40
Polymyositis/dermatomyositis	35
Discoid lupus	15

Monitoring

- If a diagnosis of an autoimmune disease has been established, there is rarely any need to repeat the ANA, as ANA titers do not typically correspond to disease activity.

INTERPRETATION

- ANA results should not be interpreted in isolation—the entire clinical picture must be considered.
- Up to 30% of healthy individuals may have a positive low-titer (1:40) ANA.
- Around 5% of healthy individuals may have a positive high-titer (1:160 or higher) ANA.
- The frequency of false-positive ANA results increases with age, especially in women.[9]
- In general, an ANA titer 1:80 or lower (by IFA) or 3.0 or lower (by EIA) is considered negative unless there is strong clinical suspicion of, or confirmatory evidence for, an associated autoimmune disease.
- Immunofluorescence staining patterns can be helpful in terms of diagnosis when considered as part of the entire clinical picture. Table 23.2 lists common patterns and the diseases with which they are associated.[10]

FOLLOW-UP

Patients with a positive ANA and clinical presentation consistent with autoimmune disease should be referred to the appropriate specialist for follow-up testing, which may include:

- Double-stranded DNA, crithidia testing (rheumatologic diseases)
- Solid-phase assays/ENA panel (rheumatologic diseases; see Chapter 69 "Extractable Nuclear Anitgen [ENA] Antibodies")
- Anti-smooth muscle antibody, liver–kidney microsomal type 1 antibody, serum protein electrophoresis, quantitative immunoglobulins, liver enzymes (autoimmune hepatitis)

TABLE 23.2: COMMON ANTINUCLEAR ANTIBODY PATTERNS AND ASSOCIATED DISEASES	
Speckled	Systemic lupus erythematosus, mixed connective tissue disease, systemic sclerosis, primary Sjögren's, polymyositis
Homogenous	Systemic lupus erythematosus, drug-induced lupus
Peripheral	Systemic lupus erythematosus, systemic sclerosis
Nucleolar	Systemic sclerosis, polymyositis
Centromere	Limited systemic sclerosis

Source: Data from Kumar Y, Bhatia A, Minz RW. Antinuclear antibodies and their detection methods in diagnosis of connective tissue diseases: a journey revisited. *Diagn Pathol.* 2009;4:1. doi:10.1186/1746-1596-4-1.

- Antimitochondrial antibody, alkaline phosphatase, liver function tests, lipid panel (primary biliary cholangitis)
- Thyroid peroxidase antibodies, thyroid-stimulating hormone receptor antibodies, thyroglobulin antibodies (autoimmune thyroiditis)
- Imaging of affected organs/glands/joints
- ECG, echocardiogram, pulmonary function tests (primary pulmonary hypertension)
- Biopsy of rash (lupus or dermatomyositis), muscle (polymyositis), liver (hepatitis, cholangitis)
- Schirmer's test and/or minor salivary gland biopsy (Sjögren's syndrome)
- Ophthalmology consult (in JIA patients to evaluate for uveitis)

Do not order autoantibody panels unless there is a positive ANA result and evidence of rheumatic disease. If the ANA is negative, subserologies are typically negative with the exception of anti-Jo$_1$, which can be positive in some forms of myositis, or occasionally, anti-SSA, in the setting of lupus or Sjögren's syndrome.[11]

PEARLS & PITFALLS

- It is not appropriate to order an ANA simply because a patient complains of "fatigue" or "joint pain" and has no other signs or symptoms of autoimmune disease.
- Approximately 1% of the adult U.S. population has an autoimmune disease that can be associated with a positive ANA and approximately 5% of the U.S. population is ANA positive. This means that the vast majority of patients with a positive ANA do not have an autoimmune disease.
- Many healthy individuals have a positive ANA.
- Results can vary widely depending on what method is used by the laboratory, even down to the strength of the UV bulb in the fluorescent microscope used in IFA.[3]
- A false positive ANA can cause years of anxiety and/or unnecessary testing or treatment for patients.
- If an autoimmune disease is suspected and a referral to the appropriate specialist (e.g., rheumatologist, endocrinologist, gastroenterologist) is possible, it is generally favorable to refer **before** testing (i.e., leave the testing to the specialist).
- If a referral to a specialist is not possible (e.g., financial issues, insurance issues, geographic issues) the only reasons to order an ANA are if there is very strong suspicion for and physical findings consistent with one of the diseases in Table 23.1.

PATIENT EDUCATION

- https://www.rheumatology.org/I-Am-A/Patient-Caregiver/Diseases-Conditions/Antinuclear-Antibodies-ANA
- https://www.mayoclinic.org/tests-procedures/ana-test/about/pac-20385204
- https://www.racgp.org.au/afp/2013/october/antinuclear-antibody-test/

RELATED DIAGNOSES AND ICD-10 CODES

Raised antibody titer	R76.0	Graves'/Hashimoto's	E05.00/E06.3
Mixed connective tissue disease	M35.1	Rheumatoid arthritis	M06.9
Systemic lupus erythematosus	M32.9	Juvenile idiopathic arthritis	M08.20
Systemic sclerosis	M34	Raynaud's syndrome	I73.00
Drug-induced lupus	M32.0	Idiopathic pulmonary hypertension	I27.0
Autoimmune hepatitis	K75.4	Polymyositis/dermatomyositis	M33.2
Primary biliary cholangitis	K83.01	Discoid lupus	L93.0
Sjögren's syndrome	M35.0		

REFERENCES

Full list of references can be accessed through Springer Publishing Company Connect™ at the following link: http://connect.springerpub.com/content/reference-book/978-0-8261 -8843-4/part/part03/toc-part/ch023

24. ANTISTREPTOLYSIN O TITER

Kathryn Deshotels

PHYSIOLOGY REVIEW

The immune system consists of mechanisms to protect the human cells by destroying pathogenic organisms, such as bacteria, fungi, viruses, and parasites. The immune system has two types of responses: an antigen-specific adaptive immune response and an innate immune response.[1,2] An antigen is a molecule that initiates the productions of an antibody and causes an immune response. These antigens are proteins, peptides, or polysaccharides. Lipids and nucleic acids may combine with those molecules and form more complex antigens that are potent bacterial toxins. Bacterial toxins may be exotoxins or endotoxins. Exotoxins are immediately released but the endotoxins are not released until the bacteria is killed by the immune system. It is these toxins that cause damage to the host and signs and symptoms of disease.[1,2]

Streptococci are a gram-positive bacterium. Streptococci are made of several immunologic groups. Groups C, G, and A produce an enzyme, streptolysin O. Streptolysin O is a toxin that causes hemolysis to red blood cells.[3] When the body is infected with Streptococci A, G, or C, it produces antibodies to the toxin called antistreptolysin O (ASO). Group A Streptococci (GAS), also called *Streptococcus pyogenes*, are the primary cause for the elevation in ASO titers. Untreated or undertreated GAS may cause several post-infectious immunologically mediated sequela, such as acute rheumatic fever (ARF), post-streptococcal reactive arthritis, pediatric autoimmune neuropsychiatric disorder (PANDAS), and post-streptococcal glomerulonephritis (PSGN). Although rare, these conditions are typically thought to be an autoimmune, inflammatory reaction to an acute pharyngitis or skin infection (e.g., impetigo) caused by GAS.[4] Following a GAS infection, the mean latent period for ARF is 18 days, post-streptococcal reactive arthritis is 7 to 10 days, PANDAS is 4 to 6 weeks, and PSGN is 12 days.[5]

OVERVIEW OF LABORATORY TEST

ASO titer (CPT code 86060) is a laboratory test that is performed on the serum.[4,6] This test detects and quantifies the existence of ASO. Levels are measured in Todd units. Todd units are the reciprocal of the highest dilution of test serum at which there continues to be neutralization of a standard preparation of streptolysin O. Levels rise within 1 to 3 weeks after infection, peak at 3 to 5 weeks, and return to unremarkable levels after 6 to 12 months.[1] Anti-deoxyribonuclease B (anti-DNase B) is another antibody produced by the body with GAS infections. Ordering both ASO and anti-DNase B is recommended to improve sensitivity.[4,7,8] Consequently, these tests can provide evidence of a recent streptococci infection and be used to guide treatment. Over 80% of patients with acute rheumatic fever and 95% of patients with acute glomerulonephritis due to streptococci have elevated levels of ASO.[6]

INDICATIONS

Screening
■ Universal and targeted screenings for ASO are not recommended.[8]

Diagnosis and Evaluation
■ Given the delay in the rise of the ASO titer, it should not be used to diagnose an uncomplicated acute pharyngitis.[1,9]
■ Diagnostic testing should be considered in individuals where there is a concern for a post-streptococcal complication including:
  ● ARF[9]
  ● Post-streptococcal reactive arthritis
  ● Scarlet fever
  ● Streptococcal toxic shock syndrome
  ● PSGN
  ● Pediatric autoimmune neuropsychiatric disorder associated with group A streptococci (PANDAS)
■ Suspected or known untreated, undertreated streptococcal A infections, as well as patients with the following symptoms/signs[1, 8–13]:
  ● Arthralgia in children[10]
  ● New-onset of tics, obsessive compulsive disorder, or choreiform in children (PANDAS)
  ● Polyarthralgia in adults[2]
  ● Sore throat and fever
  ● Red, fine papular rash (sandpaper) on the trunk[4]

- Tender, red bumps found symmetrically on the shins (i.e., erythema nodosum)
- Decreased urine output, rust-colored urine, hematuria[8]
- Proteinuria[4]
- Acute edema[7,9]
- Pyoderma or cellulitis
- Signs or symptoms of impetigo[4]
- New-onset heart murmur[4]
- Echocardiogram findings of rheumatic heart disease[4]
- Carditis[2]

■ Anti-DNase B should be ordered along with the ASO titer.[7]

Monitoring

■ If the ASO is positive, it should be repeated in 10 to 14 days.[3,7]

INTERPRETATION

■ ASO titers are collected to determine the presence of streptococcal infection. If symptoms of a post-streptococcal complication are present, an ASO titer can assist with confirming diagnosis. Although it detects Group A, C, and G, clinical usefulness is in the identification of GAS to then guide treatment.[7,9]

■ Two ASO titers should be ordered 10 to 14 days apart.

- A negative result or an ASO titer that is at a very low level generally means the individual did not have a recent streptococcal infection. Sensitivity improves with a negative anti-DNase B result or an additional negative ASO titer result from 10 to 14 days after the initial negative titer.[7]
- A positive result or elevated titer means that the individual likely had a recent streptococcal infecton. Similar to a negative result, sensitivity improves if there is a positive anti-DNase B result or an additional positive ASO titer result 10 to 14 days later. A four-fold increase between the two titers is evidence of a previous streptococcal infection.[7]

■ A negative ASO does not exclude the diagnosis of ARF or PSGN.[7]

■ Table 24.1 provides a summary of normal laboratory values for ASO.[1,7,9]

FOLLOW-UP

Additional testing may be required and will vary based on the final diagnosis.

PEARLS & PITFALLS

■ ASO titers may result in a false negative while taking antibiotics.

■ A false positive result may occur in liver disease, high lipoprotein, or tuberculosis.

■ An elevated ASO may be found in healthy carriers.

■ Repeat testing is recommended after 10 days.[1,3]

■ ASO is performed on serum and collected in a red topped tube. Avoid agitation of the tube so as not to hemolyze the sample.[1]

■ Corticosteroids can reduce the ASO titer levels.[10]

TABLE 24.1: ANTI-STREPTOLYSIN O TITER INTERPRETATIONS	
AGE	**INTERVAL**
Adult	<160 Todd unit/mL
6 months to 2 years	<50 Todd units/mL or
2 to 4 years	<160 Todd units/mL or
5 to 12 years	170 to 330 Todd units/mL
Acute rhematic fever or acute post-streptococcal glomerulonephritis	>500 Todd units

Notes: The above reference intervals may vary slightly from between laboratories.
An elevated ASO titer should be made compared with age-matched controls in the same geographic location.

Source: Data from Sen ES, Ramanan AV. How to use antistreptolysin O titer. *Arch Dis Child Educ Pract Ed.* 2014;99(6):231–238. doi:10.1136/archdischild-2013-304884

■ Specificity is 80% to 85% and many have strep A, but no disease. Therefore, a positive result does not mean disease and a negative result does not rule it out. Clinical presentation, additional diagnostics, and repeat testing should be considered.[4,12,13]

■ Skin infections have a poor ASO response.

PATIENT EDUCATION

■ https://labtestsonline.org/tests/antistreptolysin-o-aso
■ https://www.mayocliniclabs.com/test-catalog/Overview/80205

RELATED DIAGNOSIS AND ICD-10 CODES

Streptococcal pharyngitis	J02.0	Acute glomerulonephritis	N00
Streptococcal infection, unspecified site	A49.1	Toxic shock syndrome	A48.3
Acute rheumatic fever	I01	PANDAS	B95.0
Scarlet fever	A38	Bacterial endocarditis	I33
Rheumatic heart disease	I09.9		

REFERENCES

Full list of references can be accessed through Springer Publishing Company Connect™ at the following link: http://connect.springerpub.com/content/reference-book/978-0-8261 -8843-4/part/part03/toc-part/ch024

25. ANTITHROMBIN III

John Prickett

PHYSIOLOGY REVIEW

Antithrombin III (AT III, antithrombin, AT, or heparin cofactor I) is an endogenously occurring, hepatic synthesized anticoagulation factor responsible for the inactivation of FIXa and FXa.[1,2] It has two primary binding sites that are important for its biologic activity—a reactive center loop and a heparin binding site. The reactive center loop is responsible for binding to serine proteases (FII, FIXa, and FXa) and deactivation of these is a relatively slow process. Conformational changes occur when bound to heparin and can expedite the process a 1000-fold.[3] It is believed that AT III binding to naturally occurring heparin sulfate, which is generated by an intact endothelium, helps to maintain fluidity of blood; it may also reduce platelet adherence to fibrinogen.[4,5]

Deficiencies of AT III may be due to inheritance of mutations of the *SERPINC1* gene on chromosome 1 or may be acquired due to other conditions or medications.[6] Inheritance occurs in an autosomal dominant pattern with variable penetration. The presence of deficiency due to inheritance has been associated with hypercoagulability while the meaning of deficiency due to other conditions is less clear. While hundreds of mutations have been described, they can be categorized as type I (quantitative defects that present with deficiency) or type II (qualitative defects that represent a decrease in AT III function despite normal levels).[7,8] Homozygous type I AT III mutations have not been described in humans but have been found to be lethal in mice.[4] The incidence of heterozygous mutations is felt to be generally about one in 5,000 to one in 500 (0.02% to 0.2%) in the general population and imparts a 16% overall risk of thrombosis, particularly in pregnancy.[9–12] Exogenous AT III products exist and include Thrombate III, an antithrombin concentrate derived from pooled human plasma, and recombinant human antithrombin produced from the milk of transgenic goats (rhAT, ATryn). Causes of acquired AT III deficiency include liver disease, malnutrition, nephrotic syndrome, ECMO, heparin use, consumptive processes (DIC, microangiopathies with thrombosis, malignancy, or hematologic transfusion reactions), and some medications.[13–,15]

OVERVIEW OF LABORATORY TEST

AT III deficiency can be assessed by either a functional assay (AT-heparin cofactor assay) (CPT code 85300) or immunoassay. The functional assays are more commonly used as the initial test as they allow for determination of clinically relevant deficiencies. Functional assays are reported as a percent of AT III activity based on the laboratory test's normal reference range and are recommended.[1,16–18] Immunoassays (i.e., ELISA) (CPT code 85301) are best utilized as confirmatory testing once a deficiency has been established, but do not detect type II defects.

INDICATIONS

Screening
Universal or targeted screenings are not recommended.
Targeted screenings should be considered in individuals with the following:

- Strong family history of pathologic thromboses (more than two other symptomatic family members), and/or
- Known family history of AT III deficiency in a first-degree relative

Testing for AT III in unselected patients presenting with their first episode of venous thromboembolism (VTE) is not indicated as it does not reduce recurrence of VTE.

Diagnosis and Evaluation
Testing for AT III deficiency can be considered in the following:

- First VTE when younger than 40 years old
- VTE in an unusual location (portal, mesenteric, or cerebral vein)
- Recurrent VTE
- Pregnant women with a previous VTE due to a minor provoking factor (e.g., travel),
- Asymptomatic pregnant women with a family history of venous thrombosis in a first-degree relative that was unprovoked, or provoked by pregnancy, oral contraceptive use, or a minor provoking factor,
- Poor response to heparin therapy, and/or
- Prior to use of ECMO or L-aspariginase therapy
- Choosing Wisely® Guidelines suggest that AT III should not be tested in the setting of an active clotting event or other acute illness, and should not be tested within 4 to 6 weeks of taking anticoagulant medications (particularly anti-vitamin K antagonists).[19]

Monitoring
- No routine monitoring of AT III is recommended except when exogenous AT III is used as treatment.
- In individuals who have indeterminate levels or levels felt to be the result of transient state, serial testing may be indicated until baseline level obtained. If mutation is suspected, repeating once to verify is a common practice and recommended.[18]

INTERPRETATION
- Immunoassays:
  - Immunoassays can be helpful to subtype AT III deficiencies and may be used in confirmatory testing after functional assays detect clinically relevant antithrombin deficiencies.[20]

TABLE 25.1: REFERENCE VALUES FOR ANTITHROMBIN III FUNCTIONAL ASSAYS	
	AT III VALUES*
Normal intervals (% activity)	80% to 100%
• Adults	35% to 40%
• Infants	
Abnormal interval (% activity)	<80%
AT III deficiency	40% to 60%
Heterozygous SERPINC1 mutation	

*Values vary by laboratory. Each laboratory determines its own laboratory-specific reference range according to the methods and equipment used in the laboratory.

- Increased levels of AT III are not considered clinically significant (Tables 25.1 and 25.2).

FOLLOW-UP

- AT III levels should be retested in cases where there is a question about the validity of initial testing and in cases where exogenous AT III are being utilized as part of treatment. A low level should be confirmed with one or more separate samples.[18]
- Depending on the patient presentation and risk factors, AT III is typically ordered with other tests for hypercoagulation including but not limited to: prothrombin time (PT), aPTT (partial thromboplastin time), homocysteine, protein C, protein S, factor V Leiden, prothrombin gene mutation, lupus anticoagulant, antiphospholipid antibodies, and antithrombin.

PEARLS & PITFALLS

- Timing of testing related to acute thrombosis, medications, or acute illness may have a major effect on functional assays.[17]
- The risk of thrombosis due to AT III deficiency (odds ratio [OR] of 16.3%) is much higher than with protein S or protein C deficiencies (ORs 5.4 and 7.5).[12]
- The risk of thrombosis is particularly high for individuals with AT III deficiency during pregnancy.[21,22]
- There is insufficient evidence to support exogenous AT III substitution in critically ill patients including those with sepsis and DIC. It may induce harm in preterm infants with intraventricular hemorrhage and respiratory distress syndrome.[23–25]

TABLE 25.2: INTERPRETATION OF TYPES OF ANTITHROMBIN III DEFICIENCY		
TYPE OF AT III DEFICIENCY	**ANTITHROMBIN ACTIVITY**	**ANTITHROMBIN ANTIGEN**
Type I	Decreased	Decreased
Type II	Decreased	Normal

PATIENT EDUCATION

- https://rarediseases.info.nih.gov/diseases/6148/hereditary-antithrombin-deficiency#:~:text=Treatment,-Listen&text=Once%20a%20patient%20 with%20hereditary,continued%20for%203%2D6%20months
- https://rarediseases.org/rare-diseases/antithrombin-deficiency/
- https://www.stoptheclot.org/news/antithrombin-deficiency/

RELATED DIAGNOSES AND ICD-10 CODES

Other primary thrombophilia (antithrombin III deficiency, hypercoagulable state NOS, primary hypercoagulable state NEC, primary thrombophilia NEC, protein C deficiency, protein S deficiency, thrombophilia NOS)	D68.59

REFERENCES

Full list of references can be accessed through Springer Publishing Company Connect™ at the following link: http://connect.springerpub.com/content/reference-book/978-0-8261 -8843-4/part/part03/toc-part/ch025

---

26. ARTERIAL BLOOD GASES

Carolyn McClerking

PHYSIOLOGY REVIEW

An arterial blood gas (ABG) is a useful analytical tool to assess the blood partial pressure of gas and acid–base content.[1] Valuable information that can be obtained from blood gas analyses include comprehension of circulatory, metabolic, and respiratory disorders.[2] The different types of acid–base disorders are metabolic acidosis, metabolic alkalosis, respiratory acidosis, and respiratory alkalosis.[3] The four primary components of ABG are: pH (or hydrogen ions), carbon dioxide (PCO_2), oxygen (PaO_2), and bicarbonate (HCO_3).[4] The pH directly measures H+ ions in the blood and represents acidity/alkalinity of the blood.[4] PaO_2 is the direct measure of volume of dissolved oxygen in the blood.[4] $PaCO_2$ measures the amount of CO_2 dissolved in arterial blood and HCO_3 represents the metabolic system.[4]

As an individual loses or gains bicarbonate, the blood will become more acidic or more basic. The determinants of acid–base balance are: (a) respiratory (acid/CO_2), which responds quickly to changes in pH, and (b) renal (base/HCO_3), which responds in hours to days to pH changes.[4] Alterations in bicarbonate are influenced by metabolic processes (lactic acidosis, diarrhea, vomiting).[5] In order to determine the cause of metabolic acidosis, an anion gap can be calculated.[3] The anion gap is defined as the difference between the measured serum cations and measured anions.[3] An elevation in the anion gap occurs when there is a loss of bicarbonate. This loss is a result of bicarbonate combining with a hydrogen ion previously attached to a conjugate base.[3,5] Examples of diseases that cause high anion gap metabolic acidosis are renal failure, lactic acidosis, and keto-acidosis.[4] Renal tubular acidosis and diarrhea are conditions that cause a normal anion gap metabolic acidosis.[4] Respiratory processes influence alterations in $PaCO_2$ (chronic respiratory disease, increased ventilation due to hypoxia).[5] Causes of arterial hypoxemia and hypercapnia include: reduction in inspired PO_2, hypoventilation, ventilation/perfusion mismatch, diffusion limitation, shunting, and pulmonary arterial PO_2 reduction.[5] The major issue surrounding abnormalities in ABG center around hypoxemia and hypercapnia.[2,5]

OVERVIEW OF LABORATORY TEST

ABG (CPT code 82803) is indicated for critically ill individuals with pathophysiologic changes that affect acid–base balance.[6] Several preanalytical considerations are important due to the critical role in ABG results. These factors include appropriate identification of patient, utilization of appropriate sample containers, ensuring precise sampling techniques, and minimization of time between sample collection and analysis.[6,7] Other variables that can lead to erroneous ABG results include incorrect FiO_2, temperatures and barometric pressures as well as sample dilution and moderate leukosytosis.[1,7]

The most common site for arterial puncture is the radial artery; however, brachial and femoral arteries can be used to collect blood specimens as well.[8] The sample used for ABG should be whole blood and must be placed on ice and evaluated immediately. Blood gas samples are analyzed by automated blood gas analyzers and results should be available within 15 minutes after collection.[9]

INDICATIONS

Screening
- Universal screening for ABG is not recommended.
- Target screening for ABG is recommended for conditions predisposing individuals to acid–base disturbances.
- Consider screening patients with the conditions outlined in Box 26.1.

Diagnosis and Evaluation
Testing ABGs should be considered in the following individuals:
- Evaluate for ventilator management[10]
- Acute respiratory distress[11]
- Decreased responsiveness[12]
- Used to quickly evaluate other critical laboratory tests (electrolytes, hemoglobin and hematocrit, lactate)[13]
- Used to evaluate other signs/symptoms that could be related to alterations in acid–base (Table 26.1)[14]

Monitoring
- ABGs should be monitored if there is a change in the patient's status who is on a ventilator or with chest x-ray changes[15,16]

Box 26.1: Disorders of Acid–Base

Anxiety	Fat embolism
Asthma	Guillain Barre Disease
Burns	Heart failure
Chronic obstructive pulmonary disease	Illness that causes metabolic acidosis (cardiac, liver, or renal failure)
CNS depression	
Coronary artery disease	Myasthenia gravis
Diabetic ketoacidosis	Poisons or toxins
Drug overdose	Respiratory failure
	Sepsis

INTERPRETATION

Normal intervals for ABGs are found in Table 26.2.

■ Steps for determining ABG.[8,17]
  ● What is the pH? If less than 7.35 acidemia and greater than 7.45 alkalemia
  ● Determine if respiratory or metabolic. If respiratory acidosis, CO_2 will be high (greater than 45) and if metabolic acidosis, HCO_3 will be low (less than 22).
  ● If respiratory alkalosis, CO_2 will be low (less than 35), and if metabolic alkalosis, HCO_3 will be high (greater than 26).
  ● Is there compensation for the main disturbance? The opposite system works to correct the issue.
  ● Calculate the anion gap = $Na + K - Cl + HCO_3$ or $Na - Cl + HCO_3$
    ■ Normal: varies between 10 to 16 mmol/L
    ■ Level of 17 or higher represents an increased anion gap and should be evaluated to determine the cause of the elevated anion gap.
    ■ Level of 9 or lower represents a decreased anion gap.

TABLE 26.1: SIGNS AND SYMPTOMS OF ACID–BASE DISTURBANCE

RESPIRATORY ACIDOSIS (HYPOVENTILATION)	RESPIRATORY ALKALOSIS (HYPERVENTILATION)	METABOLIC ACIDOSIS	METABOLIC ALKALOSIS
Arrhythmias	Arrhythmias	Coma	Coma
Confusion	Confusion	Confusion	Depression
Dyspnea	Diaphoresis	Headache	Lethargy
Headache	Dizziness	Kussmal respirations	Muscle weakness
Shallow respirations	Lightheadedness	Nausea/vomiting	Respiratory
Tachycardia	Numbness/tingling	Skin flushing	Seizures

Source: Data from Al-Jaghbeer M, Kellum JA. Acid–base disturbances in intensive care patients: etiology, pathophysiology and treatment. *Nephrol Dial Transplant.* 2014;30(7):1104–1111. doi: 10.1093/ndt/gfu289

TABLE 26.2: NORMAL INTERVAL FOR ARTERIAL BLOOD GASES	
pH	7.35–7.45
PaO$_2$	80–100 mmHg
PaCO$_2$	35–45 mmHg
HCO$_3$	22–28 mmHg

Sources: Data from Mohammed HM, Abdelatief DA. Easy blood gas analysis: implications for nursing. *Egypt J Chest Dis Tuberc.* 2016;65(1):369–376; Sood P, Paul G, Puri S. Interpretation of arterial blood gas. *Indian J Crit Care Med.* 2010;14(2):57–64. doi:10.4103/0972-5229.68215.

■ Additional laboratory tests are needed to evaluate the anion gap; include albumin as hypoalbuminemia can cause a decreased anion gap. Creatinine can also be ordered to determine renal function.

FOLLOW-UP

■ Follow-up with pulmonary function testing for patients diagnosed with chronic obstructive lung disease.[18]

PEARLS & PITFALLS

■ A multi-center prospective observational study evaluating mechanically ventilated patients in the emergency department suggested that, although ABGs were completed on the majority of the patients, adjustments in ventilator settings were not done in individuals found to have abnormal results.[19]

■ A prospective cohort study examined the use of a protocol for ordering ABGs in critically ill patients. Implementation of the protocol resulted in decrease in the amount of ABGs ordered on a daily basis and practice transitioned to ordering based on change in patient condition as opposed to routine daily ordering.[20]

■ Being cognizant of potential erroneous issues such as type of blood container, mode of sample transportation, spurious hypoxemia, misstated FIO$_2$, compromised tissue perfusion, and cardiac output can help alleviate misinterpretation of ABG and thus improve patient outcomes and avoid excessive cost.[21]

■ In a study involving dialysis patients, results suggested serum bicarbonate and bicarbonate from blood gas analysis were comparable.[22]

■ In a small prospective study of critically ill trauma patients, venous blood gas analysis was found to be a beneficial alternative to ABG, specifically during the initial assessment.[23–25]

■ Blood gas analysis of patients admitted to the emergency department with tramadol-induced seizures exhibited a moderate correlation between amount of drug taken and severity of respiratory acidosis.[26]

■ Researchers validated the venous-to-arterial conversion (v-TAC) as a comparable method to ABG analysis, suggesting it decreased the logistic load of arterial sampling and led to improved follow-up and pain reduction.[27]

- Moderate differences in serum total carbon dioxide and blood gas bicarbonate are likely related to human error and blood gas HCO_3 (using the Henderson-Hasselbach equation) should be re-calculated to determine the source of the differences.[28]
- A study compared the differences in point of care testing and central laboratory measurements of ABG paying specific attention to turnaround time. Researchers recommended the use of point-of-care testing (POCT) over central laboratory measurement, specifically for pH analysis.[29]
- A review of the evidence supporting the use of serial arterial and venous blood gas for the management of severe diabetic ketoacidosis (DKA) remains indeterminate, specifically if the use of bicarbonate is not being used as treatment. Further evidence is warranted to determine the benefit of these interventions.[30]
- Researchers suggest venous blood gas analysis may be a beneficial substitute to ABG in individuals who present to the emergency room with psychogenic hyperventilation as the study found respiratory alkalosis and lactate levels were correlated in both groups.[31]
- The causes of non-anion gap metabolic acidosis are defined by the acronym HARD UP (Hyperalimentation, Acetazolamide, Renal Tubular Acidosis, Diarrhea, Uretoenteric fistula, and Pancreatic duodenal fistula).[32]
- The causes of anion gap metabolic acidosis are defined by the acronym MUDPILES: Methanol, Uremia (chronic kidney failure), DKA/alcoholic ketoacidosis, Propylene glycol, Infection/Iron/Isoniazid/Inborn errors of metabolism, Lactic acidosis, Ethylene, and Salicylate/Saline administration.[33]

PATIENT EDUCATION

- https://www.healthline.com/health/blood-gases#procedure
- https://www.verywellhealth.com/abg-test-results-arterial-blood-gas-testing-3156812

RELATED DIAGNOSES AND ICD-10 CODES

Other specified abnormal findings in arterial blood gas analysis   R79.81
- Synonyms: Abnormal atrial blood gas; arterial carbon dioxide; abnormal blood oxygen level

REFERENCES

Full list of references can be accessed through Springer Publishing Company Connect™ at the following link: http://connect.springerpub.com/content/reference-book/978-0-8261-8843-4/part/part03/toc-part/ch026

27. AUTOANTIBODIES IN DIABETES

Cara Harris and Kathleen Wyne

PHYSIOLOGY REVIEW

Autoantibodies signal the immune system to attack the body's own tissues. In type 1 diabetes mellitus (T1D), autoantibodies target beta cells. There is variability in the rate of beta-cell destruction, but the appearance of T1D-associated autoantibodies usually precedes the development of the clinical diagnosis by months or years. Detection of these autoantibodies indicate autoimmune destruction of the pancreatic beta cells and confirm the diagnosis of T1D. Those with the presence of two or more autoantibodies have a much higher risk of T1D than those with presence of a single autoantibody.[1-3] The five most common autoantibodies produced in T1D are glutamic acid decarboxylase antibodies (GAD-65 Ab), insulinoma associated-2 antibodies (IA-2, also abbreviated ICA512), islet cell autoantibodies (ICA), zinc transporter 8 (ZnT8), and insulin autoantibodies (IAA).

OVERVIEW OF LABORATORY TESTS

Autoantibodies in diabetes can be ordered as individual tests but are usually ordered as a combined panel (CPT code 86337). Autoantibody tests are standardized by the Diabetes Autoantibody Standardization Program (DASP) and, individually, are highly sensitive and specific assays, though the sensitivity and predictive value can be increased by checking all five antibodies simultaneously.[2,4,5] Most are widely available, validated, and standardized. Further overview of these tests is reviewed in the text that follows.

- When initially diagnosed with T1D, GAD 65Ab are present in about 70% to 80% of patients.[6] However, if positive in the absence of hyperglycemia, they only indicate risk for T1D and are not diagnostic since some individuals with positive GAD65 Ab never go on to develop T1D. GAD65Ab may also be present in type 2 diabetes mellitus (T2DM), as demonstrated by United Kingdom predictive diabetes study (UKPDS) data that found 12% of their newly diagnosed T2DM population were positive for GAD-65.[7]
- At the time of T1D diagnosis, IA2 autoantibodies are present in about 54% to 75% of patients and ICA autoantibodies are detected in 69% to 90%.[8]
- ZnT8 Ab are the most recent antibody to be standardized and are detected in 60% to 80% of patients at the onset of T1D.[3] When detected, they are predictive of need for future insulin therapy.[9] ZnT8 is rarely found as the only autoantibody present.
- IAAs are found at the time of T1D diagnosis in about 70% of children. Studies in children have shown that higher IAA titer levels predict more likely progression to T1D. These antibodies can be detected before insulin

is started but may also not result positive until after a brief period of treatment with exogenous insulins.[6,8] IAA has some variability and is the least specific Ab. More reliable, improved measurements are becoming available with this test.[4,10]

INDICATIONS

Screening

■ Antibodies for T1D are not recommended as universal screening but may be used in research trials.
■ Antibodies for T1D may be used for targeted screening of patients genetically predisposed to T1D (first- or second-degree relatives of people with T1D) as antibodies often can be detected before the onset of symptoms. If results are positive, counseling on risk of T1D and a monitoring plan is warranted. Negative results do not exclude a possibility of future T1D diagnosis.[1,4]

Diagnosis and Evaluation

■ Autoantibodies are used to evaluate for and assist in diagnosis of T1D.[1,4]
■ Autoantibodies may especially be used in adult patients with hyperglycemia when trying to differentiate between T1D and T2DM. Situations that make T1D more likely than T2DM (and would warrant testing) include hyperglycemia in the presence of normal body mass index, uncontrolled hyperglycemia despite being on several oral agents, variable glucose control, and no family history of T2DM.[1,4]

Monitoring

■ Autoantibodies are not used for monitoring of T1D.[2,4]

INTERPRETATION

■ It is recommended to follow reference intervals provided by the clinician's local laboratory. A normal finding is low or undetectable.
■ Positivity for autoantibodies supports the diagnosis of T1D and expect that at some point these patients will need insulin therapy.[9]
■ Follow-up testing to confirm or refute a diagnosis of T1D is not indicated. The risk of a false negative exists but is small at 4% or less.[4]
■ Multiple antibody positivity, regardless of the autoantibody tested, results in a certainty of T1D.[4,5] However, there is no consensus on the minimum number of antibodies needed to achieve this certainty of T1D. If one autoantibody is present there is a 17% likelihood of T1D; with two, there is a 39% likelihood; and with three, there is a 70% likelihood.[2,4]
■ The evidence is unclear regarding the significance of positivity in a single autoantibody. There are cases of T1D where a patient might only have one positive autoantibody,[2,4] and there are cases where some do not progress to T1D. However, one antibody in the context of hyperglycemia and/or diabetic ketoacidosis (DKA) is diagnostic of T1D.[4,10]

FOLLOW-UP

- Patients with T1D are prone to other autoimmune disorders such as Graves' disease, Hashimoto's thyroiditis, primary adrenal insufficiency (Addison's disease), vitiligo, pernicious anemia, autoimmune hepatitis, inflammatory bowel disease, and celiac disease.[11] If patients demonstrate signs and symptoms, testing for these conditions is warranted.
- In the presence of an uncertain diagnosis, additional testing for T1D can be done with human leukocyte antigen (HLA) gene loci testing. These genetic markers have been identified to be highly associated with T1D.[1,6,9,12]
- C-peptide may clarify the clinical picture. Low c-peptide along with multiple positive autoantibodies provides a high certainty of T1D.[2–4,6,8,12,13]

PEARLS & PITFALLS

- T1D can occur at any age but has a bimodal distribution with peak diagnoses at ages 18 years old and younger, as well as 40 years old and older.[4,12]
- The term "latent autoimmune diabetes of adulthood" (LADA) has been used to identify T1D that presents in older adults (older than 35 years) after a 5- to 10-year honeymoon period. When T1D is diagnosed prior to age 35 years, there is usually a 1- to 2-year honeymoon period.[1,4,8]
- Insulin deficiency is a serious condition and must be identified as early as possible. Correct diagnosis is paramount. Without insulin, hyperglycemia occurs and the patient could develop DKA, which can result in risk of death.[11]
- Over 90% of patients with T1D will test positive for one or more autoantibodies.[2]
- Fewer than 10% of patients with T1D will only test positive for one autoantibody.[3,9]
- There are still patients who clinically appear to have T1D but are antibody negative. This has led to ongoing research to identify additional autoantibodies related to T1D, such as tetraspanin-7.[13]

PATIENT EDUCATION

- https://www.niddk.nih.gov/health-information/diabetes/overview/what-is-diabetes/type-1-diabetes

RELATED DIAGNOSES AND ICD-10 CODES

Type 1 diabetes mellitus	E10
Hyperglycemia	R73.9

REFERENCES

Full list of references can be accessed through Springer Publishing Company Connect™ at the following link: http://connect.springerpub.com/content/reference-book/978-0-8261-8843-4/part/part03/toc-part/ch027

28. ARTHROCENTESIS ANALYSIS

Zachary Stutzman

PHYSIOLOGY REVIEW

There are three types of joints in the body: synarthrotic (immovable), amphiarthrotic (slightly movable), and diarthrotic (freely movable). This section will focus on the diarthrotic joints as these are the only ones with synovial fluid. Synovial fluid is a lubricating fluid that reduces friction and encourages the free movement of the joint.[1] There are a variety of types of diarthrotic joints, but the ones most commonly associated with arthrocentesis are the knee, hip, shoulder, and ankle. Occasionally, interphalangeal and carpal joints will be aspirated, although this is fairly uncommon.

Every synovial joint is lined with a thick, fibrous capsule that encloses the joint. Inside of the capsule, there is synovial fluid that is produced by the synovium tissue lining the joint. This fluid acts as a natural lubricant for the joint and also allows for the transfer of nutrients and inflammatory mediators from the blood into the joint environment.[1] The synovial fluid is an ultrafiltrate of plasma with glucose and uric acid levels equal to plasma levels and protein levels approximately one-third of that seen in plasma in a normal functioning joint.[1]

Few studies have been done looking at the normal amount of fluid present in joints. In the knee, a healthy joint has approximately 4 mL of synovial fluid; however, when effusion is present, 60 to 100 mL is not uncommon to aspirate. In the shoulder, one study looked at pathologic rotator cuff tears prior to surgery, finding small tears had less than 1 mL of fluid in the joint, while large tears had around 6 mL of fluid.[2] Studies looking at the hip joint in adolescents found around 2 to 3 mL with a slight variation based on sex. Males tended to have around 0.5 mL more fluid.[3]

OVERVIEW OF LABORATORY TESTS

Laboratory tests ordered in a typical arthrocentesis evaluation would include:

- Gram stain CPT code 37008 – capped syringe
- Cell count CPT code 89051 (lavender)
- Crystal analysis CPT code 89060 (green top)
- Culture CPT code 87070 – capped syringe

Gram stain (CPT code 37008) is used to determine the cell wall physiology of bacteria. It is one of the most common tests used to differentiate between varieties of bacteria. The abundance of peptidoglycan in the cell wall is the differentiator; those walls with high levels of peptidoglycan are considered gram positive and will stain purple. Those without high levels are considered gram negative and will stain pink.[4]

Cell count analysis (CPT code 89051) involves manually counting the number of white blood cells per mL. This provides information about the type of reaction the body is having, whether it is inflammatory or a reaction to an infection. The cell count will also give the percent of neutrophils, which are the white blood cells responsible for killing most bacteria. Neutrophils act as a first line of defense and will be elevated in the presence of an infection.

Crystal analysis (CPT code 89060) is performed using polarized light microscopy. The fluid will be analyzed for the presence of crystals. If crystals are found, the birefringence of the crystals will be determined. Birefringence is a property describing the refractivity of light on the crystals. Negatively birefringent crystals indicate gout and positively birefringent indicate pseudogout.[5]

If infection is suspected, aspirate should also be sent for a bacterial culture (CPT code 87070). The laboratory will attempt to grow organisms from the aspirate in a variety of conditions, providing additional information as to which organism is causing the infection. Along with cultures, samples are often sent for sensitivities, where the organisms will be placed near specific antibiotics to trial if certain antibiotics inhibit growth or lead to the bacterium dying.

Sensitivities and specificities will vary based on the test, setting, and organism. When infection is the etiology, sensitivity and specificity values are dependent on the type of pathogen, and whether it is a native joint or a prosthesis. As a general rule, Gram stain sensitivity has been reported to be quite low, around 17%, but the specificity is much higher, around 99%. In the setting of infection, the white count has a high sensitivity and specificity, 94% and 97%, respectively. Synovial fluid analysis for joint crystals has a sensitivity of 84% and a specificity of 100%. If the specimen is collected too early in a flare, crystals may be absent.[5,6]

INDICATIONS

Screening
- There is no evidence for universal or targeted screenings for joint fluid analysis.

Diagnosis and Evaluation
Arthrocentesis and synovial fluid analysis should be used to diagnose the cause of the synovial fluid formation and to differentiate inflammatory from non-inflammatory causes. It should be considered for either an acutely painful joint or persistent joint effusion. Common conditions that warrant arthrocentesis and synovial fluid analysis are:

- Septic joint
- Gout/pseudogout
- Hemorrhagic joint
- Trauma
- Rheumatic disease
- Tumor

Monitoring
- If the joint is infected, consider serial aspirations and blood work to ensure the infection has cleared before proceeding with elective surgical procedures.

INTERPRETATION

Table 28.1 is a distillation of the most investigated aspects of synovial fluid analysis. Typically, a gross visualization should be documented at the time of aspiration, commenting on color and consistency. Normal joint fluid is straw colored and a clinician should be able to see through it. Richer yellow colors and increased cloudiness are both possible signs of pathology.

Increased protein levels in joint fluid is seen in ankylosing spondylitis, Crohn disease, gout, and psoriasis.

The white blood cell (WBC) count itself can be used for screening for the absence of microcrystals in synovial fluid. The cutoff of fewer than 1,650 WBC/mm³ accurately predicts the absence of crystals, thus reducing the need for polarized light microscopy. This leads to a simplified and shortened laboratory analysis of synovial fluid and a reduction in laboratory turnaround time.[7]

FOLLOW-UP

- If infection is suspected, serum erythrocyte sedimentation rate (ESR), C-reactive protein (CRP), and complete blood count (CBC) should be performed. CRP has been shown to be a reliable independent marker for differentiating septic arthritis, crystal arthropathy, and normal/arthritic joints in the adult population. For patients with CRP lower than 90 mg/L, septic arthritis is rare.[8]

TABLE 28.1: SYNOVIAL FLUID ANALYSIS

CATEGORY	VISUAL	VISCOSITY	CELL COUNT	GLUCOSE BLOOD:SF	OTHER
Normal	Straw, clear	High	<150 WBC <25% neutrophils	0–10	
Non-inflammatory (osteoarthritis)	Yellow, mild cloudy	Decreased	<1,000 WBC <30% neutrophils	0–10	
Inflammatory (arthritic flare, rheumatoid arthritis, psoriatic arthritis)	White/gray/ yellow Cloudy, turbid	Absent	<100,000 WBC >50% neutrophils	0–4	
Septic (infection)	White/gray/ green/yellow Cloudy, purulent	Absent	50K–200,000 WBC >90% neutrophils	20–100	+ cultures
Crystal induced (gout, pseudogout)	White Cloudy, turbid, milky, opaque	Absent	500–200,000 WBC <90% neutrophils	0–80	+ crystals
Hemorrhagic (fracture, trauma)	Sanguinous, red/brown	Absent	50–10,000 WBC <50% neutrophils	0–20	RBCs present

RBCs, red blood cells; WBC, white blood cell.

Sources: Data from Seidman AJ, Limaiem F. Synovial fluid analysis. [Updated 2020 Oct 27]. In: *StatPearls* [Internet]. StatPearls Publishing; 2021. https://www.ncbi.nlm.nih.gov/books/NBK537114/; Courtney P, Doherty M. Joint aspiration and injection and synovial fluid analysis. *Best Pract Res Clin Rheumatol.* 2009;23(2):161–192. doi:10.1016/j.berh.2009.01.003

- For the diagnosis of periprosthetic joint infection, the most frequently studied synovial fluid markers are C-reactive protein, leukocyte esterase, interleukin-6, interleukin-1β, α-defensin, and interleukin-17. All of these tests have high diagnostic utility and should be considered to rule in and/or rule out periprosthetic joint infection.[9]
- If trauma is implicated, obtain necessary imaging, x-ray, and MRI, if warranted.

PEARLS & PITFALLS

- For knee arthrocentesis, the patient should be supine, not seated, which leads to more reliable fluid collection.[10]
- Evidence is mixed on the need for ultrasound guidance for the knee during the procedure but is necessary for the hip and shoulder.
- Do not aspirate through an area of skin infection or if a tumor is suspected.
- As always, a proper history and physical examination should be performed and be correlated to the need for an arthrocentesis analysis.
- Ethyl chloride can be used to numb skin before a procedure with little worry for affecting cultures or increasing risk of seeding infection.[11] When aspirating, it is important to obtain the sample in a sterile fashion, as to not seed infection into a joint. It is also important to ensure any cultures that are sent for diagnostic purposes are not cross-contaminated as this could lead to unnecessary workup or treatment.

PATIENT EDUCATION

- https://my.clevelandclinic.org/health/treatments/14512-arthrocentesis -joint-aspiration
- https://www.medicinenet.com/joint_aspiration/article.htm

RELATED DIAGNOSES AND ICD-10 CODES

Infected native joint	M00.9
Gouty arthropathy	M10.0_
Hemarthrosis	M25.00
Rheumatoid arthritis	M05.9
Infection and inflammatory reaction due to unspecified internal joint proesthesis	T84.50XA

REFERENCES

Full list of references can be accessed through Springer Publishing Company Connect™ at the following link: http://connect.springerpub.com/content/reference-book/978-0-8261 -8843-4/part/part03/toc-part/ch028

29. BETA HYDROXYBUTYRATE

Carolyn McClerking and Kelly Small Casler

PHYSIOLOGY REVIEW

Beta hydroxybutyrate (BHB) is the largest and most common of three ketone bodies that exist in mammals. Approximately 78% of ketone bodies are in the form of BHB.[1] The other 20% and 2% are from acetoacetate and acetone, respectively.[1,2] Ketone bodies are tiny molecules produced mainly in the liver from fats. They are present in the bloodstream during periods of low-calorie intake, extensive exercise, and carbohydrate restriction.[2] The inability of the body to utilize carbohydrate and properly store glycogen leads to an increased production of acetoacetate in peripheral tissues.[3] The elevated acetoacetate then accumulates in the blood, where there is partial conversion to acetone.[2,3] The significant part of acetoacetate that remains is transformed to BHB.[3,4]

OVERVIEW OF LABORATORY TESTS

BHB (CPT code 82010) is used in the evaluation of diabetic ketoacidosis (DKA), since it is the main ketone that occurs and is responsible for acidosis.[5] DKA is a primary cause of morbidity in patients with diabetes, particularly insulin-dependent diabetes, and is considered a medical emergency.[3,5] Patients with DKA present with ketosis, metabolic acidosis, and lactic acidosis.[6] Laboratory assessment of plasma BHB has been the traditional method to evaluate levels of ketosis. New point of care (POC) tests using venous or capillary whole blood are becoming more common and provide comparable accuracy to methods that use plasma.[7,8] However, further study is being conducted to determine if capillary and venous whole blood samples require different reference limits for identifying DKA.[8] POC tests offer numerous advantages including reduction in hospital admissions, improved recovery time, and decreased emergency room evaluation.[9,10]

Other methods can complement the use of BHB including urine ketone testing through urine dipstick nitroprusside reaction. This method of evaluation provides a semi-quantitative measure of acetoacetate; however, it does not measure BHB, the primary cause of ketosis.[11] Another method, nuclear magnetic resonance (NMR) spectroscopy, is being studied and can determine the concentrations of all three ketones.[12]

INDICATIONS

Screening
- Universal screening for BHB is not recommended.
- Targeted screening with serum BHB may be used in conditions where patients are at high risk of ketosis (Box 29.1).[10,13–15]

Box 29.1: Disorders Predisposing Individuals to Ketosis

Elevated ion gap
High metabolic rate and increased energy demand
Inborn errors of metabolism
Ketogenic diet
Pregnancy

Sources: Data from Depczynski B, Lee ATK, Varndell W, Chiew AL. The significance of an increased beta-hydroxybutyrate at presentation to the emergency department in patients with diabetes in the absence of a hyperglycemic emergency. *J Diabetes Res*. 2019;2019:7387128. doi:10.1155/2019/7387128; Kanikarla-Marie P, Jain SK. Hyperketonemia and ketosis increase the risk of complications in type 1 diabetes. *Free Radic Biol Med*. 2016;95:268–277. doi:10.1016/j.freeradbiomed.2016.03.020; Misra S, Oliver NS. Utility of ketone measurement in the prevention, diagnosis and management of diabetic ketoacidosis. *Diabet Med*. 2015;32(1):14–23. doi:10.1111/dme.12604; Noor N, Basavaraju K, Sharpstone D. Alcoholic ketoacidosis: a case report and review of the literature. *Oxf Med Case Reports*. 2016;2016:31–33. doi:10.1093/omcr/omw006

Diagnosis and Evaluation

■ Used in the evaluation of patients with hyperglycemia and suspected new-onset type 1 diabetes.[16,17]
■ Used in the evaluation of new-onset mental status changes.[18]
■ May be used to evaluate for hyperinsulin hypoglycemic conditions.[19]
■ Used to evaluate signs and symptoms that could be due to ketosis (Box 29.2).

Monitoring

■ Measuring ketone bodies such as BHB is useful in monitoring the response to DKA treatment.[3] BHB may be monitored as frequently as every 1 to 4 hours.[20]

Box 29.2: Signs and Symptoms of Ketosis

■ Abdominal pain
■ Flushed skin
■ Fruity or acetone breath
■ Lethargy
■ Mental status changes
■ Nausea
■ Tachycardia
■ Tachypnea
■ Vomiting

Sources: Data from Diabetes Canada Clinical Practice Guidelines Expert Committee, Goguen J, Gilbert J. Hyperglycemic emergencies in adults. *Can J Diabetes*. 2018;42(suppl 1):S109–S114. doi:10.1016/j.jcjd.2017.10.013; Jensen NJ, Nilsson M, Ingerslev JS, et al. Effects of β-hydroxybutyrate on cognition in patients with type 2 diabetes. *Eur J Endocrinol*. 2020;182(2):233–242. doi:10.1530/EJE-19-0710; Sass JO, Fukao T, Mitchell GA. Inborn errors of ketone body metabolism and transport:an update for the clinic and for clinical laboratories. *J Inborn Errors Metabol Screen*. 2018;6:2326409818771101.

INTERPRETATION

- Reference interval: 0.02 to 0.27 mmol/L[21]
- BHB levels 3.0 mmol/L or higher (children) and 3.8 mmol/L or higher (adults) were suggested as reference limits for diagnosis of DKA by one study.[22]

FOLLOW-UP

- Evaluate electrolytes including sodium, potassium, magnesium, and phosphate since abnormal levels are often seen in acidotic states.[23]
- In the setting of elevated BHB, use history, physical examination, and follow-up testing to focus evaluation on the differential diagnoses of alcoholic ketoacidosis, DKA, and inborn errors of metabolism.[10,13–15]
- Arterial blood gas (ABG), glucose, and anion gap (basic metabolic panel) can be performed to help clarify the clinical picture. Findings suggestive of DKA include arterial pH 7.25–7.30 or lower, bicarbonate levels 15–18 mEq/L or lower, and/or anion gap greater than 10 with glucose greater than 250 mg/dL. Serum osmolality may also help clarify the clinical picture but is variable in DKA.[17]

PEARLS & PITFALLS

- Evidence suggests there is a link between patient survival in sepsis and levels of BHB. Specifically, one study found BHB levels were more valuable in predicting mortality in the ICU than SOFA (sequential sepsis-related organ failure assessment) and APACHE II (acute physiologic and chronic health evaluation) scores.[24]
- In a retrospective study evaluating the ability of BHB to predict outcomes in patients with type 1 diabetes, there was no association between use of BHB and patient outcome.[14] Other studies have found that using BHB over urine acetoacetate testing improves outcomes in patients presenting with DKA.[9,25]
- In one cross-sectional study, BHB levels were noted to be increased in patients with type 2 diabetes mellitus.[12]
- Some evidence suggests an association between maternal ketosis and abnormal fetal central nervous system development. Although there are no current guidelines for routine ketone monitoring in patients with gestational diabetes, researchers argue monitoring should be considered.[26]
- Breath acetone tests are being studied as a less invasive alternative to BHB in evaluating patients with suspected DKA. More research is needed.[27]
- Some POC devices for BHB are less accurate in the setting of anemia, elevated ascorbic acid, and severe ketoacidosis (BHB greater than 5 mmol/L). Clinicians should be familiar with the limitations of the device being used in their organization.[20,28]
- Hyperosmolar hyperglycemic state (HHS) is another metabolic complication of diabetes besides DKA that can cause small increases in BHB and urine ketone testing. Arterial pH is ususually greater than 7.30 and HCO_3 is greater than 18 mEq/L in these patients. Serum osmol is often greater than 320 mOsm/kg and glucose is greater than 600 mg/dL.[17]

PATIENT EDUCATION

■ https://medlineplus.gov/lab-tests/ketones-in-blood

RELATED DIAGNOSES AND ICD-10 CODES

Other specified abnormal findings of disorders of ketone metabolism	E71.32

REFERENCES

Full list of references can be accessed through Springer Publishing Company Connect™ at the following link: http://connect.springerpub.com/content/reference-book/978-0-8261 -8843-4/part/part03/toc-part/ch029

---

30. BILIRUBIN

Kelly Small Casler, Pam Kibbe, and Amanda Chaney

PHYSIOLOGY REVIEW

Bilirubin formation begins at the end of red blood cell (RBC) life after the breakdown of RBC into heme and globin by the reticuloendothelial system in the spleen. Heme is converted to bilirubin, after which bilirubin is released into the bloodstream and pairs with albumin. Bilirubin in this form is considered unconjugated. It is transported to the liver by albumin, after which it is combined with glucuronic acid by the hepatocytes. At this point the bilirubin is now conjugated, water soluble, and incorporated into bile (Figure 30.1).[1,2] As bile is secreted into the intestines, it is broken down into urobilinogen and either excreted with feces or reabsorbed back into the liver or by the kidneys where it is excreted in the urine.[2,3] Bilirubin levels become high in the setting of hepatocellular injury (inability to conjugate bilirubin), hemolysis (excess breakdown of RBC), or cholestatic problems (bile cannot be excreted from the liver).[3] Newborns commonly experience a physiologically normal and temporary hyperbilirubinemia state related to liver immaturity and polycythemia at birth. A small amount of newborns may have pathophysiologic hyperbilirubinemia, and for these newborns, hyperbilirubinemia can become extreme and cross the blood-brain barrier, causing a risk of bilirubin encephalopathy and kernicterus.[4]

OVERVIEW OF LABORATORY TESTS

Bilirubin is most commonly measured through serum samples using electrophoresis or enzyme-based laboratory methods.[4] Total serum bilirubin (TSB) (CPT code 82247) levels are most commonly assessed as part of a comprehensive metabolic panel or liver profile test (formally called liver function test) and include a total amount of bilirubin that is both conjugated and unconjugated.

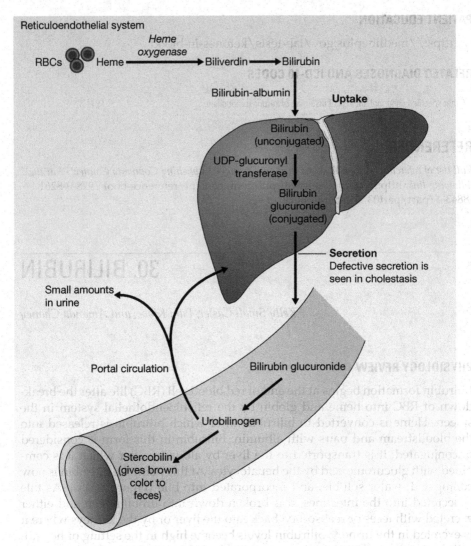

FIGURE 30.1. The formation of bilirubin. Bilirubin is constantly generated from heme released upon breakdown of aging RBCs by the reticuloendothelial system. Unconjugated (indirect) bilirubin is initially hydrophobic and nonpolar, and travels in the circulation bound to albumin. Hepatocytes take up bilirubin and conjugate it to glucuronic acid. Conjugated (direct) bilirubin glucuronide is hydrophilic and is secreted into the bile. In the gut, bacteria further metabolize bilirubin to urobilinogen, a fraction of which is reabsorbed and ultimately excreted by the kidneys. Much of the remaining urobilinogen is converted to stercobilin and is excreted in the feces, adding the characteristic brown color. RBCs, red blood cells; UDP, uridine 5′-diphospho-glucuronosyltransferase. *Source:* Andres J, Diamond A, Miller KA, et al. Liver. In Tkacs NC, Herrmann LL, Johnson RL, eds. *Advanced Physiology and Pathophysiology: Essentials for Clinical Practice*. Springer Publishing Company; 2020, Fig. 14.8.

If desired, conjugated (direct) bilirubin levels can also be ordered (CPT code 82248), which provides a TSB and also reports the amount of conjugated versus unconjugated (indirect) bilirubin. Bilirubin levels in newborns can also be assessed transcutaneously (transcutaneous bilirubin, TcB). Correlation of TcB to TSB is 83%, and accuracy with TcB can vary based on the brand of device used. TcB can also underestimate TSB in newborns of color. In one study, TcB underestimated TSB by up to 3 mg/dL.[5-7] However, TcB evaluation can decrease healthcare costs and provider burden and is more acceptable to parents related to reduced need for frequent heel sticks.[8,9]

INDICATIONS
Screening
- Universal screening of bilirubin (serum or transcutaneous) is recommended at the time of newborn metabolic screening by the majority of guidelines as a way to prevent bilirubin encephalopathy.[10-12] However, the United States Preventive Services Task Force (USPSTF) and other researchers conclude that data is insufficient to recommend this practice.[13,14]

Diagnosis and Evaluation
- In newborns, TSB and *conjugated bilirubin (CB)* are used to evaluate jaundice that appears in the first 24 hours of life.[11]
- In infants with persistent hyperbilirubinemia/jaundice and older than 2 weeks (bottle fed) or 3 weeks (breastfed or preterm) TSB and conjugated (direct) bilirubin are evaluated to rule out cholestasis[11,15] TSB and CB should also be evaluated if newborn hyperbilirubinemia is crossing percentiles of risk zones (see interpretation section).
- In pediatric and adult patients, TSB and CB are used to evaluate cases of jaundice.

Monitoring
- TSB or TcB is used to monitor newborn bilirubin levels and need for/response to phototherapy treatment for hyperbilirubinemia.[16] Levels that require phototherapy will vary based on the newborn's history (https://pediatrics.aappublications.org/content/114/1/297).
- Frequency of testing is usually every 24 to 48 hours if on phototherapy[17] but will vary based on newborn age, risk factors for hyperbilirubinemia, gestational age at birth, length of phototherapy treatment, and prior bilirubin level. Infants younger than 38 weeks' gestation or with risk factors may need more frequent monitoring due to higher risk of severe hyperbilirubinemia.[11] Guidance on frequency of bilirubin monitoring is offered at https://bilitool.org/ (BiliTool).
- In adults, bilirubin is often used with other parameters to determine prognosis of chronic liver disease (Table 30.1).

INTERPRETATION
- Reference interval after neonatal period: 0.3 to 1.9 mg dL.[4]
- The "normal" reference interval for newborn bilirubin levels is highly variable and is based on age in hours, risk factors for hyperbilirubinemia,

TABLE 30.1: USE OF BILIRUBIN FOR PROGNOSIS IN CHRONIC LIVER DISEASE		
NAME OF RESOURCE	ROLE	OTHER PARAMETERS USED TO CALCULATE
Child Turcotte-Pugh Calculator	Prognosis: Determine severity of cirrhosis	Presence of ascites, encephalopathy, bilirubin, albumin, INR
Link: https://www.hepatitisc.uw.edu/page/clinical-calculators/ctp		
MELD-Na	Prognosis: determines prognosis in end-stage liver disease and eligibility for receiving liver transplant	Serum bilirubin, INR, need for dialysis, serum sodium
Link: https://www.hepatitisc.uw.edu/page/clinical-calculators/meld		

INR, international normalized ratio.

and history/physical examination findings. It is recommended that clinicians utilize BiliTool (https://bilitool.org/) to guide interpretation of newborn bilirubin levels.[11] Of particular note is to determine the patient's risk zone based on initial TSB (https://pediatrics .aappublications.org/content/pediatrics/114/1/297/F2.large.jpg). If subsequent TSB levels place the newborn in a different risk zone than initial, the infant is more at risk for needing phototherapy.

■ If more than 20% of TSB is conjugated or if CB is 2.0 mg/dL or greater, there is a strong likelihood of cholestatic problems and further evaluation is needed.[18] In one study with newborns, a CB of 2.0 mg/dL or greater had a positive likelihood ratio for hepatobiliary disease of 17.6.[19] For severe CB elevations (greater than 3 to 6 mg/dL) consider the possibility of congenital disorders.[20]

FOLLOW-UP

■ For persistent elevations in TSB or if there is concern for hepatobiliary disease, a conjugated (direct) bilirubin is ordered.[20] A normal conjugated (direct) bilirubin with an elevated TSB rules out conditions that cause cholestasis/biliary occlusion and would move the differential diagnosis focus to problems of bilirubin conjugation (Gilbert's syndrome) or hemolytic anemia.[20]

■ In infants with severe enough hyperbilirubinemia to require phototherapy (and especially if infants are slow to respond to phototherapy), consider testing for glucose-6-phosphate dehydrogenase (G6PD) deficiency, especially in infants at risk due to genetic heritage (African, Black, Mediterranean, Arabian, Southeast Asian, Middle Eastern).[11]

■ In newborns with hyperbilirubinemia, consider evaluating for sepsis/ infection, especially if CB is greater than 0.5 mg/dL.[11,19]

■ On patients with hyperbilirubinemia severe enough to need hospital admission, evaluate the serum albumin level.[11]

■ In newborns with elevated CB, extensive workup is usually needed. Assessment should include evaluation for thyroid disorders (thyroid-stimulating hormone), alpha-1 antitrypsin deficiency, hemolytic anemia, sepsis (complete blood count and urinalysis), liver failure (international normalized ratio, albumin, platelets), and congenital conditions (imaging often needed).

- Refer patients with CB levels greater than 1.0 mg/dL to pediatric gastroenterology.[15]
- In pediatric and adult patients with elevated bilirubin and other markers of cholestasis (elevated alkaline phosphatase), right upper quadrant imaging should be performed to assess for biliary tract problems.[21]
- Consider the liver transaminases when interpreting bilirubin levels. Isolated bilirubin elevations, especially without an alkaline phosphatase (ALP) elevation, would be suspicious for conditions that cause unconjugated hyperbilirubinemia (e.g., hemolysis, Gilbert's syndrome). If ALP is elevated, conjugated hyperbilirubinemia is more likely, and the problem is likely due to cholestatic problems. Table 30.2 compares causes of unconjugated versus conjugated hyperbilirubinemia. If aspartate

TABLE 30.2: UNCONJUGATED VERSUS CONJUGATED CAUSES OF HYPERBILIRUBINEMIA

UNCONJUGATED (INDIRECT)	CONJUGATED (DIRECT)
Hemolysis	Inherited conditions of bilirubin transport
Inherited: sickle cell disease, spherocytosis, G6PD deficiency	Congenital disorders (e.g., Dubbin-Johnson syndrome, Rotor's syndrome)
Acquired: hypersplenism, DILI, parasitic infections, immune mediated	Advanced cirrhosis/liver failure
Ineffective erythropoiesis: increase bilirubin production	Cholestasis/bile duct occlusion (tumor, primary biliary cirrhosis)
Nutrition deficiencies (folate and cobalamin)	Sepsis
Thalassemia	Hepatitis
Defects of bilirubin conjugation (Gilbert's)	
Inherited: Cigler-Najjar syndrome	
Physiologic jaundice of newborn/breast milk jaundice	
Hematoma	
Blood transfusion	
Drug-induced liver injury	
Hypothyroidism (causes decreased conjugation)	

DILI, drug-induced liver injury.

Sources: Data from Agrawal S, Dhiman RK, Limdi JK. Evaluation of abnormal liver function tests. *Postgrad Med J.* 2016;92(1086): 223–234. doi:10.1136/postgradmedj-2015-133715; Giannini EG. Liver enzyme alteration: a guide for clinicians. *Can Med Assoc J.* 2005;172(3):367–379. doi:10.1503/cmaj.1040752; McCance KL, Huether SE, Brashers VL, Rote NS, eds. *Pathophysiology: The Biologic Basis for Disease in Adults and Children.* 8th ed. Mosby; 2019; Pollock G, Minuk GY. Diagnostic considerations for cholestatic liver disease: causes of cholestasis. *J Gastroenterol Hepatol.* 2017;32(7):1303–1309. doi:10.1111/jgh.13738; Schreiner AD, Rockey DC. Evaluation of abnormal liver tests in the adult asymptomatic patient. *Curr Opin Gastroenterol.* 2018;34(4): 272–279. doi:10.1097/MOG.0000000000000447.

aminotransferase (AST) and alanine aminotransferase (ALT) elevations are seen, intrahepatic causes of hyperbilirubinemia might be considered such as cirrhosis, hepatitis, or sepsis.

PEARLS & PITFALLS

- Errors are common in the visual estimation of presence/absence of jaundice especially in newborns of color. Be sure to also rely on history.
- Bilirubin is usually greater than 3.0 mg/dL before jaundice/icterus can be visualized.[11,15]
- Stool pigment visualization is critical to evaluation and differential of prolonged jaundice/hyperbilirubinemia. Stools normally have a yellow color in newborn infants and brown color in children and adults. Acholic (pale, clay colored) stools are a particular concern for disorders of the biliary tract.[15]
- Although there is a slight difference, the terms "conjugated bilirubin" and "direct bilirubin" are sometimes used interchangeably.[19,22] Technically, direct bilirubin includes conjugated bilirubin and delta bilirubin, an extremely small fraction of conjugated bilirubin that is bound with albumin.[19,22] In contrast, conjugated bilirubin is technically only bilirubin conjugated with glucuronic acid.
- Kernicterus is seen with bilirubin levels of 40 mg/dL or greater[16] and is rare if bilirubin is less than 25 mg/dL.[23]
- Point-of-care evaluation of bilirubin presents similar accuracy to laboratory-based measurement of TSB.[24,25]
- Newborns with TSB levels that rise faster than an average of 0.2 mg/dL per hour warrant closer monitoring and are more likely to have hyperbilirubinemia that requires phototherapy.[17,26]
- In infants with severe hyperbilirubinemia, phototherapy can decrease bilirubin levels by 30% to 40% over 24 hours.[17]
- Assessing bilirubin and platelet level is useful to predict outcomes in acute or chronic liver failure.[27]
- Gilbert's syndrome (GS) is a benign condition causing hyperbilirubinemia in 5% to 10% of the population.[20] TSB is always less than 5 mg/dL in these patients,[20] and some with GS may have normal bilirubin levels.[28] GS does not cause elevations in AST, ALT, or ALP.
- CB is water soluble and, therefore, is excreted in urine. When bilirubin elevations are seen on UA, it usually is a sign of conjugated hyperbilirubinemia.

RELATED DIAGNOSES AND ICD-10 CODES

Neonatal jaundice	P59.9
Hyperbilirubinemia	E80.6

REFERENCES

Full list of references can be accessed through Springer Publishing Company Connect™ at the following link: http://connect.springerpub.com/content/reference-book/978-0-8261-8843-4/part/part03/toc-part/ch030

31. BLOOD TYPING AND RH

Kelli M. Hiller and Rachel M. Donner

PHYSIOLOGY REVIEW

There are four major blood groups: A, B, O, and AB. Each blood group is determined by the presence or absence of two antigens. These antigens, A and B, are carbohydrate structures located on the red blood cell (RBC) (and other cells in the body).[1-3] In addition to antigens, individuals will have antibodies to the A and B antigens not present on their own RBCs, anti-A and anti-B, respectively. An antibody is a protein that is produced by immune cells (plasma cells) in response to a stimulus.[4] ABO antibodies are naturally occurring and develop in patients approximately 6 months after birth (with variation depending on the infant's immune system).[3] See Figure 31.1.

In addition to the A and B antigens, a protein, termed the Rh factor, is either absent or present on each RBC. If the Rh factor is present, it is (+) and if the Rh factor is absent, it is (−). The Rh system consists of the D antigen (also referred to as Rhesus factor) to determine if a patient or a donor is Rh positive or negative.[5] Unlike the ABO system, Rh-negative patients do not have naturally

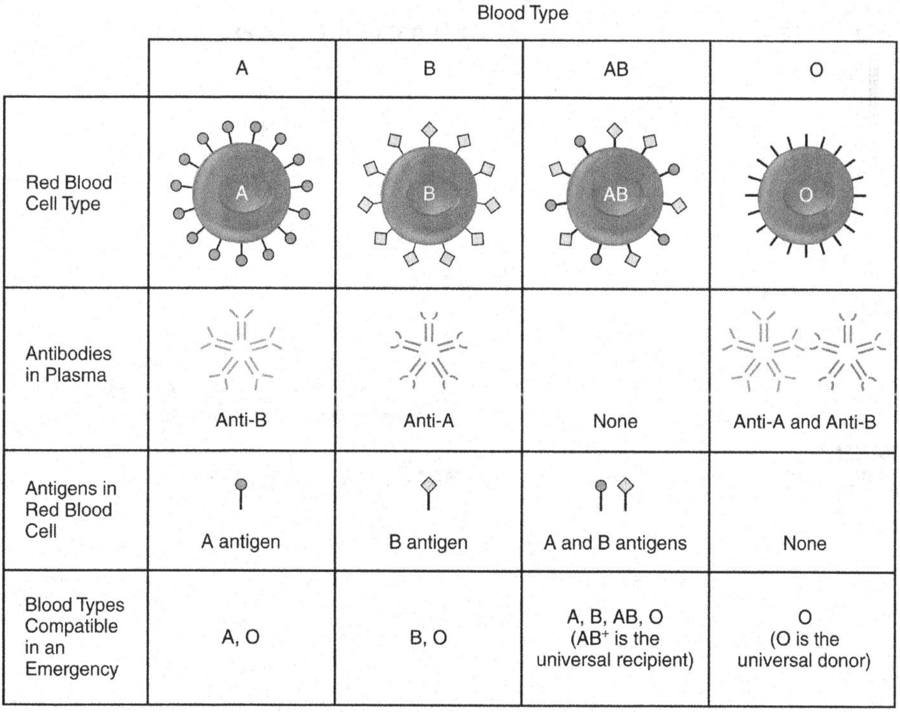

Blood Type

	A	B	AB	O
Red Blood Cell Type				
Antibodies in Plasma	Anti-B	Anti-A	None	Anti-A and Anti-B
Antigens in Red Blood Cell	A antigen	B antigen	A and B antigens	None
Blood Types Compatible in an Emergency	A, O	B, O	A, B, AB, O (AB⁺ is the universal recipient)	O (O is the universal donor)

FIGURE 31.1. Blood type groups. *Source:* OpenStax College.

occurring antibodies to the D antigen but can develop anti-D upon exposure to Rh-positive blood. ABO/Rh blood grouping is performed to type blood donors, as pre-transfusion testing for patients, for cross-matching and selection of compatible blood units, and for fetal maternal care.[3]

OVERVIEW OF LABORATORY TESTS

Laboratory testing for the ABO blood group system is determined by evaluating the presence or absence of A and B antigens (forward typing) (CPT code 86900) as well as the presence or absence of their corresponding antibodies (reverse typing) (CPT code 86904). Testing for the Rh blood group system evaluates the presence or absence of the D antigen (CPT code 86901). These tests are utilized to type donor blood, select compatible units of blood and plasma, and evaluate fetal/maternal compatibility (Tables 31.1 and 31.2).[3]

Plasma donor compatibility matching will be different from red cell selection due to the presence in anti-A and/or anti-B present in plasma.[3,6]

Rh-positive patients can receive Rh-positive and Rh-negative blood products. Rh-negative patients should only receive Rh-negative RBCs to prevent sensitization to the D antigen and production of anti-D.[3,6] Refer to Chapter 50, "Coombs' Test," for further detail.

TABLE 31.1: RED BLOOD CELL COMPATIBILITY CHART

PATIENT BLOOD TYPE	RED CELL DONOR BLOOD TYPE			
	A	B	0	AB
A	Compatible	X	Compatible	X
B	X	Compatible	Compatible	X
0	X	X	Compatible	X
AB	Compatible	Compatible	Compatible	Compatible

TABLE 31.2: PLASMA COMPATIBILITY CHART

PATIENT BLOOD TYPE	PLASMA DONOR BLOOD TYPE			
	A	B	0	AB
A	Compatible	X	X	Compatible
B	X	Compatible	X	Compatible
0	X	X	Compatible	Compatible
AB	X	X	X	Compatible

INDICATIONS

Screening

■ Universal screening of blood type and Rh factor occurs on all blood donations.

■ Targeted screenings of blood type and Rh factor should occur with the following:

● Pregnancy

▪ Blood typing to establish the need for Rh immune globulin (RHIG) in Rh-negative mothers (Rh-negative mothers should receive RHIG at 22 weeks' gestation and post-delivery if infant cord blood types Rh positive)[3,6,7]

▪ ABO/Rh testing of infant blood to determine if maternal/fetal incompatibility is present and monitor for hemolytic disease of the fetus and newborn (HDFN)[7,8]

● Preoperative

▪ The Joint National Commission requires screening of ABO group and Rh type before surgery begins and requires the development of a formal protocol to ensure that patients have blood testing completed prior to surgery start time.[9]

▪ Operations where the median estimated blood loss (EBL) is less than 50 mL, there is a historically low fraction of transfusion use, and there is a low transfusion index should not require preoperative blood type and screen.[10,11]

● Pre-transfusion

● Neonatal exchange transfusion

● Neonatal transfusion

● Donor compatibility

● Hematopoietic stem cell transplant compatibility

● Organ transplantation compatibility (most allografts do not need ABO compatibility)

Diagnosis and Evaluation

■ Testing for blood type and Rh factor should be considered in the following individuals and circumstances[3]:

● Transfusion reaction investigations (symptoms can be mild or severe)

▪ Mild as seen in an allergic reaction. Symptoms include hives and itching. Fever can be an insignificant response or significant response and should be monitored.

▪ Severe as seen in an acute immune hemolytic reaction. Symptoms include nausea, fever, chills, lower back pain, chest pain, and dark urine.

Monitoring

■ Once a blood type and Rh factor are established, no further monitoring is needed.

INTERPRETATION

▪ Tables 31.3 and 31.4 summarize the interpretation of test results.

TABLE 31.3: ABO GROUP TYPE INTERPRETATION

BLOOD GROUP	FORWARD GROUP			REVERSE GROUP	
	ANTI-A	ANTI-B	ANTI-A,B	A1 CELLS	B CELLS
A	+	0	+	0	+
B	0	+	+	+	0
AB	+	+	+	0	0
O	0	0	0	+	+

+ = agglutination present; 0 = no agglutination present.

TABLE 31.4: RH GROUP TYPE INTERPRETATION

BLOOD GROUP	ANTI-D
Rh positive	+
Rh negative	0

+ = agglutination present; 0 = no agglutination present.

FOLLOW-UP

Maternal Testing

Follow-up testing with maternal IgG anti-A/B titers is needed in the event of fetal maternal incompatibility. These levels are significantly associated with the risk of ABO hemolytic disease in newborns and the need for invasive intervention for antibody titers of 512 and above.[12]

Fetal/Newborn Testing

Follow-up testing is recommended in the case that a fetal maternal incompatibility exists. The fetus should be evaluated for bilirubin levels and lung maturity. Using maternal antibody screens/titers and a Liley graph in conjunction with the following follow-up tests, clinicians can evaluate safety and a need for early delivery if applicable.[8,13-16]

Follow-up tests to consider include:
- Amniocentesis
- Lamellar bodies
- Lecithin-to-Sphingelomyelin ratio
- Liley graph
- ABO discrepancy investigations
- Erythropoietin
- Direct antiglobulin testing (DAT) to monitor hemolytic anemia

PEARLS & PITFALLS

- In some emergency situations, it may be necessary to switch transfused blood to a non-Rh match. Usually this is done when a patient (of non-childbearing age) is Rh negative and is being transfused with multiple units of blood.[3,17,18]
- Emergency release is utilized in situations where waiting for cross-matched blood puts the patient at risk of death. These situations include events like massive traumas, gunshots, and aneurysm rupture. Physicians must sign an emergency release form.[13]
- The H system is the precursor for all ABO antigens and is present in all normal individuals. In some cases, patients present with no H antigen and subsequent antibodies to A and B antigens in addition to H antigens, which makes the search for compatible blood incredibly difficult.[3,19,20]
- When selecting blood products for transfusion, clinicians should exercise caution when choosing when to transfuse. Transfusions pose minimal risks, but in patients who have underlying medical conditions, it can pose a greater risk. Care should be taken to avoid circulatory overload, immune stimulation, and iron overload.[21]
- Humans do not have a sufficient mechanism to remove iron from the body. Clinicians should avoid transfusions for iron deficiency in a hemodynamically stable patient to avoid iron-overload and subsequent organ damage.[21]

PATIENT EDUCATION

- https://stanfordbloodcenter.org/donate-blood/blood-donation-facts/blood-types
- https://www.acog.org/womens-health/faqs/the-rh-factor-how-it-can-affect-your-pregnancy

RELATED DIAGNOSES AND ICD-10 CODES

Encounter for blood typing	Z01.83
Unspecified transfusion reaction	T80.92

REFERENCES

Full list of references can be accessed through Springer Publishing Company Connect™ at the following link: http://connect.springerpub.com/content/reference-book/978-0-8261-8843-4/part/part03/toc-part/ch031

32. BLOOD UREA NITROGEN, CREATININE, AND GLOMERULAR FILTRATION RATE (BASIC METABOLIC PANEL)

Kelly Small Casler, Kristopher R. Maday, and Joelle D. Hargraves

PHYSIOLOGY REVIEW

The kidney is essential in maintaining fluid and electrolyte homeostasis and eliminating metabolic waste, such as creatinine and urea. Creatinine is a by-product of muscle metabolism and the breakdown of creatine. People with larger muscles produce more creatinine, since the amount of creatinine produced is related to the mass of the muscle.[1] Breakdown of protein by the liver produces urea, after which urea binds with nitrogen and is carried in the blood to the kidneys to be filtered and excreted. Glomerular filtration rate (GFR) reflects how much blood is filtered by the glomeruli each minute.

OVERVIEW OF LABORATORY TESTS

Blood urea nitrogen (BUN) measures the amount of urea in the blood that is bound to nitrogen. When levels are elevated, it is termed "azotemia." BUN:Cr ratio is a traditional method of assessing the differential diagnosis for elevated BUN or creatinine, but this ratio is not rooted in much evidence.[2] GFR can be directly measured or estimated. Although measured GFR is the best representation of kidney function, it can only be obtained by time-intensive laboratory methods in the inpatient setting.[1,3] Therefore, estimated GFR (eGFR) is used and is determined using equations incorporating plasma creatinine levels. Table 32.1 summarizes these equations.[1,4] GFR can also be estimated using cystatin or creatinine clearance (CrCl), a method that compares urine creatinine with plasma levels of creatinine.[1]

INDICATIONS

Screening
- There is limited evidence to recommend universal screening of BUN, Cr, and eGFR,[9] but routine, universal screening (no interval suggestion is made) is recommended by the American Society of Nephrology based on expert consensus.[10]
- The United States Preventive Services Task Force (USPSTF) and the American College of Physicians both found insufficient evidence to recommend universal screening.[11,12]
- Other groups recommend screening only for patients who are at risk of chronic kidney disease (Box 32.1).[11,13,14]

TABLE 32.1: SUMMARY OF GLOMERULAR FILTRATION RATE ESTIMATION METHODS

	POPULATIONS WHERE ESTIMATION IS MOST RELIABLE	ADVANTAGES	DISADVANTAGES
Modification of Diet in Renal Disease Study Equation (MDRD)	• Nonhospitalized, nonpregnant patients between the ages of 18 and 85 years • Patients of African, European, and Asian genetic heritage • Kidney transplant recipients • Patients with or without CKD or diabetes	Does not require weight; better to use for older adult patients since it incorporates age	Underestimates GFR when above 60 mL/min/1.73 m²; may underestimate GFR in T2DM
Chronic Kidney Disease Epidemiology Collaboration (CKD-EPI$_{cr}$)*	• Nonhospitalized, nonpregnant patients between the ages of 18 and 97 years • Patients of African, European, and Asian genetic heritage	Recommended by KDIGO[5]	May underestimate GFR in T2DM. More accurate estimate of GFR compared to MDRD[6,7]
Schwartz formula	Hospitalized or nonhospitalized patients under the age of 18	Has a quick bedside estimate calculation Developed for children[8]	Overestimates GFR when used with creatinine instead of cystatin C

Note: A calculator for these estimation methods can be found at https://www.kidney.org/apps/professionals/egfr-calculator

CKD, chronic kidney disease; GFR, glomerular filtration rate; KDIGO, Kidney Disease Improving Global Outcomes; T2DM, type 2 diabetes mellitus.

Source: Data from National Kidney Foundation. *Frequently asked questions about GFR estimates.* Published 2014. https://www.kidney.org/sites/default/files/docs/12-10-4004_abe_faqs_aboutgfrrev1b_singleb.pdf.

Box 32.1: Risk Factors for Chronic Kidney Disease

■ Age older than 60 years
■ Autoimmune disease
■ Diabetes or hypertension
■ Family history of kidney disease
■ Male sex
■ Prior acute kidney injury

Sources: Data from Inker LA, Astor BC, Fox CH, et al. KDOQI US commentary on the 2012 KDIGO clinical practice guideline for the evaluation and management of CKD. *Am J Kidney Dis.* 2014;63(5):713–735. doi:10.1053/j.ajkd.2014.01.416; Kazancioğlu R. Risk factors for chronic kidney disease: an update. *Kidney Int Suppl.* 2013;3(4):368–371. doi:10.1038/kisup.2013.79; Saunders MR, Cifu A, Vela M. Screening for chronic kidney disease. *JAMA.* 2015;314(6):615–616. doi:10.1001/jama.2015.9425.

Diagnosis and Evaluation

■ BUN, creatinine, and eGFR are indicated with signs and symptoms of kidney impairment including but not limited to edema, decreased urine output, altered mental status, hypertension, pruritis, shortness of breath, or changes in mental status.

Monitoring

- Monitoring is indicated when using renally excreted medications, specifically:
  - Baseline eGFR level and yearly monitoring (more often if eGFR is abnormal) is recommended with direct oral anticoagulants.[15]
  - Baseline levels are recommended for heart failure patients on antimineralcorticoids.[16]
  - Baseline levels are recommended before initiating angiotensin-converting enzyme inhibitor (ACE-I) or angiotensin receptor blocker (ARB) therapy and at 1 to 2 weeks after dose initiation or change.[5,14]
  - Baseline levels are recommended before initiating biguanide therapy. If eGFR is 60 or more, monitor yearly. If less than 59, monitor every 6 months.[17]
- Regular monitoring is indicated in patients with renal transplant.
- For patients with established CKD, annual monitoring for progression using creatinine and eGFR is recommended. Urine albumin and creatinine ratios should be completed concurrently.[14]
- Yearly monitoring is recommended for patients with type 2 diabetes mellitus or type 1 diabetes for greater than 5 years. Twice yearly monitoring is recommended for these patients if eGFR is lower than 60.[18]
- BUN may be monitored during supplemental nutrition to detect potential protein overload.[19]

INTERPRETATION

Reference intervals and limits are listed in the text that follows.

- BUN 7 to 23 mg/dL[20]
- Creatinine
  - Men ages 18 and older: 0.67 to 1.19 mg/dL[21]
  - Women ages 18 and older: 0.51 to 1.02 mg/dL[21]
  - Pregnancy: 0.4 to 0.6 mg/dL
  - Pediatric reference intervals vary widely based on age.[21]
- eGFR (also see Table 32.2)
  - Normal eGFR is 60 mL/min/1.73 m² or more.[5,20]
- BUN:Cr ratio 10:1 to 20:1

Additional interpretation guidance:

- eGFR lower than 60 mL/min/1.73 m² is suspicious for CKD, but must persist for 90 days or more before diagnosis.[5,14]
- 48-hour increases in Cr by 0.3 mg/dL or more or increases in Cr of 1.5 times baseline or more defines acute kidney injury.[22]
- Traditionally, a BUN:Cr ratio of 20:1 or more suggested a prerenal problem and less than 10:1 suggested a renal or postrenal problem. However, the evidence for the BUN:Cr ratio association with diagnoses is lacking.[2]

FOLLOW-UP

- If clinicians doubt the accuracy of the eGFR based on creatinine (CKD-EPI$_{cr}$), cystatin-C can be ordered and used to calculate eGFR

TABLE 32.2: INTERPRETATION OF GLOMERULAR FILTRATION RATE AND ASSOCIATION TO CHRONIC KIDNEY DISEASE

GFR LEVEL	INTERPRETATION	GFR CATEGORY	ACTION
≥ 90 mL/min/1.73 m²	Normal or high	1*	Refer if albuminuria >300 mg/g or other concerns. Albuminuria >30 mg/g warrants close monitoring.
60–89 mL/min/1.73 m²	Mildly decreased	2*	Refer if albuminuria >300 mg/g or other concerns. Albuminuria >30 mg/g warrants close monitoring.
45–59 mL/min/1.73 m²	Mild to moderately decreased	3a	Refer if albuminuria >300 mg/g or other concerns. Albuminuria >30 mg/g warrants close monitoring.
30–44 mL/min/1.73 m²	Moderately to severely decreased	3b	Refer if albuminuria >300 mg/g or other concerns. Albuminuria >30 mg/g warrants close monitoring.
15–29 mL/min/1.73 m²	Severely decreased	4	Refer
<15 mL/min/1.73 m²	Kidney failure	5	Refer

*CKD is diagnosed if albuminuria or structural disease is present.

CKD, chronic kidney disease; GFR, glomerular filtration rate.

Source: Data from KDIGO 2017 clinical practice guideline update for the diagnosis, evaluation, prevention, and treatment of chronic kidney disease–mineral and bone disorder (CKD-MBD). *Kidney Int Suppl.* 2017;7(1):1–59. doi:10.1016/j.kisu.2017.04.001

(CKD-EPI$_{cys}$). If CKD-EPI$_{cys}$ is lower than CKD-EPI$_{cr}$ patients are at risk for worse outcomes. If CKD-EPI$_{cys}$ ends up being higher than CKD-EPI$_{cr}$ this is reassuring. Alternatively, clinicians could calculate eGFR based on both cystatin and creatinine (CKD-EPI$_{cys-cr}$), which tends to average out the imperfections in both cystatin- and creatinine-based eGFR.[23]

- ACE-I or ARB therapy should be discontinued if the eGFR declines more than 30% from baseline over the first 4 months. In these instances, workup for underlying renal disease should be considered.[5,24]
- When creatinine-based eGFR is 45 to 59 mL/min/1.73 m² for 90 days or longer, follow up with a cystatin-C–based eGFR (due to better sensitivity/specificity) to confirm CKD and prevent overdiagnosis of CKD.[5,25]
- To assess severity or for presence of CKD, order an albumin-to-creatinine ratio (ACR) in patients with eGFR lower than 60 mL/min/1.73 m² and in patients with eGFR of 60 mL/min or more if clinical suspicion is high.[5,25]
- In patients with CKD and GFR lower than 60 mL/min/1.73 m², calcium, phosphorus, and parathyroid hormone should be evaluated to assess for metabolic bone disease.[26]

PEARLS & PITFALLS

■ The complexity surrounding the role of race in CKD risk goes beyond biologic factors. Therefore, the appropriateness of using Black race as a coefficient in eGFR calculations is being reconsidered and extensively evaluated.[27]

■ In patients with extremes of muscle mass (body builders, sarcopenia, amputation), eGFR is more accurate when calculated using cystatin and not creatinine.[28]

■ Rapid drops of eGFR are defined as more than 5 mL/min/1.73 m² per year.[5]

■ Serum creatinine does not have adequate sensitivity to predict renal function in most patients. eGFR should be used.[29]

■ Patients with elevated BUN without changes in creatinine need to be evaluated for gastrointestinal bleeding.[30,31]

■ Creatinine levels can be influenced by levels of dietary meat intake.[1]

■ CKD can be diagnosed in the presence of albuminuria or abnormalities in kidney structure, even with a normal GFR.[14,22]

■ During the first 2 months of therapy with ARB/ACE-Is, patients may have a creatinine rise up to 30% from baseline. As long as the creatinine does not increase past 30% of baseline, therapy with ACE-I/ARBs do not necessarily have to be discontinued.[18,32]

■ Rapid changes in creatinine are concerning.[33]

■ Some medications like trimethoprim-sulfamethoxazole and histamine 2 blockers can spuriously raise the creatinine value by as much as 0.5 mg/dL.[33] Confirm suspicion of this event by looking for BUN levels to stay stable.[33]

■ BUN and creatinine levels will usually increase concurrently when there is a decrease in GFR.[33]

■ A GFR less than 60 mL/min/1.73 m² is a certain, but not only, indicator of CKD. Proteinuria with a GFR greater than 60 mL/min/1.73 m² can also indicate CKD.[33]

■ eGFR calculations are less accurate when GFR is greater than 60 mL/min/1.73 m².[3]

■ Serum creatinine is a specific but not sensitive test. There may be up to 50% impairment in kidney function before the serum creatinine rises.[20]

■ In one study, eGFR lower than 60 mL/min per 1.73 m² was associated with risk for postoperative acute kidney injury.[34]

■ Serum creatinine should be interpreted in the context of the patient's age, sex, and muscle mass.[33]

■ Cystatin-based eGFR is more accurate in inpatients.[23]

■ Research regarding BUN:Creatinine ratio has shown it is not useful for:
  ● Distinguishing prerenal azotemia from acute tubular necrosis.[35]
  ● Differentiating prerenal from intrarenal causes of AKI.[36]
  ● Distinguishing prerenal from other causes of AKI.[37]
  ● Predicting hydration. Serum osmolality is better used in cases where laboratory support is needed in determining hydration.[38]
  ● Suggesting mortality risk in critical care patients. Traditionally a BUN:Cr greater than 20 had been associated with less mortality risk in AKI, but a 2012 study found the opposite was true.[39]

- In 2018, multiple organizations developed a new laboratory order, the "Kidney Profile," which includes a serum creatinine with an eGFR and a urine ACR.[40] This order set is most useful for monitoring patients with CKD.
- Use creatinine reference intervals based on gender identity for transgender patients on gender-affirming hormone therapy for 6 months or greater. For transgender patients not on gender-affirming hormone therapy or using it for less than 6 months, use creatinine reference intervals for gender at birth.[41,42]
- Because transgender patients have not been included in studies regarding accuracy of calculations for eGFR, clinicians should consider the imprecisions of estimates when interpreting levels in these patients. It may be beneficial to calculate estimates using the calculations for both males and females and determine a range that reflects the potential eGFR for the patient.[41,42] When in doubt, directly measure GFR or creatinine clearance.
- Traditionally, medication dosing recommendations for renal impairment followed CrCl. More recently, eGFR is being used in lieu of CrCl to guide medication dosing decisions. Although eGFR may overestimate CrCl,[43] the consensus is that there is generally good concordance between eGFR equations and CrCl when compared to measured GFR.[44–47] Concordance does seem to fluctuate at extremes of age or body weight, however.[48] Therefore, in patients requiring pharmacotherapy with narrow therapeutic index medications or medications with high risk for nephrotoxicity, consider measuring CrCl if eGFR seems imprecise.[46]

PATIENT EDUCATION

- https://www.niddk.nih.gov/health-information/kidney-disease/chronic-kidney-disease-ckd/tests-diagnosis

RELATED DIAGNOSES AND ICD-10 CODES

Azotemia	R79.89
CKD, GFR stage 1	N18.1
CKD, GFR stage 2	N18.2
CKD, GFR stage 3a	N18.31
CKD, GFR stage 3b	N18.32
CKD, GFR stage 4	N18.4
CKD, GFR stage 5	N18.5

REFERENCES

Full list of references can be accessed through Springer Publishing Company Connect™ at the following link: http://connect.springerpub.com/content/reference-book/978-0-8261-8843-4/part/part03/toc-part/ch032

33. BRAIN NATRIURETIC PEPTIDE

LouAnn B. Bailey and Kelly Small Casler

PHYSIOLOGY REVIEW

In concert with the renin-angiotensin-aldosterone system, natriuretic peptides from the heart are responsible for homeostasis of the cardiovascular system.[1] Atrial natriuretic peptide was the first natriuretic peptide to be discovered, being named as such because it was found in large concentrations in the atria. Brain natriuretic peptide (BNP) was the next peptide to be discovered, and was so named to distinguish it from ANP and because it was identified in the brain, in addition to the heart.[2] Unlike ANP, BNP is primarily secreted by the ventricles. Stretch of the myocardial wall from increased volume or pressures triggers release of a precursor peptide that either becomes NT-proBNP or BNP.[3,4] BNP is biologically active as a hormone and has a short half-life (20 minutes) whereas NTproBNP is not biologically active and has a long half-life (120 minutes).[5] NTproBNP also circulates in much greater amounts compared to BNP, leading to it becoming the more preferred method of measurement.[6,7]

OVERVIEW OF LABORATORY TESTS

BNP and NT-proBNP testing (CPT code 83880) provide a means to evaluate for heart failure in patients who present with symptoms of acute dyspnea.[8] Normally, circulating BNP and NT proBNP levels are very low. However, when elevated, they can be a strong predictor of heart failure and, if significantly or persistently elevated, can also predict morbidity and mortality.[9,10] Beyond heart failure, BNP and or NT-proBNP can be elevated in other cardiac and noncardiac causes (Table 33.1[8,11–16]).

INDICATIONS

Screening
- BNP and/or NTproBNP are not used for universal screening.
- BNP and/or NT proBNP may be used to screen at-risk patients who are at risk to develop heart failure due to hypertension, diabetes mellitus, metabolic syndrome, and atherosclerotic cardiovascular disease. The optimum way to deliver this kind of screening in a cost-effective manner is still being discussed. Additionally, to make this kind of screening impactful to patient outcomes, clinicians would need to prioritize treatment maximization for these patients.[11,17–20]

Diagnosis and Evaluation
- This is used with history and physical findings to evaluate for heart failure in patients with acute dyspnea.[11,19]

TABLE 33.1: CONDITIONS OTHER THAN HEART FAILURE THAT CAN CAUSE ELEVATED BNP	
CARDIAC	**NONCARDIAC**
Acute coronary syndrome	Advanced age
Anemia	Bacterial sepsis
Atrial fibrillation/flutter	COPD
Cardiotoxic drugs	Medications (sacubitril/valsartan)
Cardioversion	Obstructive sleep apnea
Hypertrophic cardiomyopathy	Pulmonary edema
Left ventricular hypertrophy	Pulmonary embolism
Myocarditis	Pulmonary hypertension
Pericardial disease	Renal failure/CKD
	Severe burns
	Severe pneumonia
Valvular heart disease	Stroke

BNP, brain natriuretic peptide; CKD, chronic kidney disease; COPD, chronic obstructive pulmonary disease.

Monitoring

- Can be used to monitor a patient's response to heart failure treatment. The optimum way to use BNP/NT-proBNP for monitoring in this manner is still be studied.[11,19,21]
- BNP/NT-proBNP levels on admission can provide prognosis for hospital course (higher levels = worse outcomes). The improvement of levels greater than 30% from admission has been associated with better outcomes after hospital discharge for patients with both acute and chronic heart failure.[11,19,22]
- BNP/NT-proBNP levels have been used to determine prognosis in patients with underlying cardiac disease and COVID-19 infection.[23,24]
- BNP/NT-proBNP levels offer some insight into prognosis after cardiac surgery, but perform weakly for this indication.[25]

INTERPRETATION

- The interpretation of BNP/NT-proBNP is summarized in Table 33.2.[8,12,26–28]
- An elevated BNP/NT-proBNP does not always equate to heart failure. Be sure to consider conditions listed in Table 31.1 during interpretation.

FOLLOW-UP

- 12-lead electrocardiogram should be obtained to complement the patient's evaluation and to evaluate for acute coronary syndrome (ACS), atrial arrhythmias, and changes indicative of pulmonary embolism (PE).

TABLE 33.2: REFERENCE LIMITS AND INTERPRETATION FOR BNP/NT-PROBNP IN PATIENTS WITH DYSPNEA

BRAIN NATRIURETIC PEPTIDE	NT-PROBNP		INTERPRETATION
<100 pg/mL	<300 pg/mL		HF unlikely
100–400 pg/mL			Indeterminate. Use clinical judgment
>400 pg/mL (reference limits based on age)	Age ≤50 years	>450 pg/mL	HF likely
	Age 50–75 years	>900 pg/mL	
	Age >75 years	> 1800 pg/mL	

BNP, brain natriuretic peptide; HF, heart failure.

- Echocardiogram is useful to evaluate left ventricular function, right ventricular function, valvular health, pulmonary pressures, and left ventricular end-diastolic pressures. Echocardiogram is required to confirm HF in a patient with elevated BNP/NT-proBNP related to the low specificity (80%[28]) of BNP.[16,29]
- The basic metabolic panel is used to evaluate renal function and rule out chronic kidney disease/renal failure as a cause of elevated BNP/NT-proBNP.
- Chest radiography is used to evaluate for cardiac size, evidence of lung disease, and evidence of underlying congestion/fluid excess.

PEARLS & PITFALLS

- There is no easy conversion factor between NT proBNP and BNP and the values cannot be used interchangeably.[27,30] There is also significant variability from laboratory to laboratory. Generally, levels performed at alternate sites are, therefore, unable to be compared accurately.[27]
- Always correlate the level of BNP/NT-proBNP with clinical examination and history. However, remember that the seminal Breathing Not Properly study noted that BNP/NT-proBNP performed stronger than history/physical for diagnosis of HF in acutely dyspneic patients.[31]
- Remember to correlate age, renal dysfunction, chronic disease, and obesity with levels of BNP and/or NT-proBNP.
- Because neprilysin breaks down BNP, pharmacotherapy with angiotensin-receptor-neprilysin inhibitors (ARNI) can result in persistently increased BNP levels but not NT-proBNP levels.[13,14]
- Heart failure with preserved ejection fraction (HFpEF) and obesity can result in lower levels of BNP/NT-proBNP than expected.[11,22,26,30] Patients with obesity may need reference limits 50% lower than patients without obesity.[16]
- Race and sex do not seem to influence BNP/NT-proBNP interpretation, although more research is needed.[27,32]
- In a study of patients presenting to the emergency department with dyspnea and a NT-proBNP lower than 300 pg/mL, the negative likelihood ratio for HF was 0.09.[26]

- The diagnostic accuracy of NT proBNP and BNP is similar (greater than 90% sensitivity for both)[28] and guidelines support the use of either test, though there is some evidence that NT proBNP may pick up on earlier heart failure.[6,7,33,34] Additionally, one study showed poor concordance between the two (i.e., a patient might test negative for HF by one method but positive by the other), but neither test outperformed the other.[29] Further research is likely needed.
- Point-of-care testing for BNP/NT-proBNP is available but lacks adequate sensitivity or specificity for clinical use at this time.[35] Additionally, use of this testing method for home monitoring to identify early clinical deterioration is being investigated.[36]
- Future research is aimed at the predictive ability of multiple biomarkers for prognosis. Galectin-3 and soluble ST2 receptor reflect myocardial stress and fibrosis and may provide additional information on prognosis since BNP/pro-NTBNP only looks at myocardial stretch.[11,37–39] Mr-pro-ANP is another natriuretic peptide that is currently rarely used due to its inability to outperform BNP/pro-NT BNP.[27] However, research is ongoing regarding the usefulness of Mr-pro-ANP in diagnosis of HFpEF where it might be more accurate compared to BNP/pro-NT BNP.[40]

PATIENT EDUCATION

- https://labtestsonline.org/tests/bnp-and-nt-probnp

RELATED DIAGNOSES AND ICD-10 CODES

Hypertensive heart disease with heart failure	I11.0
Unstable angina	I20.0
Left ventricular failure, unspecified	I50.1
Acute systolic (congestive) heart failure	I50.21
Chronic systolic (congestive) heart failure	I50.22
Acute diastolic (congestive) heart failure	I50.31
Chronic diastolic (congestive) heart failure	I50.32
Right heart failure	I50.810
Acute right heart failure	I50.811
End-stage heart failure	I50.84
Other heart failure	I50.89
Heart failure unspecified	I50.9
Dyspnea, unspecified	R06.00
Orthopnea	R06.01

Shortness of breath	R06.02
Acute respiratory distress	R06.03
Other forms of dyspnea	R06.09
Wheezing	R06.2
Tachypnea, not elsewhere classified	R06.82
Other abnormalities of breathing	R06.89
Generalized edema	R60.1

REFERENCES

Full list of references can be accessed through Springer Publishing Company Connect™ at the following link: http://connect.springerpub.com/content/reference-book/978-0-8261 -8843-4/part/part03/toc-part/ch033

34. C-REACTIVE PROTEIN

Dayna Jaynstein

PATHOPHYSIOLOGY REVIEW

C-reactive protein (CRP) is an acute-phase reactive protein synthesized by the liver.[1] Levels of CRP elevate in response to inflammatory, traumatic, and infectious processes, and can be used to evaluate both acute and chronic illness. During a systemic inflammatory insult, activation of the immune system results in release of interleukin-6 by macrophages and T cells. As part of this cytokine response, CRP is synthesized and released by hepatocytes.[2] Additional CRP is released by endothelial cells, adipose tissue, and myocytes.[3] Once in the serum, CRP binds to polysaccharides activating the complement system.[4]

C-reactive protein was the first acute-phase protein to be described and continues to be highly utilized in clinical medicine.[4] A wide range of acute and chronic inflammatory conditions including bacterial, protozal, or fungal infections; tissue injury and necrosis; rheumatic and other inflammatory diseases; and malignancy can all elevate CRP levels. CRP is a very sensitive test but lacks specificity.

CRP is the first acute-phase reactant to elevate.[5] Trace amount of CRP, less than 0.8 mg/L, is found in all individuals; however, CRP levels rapidly increase following tissue insult or injury and double every 6 to 8 hours; peaking at 36 to 50 hours.[2] The plasma half-life of CRP is roughly 19 hours.[2] Therefore, continued trending of CRP levels can provide indication of increasing or resolving inflammation, or maintain at above normal levels indicating chronic inflammation.

Elevated levels of CRP not only act as a biomarker of inflammation, but CRP also decreases the production of nitrous oxide, activates endothelium-1 receptors, and increases LDL oxidization, all leading to endothelial dysfunction promoting athrosclerosis.[3] It is for these reasons that research has focused on CRP levels as markers of cerebrovascular risk.

OVERVIEW OF LABORATORY TESTS

A CRP level can be easily obtained from a venous blood sample. There are two distinct tests: a CRP and a high-sensitivity CRP (hs-CRP). The standard CRP test is classically used in the evaluation of patients with suspected acute or chronic inflammatory, traumatic, or infectious processes and measures the serum level of CRP within the range of 8 to 1,000 mg/L (0.8 to 100 mg/dL). The hs-CRP detects even lower levels (0.3 to 10 mg/L) and is specifically used for prognostic cardiovascular risk assessment. Point-of-care CRP testing is also available.

INDICATIONS
Screening
- Multiple studies have demonstrated that elevated hs-CRP is an independent risk factor for cardiovascular disease but no universal screening recommendations exist.[6-8]
  - The United States Preventive Services Task Force determined there is insufficient evidence to recommend the routine use of hs-CRP in determining the risk assessment of CVD.[9]
  - The American Heart Association and U.S. Centers for Disease Control and Prevention (CDC) have both defined risk groups based on hs-CRP levels, but agree that universal screening is not recommended.[10]

Diagnosis and Evaluation
- Elevated CRP levels can be seen in any process that leads to an immune response.
- Increased levels of CRP have been found in patients with appendicitis, pancreatitis, cholecystitis, septic joints, and meningitis.[11]
- Some research has demonstrated that CRP does not consistently rise, or rises to lower levels, in viral infections. Therefore, CRP can be helpful in differentiating bacterial from viral infections.[5,12,13]
- Several studies have evaluated the use of CRP as a point-of-care test to diagnose infection in an effort to improve antibiotic stewardship:
  - A systematic review by Verbakel et al. analyzed data from 11 randomized controlled trials (RCTs) and eight non-RCT studies and found that POC CRP levels reduced immediate antibiotic prescribing in both adults and children.[14]
  - A 2019 RCT demonstrated that the use of POC CRP testing significantly reduced the number of antibiotic prescriptions written for patients with COPD exacerbations without increased harm.[15]

Monitoring

■ CRP is the first acute-phase reactant to rise and reliably decreases as inflammation subsides. Therefore, trended CRP levels can be used to monitor improvement of inflammatory states.

■ CRP levels can be used to evaluate therapeutic response in patients being treated for acute as well as chronic, including autoimmune, diseases.[4]

■ Cancer research has demonstrated the potentional prognostic value of CRP levels. Baseline CRP levels have predicted mortality in patients with non-operable lung cancer.[16] hs-CRP levels have been associated with increased mortality in patients with breast, lung, and renal cell carcinomas.[17]

■ CRP is used to monitor severity of illness in patients hospitalized with SARS-CoV-2 infection.[18]

INTERPRETATION

Standard CRP test[2,5]:

■ CRP levels less than 0.8 mg/L are considered normal.

■ Results between 0.8 to 10 mg/L are considered abnormal and may prompt further investigation.

■ Levels greater than 10 mg/L are considered significantly elevated and should prompt further investigation.

hs-CRP test[7,10,17]:

■ hs-CRP tests measure CRP levels between 0.5 to 10 mg/L.

■ The AHA and CDC have defined the following risk groups for future CVD:
  ● Low risk: less than 1.0 mg/L
  ● Moderate risk: 1.0 to 3.0 mg/L
  ● High risk: greater than 3.0 mg/L

■ Elevated levels of CRP are sensitive but not specific. Therefore, an elevated CRP is not truly indicative of any one disease process.

■ Factors that have been associated with increased CRP levels include cigarette smoking, estrogen and progesterone use, advanced age, hypertension, diabetes, and obesity.[5]

■ Factors that have been associated with decreased CRP levels include niacin and statin therapy, steroid and NSAID use, physical activity, and moderate alcohol consumption.[19-21] Further, since CRP is synthesized by hepatocytes, patients with liver failure will produce lower levels of CRP.[22]

FOLLOW-UP

■ Isolated CRP levels can be indicative of many disease processes and more focused laboratory assessment may be needed to determine the cause of CRP elevation. Monitoring of CRP levels can be helpful in determining therapeutic response.

PEARLS & PITFALLS

- Women tend to have higher levels than men, and Black individuals have higher levels than Caucasians.[23]
- CRP levels are nonspecific. Clinicians need to critically evaluate if additional workup into the cause of CRP levels is necessary.
- CRP levels should not be ordered in all patients with suspected inflammatory, traumatic, or infectious disease. Clinicians should have an understanding of the utility and limitations of CRP levels when deciding if a CRP level should be obtained.
- A normal CRP level does not always indicate the absence of inflammation. Several studies have demonstrated normal levels in patients with RA.[24,25]
- CRP is a more sensitive indicator of acute inflammation than erythrocyte sedimentation rate (ESR); therefore, a CRP should be ordered in the evaluation of acute inflammation.[26]
- Clinicians might consider POC CRP testing when deciding if immediate antibiotic prescribing is necessary.[14,15]

PATIENT EDUCATION

- https://www.mayoclinic.org/tests-procedures/c-reactive-protein-test/about/pac-20385228

RELATED DIAGNOSES AND ICD-10 CODES

- None

REFERENCES

Full list of references can be accessed through Springer Publishing Company Connect™ at the following link: http://connect.springerpub.com/content/reference-book/978-0-8261 -8843-4/part/part03/toc-part/ch034

35. CALCITONIN AND PROCALCITONIN

Carolyn McClerking

PHYSIOLOGY REVIEW

Procalcitonin, a peptide precursor of calcitonin, is a biomarker with several important functions in clinical practice. As a biomarker, procalcitonin is commonly used in determining the diagnosis of sepsis, assisting in evaluating the severity of the disease, and guiding antibiotic treatment. Procalcitonin, which is a component of the sepsis inflammatory cascade, can also be beneficial in distinguishing between bacterial and viral infections.[1] Procalcitonin levels are usually decreased in viral infections and increased in bacterial infections. However, other conditions such as trauma, renal dysfunction, and autoimmune disorders may also cause elevated procalcitonin levels as well.[2] This can be particularly important when patients with advanced age present with symptoms of possible infection. Careful analysis of patient comorbidities combined with laboratory evaluation of procalcitonin offers assistance in identifying accurate diagnoses.[1,3,4]

Calcitonin is a peptide hormone produced by the thyroid and is responsible for metabolizing calcium and phosphate.[5] Calcitonin also has a role in decreasing the level of calcium in the blood and preventing osteoclastic activity in the bone.[5] In addition, calcitonin serves as a tumor marker for diagnosis of medullary thyroid carcinoma.[5] There is an increase in the level of calcitonin during pregnancy and lactation; however, the baseline level is higher in males than in females.[5] Calcitonin levels may also decrease with age.[5]

OVERVIEW OF LABORATORY TEST

Procalcitonin (CPT code 84145) was initially found in a cell line from a medullary thyroid carcinoma.[6] Procalcitonin is normally cleaved by a specific protease, and thus levels of procalcitonin are generally low or undetectable. However, in conditions such as severe sepsis, levels can exceed 900 ng/mL.[7] During this time period, procalcitonin can increase very rapidly, usually within 2 to 6 hours. The level plateaus after approximately 6 to 12 hours and remains elevated for approximately 2 days.

The introduction of point-of-care testing (POCT) for procalcitonin is important due to the presentation of sepsis in both primary and acute care settings. Some advantages of POCT for procalcitonin include easier preanalytical process, simplified sample collection, faster diagnosis, and earlier institution of treatment.[7] Procalcitonin is measured by lateral flow immunochromatography and requires an incubation period of approximately 30 minutes. Once processed, results are usually available within 1 hour of obtaining the sample.[8]

Calcitonin (CPT code 82308) measurement can be completed through several different methods.[9] The initial method included measurement by radioimmune assay (RIA) through the use of polyclonal antibodies. However, due to the decreased specificity and sensitivity, the RIA was subsequently replaced with two-sided immune radiometry assays.[10] More recently, there has been a transition from radiolabeled systems to fluorescence and chemiluminescence tests.[10] The chemiluminescence test (ILMA) identifies the monomeric form of serum calcium and allows for earlier detection of medullary thyroid cancer (MTC).[11] The latest development for measurement of serum calcitonin is electrochemiluminescence immunoassay (ECLIA).[12] The ECLIA is valuable as the decreased test time and wider reference range allows for faster diagnosis of calcitonin-associated diseases.[12]

INDICATIONS

Screening

- Universal screening for procalcitonin and calcitonin is not recommended.
- Use of targeted serum calcitonin screening to complement ultrasound and fine needle aspiration in the routine diagnosis of thyroid nodules is controversial.[13]

Diagnosis and Evaluation

Procalcitonin

Procalcitonin is not diagnostic itself but is used as a clinical marker in a myriad of conditions to assist with diagnosis. Choosing Wisely guidelines recommend against procalcitonin testing without an established evidence-based protocol.[14]

It is used in the evaluation of children with the following conditions[15-21]:

- Mild to moderate bacterial infections
- Urinary tract infection and kidney involvement
- Neutropenic patients with bacterial infection
- Septic shock risk stratification
- Non-infectious systemic inflammation
- Pulmonary aspiration
- Pancreatitis
- Trauma

Procalcitonin is used in the evaluation of adults with the following conditions:

- Bacterial sepsis[22,23]
- Has been used to determine bacterial versus viral conditions including meningitis and pneumonia; however, a recent meta-analysis suggested procalcitonin did not offer instant information on whether an infection was bacterial or viral, nor whether antibiotics should be initiated if infection was bacterial or held if viral.[24-27]
- Used in treatment guidance and evaluation of therapeutic response to antibiotic therapy[25-28]

Calcitonin

- The main clinical utility of calcitonin is to identify C-cell hyperplasia and medullary thyroid cancer (MTC).[13,29-31]

Monitoring

Procalcitonin

- Monitor procalcitonin levels for patients who are critically ill in the intensive care unit to determine efficacy and safety of procalcitonin-guided treatment; however this recommendation is controversial.[32,33]
- Monitor for patients with severe gram-negative rod bacteremia.[34]
- Studies suggest that procalcitonin-guided therapy is useful in reducing the exposure to antibiotics as well as length of treatment.[35-37]
- Monitoring serial procalcitonin is recommended in predicting efficacy of treatment and prognosis for patients with community-acquired pneumonia.[38,39]
- Serial procalcitonin levels, in addition to individualized care, are proposed as an appropriate measure to guide treatment for and adaptation of antibiotics for septic patients.[40]

Calcitonin

- Routine calcitonin measurement in combination with pentagastrin stimulation detects MTC in a good proportion of individuals with nodular thyroid disease.[41]
- The assessment of calcitonin provides a sensitive marker for progression and aggressiveness of metastatic MTC.
- A study evaluating the value of monitoring calcitonin during follow-up for neuroendocrine tumors concluded further studies are needed to offer a recommendation of confirmation.[42]

INTERPRETATION

- Current reference ranges for antibiotic stewardship should be reviewed (Table 35.1)[36,39]
- There is currently no single test that provides an accurate diagnosis of sepsis.[1,43–45]
- There is insufficient evidence to support the use of procalcitonin-guided antibiotic therapy to decrease mortality, mechanical ventilation, or duration of antibiotic therapy for septic patients (evidence very low to moderate quality and sample power per outcome insufficient).[46]
- A study found the use of procalcitonin in guiding antimicrobial treatment in patients diagnosed with acute respiratory infections decreased exposure to antibiotics and improved patient survival.[36,37]
- A task force appointed by the American Thyroid Association provided recommendations for calcitonin: "falsely high or low serum Calcitonin levels might occur with a variety of clinical diseases other than MTC" (Box 35.1).[47]
- The task force also recommended: "in interpreting serum calcitonin data, …Calcitonin levels are markedly elevated in children under 3 years of age, especially under 6 months of age… higher in males compared with females."[47]

TABLE 35.1: REFERENCE INTERVAL FOR PROCALCITONIN AND CALCITONIN

REFERENCE INTERVAL FOR PROCALCITONIN	REFERENCE INTERVAL FOR CALCITONIN
<0.1 ug/L: Very unlikely bacterial infection	• Diagnosis of medullary thyroid cancer (MTC)
0.1–0.25 ug/L: Unlikely bacterial infection	○ <10 ng/L: Normal
>0.25–0.5 ug/L: Likely bacterial infection	○ 10–100 ng/L: Intermediate
>0.5 ug/L: Very likely bacterial infection	○ >100 ng/L: Suspected MTC
	• Follow-up monitoring
	○ <10 ng/L: No residual tumor tissue
	○ 10–150 ng/L: Possible local disease
	○ >150 ng/L: Possible distant metastasis

Sources: Data from Sager R, Kutz A, Mueller B, Schuetz P. Procalcitonin-guided diagnosis and antibiotic stewardship revisited. *BMC Med.* 2017;15(1):15; Schuetz P, Bolliger R, Merker M, et al. Procalcitonin-guided antibiotic therapy algorithms for different types of acute respiratory infections based on previous trials. *Expert Rev Anti Infect Ther.* 2018;16(7):555–564.

Box 35.1: Other Causes of Elevated Calcitonin

- Beta-blockers
- Chronic autoimmune thyroiditis
- Glucocorticoids
- Goiters
- Hypercalcemia
- Hypergastreinemia
- Omeprazole
- Papillary and follicular carcinomas
- Presence of heterophilic antibodies
- Neuroendocrine tumors
- Renal insufficiency

FOLLOW-UP

- Additional testing may be necessary based on the determined diagnosis.

PEARLS & PITFALLS

Procalcitonin

- Procalcitonin was compared to calcitonin as a promising marker for managing patients with medullary thyroid cancer. Procalcitonin was found to be useful in distinguishing medullary thyroid carcinoma in patients with current disease from those without evidence of disease. Therefore, this study recommended using procalcitonin as a complement to calcitonin to follow-up patients with a history of medullary thyroid carcinoma.[48]
- Admission procalcitonin may serve as a risk-stratifying tool for adverse events in critically ill patients.[39,49]
- Evidence suggests elevated procalcitonin in patients with acetaminophen toxicity may be related to inflammation associated with cytokine release from hepatic damage[49]
- There is growing evidence looking at the role of procalcitonin as a diagnostic marker for COVID-19 and its implications[50]
- Several studies continue to debate the utility of procalcitonin for the diagnosis of bacterial infections[51–53]
- Incorporating procalcitonin with quick sequential organ failure assessment (qSOFa) may assist in better identifying patients in certain risk groups, thereby enhancing the ability to determine risk of short-term mortality.[54]
- Studies suggest serum procalcitonin is a predictor of mortality in individuals diagnosed with ventilator-associated pnuemonia[55,56]
- Procalcitonin can offer reduction in the length of antibiotic therapy in children with upper respiratory infections, fever, and pneumonia[57]
- Procalcitonin exhibits greater specificity than other proinflammatory markers.[58]

Calcitonin

■ A study found that it was common for patients with chronic kidney disease on dialysis to have basal calcitonin levels greater than 10 mg/mL.[59]

■ There should be a high likelihood of MTC in patients with nodular disease who have hypercalcitoninemia, even with a diagnosis of Hashimoto thyroiditis.[60]

■ The identification of "macrocalcitonin" (present in the calcitonin immunoassay) may assist providers in minimizing the number of diagnostic studies and treatment needed during ongoing medullary thyroid cancer follow-up.[61]

■ After over a half century since its discovery, the specific role of calcitonin remains indefinable.[5]

PATIENT EDUCATION

■ https://medlineplus.gov/lab-tests/procalcitonin-test
■ https://labtestsonline.org/tests/procalcitonin
■ https://www.labtestsonline.org.au/learning/test-index/calcitonin
■ https://www.hormone.org/your-health-and-hormones/glands-and
-hormones-a-to-z/hormones/calcitonin

RELATED DIAGNOSES AND ICD-10 CODES

Other specified abnormal findings of blood chemistry	R79.89
Malignant neoplasm of thyroid gland	C73
Hyposecretion of calcitonin	E07.0

• Synonyms: PCT, sepsis, sepsis procalcitonin, calcitonin, thyrocalcitonin

REFERENCES

Full list of references can be accessed through Springer Publishing Company Connect™ at the following link: http://connect.springerpub.com/content/reference-book/978-0-8261 -8843-4/part/part03/toc-part/ch035

36. CALCIUM, IONIZED

Carolyn McClerking

PHYSIOLOGY REVIEW

As the fifth most abundant cation, calcium plays a vital role in the body's numerous functions, with the most important being mineralization of bone.[1] Over 99% of calcium is stored in bone and the remaining non-osseous calcium is regulated by a combination of hormones (parathyroid hormone and

1,25-dihydroxyvitamin D) and receptors (bones, kidneys, and digestive tract).[2] Non-osseous calcium exists in three physiologic states: free or ionized calcium (40%), ionic-bound (10%) and protein-bound (50%). Non-osseous calcium is important in signaling pathways as well as muscle contraction and transmission of nerve impulses. Ionized calcium levels are highly regulated and can be potentially toxic outside the physiologic range.[1,2]

OVERVIEW OF LABORATORY TEST

Ionized calcium (CPT code 82330) is the most active form of calcium. Ionized calcium is measured using ion selective electrodes.[3] Although ionized calcium has been useful in the acute clinical setting, the restrictions in sample handling requirements as well as preanalytical conditions have limited its use in the laboratory. These preanalytical conditions include such things as anticoagulant choice, pH dependence, oxygen supply, and diet.[3] The decision to use total versus ionized calcium in clinical practice has been the focus of several studies over the past several years.[4] Results suggest ionized calcium is superior and total calcium is less reliable in critically ill patients.[4,5] It is also more useful in patients with conditions listed in Box 36.1. However, experts warn against overordering of ionized calcium and considering whether daily monitoring is truly needed since evaluation of ionized calcium costs approximately 30 times more than evaluating total calcium and requires more laboratory resources.[1]

INDICATIONS

Screening

- Targeted screening of iCa may be appropriate in patients at risk for hyper/hypocalcemia from conditions where total serum calcium levels have been found to be normal, despite alterations in calcium homeostasis (Box 36.1).
- Chronic kidney disease (CKD) guidelines generally recommend using total, rather than ionized, calcium to screen most patients with glomerular filtration rate (GFR) lower than 60 mL/min/1.73 m^2 for hypercalcemia.[6,7] In patients with GFR lower than 30 to 45 mL/min/1.73 m^2, ionized calcium may be more accurate.[1] Patients with GFR lower than 15 should be screened monthly and those with GFR lower than 30 should be screened every 3 months.[7]

Diagnosis and Evaluation

- Used to evaluate individuals with signs/symptoms of hypo/hypercalcemia (Table 36.1) when total calcium levels are suspected to be inaccurate (Box 36.1).[8]

Monitoring

- Ionized calcium may be used to monitor calcium status in patients with parathyroid disease.[9,10]

Box 36.1: Disorders Where Ionized Calcium May Be More Accurate Than Total Calcium

Certain medications#

Hypoalbuminemia

Thyroidectomy-induced hypoparathyroidism

Malignancy/multiple myeloma

Multiple myeloma

Osteomalacia

Pancreatitis

Plasmapheresis, chelation, or blood transfusion

Sepsis

Severe cardiovascular disease*

Severe chronic kidney disease^

Severe metabolic derangement (pH>7.5 or <7.3)

#Cisplatin,5-fluorouracil, leucovorin, mithramycin, bisphosphonates, phosphate containing preparations, calcitonin.
*Ventricular arrhythmias, left ventricular systolic function, QTc prolongation.
^GFR less than 30 mL/min/1.73 m² and/or renal replacement therapy.

Sources: Data from Baghdadi T, Farzan M, Mortazavi S, Pirabadi N, Farhoud A. Frequency of osteomalacia in elderly patients with hip fracture. *J Orthop Spine Trauma.* 2016;2(1):e4936. https://jost.tums.ac.ir/index.php/jost/article/view/29; Hamroun A, Pekar J-D, Lionet A, et al. Ionized calcium: analytical challenges and clinical relevance. *J Lab Precis Med.* 2020;5:22. doi:10.21037/jlpm-20-60; Mirrakhimov AE. Hypercalcemia of malignancy: an update on pathogenesis and management. *N Am J Med Sci.* 2015;7(11):483–493. doi:10.4103/1947-2714.170600; Newman D, Siontis K, Chandrasekaran K, Jaffe A, Kashiwagi D. Intervention to reduce inappropriate ionized calcium ordering practices: a quality-improvement project. *Perm J.* 2015;19:49–51. doi:10.7812/TPP/14-108; Payne ME, Pierce CW, McQuoid DR, Steffens DC, Anderson JJ. Serum ionized calcium may be related to white matter lesion volumes in older adults: a pilot study. *Nutrients.* 2013;5(6):2192–2205. doi:10.3390/nu5062192; Reid IR, Birstow SM, Bolland MJ. Calcium and cardiovascular disease. *Endocrinol Metab (Seoul).* 2017;32(3):339–349. doi:10.3803/EnM.2017.32.3.339; Smith JD, Wilson S, Schneider HG. Misclassification of calcium status based on albumin-adjusted calcium: studies in a tertiary hospital setting. *Clin Chem.* 2018;64(12):1713–1722. doi:10.1373/clinchem.2018.291377; Tee MC, Holmes DT, Wiseman SM. Ionized vs serum calcium in the diagnosis and management of primary hyperparathyroidism: which is superior? *Am J Surg.* 2013;205(5):591–596; discussion 596. doi:10.1016/j.amjsurg.2013.01.017; Wang B, Li D, Gong Y, Ying B, Cheng B. Association of serum total and ionized calcium with all-cause mortality in critically ill patients with acute kidney injury. *Clinica Chimica Acta.* 2019;494:94–99. doi:10.1016/j.cca.2019.03.1616; Yap E, Roche-Recinos A, Goldwasser P. Predicting ionized hypocalcemia in critical care: an improved method based on the anion gap. *J Appl Lab Med.* 2019;5(1):4–14. doi:10.1373/jalm.2019.029314; Zagzag J, Hu MI, Fisher SB, Perrier ND. Hypercalcemia and cancer: differential diagnosis and treatment. *CA Cancer J Clin.* 2018;68(5):377–386. doi:10.3322/caac.21489.

INTERPRETATION

- The reference interval for ionized calcium is 4.4 to 5.4 mg/dL.[11]
- Underlying etiologies for levels above or below the reference limits are found in Table 36.2.

TABLE 36.1: SIGNS AND SYMPTOMS OF HYPO- OR HYPERCALCEMIA

HYPOCALCEMIA	HYPERCALCEMIA
Confusion	Abdominal pain
Depression	Bone pain
Fatigue	Coma
Muscle weakness	Constipation
Memory loss	Drowsiness
Paresthesia	Headache
QT prolongation	Hypertension
Seizures	Nausea
Tetany	Vomiting
	Weakness

Source: Data from Turner JJO. Hypercalcaemia—presentation and management. *Clin Med (Lond).* 2017;17(3):270–273. doi:10.7861/clinmedicine.17-3-270.

TABLE 36.2: ETIOLOGIES FOR ABNORMALITIES OF IONIZED CALCIUM

IONIZED HYPERCALCEMIA	IONIZED HYPOCALCEMIA
Acidotic states	Alkalotic states
Hyperparathyroidism	ESRD and hemodialysis (due to citrate)
Hypervitaminosis D	Hypoparathyroidism
Malignancy	Multiple blood transfusions
Multiple myeloma	Pancreatitis
	Pharmacotherapy with heparin
	Thiazide diuretics
	Severe critical illness (sepsis, burns)
	Vitamin D deficiency

ESRD, end-stage renal disease.

Sources: Data from Baghdadi T, Farzan M, Mortazavi S, Pirabadi N, Farhoud A. Frequency of osteomalacia in elderly patients with hip fracture. *J Orthop Spine Trauma.* 2016; 2(1):e4936. https://jost.tums.ac.ir/index.php/jost/article/view/29; Payne ME, Pierce CW, McQuoid DR, Steffens DC, Anderson JJ. Serum ionized calcium may be related to white matter lesion volumes in older adults: a pilot study. *Nutrients.* 2013;5(6):2192–2205. doi:10.3390/nu5062192; Rao LV, Snyder LM, Wallach JB. *Wallach's Interpretation of Diagnostic Tests.* Lippincott Williams & Wilkins; 2021; Reid IR, Birstow SM, Bolland MJ. Calcium and cardiovascular disease. *Endocrinol Metab (Seoul).* 2017;32(3):339–349. doi:10.3803/EnM.2017.32.3.339; Tee MC, Holmes DT, Wiseman SM. Ionized vs serum calcium in the diagnosis and management of primary hyperparathyroidism: which is superior? *Am J Surg.* 2013;205(5):591–596; discussion 596. doi:10.1016/j.amjsurg.2013.01.017; Wang B, Li D, Gong Y, Ying B, Cheng B. Association of serum total and ionized calcium with all-cause mortality in critically ill patients with acute kidney injury. *Clinica Chimica Acta.* 2019;494:94–99. doi:10.1016/j.cca.2019.03.1616; Zagzag J, Hu MI, Fisher SB, Perrier ND. Hypercalcemia and cancer: differential diagnosis and treatment. *CA Cancer J Clin.* 2018;68(5):377–386. doi:10.3322/caac.21489.

FOLLOW-UP

- Consider an electrocardiogram to evaluate heart function.[12]
- Calcium homeostasis is largely influenced by kidney function and levels of phosphorus, vitamin D, and magnesium. Therefore, evaluation of estimated

GFR, vitamin D, phosphorus, and magnesium will help clarify the clinical picture when calcium levels are abnormal.[12]

■ Urine calcium, phosphate, and cAMP may be used to determine etiology of persistent hypocalcemia.[13]

PEARLS & PITFALLS

■ A total calcium/iCa ratio is sometimes used to monitor for citrate accumulation during continuous venovenous hemofiltration (CVVH). Citrate accumulation causes a rise in the ratio. However, in one study, metabolic alkalosis/acidosis, hyper/hypophosphatemia, hypo/ hyperalbuminemia, and severity of critical illness were found to also influence the ratio, so elevations may not be specific to citrate accumulation.[14]

■ There are studies that question the rationale for measurement of iCa and whether its use meaningfully influences patient outcomes.[15] However, the association of iCa with health outcomes has been a focus of recent research:
  ● Patients admitted with iCa lower than 4.8 mg/dL had an increased risk for intubation.[16]
  ● Decreased iCa was associated with risk of hematoma expansion in patients with hypertensive intracerebral hemorrhage.[17]
  ● Decreased iCa was a major predictor of mortality for critically ill patients with acute kidney injury.[18,19]
  ● An elevated iCa level in patients requiring cardiopulmonary resuscitation was associated with a more likely return of spontaneous circulation (ROSC).[20]
  ● Increased iCa levels in patients undergoing congenital cardiac surgery and cardiopulmonary bypass were found to have longer lengths of stay in the intensive care unit.[21]

■ Patients with cancer who present with an elevated calcium should be evaluated immediately as this form of secondary hypercalcemia can be fatal if not treated appropriately.[22,23]

PATIENT EDUCATION

■ https://account.allinahealth.org/library/content/49/150492

RELATED DIAGNOSES AND ICD-10 CODES

Other specified abnormal findings of blood chemistry	E83.51

REFERENCES

Full list of references can be accessed through Springer Publishing Company Connect™ at the following link: http://connect.springerpub.com/content/reference-book/978-0-8261 -8843-4/part/part03/toc-part/ch036

37. CANCER ANTIGEN 125

Karen Hande and Taylor Butler

PHYSIOLOGY REVIEW

The human cancer antigen 125 (CA 125) is a large transmembrane glycoprotein derived from both coelomic (pericardium, pleura, peritoneum) and müllerian (fallopian tube, endometrial, endocervical) epithelia.[1,2] Also known as mucin 16 (MUC16), the CA 125 protein in humans is encoded by the *MUC16* gene. CA 125 is overexpressed in epithelial ovarian cancer cells and plays a major role in the pathogenesis of ovarian cancer.[3]

Ninety-five percent of ovarian malignancies are epithelial while the remainder arise from other ovarian cell types (germ cell tumors, sex cord-stromal tumors).[4] High-grade epithelial ovarian, fallopian tube, and peritoneal carcinomas share clinical behavior and treatment and possible shared pathogenesis.[5] This group of malignancies, considered as one clinical entity, is termed epithelial ovarian cancer (EOC). CA 125 is the only biomarker recommended for clinical use in the diagnosis and management of EOC.[6] While CA 125 may detect EOC, it does not determine if a woman has it.

OVERVIEW OF LABORATORY TESTS

Laboratory evaluation of cancer antigen 125 status can be assessed by the quantitative immunoassay from blood serum CA 125 (C56.9). CA 125 increases when a woman has EOC. A number of noncancerous conditions can also cause elevations.[6]

INDICATIONS

Screening

- The United States Preventive Services Task Force (USPSTF)[7] recommends against screening for EOC in asymptomatic women who are not known to have a high-risk hereditary cancer syndrome.
- There is moderate or high certainty that EOC screening has no net benefit or that the harms outweigh the benefits.[7,8]
- All screening strategies are associated with a high rate of false-positive tests and a risk of harm from invasive testing.[7,8]
- Adequate evidence supports that screening for ovarian cancer does not reduce ovarian cancer mortality.[7,8]
- After reviewing a family history to identify high- versus average-risk women, high-risk individuals (including those with BRCA mutations) should have targeted EOC screening that includes the serum tumor marker, CA125, and vaginal ultrasonography.[7,8]

Diagnosis and Evaluation

- Following a full clinical assessment, measurement of serum CA 125 is routinely used to aid diagnosis but is not diagnostic in isolation.[7,8]
- Patients with ovarian cancer confined to the ovary may have few or no symptoms, making clinical diagnosis of early EOC more difficult. Symptoms are most commonly seen with advanced disease.[9]
- In comparison to women in the general population, women with EOC, even in the early stages,[10-14] are much more likely to experience abdominal bloating, pelvic or abdominal pain, difficulty eating or feeling full quickly, and urinary frequency or urgency.[9,10,15]
- Women who experience these symptoms almost daily for more than 2 weeks should see a women's health clinician. Early-stage diagnosis is associated with an improved prognosis.[9]
- In advanced EOC, ascites and abdominal masses lead to increased abdominal girth, bloating, nausea, anorexia, dyspepsia, and early satiety. Extension of disease across the diaphragm to the pleural cavities can produce pleural effusions and the development of respiratory symptoms. Patients may become aware of an abdominal or nodal mass either in the inguinal region, axillae, or the supraclavicular fossa.[9]

Monitoring

- Serial tests should be done by using the same laboratory to monitor CA 125 levels.[6]
- The role of CA 125 in surveillance of EOC remains controversial.
- National Comprehensive Cancer Network (NCCN) guidelines recommend monitoring women who have completed treatment for EOC using CA 125, or other tumor markers, at every visit, if these markers were elevated at the initial presentation.[16]
- The Society of Gynecologic Oncology (SGO) suggests CA 125 be considered "optional" in the surveillance of patients with EOC.[17]

INTERPRETATION

- Normal value for CA 125 assay is 35 units/mL or less.
- Absolute CA 125 cutoffs remain clinically arbitrary, particularly for premenopausal patients. Some experts suggest that normal values may range from 20 to 200 units/mL; these variations take into consideration elevations in serum due to a variety of benign and malignant gynecologic and non-gynecologic conditions that can elevate CA 125 leading to false-positive results.[6] See Table 37.1 for clinical cutoffs for referral.
- CA 125 testing alone has a low sensitivity, particularly for early-stage ovarian cancer, and a low overall specificity. The specificity is particularly low in premenopausal patients.[6]
- CA 125 sensitivity for ovarian cancer ranges from 69% to 87%, and the specificity ranges from 81% to 93% in postmenopausal women with an adnexal mass.[6]

TABLE 37.1: REFERRAL OF WOMAN WITH A PELVIC MASS TO A GYNECOLOGIC ONCOLOGIST: AMERICAN COLLEGE OF OBSTETRICIANS AND GYNECOLOGISTS GUIDELINES	
REFER IF ANY ARE PRESENT	
Premenopausal women	Very elevated CA 125 level
	Ascites
	Evidence of abdominal or distant metastases
Postmenopausal women	Elevated CA 125 level
	Ascites
	Nodular or fixed pelvic mass
	Evidence of abdominal or distant metastases

Source: Data from American College of Obstetricians and Gynecologists. *Evaluation and management of adenxal masses.* https://www.acog.org/clinical/clinical-guidance/practice-bulletin/articles/2016/11/evaluation-and-management-of-adnexal-masses

- CA 125 sensitivity was 50% to 74%, and the specificity was 69% to 78% in premenopausal women with an adnexal mass.[6]
- CA 125 may vary (35 units/mL or more) with other factors in women without ECO such as age 60 years or older and a history of cigarette smoking.[18]
- CA 125 is significantly less likely to be elevated in women who are obese (body mass index 30 kg/m^2 or more) or who have had a hysterectomy.[6]
- There can be many other malignant and nonmalignant conditions that can cause an elevated CA 125 level. See Table 37.2 for a list of these conditions.

FOLLOW-UP

- Women in whom there is a high suspicion of EOC should be referred to a gynecologic oncologist.[18]
- Ultrasonography of the abdomen and pelvis is usually the first imaging investigation recommended for women in whom EOC is suspected.[16]
- National Comprehensive Cancer Network Guidelines recommend women with an initial elevated CA 125 level to repeat CA 125 level or other tumor makers.[16]

PEARLS & PITFALLS

- There is no evidence that supports the impact of serial CA 125 values on overall survival.[19,20]
- CA 125 did not reduce mortality due to ovarian cancer when studied as a possible screening test in the randomized Prostate, Lung, Colon, Ovarian Cancer (PLCO) Screening Trial.[21]
- CA 125 is the most commonly used laboratory test for the evaluation of EOC, but the test has several shortcomings. The diagnostic performance of CA 125 is limited, particularly for early-stage disease and is mainly useful in postmenopausal women.[6]

TABLE 37.2: CONDITIONS ASSOCIATED WITH AN ELEVATED CA 125

GYNECOLOGIC CANCER	BENIGN GYNECOLOGIC CONDITIONS	NONGYNECOLOGIC CANCERS	NONGYNECOLOGIC CONDITIONS
Endometrial	Adenomyosis	Breast	Ascites
Epithelial ovarian	Benign ovarian neoplasm	Colon	Appendicular abscess
Fallopian tube	Endometriosis	Gallbladder	Cirrhosis and other liver disease
Primary peritoneal	Functional ovarian cysts	Hemotologic malignancies	Colitis
	Meig syndrome	Liver	Cystic fibrosis
	Menstruation	Lung	Diverticulitis
	Ovarian hyperstimulation	Pancreas	Heart failure
	Pelvic inflammatory disease		Myocardial infarction
	Pregnancy		Myocardiopathy
	Uterine leiomyomas		Pancreatitis
			Pleural effusion
			Pneumonia
			Pulmonary embolism
			Recent surgery
			Renal insufficiency
			Sarcoidosis
			Systemic lupus erythematosus
			Tuberculosis peritonitis
			Urinary tract infection

Sources: Data from Buamah P. Benign conditions associated with raised serum CA-125 concentration. *J Surg Oncol.* 2000;75(4): 264–265. doi:10.1002/1096-9098(200012)75:4<264::aid-jso7>3.0.co;2-q; Miralles C, Orea M, España P, et al. Cancer antigen 125 associated with multiple benign and malignant pathologies. *Ann Surg Oncol.* 2003;10(2):150–154. doi:10.1245/aso.2003.05.015; Moss EL, Hollingworth J, Reynolds TM. The role of CA125 in clinical practice. *J Clin Pathol.* 2005;58(3):308–312. doi:10.1136/ jcp.2004.018077.

- Its utility to detect early disease is questionable as it is elevated only in about 50% of patients with the International Federation of Gynecology and Obstetrics stage I disease.[6]
- In advanced EOC disease, CA 125 is elevated in about 85% of patients.[6]
- There is also a growing body of evidence that CA 125 is being used as a marker for heart failure and pancreatic cancer.[22,23]

PATIENT EDUCATION

- https://www.ucsfhealth.org/education/taking-charge-how-is-ovarian-cancer-diagnosed
- https://www.ucsfhealth.org/education/taking-charge-screening-for-ovarian-cancer
- https://www.nccn.org/patients/guidelines/content/PDF/ovarian-patient.pdf

RELATED DIAGNOSES AND ICD-10 CODES

Screening for malignant neoplasm of ovary	Z12.73
Personal history of malignant neoplasm of ovary	Z85.43
Personal history of malignant neoplasm of other female genital organs	Z85.44
Generalized intra-abdominal and pelvic swelling, mass, and lump	R19.07
Elevated cancer antigen 125	R97.1

REFERENCES

Full list of references can be accessed through Springer Publishing Company Connect™ at the following link: http://connect.springerpub.com/content/reference-book/978-0-8261-8843-4/part/part03/toc-part/ch037

---

38. CARBAMAZEPINE/TEGRETOL LEVELS

Carol D. Campbell

PHYSIOLOGY REVIEW

Carbamazepine, 5H-dibenz(bf)azepine-5-carboxamide, an iminostilbene compound also identified by its most common brand name, Tegretol, is one of the most frequently prescribed anticonvulsant medications.[1,2] It has U.S. Food and Drug Administration (FDA) approval for the treatment of epilepsy and other seizure disorders, trigeminal neuralgia, and bipolar disorder. Carbamazepine exerts its primary effects through production of frequency- and voltage-dependent blockade of sodium channels. It extensively induces the CYP450 system, primarily by CYP3A4, but also CYP3A5, CYP1A2, CYP2B6, and CYP2C9.[3] It is metabolized into carbamazepine-10,11-epoxide, an active metabolite by CYP3A4. Carbamazepine is also a powerful inducer of auto-induction and hetero hepatic enzymes that are extensively metabolized in the liver and cause several clinically relevant medication interactions. Auto-induction results in carbamazepine's metabolism becoming more effective as the duration of treatment increases; its half-life is initially 26 to 65 hours but after several weeks decreases to 12 to 17 hours.

OVERVIEW OF LABORATORY TESTS

Laboratory evaluation of carbamazepine can be assessed by carbamazepine, total, serum (CPT code 80156); carbamazepine, free, serum (CPT code 80157); and carbamazepine-10, 11 epoxide, serum/plasma (CPT code 80161). In most cases, a carbamazepine total serum level should be ordered. A carbamazepine free serum level should be ordered with suspected medication interactions, when making medication dosage adjustments in uremic patients, and when the total carbamazepine level is within the expected reference range, but the patient is experiencing side effects.[4] A carbamazepine epoxide metabolite level should be ordered if signs of toxicity are present.

INDICATIONS

Screening

- There is no evidence recommending universal screening/monitoring of carbamazepine levels in the general population.
- The U.S. FDA recommends genetic pre-screening for the HLA-B*15:02 allele before prescribing carbamazepine to patients of Asian descent as those positive for HLA-B*15:02 may be at increased risk for Stevens-Johnson Syndrome/toxic epidermal necrolysis (SJS/TEN).[5]
- Targeted screening is recommended for patients receiving carbamazepine treatment to optimize treatment outcomes, to provide the clinician with an indicator for adjusting medication dosages based on serum reference ranges, to help in assessing adherence to treatment in the context of breakthrough or uncontrolled seizures, and in diagnosing toxicity.[4,6]

Diagnosis and Evaluation

- Carbamazepine therapy should be evaluated in the treatment of epilepsy and other seizure disorders, trigeminal neuralgia, and bipolar disorder.[4]
- Long-term use of carbamazepine is associated with aplastic anemia, bone marrow depression, exfoliative dermatitis, hepatitis, hyponatremia, hypothyroidism, leukopenia, neuroleptic malignant syndrome, renal disease, Stevens-Johnson syndrome, and toxic epidermal necrolysis.[1,3]
- Signs and symptoms of carbamazepine toxicity include hyponatremia, hypotension, leukopenia, respiratory depression, seizures, stupor, and possible coma.[1,3]

Monitoring

- High levels of evidence (systematic reviews) recommend therapeutic drug monitoring (TDM) for anticonvulsants such as carbamazepine.[2,6,7]
- Monitor serum levels for achievement of a steady state after initiating carbamazepine therapy, changing dosages, switching to another medication formulation, substituting a generic brand, and after starting or stopping a CYP3A4 inducer or inhibitor.[4,6]
- Monitoring of trough levels is recommended to maintain consistency.[4]
- TDM may be particularly beneficial with children and adolescents, older adults, in pregnancy, in individuals with intellectual disabilities, and in individuals with substance abuse disorders.[6]

- Review Table 38.1 for additional information and monitoring considerations.

INTERPRETATION

- The generally accepted total carbamazepine reference interval is between 4 and 12 mcg/mL. However, response to carbamazepine is variable, and reference ranges should be individualized for each patient as they are not always correlated with therapeutic response.[4]
- Presently, there is a lack of agreement on toxicity references. Table 38.2 provides the most used guidelines and evidence for interpretation of carbamazepine levels.

FOLLOW-UP

- Refer to Table 38.1.

PEARLS & PITFALLS

- Absorption of carbamazepine is slow and often unpredictable.[8]

TABLE 38.1: RECOMMENDED MONITORING FOR CARBAMAZEPINE THERAPY

Initial monitoring	CBC, LFTs, renal function, electrolytes, thyroid function: T_3, T_4, TSH, urinalysis, BUN, height, weight
Monthly monitoring for 3 months then annually	CBC, LFTs, renal function, electrolytes, thyroid function: T_3, T_4, TSH, urinalysis, BUN, height, weight
Carbamazepine monitoring	Check carbamazepine level • If initiating therapy, every 2 to 4 weeks for 2 months, then every 3 to 6 months during therapy • If initiating carbamazepine therapy, changing dosages, switching to another medication formulation, substituting a generic brand, and after starting or stopping a CYP3A4 inducer or inhibitor • If nonadherence, side effects, or toxicity suspected

BUN, blood urea nitrogen; CBC, complete blood count; LFTs, liver function tests; TSH, thyroid-stimulating hormone.

Source: Stahl SM. *Stahl's Essential Psychopharmacology: Prescriber's Guide.* 7th ed. Cambridge University Press; 2021; Hiemke C, Bergemann N, Clement HW, et al. Consensus guidelines for therapeutic drug monitoring in neuropsychopharmacology: update 2017. *Pharmacopsychiatry.* 2018;51(1-02):9–62. doi:10.1055/s-0043-116492.

TABLE 38.2: INTERPRETATION OF CARBAMAZEPINE

TEST	REFERENCE INTERVAL
Total carbamazepine	4–12 mcg/mL
Toxicity	>12 mcg/mL
Free carbamazepine	1–3 mcg/mL
Toxicity	>4 mcg/mL
Carbamazepine epoxide metabolite	0.4–4 mcg/mL
Toxicity	>8 mcg/mL

- Black box warnings for carbamazepine include aplastic anemia, agranulocytosis, SJS, and TEN.[1]
- The most common side effects of carbamazepine include ataxia, diarrhea, dizziness, drowsiness, headache, nausea, rash, and vomiting.[3,8]
- Coadministration of other anticonvulsant medications can significantly increase serum carbamazepine levels.[9]
- Carbamazepine dosages correlate poorly with serum levels. Dosages and serum levels also vary depending on sex, age, or race (i.e., females, children, and individuals of African descent often require increased dosages compared with Caucasian males to reach comparable serum levels).[10]
- Carbamazepine should be avoided in the first trimester of pregnancy as it can cause growth deficiencies, fetal malformations, and developmental delays. Although, with its teratogenicity being considered significantly lower than other anticonvulsants, it is a preferred anticonvulsant in pregnancy.[11]
- Folate supplementation should be initiated in females of childbearing age with those on carbamazepine therapy receiving at least 0.4 mg per day.[12]
- Carbamazepine's mild anticholinergic properties increases the risk of delirium in the older adult population, which can lead to constipation, increased intraocular pressure, and urinary retention.[3,13]

PATIENT EDUCATION

- https://www.mskcc.org/pdf/cancer-care/patient-education/carbamazepine-01
- https://www.appi.org/docs/dulcan/APA-Publishing_Dulcan_Understanding-Medications_md12_Carbamazepine.pdf

RELATED DIAGNOSES AND ICD-10 CODES

Complex partial seizures	G40.209
Generalized tonic-clonic seizures	G40.3
Trigeminal neuralgia	G50.0
Bipolar disorder • current episode, acute mania • current episode, mixed	• F31.10 • F31.60

REFERENCES

Full list of references can be accessed through Springer Publishing Company Connect™ at the following link: http://connect.springerpub.com/content/reference-book/978-0-8261-8843-4/part/part03/toc-part/ch038

39. CARBOXYHEMOGLOBIN

Lynne M. Hutchison

PHYSIOLOGY REVIEW

Carboxyhemoglobin (COHb) is formed by combining carbon monoxide (CO) and hemoglobin (Hgb).[1] Carbon monoxide is an odorless, colorless gas which can rapidly diffuse through the alveolar membrane and has a 200 to 300 times greater ability to bind with hemoglobin than oxygen. Higher than normal levels of CO cause a leftward shift in the position of the oxyhemoglobin dissociation curve, which reduces oxygen transport capacity, leading to reduction in oxygen released in peripheral tissues.[2] In addition, when CO displaces oxygen at the binding sites, the hemoglobin molecule is changed to more tightly bind any remaining oxygen. Less oxygen is available for tissue cell use. This combination of events results in hypoxemia.[3]

OVERVIEW OF LABORATORY TESTS

This test is used to measure the amount of carboxyhemoglobin (CPT code 82375)[4] in the blood, which is an indirect measure of carbon monoxide (CO) poisoning. The specimen, if collected in a lavender (EDTA) or green (heparin) top tube, is relatively stable for up to 2 weeks.[5] Blood collection sample source can be venous or arterial. It is also important to collect the blood specimen before starting oxygen therapy if possible.[5]

INDICATIONS

Screenings
- Universal or targeted screenings are not recommended.[6]

Diagnosis and Evaluation
Obtaining a COHb level is appropriate in patients with suspected CO poisoning or unexplained lethargy, headache with nausea, vertigo, coma, or convulsions.[7] This test is routinely ordered in patients who have been exposed to smoke, exhaust fumes, fires, and chemical explosions.[7]

Monitoring
- Abnormal carboxyhemoglobin test results should be followed up with repeat levels. Repeated testing is often ordered to evaluate the effectiveness of treatment therapies.[6]

INTERPRETATION

- Reference intervals vary per diagnostic laboratory setting and are reported as the percent of CO saturated Hgb. Ranges also vary based on smoking status. See Table 39.1 for reference intervals.

TABLE 39.1: REFERENCE INTERVAL(S) FOR CARBOXYHEMOGLOBIN

Nonsmoker	<2% of total Hgb
Average smoker	4–5% of total Hgb
Heavy smoker	8–12% of total Hgb
Potentially toxic	>15% of total Hgb

Source: Quest Diagnostics. Carboxyhemoglobin. Quest Diagnostics website. https://testdirectory.questdiagnostics.com/test/test-detail/309/carboxyhemoglobin-blood?cc=MASTER.

TABLE 39.2: RELATIONSHIP OF SYMPTOMS OF CARBON MONOXIDE POISONING TO LEVEL OF Hgb SATURATION

CARBOXYHEMOGLOBIN RESULT	SYMPTOMS*
10%	Slight difficulty breathing, may be asymptomatic
20%	Throbbing headache, dyspnea, nausea
30%	Impaired mental judgment, irritable, vision changes
40%	Confusion, weakness, lethargy, syncope
50%	Loss of consciousness, seizures
60%	Comatose, cardiopulmonary failure
>60%	Death

* Symptoms and outcomes do not always match level of carbon monoxide (CO) saturation of hemoglobin.

Source: Pagana KD, Pagana TJ. *Mosby's Manual of Diagnostic and Laboratory Tests.* 6th ed. Elsevier; 2018; Evidence-Based Medicine Consult. Lab test: Carboxyhemoglobin. EBM Consult Website. https://www.ebmconsult.com/articles/lab-test-carboxyhemoglobin-level.

- There are published references linking the percent of CO saturation of Hgb to symptoms and severity, although Level 2 evidence does not exist. Commonly used symptom-based guidelines are reviewed in Table 39.2.

FOLLOW-UP

- Consider ordering arterial blood gases, toxicology screens, pregnancy testing, and cardiac biomarkers (troponin, creatine kinase MB isoenzyme [CK-MB])[5] as part of a symptom-based workup. Lactic acid levels are used to differentiate CO poisoning from cyanide poisoning.[9]

PEARLS & PITFALLS

- Obtain a thorough patient history for possible exposures to CO.[5]
- Fetal hemoglobin has a higher affinity for CO and is typically about 30% higher than maternal levels.[8]
- Be cognizant that symptoms and outcomes do not always match level of CO saturation of hemoglobin. CO will be present in smokers. There is no difference

in laboratory results based on age, smoking status, or sex. The main clinical utility of COHb is determining the presence of carbon monoxide exposure.[10]

■ Pulse oximetry is not an accurate measure of carboxyhemoglobin levels.[11,12]

■ Total blood carbon monoxide (TBCM) is another viable alternative to carboxyhemoglobin for measuring CO. Some evidence suggests that TBCM has greater validity as a diagnostic marker for CO and also has more sample stability in various storage conditions.[13]

PATIENT EDUCATION

■ https://www.cdc.gov/co/pdfs/Flyer_Danger.pdf
■ https://www.cdc.gov/co/guidelines.htm
■ https://www.cdc.gov/co/faqs.htm

RELATED DIAGNOSES AND ICD-10 CODES

Poisoning (accidental) by carbon monoxide	V93.89[14]
Toxic effect of carbon monoxide	T58.8X2A[15]

REFERENCES

Full list of references can be accessed through Springer Publishing Company Connect™ at the following link: http://connect.springerpub.com/content/reference-book/978-0-8261 -8843-4/part/part03/toc-part/ch039

40. CARCINOEMBRYONIC ANTIGEN

Taylor Butler and Karen Hande

PHYSIOLOGY REVIEW

Carcinoembryonic antigen, better known as CEA, is an oncofetal antigen that is most commonly seen in humans at birth (Figure 40.1). CEA levels tend to be minimal or absent in most adults.[1] During fetal growth, CEA is responsible for the promotion of maternal tolerance toward the embryo and the cell proliferation and differentiation of the fetus.[2] Gold and colleagues demonstrated in 1965 that CEA was elevated in animal models exposed to colonic carcinomata, which started the exploration of utilizing CEA as a tumor marker.[3] This tumor-specific antigen is produced by the primary tumor in the blood. CEA inhibits the regulation of cancer cell growth and suppresses pro-inflammatory cytokines to decrease host defenses.[2] High levels of CEA may indicate progressive disease because CEA protects circulating cancer cells from death, inhibits protective macrophages in the liver, and upregulates adhesion of micrometastasis.[4]

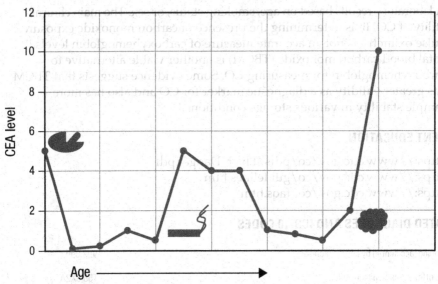

FIGURE 40.1. Carcinoembryonic antigen (CEA) physiology.

OVERVIEW OF LABORATORY TESTS

Laboratory evaluation of CEA status can be assessed by carcinoembryonic antigen (CPT code 82378). CEA may be detected in human sera and is usually a quantitative immunoassay from blood serum. These are usually conducted using electrochemiluminescence immunoassays and amperometric immunoassays. It may also be tested in body fluids and tissue biopsies. It is recommended that the same method is used to serially monitor patients, in combination with a history, physical, and other diagnostic procedures (e.g., colonoscopy or computed topography of the chest, abdomen, and pelvis).[5]

INDICATIONS

Screening

- The United States Preventive Services Task Force (USPSTF) has no recommendations for the routine utilization of CEA for universal cancer screening.[6]
- The National Comprehensive Cancer Network (NCCN) provides no recommendation for utilizing CEA for the screening of colorectal cancer.[7]
- NCCN provides no recommendation for CEA screenings with a high risk of colorectal cancer (e.g., Lynch syndrome, familial adenomatous polyposis, BRCA mutations, etc.)[7,8]
- It is not recommended to use CEA for a single diagnostic method or screening because of its low sensitivity (46%) and specificity.[9]

Diagnosis and Evaluation

There are up to 49 different differential diagnoses for CEA elevations. These include malignant and nonmalignant conditions. The most common malignant condition is colorectal adenocarcinoma, but CEA may be elevated with lung cancer, medullary thyroid cancer, gastric cancer, and pancreatic cancer, among others.[5] There is emerging evidence that CEA can be combined with other tests to increase the diagnostic specificity and sensitivity, but more evidence is needed to determine applicability in clinical practice.[10] A colon score, comprised of CEA, cancer antigen 19-9 (CA19-9), cytokeratin 1 (CK1), and mucin-1 (MUC1), was shown to be increased in patients with active colon adenocarcinoma versus benign growth and healthy controls. Some nonmalignant conditions that may elevate CEA include adenoma, infection, peptic ulcer disease, inflammatory bowel disease, cirrhosis, pancreatitis, hypothyroidism, and biliary obstruction. Social history is important to assess as smoking may lead to mild elevations of CEA.[5]

Monitoring

- American Society of Clinical Oncology/Cancer Care Ontario and NCCN recommend monitoring CEA levels at the diagnosis of colorectal cancer and every 3 to 6 months for 2 years, and then every 6 months for years 2 to 5.[7,11]
- The NCCN recommends against continuing CEA levels 5 years after curative surgery.[12,13]
- Choosing Wisely and the Society of Surgical Oncology recommends CEA as the only routine blood work utilized during surveillance of resected colorectal cancer.[14] Levels should return back to normal within 1 to 4 months after removal of the malignant tissue.

INTERPRETATION

- Presently, there is a lack of guideline recommendations on cutoff values for further screening of CEA. Table 40.1 provides recommendations based on the results from the Cochrane Database analysis on CEA surveillance monitoring and a review article by Perkins et al. on serum tumor markers.[15,16]
- The sensitivity for early colon cancer risk is low (4% at stage 1) but increases with an increasing stage of disease. CEA has a pooled sensitivity of 68% to 82% for colorectal cancer recurrence depending on the cutoff, but has a high specificity with a cutoff of 10 ng/mL.[16]

FOLLOW-UP

- Serial CEA elevations should be followed up with a physical examination, colonoscopy, and CT with contrast of the chest/abdomen/pelvis; consider a PET/CT if workup is negative or as clinically indicated[12,13]
- Testing CEA can also be clinically useful for assessing the effectiveness of treatments including chemotherapy and radiation.

TABLE 40.1: INTERPRETATION OF CARCINOEMBRYONIC ANTIGEN*		
NORMAL	**ACTIVE SMOKER**	**MALIGNANCY****
0–2.5 ng/mL	0–5 ng/mL	>5 ng/mL

*Laboratory value alone cannot exclude malignancy.

**Indicates need for further testing, cannot be used alone.

PEARLS & PITFALLS

- CEA surveillance has shown in several large studies that it may identify recurrence of colorectal cancer (CRC) earlier but has failed to show a survival benefit to patients with CRC in remission.[17,18]
- A retrospective analysis of CEA surveillance at Memorial Sloan-Kettering Cancer Center (MSKCC) showed that 49% of patients had false-positive elevations of CEA. In this study, 46% had a true recurrence of CRC and 5% had a new primary malignancy.[19]
- The pooled sensitivity analysis of 42 studies looking at the diagnostic value of CEA was 46%, which signals low value as a screening tool.[20]
- Prognostic value of elevated CEA levels may indicate a poorer prognosis in CRC.[20]
- Other malignancies that may have CEA elevations include breast, lung, gastric, pancreatic, bladder, thyroid, head and neck, lymphoma, melanoma, and hepatic cancers.[15]

PATIENT EDUCATION

- https://www.healthline.com/health/cea
- https://www.medlineplus.gov/lab-tests/cea-test

RELATED DIAGNOSES AND ICD-10 CODES

| Malignant neoplasm of the rectum | C20 |
| Malignant neoplasm of the colon, unspecified | C18.9 |

REFERENCES

Full list of references can be accessed through Springer Publishing Company Connect™ at the following link: http://connect.springerpub.com/content/reference-book/978-0-8261-8843-4/part/part03/toc-part/ch040

41. CATECHOLAMINE TESTING

Lisa Ward

PATHOPHYSIOLOGY REVIEW

Catecholamines (cats) are produced in the adrenal medulla and sympathetic nervous system and released into the blood in response to physical or emotional stress.[1] The primary catecholamines include dopamine, epinephrine (adrenaline), and norepinephrine (noradrenaline). These three chemicals help to transmit nerve impulses in the brain, increase glucose release for energy, and dilate the bronchioles and the pupils. In addition, norepinephrine (norepi) also constricts blood vessels, causing increased blood pressure, and epinephrine (epi) increases heart rate and metabolism.[2,3] The systemically circulating fraction of the catecholamines is derived almost exclusively from the adrenal medulla. After the catecholamines are released, they are quickly broken down into inactive compounds and excreted in the urine (Figure 41.1). Metanephrines (metanephrine and normetanephrine) are the stable, inactive metabolites of the catecholamines epinephrine and norepinephrine, respectively.[3-5] Metanephrine's precursor is epinephrine and normetanephrine's (NMN) precursor is norepinephrine (Figure 41.1).

Normally, catecholamines and metanephrines are present in the body in small, fluctuating amounts that will only increase slightly during and shortly after a stressful situation[2-4] However, catecholamines and metanephrines can significantly increase in plasma and urine in patients with rare catecholamine-secreting tumors. Catecholamine-secreting tumors that arise from the adrenal medulla are called pheochromocytomas (pheos), whereas those originating from the sympathetic ganglia are called paragangliomas (PGL).[2-5]

OVERVIEW OF LABORATORY TESTS

In evaluating for pheos or PGL, laboratory evaluation of plasma-free fractionated metanephrines (CPT code 83835) and/or 24-hour urine metanephrines (CPT code 004234) are most often used. The 24-hour urine collection for metanephrines should include measurement of urinary creatinine (CPT code 82570)

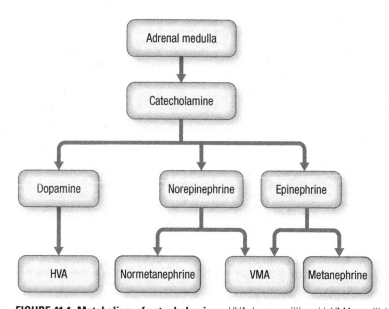

FIGURE 41.1. Metabolism of catecholamines. HVA, homovanillic acid; VMA, vanillylmandelic acid.

Sources: Data from Labtestsonline.org. 2021. Metanephrines. [online]. https://labtestsonline.org/tests/plasma-free-metanephrines; Lexicomp Online. Lab Tests and Diagnostic Procedures. UpToDate, Inc; 2019, February 25, 2021.

to verify an adequate collection.[6–8] Current practice guidelines recommend plasma samples be collected in the supine position after 30 minutes of rest;[7,9–11] however, some recent studies have shown that testing done in the seated position provided equivalent results and can be used if the patient is unable to lie supine.[9–11] A 24-hour urine metanephrines test may be difficult in children due to their inability to follow collection instructions for the entire 24-hour period. Therefore, use of plasma metanephrines to diagnose pheos in children is the preferred test.[12]

There is some evidence that plasma metanephrines are more sensitive than urine metanephrines when diagnosing pheo/PGL;[7] however, until there is data available directly comparing plasma and urine measurements, there can be no recommendation that one test is superior to the other.[7] A 24-hour urine testing measures the total amount of metanephrines released and may detect excess production that is missed with a blood test, especially if the excess is episodic.[2] Often the choice for the initial test is based on patient convenience. The advantages and disadvantages of plasma and urine metanephrine testing is summarized in Table 41.1.

TABLE 41.1: COMPARISON OF PLASMA AND URINE CATECHOLAMINES/METANEPHRINES

FACTOR	PLASMA ADVANTAGES	PLASMA DISADVANTAGES	URINE ADVANTAGES	URINE DISADVANTAGES
Clinical utility	Reflects free metanephrines produced by tumor			Does not reflect metanephrines produced by tumor
Sample collection	Single sample, more convenient	Sample must be collected on ice, centrifuged, and frozen within hours of collection	Sample collected as outpatient	24-hour collection is inconvenient to patients. Often not collected reliably. Urine metanephrines are more stable and can be processed with no urgency in an unpreserved container
Measurement		More difficult to measure than urine because plasma matrix is more complex than urine metanephrines	Less challenging to measure than plasma metanephrines	
Preparation	Easier to control diet and medication for single lab test	Sample should be collected in supine position and fasting state	Patient does not need to fast	Harder to control diet and medications over 24-hour period
Utility in CKD	Can be used in CKD			Test not useful in CKD

CKD, chronic kidney disease.

Source: Data from Davison AS, Jones DM, Ruthven S, Helliwell T, Shore SL. Clinical evaluation and treatment of phaeochromocytoma. *Ann Clin Biochem.* 2018;55(1):34–48. doi:10.1177/0004563217739931.

TABLE 41.2: EXAMPLE PATIENT PREPARATION FOR PLASMA/URINE METANEPHRINE AND CATECHOLAMINE TESTING	
1 week prior	Discontinue drugs; release epi, norepi, or dopamine or hinder their metabolism (i.e., methyldopa, bronchodilators, decongestants, appetite suppressants)
1–3 days prior	Hold medications (if medically safe to do so)
12 hours prior	Unless the purpose is drug monitoring, discontinue epi, norepi, or dopamine injections/infusions
8–12 hours prior	• Avoid caffeine, walnuts, chocolate, avocados, bananas, citrus, cheese • Minimize stress • Refrain from smoking • Refrain from exercise

Source: Data from Lexicomp Online, Lab Tests and Diagnostic Procedures. UpToDate, Inc; 2019, February 25, 2021.

Urine catecholamines can be assessed with testing 24-hour urine catecholamines (CPT code 286161) and are recommended over plasma catecholamines testing since plasma catecholamines are chemically labile and specimens must be handled carefully due to rapid metabolism and rapid oxidation upon exposure to air.[3,5] Additionally, just the stress of having blood drawn can increase catecholamine serum levels and plasma catecholamine levels may only be elevated during a period of paroxysm hypertension episode.[3] Just like metanephrine testing, the 24-hour urine collection for catecholamines should include measurement of urinary creatinine (CPT code 82570) to verify an adequate collection.[6–8] If indicated, plasma catecholamines can be assessed with testing fractionated catecholamines (CPT code 82384).

Both metanephrines and catecholamines testing are very sensitive to stress, medications, and food, and therefore, false-positive results often occur. Whether testing plasma or urine, patients must meticulously prepare for the testing for most accurate results. The ordering clinician must complete a thorough diet and medication history prior to testing to determine possible interfering agents. Recommendations for patient preparation vary between laboratories. Table 41.2 provides a summary of usual recommendations.

INDICATIONS

Screening
- Because pheos and PGL are very rare, occurring in only 0.2% to 0.6% of the population,[8,11] universal screening with catecholamines/metanephrines is generally not suggested.
- Screening with plasma or urine metanephrines is appropriate in patients with predisposition to hereditary pheos or PGL or past history of pheos or PGL.[8,11] However, the Endocrine Society recommends using plasma metanephrines to screen patients at high risk for pheos or PGL (predisposing genetic syndromes or family history of pheo//PGL)[3,7] and urine metanephrines if screening is needed in patients who do not meet high-risk guidelines[5,6] or when there is a low index of suspicion.[8]

■ The European Society of Endocrinology (ESE), American Association of Clinical Endocrinologists (AACE), and Korean Endocrine Society (KES) all recommend screening plasma and/or urinary metanephrines (not catecholamines) to rule out pheochromocytoma in patients with incidental adrenal adenoma.[13]

Diagnosis and Evaluation

■ The Endocrine Society recommends using plasma metanephrines in patients with persistent hypertension (HTN) or paroxysm of HTN.[3,7]

■ The European Society for Medical Oncology (ESMO) clinical practice guidelines recommend plasma or 24-hour urine fractionated metanephrines be completed to evaluate all adrenal masses and possible PGL tumors.[14]

■ In general, most clinical practice guidelines recommend plasma or 24-hour urine metanephrine testing for evaluation of pheos or PGL. Plasma fractionated metanephrines are also a good first-line test for children because obtaining a complete 24-hour urine collection is difficult.[3,8,12]

■ The most common diagnostic indications for biochemical screening with plasma or urine metanephrines are:[8,11,15]

  ● Patients with signs or symptoms of pheochromocytoma (Table 41.3)
  ● The presence of both hypertension and episodic symptoms of catecholamine excess (e.g., Palpitations/tachycardia, headache, and diaphoresis).
  ● Resistant hypertension.
  ● Incidentally identified adrenal masses.
  ● Predisposition to hereditary pheos or PGL.
  ● Assessment of recurrence of pheos or PGL.

■ Plasma and/or urine catecholamine levels may aid in the diagnosis of autonomic dysfunction/failure or autonomic neuropathy. Generally, subnormal resting plasma or urine catecholamine levels or an absent rise in catecholamine levels in response to stressful stimuli indicates possible autonomic dysfunction.[4,5]

TABLE 41.3: SIGNS AND SYMPTOMS OF PHEOCHROMOCYTOMA

COMMON SIGNS	UNCOMMON SIGNS	COMMON SYMPTOMS	UNCOMMON SYMPTOMS
Hypertension	Pallor	Headache	Nausea/vomiting
Tachycardia	Flushing	Palpitations	Visual disturbance
Reflex bradycardia	Weight loss	Anxiety	Paresthesia
Sweating	Tachypnea	Tremulousness	Faintness
Hyperglycemia	Postural hypotension	Fatigue	Abdominal complaints

These symptoms can also be seen in alcohol withdrawal, uncontrolled hypertension, cocaine use, autonomic dysfunction, and anxiety disorders.

Source: Data from Bajwa SS, Bajwa SK. Implications and considerations during pheochromocytoma resection: a challenge to the anesthesiologist. *Indian J Endocrinol Metab.* 2011;15(Suppl4):S337–S344. doi:10.4103/2230-8210.86977.

Monitoring

- The ESE recommends against repeat plasma or urine metanephrine testing in adrenal adenoma patients where the initial testing was negative. However, the AACE and KES recommends annual plasma or urine metanephrine testing for 5 years after identification of adrenal nodules greater than 3 cm.[13]
- The ESE recommends measuring plasma or urine metanephrine 2 to 6 weeks postoperatively (pheo or PGL) and then annually for 10 years.[11,16] Metanephrines testing is more sensitive than catecholamine testing for this purpose, but plasma and/or 24-hour urine catecholamine can be used.[16]
- The ESE recommends lifelong, annual plasma or urine metanephrine monitoring in patients with genetic syndromes that increase risk for developing pheo or PGL.[16]

INTERPRETATION

- Pediatric catecholamine/metanephrine levels vary from adults, often because of smaller size and pre-pubertal status.[12] Therefore, normal reference intervals observed in adults are not applicable for children.[12]

Metanephrines

- Normal values vary depending on testing laboratory and are typically based on reference intervals derived from normotensive patients.[15] Hypertensive patients have different, higher normal values and clinicians should use specific hypertensive values to interpret 24-hour urine results.[5] Examples of normal adult ranges are listed in Tables 41.4[3–5] and 41.5[3–5] and pediatric reference intervals are listed in Table 41.6
- Normal plasma metanephrines and 24-hour urine metanephrines indicate it is unlikely that a pheo or PGL is present.[2–4]

TABLE 41.4: ADULT PLASMA METANEPHRINE (nmol/L)

Normetanephrine	<0.9 nmol/L
Metanephrine	<0.5 nmol/L

Sources: Data from Lexicomp Online, Lab Tests and Diagnostic Procedures. UpToDate, Inc; 2019, February 25, 2021; Plasma metanephrine. Mayo Clinical Laboratories website. https://www.mayocliniclabs.com/test-catalog/Performance/81609; Urinary metanephrine. Mayo Clinical Laboratories website. https://www.mayocliniclabs.com/test-catalog/Performance/83006.

TABLE 41.5: ADULT 24-HOUR METANEPHRINES (mcg/24 HRS)

HORMONE	NORMOTENSIVE	HYPERTENSIVE
Normetanephrine	<600 mcg/24 hrs	<900 mcg/24 hrs
Metanephrine	<300 mcg/24 hrs	<400 mcg/24 hrs
Total metanephrine	200-700 mcg/24 hr	<1,300 mcg/24 hrs

Sources: Data from Lexicomp Online, Lab Tests and Diagnostic Procedures. UpToDate, Inc; 2019, February 25, 2021; Plasma metanephrine. Mayo Clinical Laboratories website. https://www.mayocliniclabs.com/test-catalog/Performance/81609; Urinary metanephrine. Mayo Clinical Laboratories website. https://www.mayocliniclabs.com/test-catalog/Performance/83006.

TABLE 41.6: CHILDREN 24-HOUR METANEPHRINES (mcg/24 HRS)			
AGE	METANEPHRINES	NORMETANEPHRINES	TOTAL METANEPHRINE
3–8 years	18–140 mcg/24 hr	30–160 mcg/24 hr	47–220 mcg/24 hr
9–12 years	40–180 mcg/24 hr	55–400 mcg/24 hr	100–500 mcg/24 hr
13–17 years	44–220 mcg/24 hr	60–390 mcg/24 hr	110–600 mcg/24 hr

Source: Data from Urinary metanephrine. Mayo Clinical Laboratories website. https://www.mayocliniclabs.com/test-catalog/Performance/83006.

- Small increases in metanephrines (less than 1 times the upper limit of normal) usually are due to physiologic stimuli, drugs, or improper specimen collection.[2,3]
- Moderate metanephrine elevations (1 to 3 times upper limit of normal reference range) may reflect false positive and retesting may be needed with strict patient adherence to test preparation and collected under low stress conditions.[3,11]
- Elevated metanephrines greater than 4 times upper limit of normal is strongly suggestive of pheo/PGL.[3]
- Plasma metanephrine testing has the highest sensitivity (96%) for detecting a pheochromocytoma, but it has a lower specificity (85%).[6] In comparison, a 24-hour urinary collection for metanephrines has a sensitivity of 87.5% and a specificity of 99.7%.[6]

Catecholamines

- The most useful finding with catecholamines testing is a disproportional elevation in one of the three catecholamines. The normal ratio of catecholamine levels in norepinephrine is greater than epinephrine, which is greater than dopamine.[3–5] Disruption in these ratios may indicate autonomic dysfunction., particularly if the dopamine ratio is disproportional, which may be observed in neuroendocrine tumors.[3]
- Reference intervals vary depending on age.[15] Reference intervals for adults are listed in Tables 41.7[3,4] and 41.8.[3,4] Reference intervals for children are listed in Table 41.9.[5,12]
- Small increases in catecholamines (less than 2 times the upper limit of normal) usually are due to physiologic stimuli, drugs, or improper specimen collection.[3]
- Moderate catecholamine elevations (1 to 3 times upper limit of normal reference range) may reflect false positive; retesting may be needed with strict patient adherence to test preparation and collected under low stress conditions.[3,11]
- Elevated catecholamines greater than 3 times the upper limit of normal concurrent with signs and symptoms of pheo/PGL is strongly associated with increased probability of neuroendocrine tumor, and imaging studies are indicated to locate the source.[2,3]

TABLE 41.7: ADULT 24-HOUR URINE CATECHOLAMINE (mcg/24 HRS)

Dopamine	70–450 mcg/24 hrs
Epinephrine	1–20 mcg/24 hrs
Norepinephrine	15–100 mcg/24 hrs
Urine creatinine	0.8–2 g/24 hrs

Sources: Data from Lexicomp Online, Lab Tests and Diagnostic Procedures. February 25, 2021; Plasma metanephrine. Mayo Clinical Laboratories website. https://www.mayocliniclabs.com/test-catalog/Performance/81609.

TABLE 41.8: ADULT PLASMA CATECHOLAMINE (pg/mL)

Dopamine	0–30 pg/mL
Epinephrine	10–100 pg/mL
Norepinephrine	70–800 pg/mL

Sources: Data from Lexicomp Online, Lab Tests and Diagnostic Procedures. Plasma metanephrine. Mayo Clinical Laboratories website. https://www.mayocliniclabs.com/test-catalog/Performance/81609.

TABLE 41.9: 24-HOUR URINE CATECHOLAMINE NORMAL REFERENCE VALUES (mcg/24 HRS) IN CHILDREN

AGE	NOREPINEPHRINE	EPINEPHRINE	DOPAMINE
<1 year	<11 mcg/24 hours (hrs)	<2.6 mcg/24 hrs	<86 mcg/24 hrs
1 year	1–17 mcg/24 hrs	<3.6 mcg/24 hrs	10–140 mcg/24 hrs
2–3 years	4–29 mcg/24 hrs	<6.1 mcg/24 hours	40–260 mcg/24 hrs
4–9 years	8–65 mcg/24 hrs	0.2–10 mcg/24 hrs	65–400 mcg/24 hrs
>10 years	15–80 mcg/24 hrs	0.5–21 mcg/24 hrs	65–400 mcg/24 hrs

Sources: Data from Urinary metanephrine. Mayo Clinical Laboratories website. https://www.mayocliniclabs.com/test-catalog/Performance/83006; Weise M, Merke DP, Pacak K, Walther MM, Eisenhofer G. Utility of plasma free metanephrines for detecting childhood pheochromocytoma. *J Clin Endocrinol Metab.* 2002;87(5):1955–1960. doi:10.1210/jcem.87.5.8446.

FOLLOW-UP

- Normal plasma or 24-hour urine catecholamines require no further evaluation,[2,8] except for patients being evaluated for "spells" (brief time period of experiencing symptoms). In these patients, repeat testing is needed during a "spell." If results are still normal on repeat testing, other causes of "spells" should be investigated.[8]
- Persistently elevated urine or plasma catecholamines after treatment for pheo/PGL indicate treatment was not fully effective or the tumor has returned. [2,3,11]
- Plasma and/or urine catecholamines are not the first-line test of pheo/PGL since in patients with neuroendocrine tumors, catecholamines may

only be elevated during a "spell" of symptoms, whereas increased levels of metanephrines are produced continuously.[5,7,13]

- A 24-hour urine catecholamine collection, as opposed to random urine testing, may detect cases missed by plasma testing as catecholamine secretion by pheo/PGL is typically intermittent.[2,3]
- If initial results are normal, no further evaluation is needed except for patients being evaluated for "spells." In these patients, 24-hour urine metanephrines should be repeated during a "spell." If repeat testing is normal, then other causes for the spells should be investigated.[8]
- Borderline positive plasma or urine metanephrine results may be further evaluated with a clonidine suppression test.[3,7] Clonidine is a central-acting alpha blocker and will suppress the release of catecholamines from neurons but does not affect release of catecholamines/metanephrines from a pheochromocytoma.
- Clonidine suppression test is the confirmatory test for diagnosing pheos[3] with a purported 100% specificity and 97% sensitivity.[7]
  - Clonidine suppression test protocol:[7]
    - Baseline plasma catecholamines/metanephrine are obtained.
    - Administer 0.3 mg of clonidine PO to patient.
    - Repeat plasma catecholamines/metanephrine at 3 hours post-clonidine.
    - Abnormal test includes plasma catecholamines/metanephrines; do not decrease after administration of clonidine.

PEARLS & PITFALLS

- Plasma and/or urine catecholamine testing is not the first-line test for evaluating for pheos or PGLs (metanephrines are)[3–5]; however, catecholamine testing may be appropriate if metanephrine testing is inconclusive.[5]
- In the normal population, plasma and urine MN and NMN levels are low. However, in patients with pheo or PGL, the concentrations may be significantly elevated due to the relatively long half-life of these compounds, ongoing secretion by the tumor, and the peripheral conversion of tumor-secreted catecholamines into metanephrines.[4]
- Urine catecholamines may be invalid in the presence of advanced kidney disease.[3]
- Do not perform 24-hour urine or plasma catecholamine testing on patients withdrawing from legal or illicit drugs known to cause rebound catecholamine release during withdrawal (i.e., clonidine, cocaine).[3,5]
- In general, patients with large pheo/PGL tumors produce more metanephrines because the catecholamines are metabolized within the tumor before being released, whereas small tumors are more likely to release more plasma catecholamines.[15]
- If the specimen is collected during a "spell," plasma catecholamines have a 90% to 95% diagnostic sensitivity when norepi is greater than 750 pg/mL and epi is greater than 110 pg/mL. If norepi and epi levels are lower during a "spell," a pheo is essentially ruled out.[4]

- False-positive results far outnumber true-positive results.[7] It has been estimated that 97% of hypertensive patients seen in tertiary care who have positive elevated plasma catecholamines/metanephrines will NOT have a pheochromocytoma.[15]
- Activity prior to testing is important. Recent studies show that collecting a plasma sample in a nonfasting, ambulating population can give false-positive rates of up to 30% compared with 5% in fasting, supine patients.[11]
- Several genetic syndromes can cause an increased risk of developing a pheo/PGL. These syndromes include MEN-1 and MEN-2 (multiple endocrine neoplasia), Von Hippel-Lindau syndrome (VHL), succinate dehydrogenase (SDH) mutation, neurofibromatosis (NF)1, and Carney syndrome.[2,12,15]
- Metanephrine testing is preferred over catecholamine testing because the metabolites are continuously produced within tumors by a process that is independent of catecholamine release, which for some tumors occurs at low rates or is episodic in nature.[7] Urine metanephrines are more sensitive and have more accuracy with fewer false-negative test results than urine catecholamines.[7]
- Defining the pretest probability of a pheo or PGL in an individual patient is essential to the appropriate interpretation of the results and should not be solely based on the magnitude of the increase above the reference range for laboratory values.[11]

TABLE 41.10: MEDICATIONS AND MET/CAT TESTING

↑ CATECHOLAMINES AND METANEPHRINES[3,5,6]	DECREASE 24-HOUR URINE LEVELS OF METANEPHRINES[6]	DO NOT INTERFERE WITH TESTING[4,5]
Tricyclic antidepressants	Methyltyrosine	Acetaminophen
Reserpine	Methylglucamine (present in radiocontrast media)	Atropine
Levodopa		Beta-blockers
Decongestants		Fludrocortisone
Amphetamines		Hydralazine
Buspirone		Hydrochlorothiazide
MAO inhibitors		Spironolactone
Clonidine withdrawal		Prednisone
Ethanol		
Caffeine		
Prochlorperazine		
Cocaine		
Imipramine		
ETOH withdrawal		

ETOH, ethanol; MAO, monoamine oxidase.

■ Measurements of urinary metanephrines may be invalid in patients with CKD.[8] Plasma metanephrines is the test of choice in this patient population.
■ Mercury intoxication can mimic pheo, causing both HTN and elevated plasma and urine metanephrines.[8,15]
■ Measuring plasma and/or urine metanephrines is recognized as one of the best tests for detecting pheo or PGL and is superior to testing catecholamines. Pheo tumors continuously produce metanephrines independent of catecholamine secretion (which is episodic), thus allowing for higher diagnostic sensitivity compared to catecholamine testing.[8] PGL do not typically produce catecholamines.[17] Metanephrines are more stable than catecholamines, and therefore are more sensitive and specific for detecting pheos and/or PGL.[3]
■ Some medications can interfere with catecholamine and metanephrine testing and can cause falsely elevated metanephrine levels while others can falsely decrease levels. Others do not. These are summarized in Table 41.10.

PATIENT EDUCATION

■ https://www.uhs.nhs.uk/Media/UHS-website-2019/Patientinformation/Tests/Plasma-metanephrine-test-patient-information.pdf
■ https://www.uclahealth.org/endocrine-center/catecholamine-test

RELATED DIAGNOSES AND ICD-10 CODES

Pheochromocytoma	C74.10	Adrenal nodule	E27.9
Paraganglioma	D44.7	Uncontrolled hypertension	I10

REFERENCES

Full list of references can be accessed through Springer Publishing Company Connect™ at the following link: http://connect.springerpub.com/content/reference-book/978-0-8261-8843-4/part/part03/toc-part/ch041

42. CELIAC DISEASE TESTING

Christine Colella and Kelly Small Casler

PATHOPHYSIOLOGY REVIEW

Gliadin and glutenin are the protein components of gluten, the dietary substance found in wheat, barley, and rye.[1] Celiac disease (CD), an autoimmune disease affecting one in 141 people across all races, ages, and sex, causes an immune-mediated small intestine enteropathy in response to gluten.[1-3] When exposed to gluten in the diet, the immune system of genetically susceptible individuals mistakes gluten as pathologic and produces autoantibodies to tissue-transglutaminase (enzyme used in gliadin deamidation), endomysium (connective tissue of gastrointestinal [GI] musculature), gliadin, and deamidated gliadin peptide (peptide resulting from gliadin deamidation that binds with human leukocyte antigen (HLA)-receptors of immune cells to produce the immune response).

OVERVIEW OF LABORATORY TESTS

Testing for CD involves laboratory tests to detect autoantibodies and genetic-testing for HLA serotypes that predispose individuals to CD autoimmunity. Laboratory tests for autoantibodies can be performed on blood serum as enzyme-linked immunosorbents (ELISAs) or radio assays. Recent research is focusing on point-of-care methods, although performance is not yet as good as laboratory-based methods.[4] For accuracy, laboratory tests for autoantibodies require the individual to be on a gluten-containing diet so that the immune components are produced and, subsequently, identifiable.[5]

The laboratory tests available for CD are divided into three categories: autoantibody tests, molecular tests, and small bowel biopsy. Autoantibody tests are often offered as combined "celiac panels." The algorithm in Figure 42.1 depicts a common approach to CD testing.

Autoantibody Laboratory Tests[6,7]

- **Total serum IgA (CPT code 82784):** Used to evaluate for presence of IgA deficiency, which occurs in 2% to 3% of the CD population. Since IgA deficiency can cause false-negative tissue transglutaminase (tTG) IgA antibody or endomysial antibody (EMA) results, if the IgA is low, test for deamidated gliadin peptide (DGP) IgG or tTG IgG antibody instead of TTG-IgA antibody.
- **Tissue transglutaminase IgA antibody (tTG-IgA) (CPT code 83516):** Initial test of choice in most CD workups and the most sensitive test. Sensitivity is 95% with a 98% specificity. This test can have false negatives in the presence of IgA deficiency.
- **Tissue transglutaminase IgG antibody (tTG-IgG) (CPT code 83516):** This test is usually only used in IgA-deficient individuals.
- **Anti-gliadin antibodies (AGA) IgG and/or IgA (CPT code 83516):** This antibody test is the least accurate and, therefore, rarely used.
- **Endomysial antibody (EMA) IgG and/or IgA (CPT code 86256):** This test is the most specific test available but is not as sensitive as tTG-IgA.[5] EMA IgG and/or IgA may be used if there is still high suspicion for CD, but tTG is negative. EMA IgG alone may be used in the presence of IgA deficiency.
- **Deamidated gliadin peptide (DGP) IgA and/or IgG (CPT code 83516):** DGP IgG testing is used for those with IgA deficiency, and DGP IgA/IgG testing can be used if there is still high suspicion of CD and initial tests are negative. It is also routinely used in combination with TTG-IgA for children 2 years of age or younger.

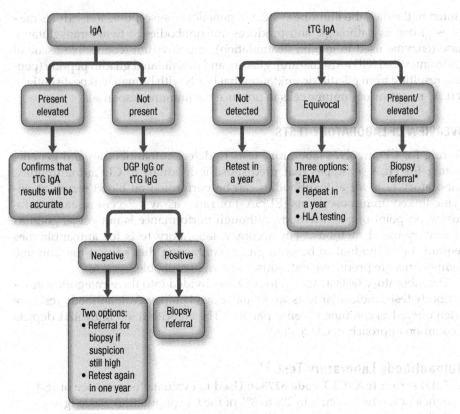

FIGURE 42.1. Common approach to testing for celiac disease. Start with simultaneous testing for both IgA and tTG IgA. *Intestinal biopsy may not be needed if tTG is greater than 10 times the upper limit of normal and confirmation is made with a positive EMA. DGP, deamidated gliadin peptide; EMA, endomysial antibody; HLA, human leukocyte antigen; tTg, tissue transglutaminase.

Molecular Laboratory Tests[6,7]

■ **HLA typing: DQ2 and DQ8 genetic markers (CPT codes 81376 and 81382):** Individuals with CD carry DQ2 and DQ8 genetic polymorphisms. Testing for the polymorphisms is used to clarify equivocal or unclear antibody testing results. The test may also be used in the case of an equivocal small bowel biopsy result. HLA typing is also useful if patients are unable to stop a gluten-free diet. The negative predictive value of the test is greater than 99% since nearly all CD patients have one of these two allotypes. However, the positive predictive value is only around 12% since this polymorphism can be seen in the general population in people who never/will never manifest CD.[7]

Small Bowel Biopsy

Small bowel biopsy is the gold-standard test. Usually, several samples are taken from the small bowel during endoscopy and examined microscopically for the characteristic changes (villi atrophy and lymphocyte infiltration) seen in CD.

INDICATIONS
Screening
- There is insufficient evidence per the United States Preventive Services Task Force (USPSTF) for CD screening.[8]
- Despite the limited evidence for screening, there is much interest on the topic, especially in children, as some research suggests that many children with CD may be undiagnosed.[9,10] Many adults are undiagnosed as well, with women more likely than men to go undiagnosed (1.42 relative risk).[11]
- Targeted screening may be appropriate even with a lack of GI symptoms for individuals with the conditions listed in Box 42.1.[12–16]

Diagnosis and Evaluation
- Testing is indicated as part of the evaluation of suspected irritable bowel syndrome or lactose intolerance and also in evaluating dyspepsia, abdominal pain, bloating, gas, flatulence, diarrhea, chronic constipation, and steatorrhea.[17]

Monitoring
- tTG and GDP are often used to evaluate success/compliance with a gluten-free diet and should be undetectable within 3 to 12 months after starting the diet.[18–20]
- A relatively new test, gluten immunogenic peptides (GIPs), can be used to monitor gluten-free diet adherence in children.[21]

INTERPRETATION
- Tests are usually reported as a titer with corresponding values of negative, weakly positive/equivocal, or positive. The higher the titer, the higher the probability of CD.[6]

FOLLOW-UP
- Traditionally, small intestine biopsy to confirm duodenal villous atrophy has been required as the follow-up test for positive antibody tests.[22] However, recent research supports that if symptoms are consistent with CD, tTG is greater than 10 times the upper limit of normal, and EMA antibody tests are positive, biopsy is not necessary for confirmation of CD in adults[23] and children.[21,24,25]
- Refer patients for gastroenterology consultation and intestinal biopsy if tTGs is 3 x ULN or higher.[20]
- If IgA deficiency is identified during the evaluation for CD, follow-up testing that considers the differential diagnosis for CD symptoms and IgA deficiency together is important. These differentials include small bowel bacterial overgrowth and common variable immunodeficiency (CVID).
- If there are negative antibody tests, but still high suspicion for CD, referral for small bowel biopsy is recommended.[6]

Box 42.1: Indications for Targeted Celiac Disease Screening

- Aphthous stomatitis
- Ataxia
- Autoimmune hepatitis
- Autoimmune thyroid disease
- Chronic constipation
- Chronic fatigue
- Delayed puberty
- Dental enamel hypoplasia
- Dermatitis herpetiformis
- Down, Turner, or William syndrome
- Early onset osteoporosis
- Elevated liver transaminases
- Failure to thrive (less than third percentile)
- First-degree relative with CD
- Hyposplenism
- Infertility
- Iron deficiency anemia
- Lupus
- Malabsorption
- Metabolic bone disease
- Microscopic colitis
- Migraine
- Neuropathy
- Psoriasis
- Selective IgA deficiency
- T1DM
- Vitamin/mineral deficiency
- Weight loss

Sources: Data from Mooney PD, Hadjivassiliou M, Sanders DS. Coeliac disease. *BMJ.* 2014;348(mar03 6):g1561–g1561. doi:10.1136/bmj.g1561; Lebwohl B, Rubio-Tapia A. Epidemiology, presentation, and diagnosis of celiac disease. *Gastroenterology.* 2021;160(1):63–75. doi:10.1053/j.gastro.2020.06.098; Oxentenko AS, Rubio-Tapia A. Celiac disease. *Mayo Clin Proc.* 2019;94(12):2556–2571. doi:10.1016/j.mayocp.2019.02.019; American Academy of Pediatrics-Section on Endocrinology. *Avoid ordering screening tests looking for chronic illness or an endocrine cause, including CBC, CMP, IGF-1, thyroid tests, and celiac antibodies, in healthy children who are growing at or above the 3rd percentile for height with a normal growth rate (i.e., not crossing percentiles) and with appropriate weight gain.* Published October 2, 2017. https://www.choosingwisely.org/clinician-lists/aap-soen-screening-tests-for-chronic-illness-or-endocrine-cause/; Hyams JS, Di Lorenzo C, Saps M, Shulman RJ, Staiano A, van Tilburg M. Functional disorders: children and adolescents. *Gastroenterology.* Published online February 15, 2016. doi:10.1053/j.gastro.2016.02.015; Hill ID, Dirks MH, Liptak GS, et al. Guideline for the diagnosis and treatment of celiac disease in children: Recommendations of the North American Society for Pediatric Gastroenterology, Hepatology and Nutrition. *J Pediatr Gastroenterol Nutr.* 2005;40(1):1–19. doi:10.1097/00005176-200501000-00001; Quigley EMM. The patient with irritable bowel syndrome-type symptoms: when to investigate and how? *Curr Opin Gastroenterol.* 2021;37(1):39–43. doi:10.1097/MOG.0000000000000686.

- Since CD may cause problems with vitamin and nutrient absorption, follow-up testing of iron, vitamin B12, vitamin D, and folate levels is recommended.[6]

■ If initial tests show a weakly positive/equivical titer, repeat testing in a year can be considered. The low titer could be a false positive, but also could be from early identification of CD. Titers would be expected to increase if a gluten-containing diet is continued.[20]

■ In patients with CD symptoms and negative CD testing, consider evaluation for non-celiac conditions that present similarly to CD: tropical sprue, small bowel overgrowth, autoimmune enteropathy, drug-associated enteropathy (olmesartan), inflammatory bowel disease, eosinophilic enteritis, malnutrition, infectious enteritis (giardiasis), and non-celiac gluten sensitivity[6]

PEARLS & PITFALLS

■ Often, the signs/symptoms of CD can be broad and nonspecific. Therefore, getting the correct diagnosis can be elusive and lengthy.[26] In some studies, CD diagnosis took up to 6 to 10 years.[2,3]

■ In patients with suspected CD, inquire about family history of CD in a first-degree relative, which heightens suspicion of CD.[27]

■ Symptoms can present as early as 6 months to 2 years of age as children start consuming gluten in their diets. The risk of dehydration and failure to thrive in the very young can lead to growth and developmental issues.[27]

■ Gluten should be consumed in the diet for 1 to 3 months before autoantibody testing.[28]

PATIENT EDUCATION

■ https://www.beyondceliac.org/celiac-disease/get-tested
■ https://celiac.org/about-celiac-disease/screening-and-diagnosis

RELATED DIAGNOSES AND ICD-10 CODES

Celiac disease	K90.0
Other malabsorption due to intolerance	K90.4
Diarrhea, unspecified	R19.7

REFERENCES

Full list of references can be accessed through Springer Publishing Company Connect™ at the following link: http://connect.springerpub.com/content/reference-book/978-0-8261 -8843-4/part/part03/toc-part/ch042

43. CELL-FREE DNA

Nancy C. Tkacs

PHYSIOLOGY REVIEW

Cell-free DNA (cfDNA) screening of a maternal blood sample leverages the power of DNA amplification by polymerase chain reaction (PCR), plus rapid DNA sequencing, to identify fetal chromosomal and genetic abnormalities as early as 10 weeks of gestational age. Aneuploidy (defined as an abnormal chromosome number—either extra chromosomes or missing chromosomes) is a relatively common occurrence, although incidence at birth may underestimate the true number, due to early pregnancy losses associated with chromosome defects. Throughout life, ongoing apoptosis of senescent cells results in release of short (approximately 200 base pair) segments of cfDNA into the circulation. During pregnancy, apoptotic cells from placental trophoblasts contribute cfDNA (approximating DNA of fetal cells, although not identical) to the maternal circulating DNA. The "fetal fraction" normally averages 10% of the maternal fraction and can be used to detect genetic and chromosomal abnormalities noninvasively.[1] Analysis of cfDNA from maternal serum is known as noninvasive prenatal testing or screening (NIPT or NIPS). Although expensive, NIPS has high sensitivity and specificity for common aneuploidies, particularly trisomy 21 (resulting in Down syndrome), and has been adopted rapidly, particularly in high resource countries. NIPS can also detect fetal Rh status and chromosomal sex. NIPS is a screening test and suspected abnormalities must be followed up by invasive confirmatory testing such as chorionic villus sampling (CVS) or amniocentesis. This is a rapidly developing field, and future applications may include fetal assessment for monogenic disorders such as sickle cell disease, cystic fibrosis, and other conditions. In another application, cancer cells also regularly undergo apoptosis, and cfDNA testing is gaining in use for genotyping cancer cells to guide chemotherapy choices.[2]

OVERVIEW OF LABORATORY TESTS

Prenatal screening using cell-free DNA is most appropriate for singleton pregnancies at and after 10 weeks gestation. Genomic sequencing used to screen for fetal trisomy 13 (Patau syndrome), 18 (Edwards syndrome), 21 (Down syndrome), and monosomy X uses CPT code 81420 (found under Genomic Sequencing Procedures and other Molecular Multianalyte Assays). DNA sequence analysis of specific sequences uses CPT code 81507 (under Multianalyte Assays With Algorithmic Analysis) to obtain risk scores of fetal aneuploidy (trisomy 13, 18, 21). Choice of one or the other test depends on the specific commercial assay provider (which varies by institution). Test providers should include the fetal fraction in the results as an indicator of validity of the assay. Tests returning a fetal fraction below 4% will not report a result in terms of

Trisomy 13, unspecified	Q91.7	Klinefelter syndrome, unspecified	Q98.4
Klinefelter syndrome karyotype 47, XXY	Q98.0	Other variants of Turner's syndrome	Q96.8
Klinefelter syndrome, male with more than two X chromosomes	Q98.1	Turner's syndrome, unspecified	Q96.9

REFERENCES

Full list of references can be accessed through Springer Publishing Company Connect™ at the following link: http://connect.springerpub.com/content/reference-book/978-0-8261 -8843-4/part/part03/toc-part/ch043

44. CEREBRAL SPINAL FLUID ANALYSIS

Carolyn McClerking

PHYSIOLOGY REVIEW

Cerebral spinal fluid (CSF) is a clear, colorless fluid that exists in two compartments, intracranial and spinal. CSF is continuously produced by the choroid plexus within the ventricles and moves via CSF pathways in the spinal cord and subarachnoid space of the brain.[1] The primary role of the CSF is to allow for buoyancy in the brain, which provides protection in case of mechanical injury.[1] The CSF is also an important supplier of essential nutrients and it assists in eliminating such materials as amino acids, neurotransmitters, and waste products of brain metabolism.[1,2] The amount of CSF produced ranges between 400 mL and 700 mL each day with the overall volume totaling nearly 150 mL.[2,3] This continual CSF secretion provides overall renewal of the CSF at least five times per day in young adults. A decrease in CSF recycling may lead to the buildup of metabolites observed in aging and neurogenerative diseases.[3] The CSF composition is firmly controlled, and any variation can offer a beneficial diagnostic tool.[3,4]

OVERVIEW OF LABORATORY TEST

Cerebral spinal fluid (CPT code 84157) is primarily obtained from lumbar puncture of the spinal canal and can be used to diagnose specific neurologic, hematologic, oncologic, and infectious diseases.[5] The location for CSF removal is generally in the area of L3–L4 or L4–L5. CSF can also be obtained via an ommaya tap or ventricular drainage.[6] The amount of CSF to be removed is dependent on patient presentation and can range between 4 mL and 6 mL. The primary tests to evaluate the CSF include cell count (CPT code 89051), protein (CPT code 84157), glucose (CPT code 82945), and cytology (CPT codes 88112 and 88108). Gram stains (CPT codes 87070, 87015, 87205, 87075) are also utilized to rule in and rule out certain conditions.

Cytology is important as it provides an idea of response to treatment of certain malignancies as well as identification of hemorrhagic and inflammatory conditions.[6,7]

INDICATIONS

Screening

- Universal screening for CSF is not recommended.
- Targeted screening with CSF is recommend for conditions that are predisposed to alterations in the central nervous system (CNS), including infections and hematologic/oncologic disorders (Box 44.1).

Diagnosis and Evaluation

CSF is often used to diagnose and evaluate the following conditions:

- Cryptococcal meningitis[8]
- Bacterial meningitis[9,10]
- Acute leukemias[11]
- Other signs and symptoms that could be due to altered CSF (Box 44.2)
  - Sporadic Creutzfeldt-Jakob disease is a type of degenerative brain disorder that can be diagnosed by laboratory assays found in the protein of CSF.[12]

Box 44.1: Disorders With Abnormalities in Cerebral Spinal Fluid

- Alzheimer's disease
- Bacterial meningitis
- Brain cancer markers
- Brain tumor mutations
- Cryptococcal meningitis
- Metastatic CNS tumors
- Neurodegenerative dementia
- Neurologic diseases
- Spinal cord trauma

CNS, central nervous system.

Sources: Rajasingham R, Wake RM, Beyene T, Katende A, Letang E, Boulware DR. Cryptococcal meningitis diagnostics and screening in the era of point-of-care laboratory testing. *J Clin Microbiol.* 2019;57(1):e01238–01218. doi:10.1128/JCM.01238-18; Tamune H, Kuki T. Cerebrospinal fluid/blood glucose point-of-care testing ratio for diagnosing bacterial meningitis in a limited medical resource setting. *Eur J Emerg Med.* 2019;26(2):145. doi:10.1097/MEJ.0000000000000558; Taniguchi T, Tsuha S, Shiiki S, Narita M. Point-of-care cerebrospinal fluid Gram stain for the management of acute meningitis in adults: a retrospective observational study. *Ann Clin Microbiol Antimicrob.* 2020;19(1):59. doi:10.1186/s12941-020-00404-9; Engelborghs S, Niemantsverdriet E, Struyfs H, et al. Consensus guidelines for lumbar puncture in patients with neurological diseases. *Alzheimers Dement.* 2017;8(1):111–126. doi:10.1016/j.dadm.2017.04.007; Pan W, Gu W, Nagpal S, Gephart MH, Quake SR. Brain tumor mutations detected in cerebral spinal fluid. *Clin Chem.* 2015;61(3):514–522. doi:10.1373/clinchem.2014.235457; Shalaby T, Achini F, Grotzer MA. Targeting cerebrospinal fluid for discovery of brain cancer biomarkers. *J Cancer Metastasis Treat.* 2016;2:176–187. doi:10.20517/2394-4722.2016.12; Ballester LY, Lu G, Zorofchian S, et al. Analysis of cerebrospinal fluid metabolites in patients with primary or metastatic central nervous system tumors. *Acta Neuropathol Commun.* 2018;6(1):85. doi:10.1186/s40478-018-0588-z; Kansal K, Irwin DJ. The use of cerebrospinal fluid and neuropathologic studies in neuropsychiatry practice and research. *Psychiatr Clin North Am.* 2015;38(2):309–322. doi:10.1016/j.psc.2015.02.002; Kwon BK, Streijger F, Fallah N, et al. Cerebrospinal fluid biomarkers to stratify injury severity and predict outcome in human traumatic spinal cord injury. *J Neurotrauma.* 2017;34(3):567–580. doi:10.1089/neu.2016.4435; Yokobori S, Zhang Z, Moghieb A, et al. Acute diagnostic biomarkers for spinal cord injury: review of the literature and preliminary research report. *World Neurosurg.* 2015;83(5):867–878. doi:10.1016/j.wneu.2013.03.012.

Box 44.2: Signs and Symptoms of Abnormal Cerebral Spinal Fluid

- Confusion
- Difficulty with speech
- Dizziness
- Hallucinations
- Fatigue
- Fever
- Nuchal rigidity
- Persistent headache
- Photophobia
- Unexplained muscle weakness

Sources: Hrishi AP, Sethuraman M. Cerebrospinal fluid (CSF) analysis and interpretation in neurocritical care for acute neurological conditions. *Indian J Crit Care Med.* 2019;23(Suppl 2):S115–s119. doi:10.5005/jp-journals-10071-23187; Benninger F, Steiner I. CSF in acute and chronic infectious diseases. *Handb Clin Neurol.* 2017;146:187–206. doi:10.1016/B978-0-12-804279-3.00012-5.

- Identification of oligoclonal bands is the hallmark of multiple sclerosis-specific changes seen in the CSF.[13]
- A standardized preanalytic protocol may be useful in measurement of Alzheimer's disease biomarkers in CSF.[14,15]

Monitoring

Certain conditions may require periodic monitoring and continued analysis of the CSF.

- Monitoring therapy for measurement of IgM oligoclonal bands in multiple sclerosis, neurosyphilis (can get reinfected on a continual basis), and tuberculosis meningitis;
- Monitoring of CSF myelin basic protein levels to determine the impact of cytotoxic intrathecal therapy for central nervous system (CNS) leukemia;
- Monitoring chronic hydrocephalus; and
- Detection of deoxyribonucleic acid (DNA) of the herpes virus for proper control of herpes simplex encephalitis.[16]

INTERPRETATION[17]

See Table 44.1 for interpretation of test results.

FOLLOW-UP

- Follow-up for signs of bleeding with complete blood count.[18]
- Follow-up for evaluation of spinal leak with neuro imaging.[18]
- Based on results of a nationwide prospective study, re-evaluating CSF in patients with an initial negative result can be beneficial in confirming a diagnosis of meningitis.[19]
- Additional testing may be completed based on the findings from the CSF analysis.

TABLE 44.1: REFERENCE VALUES FOR CEREBRAL SPINAL FLUID ANALYSIS

ANALYSIS	NORMAL INTERVAL	BACTERIAL	TUBERCULOSIS	VIRAL	FUNGAL
CSF protein	15–40 mg/dL	Elevated	Moderately elevated	Normal to mildly elevated	Normal to mildly increased
CSF white blood cell count (WBC)	0–5/cu mm (up to 30 in neonates)	10–2000/cu mm	Elevated, but <500	>100/cu mm	10–50/cu mm
Gram stain		Positive	Acid fast bacilli	Negative	Negative India for spores/fungi
CSF red blood cell (RBC)	None	Elevated	Elevated	Normal	Normal
CSF lactate	1–3 mmol/L	Elevated (>6 mmol/L)	Elevated	0–6 mmol/L	Normal
Appearance	Clear	Turbid	Turbid	Clear	Clear
CSF glucose	50–80 mg/dL (2/3 of blood glucose)	<40 mg/dL	Low	Normal to mildly less	Low to normal
Opening pressure	50–200 mmH20	Increased	Increased	Normal to elevated	Normal to mildly increased

Source: Hrishi AP, Sethuraman M. Cerebrospinal fluid (CSF) analysis and interpretation in neurocritical care for acute neurological conditions. Indian J Crit Care Med. 2019;23(Suppl 2):S115–s119. doi:10.5005/jp-journals-10071-23187.

PEARLS & PITFALLS

- Neurofilament light protein levels in CSF may predict outcome in Guillain Barré syndrome and, in addition to clinical measures, offer beneficial management decisions.[20]
- Studies suggest CSF sphingomyelin serves as a biomarker for the treatment of patients with acquired demyelinating neuropathies and may improve management.[21]
- A study found that CSF cytokine measurement determined the presence of infection as well as differentiated between viral and nonviral etiologies.[22]
- To better diagnose Alzheimer's disease, it was concluded that using CSF AB42/40 ratio as opposed to CSF AB42 alone was a better diagnostic tool.[23]
- Improvement in efficiency of diagnosing tuberculosis meningitis can be better achieved with the combination of CSF interferon gamma and the ELISPOT-technique test, T-SPOT.TB.[24]
- A study concluded that CSF plays a major role in differentiating between a group of demyelinating diseases: multiple sclerosis, neuromyelitis optic, and acute disseminated encephalomyelitis.[25]
- A meta-genomic next-generation sequencing (mNGS) test was validated in the detection of neurologic infections in the CNS.[26]

- CSF evaluation and MRI combined distinguished Creutzfeldt-Jakob disease from other prion diseases.[27]
- Evidence suggests there is no association between the volume of CSF removed from patients who received diagnostic lumbar puncture for hydrocephalus and postprocedure gait.[28]
- Data suggests serum and CSF microRNA biomarkers predict severity in spinal cord injury.[29]
- A study found a negative predictor of point-of-care (POC) glucometers to measure CSF glucose levels, specifically in the diagnosis of meningitis.[30]

PATIENT EDUCATION

- https://medlineplus.gov/lab-tests/cerebrospinal-fluid-csf-analysis
- https://www.healthline.com/health/csf-analysis#followup

RELATED DIAGNOSES AND ICD-10 CODES

Other specified abnormal findings in cerebrospinal fluid	R83.9

REFERENCES

Full list of references can be accessed through Springer Publishing Company Connect™ at the following link: http://connect.springerpub.com/content/reference-book/978-0-8261 -8843-4/part/part03/toc-part/ch044

45. CERULOPLASMIN

Kelly Small Casler

PHYSIOLOGY REVIEW

Ceruloplasmin is a copper-carrying protein synthesized by the liver and secreted by hepatocytes. It is a main transporter of copper.[1] It is also an acute phase reactant, meaning serum levels increase with inflammatory states.[1] Ceruloplasmin levels are low at birth, gradually rise during childhood, and then decrease to adult levels around puberty.[2]

OVERVIEW OF LABORATORY TEST

Serum ceruloplasmin levels (CPT code 82390) are used in the diagnostic workup of elevated liver transaminases and liver abnormalities to raise or exclude suspicion for Wilson disease (WD), a disease that results in excessive accumulation of copper in the body and increased degradation of ceruloplasmin. Serum ceruloplasmin can be measured through an enzymatic assay that measures oxidase activity (preferred) or an immunologic assay. The latter assay is less accurate.[2,3]

INDICATIONS

Screening

■ For universal screening, research is being conducted on adding the test to newborn screening panels to screen for WD, though much more research is needed.[1,4]

■ For targeted screening:
  ● Used along with other parameters to screen a first-degree relative of patients with WD who are over the age of 1 year.[1,2,5]
  ● As part of screening for WD as a possible diagnosis in unexplained liver disease in the setting of neurologic, psychiatric, or other signs and symptoms of WD (Table 45.1).[1]
  ● Used to screen for WD in patients ages 3 to 55 with an unclear cause of liver abnormalities and persistently elevated alamine aminotransferase (ALT)/ aspartate transaminase (AST). Because of the rarity of WD, ceruloplasmin is used after more common causes of ALT/AST elevation have been excluded.[1,6]
  ● Used to screen for WD in patients with liver transaminases greater than five times the upper limit of normal.[6]

Diagnosis and Evaluation

■ Not considered a diagnostic test for WD on its own and confirmatory tests will be needed to exclude/confirm suspicion of diagnosis.[6]

Monitoring

■ Conflicting opinions on use. Recommended by some guidelines every 6 months to monitor treatment response in WD,[5] while more recent research questions the usefulness of ceruloplasmin monitoring.[7]

TABLE 45.1: SIGNS AND SYMPTOMS OF WILSON DISEASE

SYSTEM	SIGNS AND SYMPTOMS
Ophthalmic	Kayser-Fleisher rings of cornea
Hematologic	Coombs'-negative hemolytic anemia
Neurologic	Ataxia, dystonia, tremor-rigidity, dysarthria, seizures, drooling
Psychiatric	Labile mood, impulsiveness, sexual exhibitionism
Hepatologic	ALP:bilirubin ratio > 1; low serum ALP, mild elevations in serum transaminases (<500 u/L), extreme hyperbilirubinemia (>17.5 mg/dL)

ALP, alkaline phosphatase.

Sources: Roberts EA, Schilsky ML. Diagnosis and treatment of Wilson disease: an update. *Hepatology.* 2008;47(6):2089–2111. doi:10.1002/hep.22261; Socha P, Janczyk W, Dhawan A, et al. Wilson's disease in children: a position paper by the Hepatology Committee of the European Society for Paediatric Gastroenterology, Hepatology and Nutrition. *J Pediatr Gastroenterol Nutr.* 2018;66(2):334–344. doi:10.1097/MPG.0000000000001787; European Association for Study of Liver. EASL Clinical Practice Guidelines: Wilson's disease. *J Hepatol.* 2012;56(3):671–685. doi:10.1016/j.jhep.2011.11.007; Poujois A, Woimant F. Wilson's disease: a 2017 update. *Clin Res Hepatol Gastroenterol.* 2018;42(6):512–520. doi:10.1016/j.clinre.2018.03.007.

INTERPRETATION

- Normal serum ceruloplasmin is greater than 0.2 g/L (20 mg/dL).
- Decreased levels of ceruloplasmin are seen in WD, Menkes disease, copper deficiency, and malnutrition.
- Elevated levels of ceruloplasmin are seen in copper toxicity.
- Levels below 0.2 g/L offer a specificity for WD of 55% to 84.5% and sensitivity for WD of 77% to 99%.[3,8]
- Lower cutoff levels have been suggested since levels below 0.1 g/L to 0.16 g/L increase sensitivity/specificity that is closer to 100% and offer a receiver operator curve of 0.956.[3,9,10]

FOLLOW-UP

- Used with other signs/symptoms and diagnostic tests (Leipzig criteria/ Wilson disease scoring system) to determine the likelihood of WD. An online calculator to assist the clinician is found at https://gastroliver.medicine.ufl. edu/hepatology/for-physicians/wilsons-disease-scoring-system/#gf_8
- A mutation/genetic analysis (ATB7B) is used if confirmation of diagnosis is needed.[5]
- Serum-free copper and urine copper complement the diagnostic process when serum ceruloplasmin is low.[5] Both serum-free copper and urine copper will be high in WD.

PEARLS & PITFALLS

- WD is very rare, occurring in only 0.003% of the population.[11]
- WD should be suspected in the presence of acute liver failure combined with hemolytic anemia and jaundice.[5]
- The predictive value of ceruloplasmin alone for WD diagnosis is too low for it to be used alone to exclude or confirm WD; ceruloplasmin should only be used for WD diagnosis along with other signs and symptoms, such as Kayser-Fleisher rings of cornea. See the link to the Leipzig criteria calculator noted earlier.[1,5]
- Normal ceruloplasmin does not exclude WD[1] as false-negative tests can occur with pregnancy, estrogen therapy, and excessive inflammation, all of which raise ceruloplasmin levels from baseline.[5]
- False positives are common; in one study, all low ceruloplasmin levels were false positives.[12] Malabsorption, familial aceruloplasminemia, WD carrier status, and severe renal disease can all cause decreased ceruloplasmin levels and, therefore, false-positive results.[5]
- In one study, the triad of low serum copper, low ceruloplasmin, and high urinary copper levels was seen in 97% of patients with WD.[13]
- In patients with WD, liver abnormalities may precede neurologic abnormalities by as much as 10 years.[5]
- The most common age range to present with signs and symptoms of WD is 6 to 30 years of age.[11]
- There is low pretest probability of WD in patients over 55 years old making ceruloplasmin testing unnecessary in these patients. Overtesting/ unnecessary testing is common in this age group.[11,12]
- Ceruloplasmin accuracy has not been established for those under 1 year of age.[2]

PATIENT EDUCATION

■ https://medlineplus.gov/lab-tests/ceruloplasmin-test

RELATED DIAGNOSES AND ICD-10 CODES

Elevated liver transaminases	R94.5
Family history of other metabolic, endocrine, or nutrition disorder (Wilson disease)	Z83.49

REFERENCES

Full list of references can be accessed through Springer Publishing Company Connect™ at the following link: http://connect.springerpub.com/content/reference-book/978-0-8261 -8843-4/part/part03/toc-part/ch045

46. CHLORIDE SWEAT TEST

Rosie Zeno and Courtney Sexton

PHYSIOLOGY REVIEW

Exocrine glands secrete substances onto an epithelial surface via a duct that originates from subepithelial exocrine tissue, including sweat, mucus, lacrimal, mammary, sebaceous, salivary, and ceruminous glands. The secretory function of exocrine glands relies on active and passive ion transport across the epithelial membrane of exocrine tissue.

Cystic fibrosis (CF) is an autosomal recessive genetic condition linked to mutations in the *cystic fibrosis transmembrane conductance regulator* (CFTR) gene that codes for the proteins essential for ion transport. CFTR gene mutations result in defective (or absent) CFTR proteins and subsequent disruption of the ion transport mechanisms vital to secretory function. The symptomatology of CF is attributed to the viscous mucus secretions of the lungs, pancreas, liver, intestines, and reproductive tract and the characteristic elevation in sweat Cl⁻ levels.

Eccrine glands are predominantly responsible for sweat production via processes mediated by sympathetic cholinergic stimulation.[1] As sweat exits through the ductal lumen, Na+ and Cl⁻ are passively reabsorbed (via epithelial Na+ channels and CFTR channels, respectively), resulting in the excretion of a hypotonic fluid through pores on the skin surface.[1,2]

OVERVIEW OF LABORATORY TESTS

The sweat Cl⁻ test is the gold standard for evaluating CFTR function and establishing a diagnosis of CF (CPT code 89230: sweat collection by iontophoresis, or CPT code 82438: chloride; other source).[3,4] The sweat chloride test is performed by dermal pilocarpine iontophoresis (cholinergic agonist) to stimulate sweat production for collection and analysis.[5] Sweat is collected for a period of 30 minutes via filter paper, gauze, or a commercial collection device with coiled tubing, then analyzed to quantify sweat Cl⁻ concentrations. Pilocarpine iontophoresis testing relies on proper collection techniques to ensure accurate results and avoid delays in diagnosis. Sweat chloride testing should only be performed in accredited facilities with CF expertise, such as an accredited CF center.[3–5]

INDICATIONS

Screening

- Universal screening for CF with sweat chloride testing has not been recommended.
- Universal newborn screening (NBS), including an assay and/or genetic analysis for CF screening, is mandated in all 50 states.[6,7] See Chapter 116.
- Sweat chloride testing is only used in the setting of a suspected CF diagnosis to evaluate CFTR function. Confirmation of CFTR dysfunction is a requisite criterion for making the diagnosis of CF or another CFTR-related diagnosis.[3,8,9]
- CFTR function should be evaluated by sweat Cl⁻ concentration in the following individuals suspected of having CF:[3,8,9]
  1. Infants with a positive NBS (or prenatal genetic test) result; they warrant prompt confirmation testing with a sweat chloride test as soon as possible.
  2. Individuals with an immediate family history of CF (sibling or parent) if previously not screened by NBS or potentially not detected (false negative).
  3. Individuals with signs or symptoms suggestive of CF that may be attributed to CFTR dysfunction (Table 46.1).

Diagnosis and Evaluation

- The probability of CF diagnosis following a positive NBS varies greatly depending on the method used, which varies from state to state, underscoring the importance of early follow-up confirmation with sweat Cl⁻ testing.[3,7]
- Differential diagnoses will vary by patient age and individual clinical presentation. Clinical manifestations of CF may share similar symptomatology with other conditions of the respiratory tract or gastrointestinal system that are unrelated to CFTR dysfunction.

TABLE 46.1: CLINICAL SIGNS AND SYMPTOMS SUGGESTIVE OF CFTR DYSFUNCTION	
INFANTS/CHILDREN	**ADULTS**
• Meconium ileus in the newborn • Failure to thrive, hyponatremia • Bronchiectasis • Chronic/recurrent lower respiratory infections • Signs of pancreatic insufficiency, recurrent pancreatitis	• Chronic/recurrent lower respiratory infections • Signs of pancreatic insufficiency, recurrent pancreatitis • Adult male infertility, azoospermia • Distal intestinal obstruction syndrome • Chronic sinusitis, nasal polyps

CFTR, cystic fibrosis transmembrane conductance regulator.

■ CFTR-related metabolic syndrome (CRMS) and cystic fibrosis, screen positive inconclusive diagnosis (CFSPID) are synonymous terms reserved for infants with a positive NBS and (1) normal sweat Cl⁻ results and 2 CFTR mutations, or (2) intermediate sweat Cl⁻ and 0–1 CFTR mutations.[3,9,10]

Monitoring

■ Sweat chloride testing is only used to establish CFTR dysfunction and diagnose CF. No regular monitoring takes place. Clinical management will vary by individual and relative to the extent of disease of the pulmonary and gastrointestinal systems.

INTERPRETATION

■ Sweat Cl⁻ results should only be interpreted with respect to individuals suspected of having CF (Table 46.2):[3,5]

FOLLOW-UP

■ Repeat sweat Cl⁻ testing for confirmation is no longer recommended for individuals with normal or diagnostic sweat Cl⁻ results.[3,4,9]
■ Infants with CRMS/CFSPD should undergo at least one repeat sweat Cl⁻ test at an accredited CF center.[3,4,9,10]
■ Individuals with intermediate sweat Cl⁻ results on two separate occasions will need further study to rule in/out a CF diagnosis through CFTR genetic analysis and/or CFTR functional analysis as intermediate sweat results are confirmatory in individuals with specific genotypes[3,4,8]
■ Newborns with diagnostic sweat Cl⁻ results should undergo CFTR genetic analysis as an important part of the diagnostic work-up to inform clinical management.[3,4,9]

PEARLS & PITFALLS

■ Clinicians should maintain suspicion for clinical symptoms consistent with CFTR dysfunction in all individuals to avoid missed diagnosis.
■ Sweat Cl⁻ testing should occur as soon as possible after a positive NBS result (as early as 48 hours of age but no later than 4 weeks of age) since disease manifestations, like malnutrition and hyponatremic dehydration, can occur in the first few weeks of life.[3,11,12]

TABLE 46.2: INTERPRETATION OF SWEAT CL⁻ CONCENTRATIONS, ALL AGES			
SWEAT CL⁻	**RESULT**	**CF DIAGNOSIS**	**REPEAT SWEAT CL⁻ TESTING**
≤ 29 mmol/L	Normal	Unlikely	Not indicated Newborns: may consider if family history is concerning or for new onset of symptoms
30–59 mmol/L	Intermediate	Possible	Recommended
≥ 60 mmol/L	Diagnostic	Diagnostic	Not recommended

- Treatment should not be delayed for any individual with a presumptive diagnosis as optimal outcomes rely on early intervention.[3,9,11]
- Obtaining an adequate specimen for sweat Cl⁻ testing is challenging but feasible for full-term infants in the first month of life. To improve likelihood of obtaining sufficient quantities of sweat, pilocarpine iontophoresis should be performed (1) bilaterally, (2) on infants weighing more than 2 kg, and (3) on at least 36 weeks' (corrected) gestational age.[3,4,5,13]
- Over 90% of new CF diagnoses in infants younger than 6 months old are detected by NBS, yet roughly 40% of *total* new CF diagnoses are reportedly not as a result of NBS.[14] It is important to maintain clinical suspicion for any individual presenting with symptoms suggestive of CFTR dysfunction as optimal outcomes rely on early intervention.

PATIENT EDUCATION

- https://www.cff.org
- https://kidshealth.org

RELATED DIAGNOSES AND ICD-10 CODES

Cystic Fibrosis[11]

• Cystic fibrosis, unspecified	E84.9
• Cystic fibrosis, with pulmonary manifestations	E84.0
• Cystic fibrosis, with other intestinal manifestations	E84.19
• Cystic fibrosis, with meconium ileus	E84.11
• Cystic fibrosis, with acute pneumothorax	E84.09
• Cystic fibrosis, with pneumothorax not otherwise specified	E84.09
• Cystic fibrosis, with hemoptysis	E84.09
• CFTR-related metabolic syndrome (CRMS), metabolic disorder unspecified	E88.89
• Cystic fibrosis, screen positive inconclusive diagnosis (CFSPID)	E88.89

CFTR-related disorder[11]

• Pancreatitis, recurrent	K85.9
• Bilateral congenital absence of the vas deferens (CBAVD)	Q55.4
• Bronchiectasis, chronic acquired	J47.9

Other[11]

• Exocrine pancreatic insufficiency	K86.81

REFERENCES

Full list of references can be accessed through Springer Publishing Company Connect™ at the following link: http://connect.springerpub.com/content/reference-book/978-0-8261-8843-4/part/part03/toc-part/ch046

47. *CLOSTRIDIUM* TESTING

Christine Colella and Kelly Small Casler

PHYSIOLOGY REVIEW

Clostridioides difficile (*C. diff*) is a spore-forming and exotoxin-producing, gram-positive, anaerobic bacterium. It is a common cause of antibiotic-associated diarrhea.[1] The toxins produced by most *C. diff* strains are responsible for many of the symptoms seen in *C. diff* infection (CDI), like profuse diarrhea. *C. diff* colonization, which is asymptomatic but still results in positive tests for the bacterium or its toxin, occurs in 8% to 10% of adults residing in hospitals or long-term care facilities.[2,3] The colonization rate among healthy adults is about 3%.[3]

OVERVIEW OF LABORATORY TESTS

Laboratory tests for *C. diff* detect the bacteria, bacterial products such as glutamate dehydrogenase (GDH), the toxins responsible for CDI symptoms, or bacterial genetic components such as the genes that encode *C. diff* toxins.[4,5] Available methods for testing are summarized in the text that follows. Depending on organizational policy, one- or two-step testing may be used (Figures 47.1 and 47.2). The asterisk indicates which tests are available as point-of-care testing.

- **Antigen detection test*** (CPT code 87493). The antigen detection test* detects GDH by immunoassay and offers rapid results, usually within 1 hour.[6] GDH is present in both toxin-producing and non–toxin-producing *C. diff* strains, so it may identify colonization and not active infection. This test is not useful alone due to lack of specificity, so it should be used in combination with other tests.[1] Most commonly, it is paired with a toxin identification test.[6,7]
- **Toxin identification tests.** These tests identify toxins that *C. diff* produces and should only be used in combination with other tests.[8] There are two types of toxin identification tests.
  - Cell cytotoxicity neutralizing assay (CCNA) (also known as tissue culture cytotoxicity) is considered the gold standard test for *C. diff*, but it is rarely used due to complexity in performing, lack of standardization, and a slow turnaround time (greater than 24 hours).[1,4,6] The test evaluates for toxin A or B cytotoxic activity and has sensitivity up to 94% and specificity up to 99% but still underperforms molecular tests and toxigenic stool culture.[1,6]
  - Enzyme immunoassays* detect toxin A, toxin B, or both toxin A and B, and are beneficial since they have a rapid turnaround time. However, the tests have a low sensitivity, which is a drawback.[1]

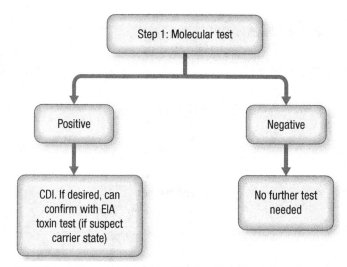

FIGURE 47.1. One test approach. CDI, *Clostridioides difficile* infection; EIA, enzyme immunoassay. *Sources:* Data from Schuetz A. Diagnosis of *C. difficile*–why so difficult? *American Association for Clinical Chemistry.* Published November 1, 2018. https://www.aacc.org/cln/articles/2018/november/diagnosis -of-c,-d-,-difficile; McDonald LC, Gerding DN, Johnson S, et al. Clinical practice guidelines for *Clostridium difficile* infection in adults and children: 2017 update by the Infectious Diseases Society of America (IDSA) and Society for Healthcare Epidemiology of America (SHEA). *Clin Infect Dis.* 2018;66(7):987–994. doi:10.1093/cid/ciy149.

- **Stool culture:** (CPT code 87081). The most sensitive test available for CDI is stool cultures, but their usefulness is limited due to a 49- to 96-hour turnaround time and poor specificity.[1] Stool cultures are also performed as toxigenic cultures where isolates from the culture are tested for toxin A or B to confirm pathogenicity. This is important since there are both toxin-producing and non–toxin-producing *C. diff* strains, but only toxin-producing *C. diff* strains cause CDI.[9]
- **Molecular tests.** Nucleic acid amplification tests (NAATs), such as polymerase chain reaction and loop-mediated isothermal amplification, provide rapid and accurate diagnosis but with a higher cost.[6,10] They test for the gene that encodes for toxin A or B.[1,6] Although they can be used as the sole test, they are usually used in partnership with other *C. diff* diagnostic tests.[5,8] Sensitivity and specificity are close to 90% as long as only symptomatic persons are tested.[6] Molecular tests are generally considered superior to toxin tests.[7]

INDICATIONS

Screening

- In general, asymptomatic patient screening is not indicated.[8] However, recent research and discussions are ongoing regarding screening for asymptomatic carrier state at time of hospital admission. This effort to identify and isolate *C. diff* carriers from noncarriers is thought to decrease the risk of hospital-acquired CDI.[11]

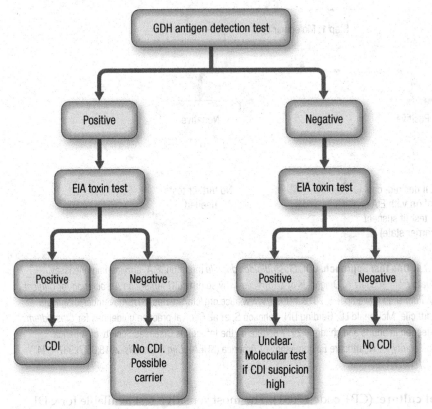

FIGURE 47.2. Two test approach with GDH antigen test and toxin EIA. CDI, *Clostridioides difficile* infection; EIA, enzyme immunoassay; GDH, glutamate dehydrogenase. *Sources*: Data from Schuetz A. Diagnosis of *C. difficile*–why so difficult? *American Association for Clinical Chemistry*. Published November 1, 2018. https://www.aacc.org/cln/articles/2018/november/diagnosis-of-c,-d-,-difficile; McDonald LC, Gerding DN, Johnson S, et al. Clinical practice guidelines for *Clostridium difficile* infection in adults and children: 2017 update by the Infectious Diseases Society of America (IDSA) and Society for Healthcare Epidemiology of America (SHEA). *Clin Infect Dis*. 2018;66(7):987–994. doi:10.1093/cid/ciy149.

Diagnosis and Evaluation

■ Testing is recommended in patients 2 years of age and older with suspicious symptoms, especially those with risk factors (Box 47.1). Suspicious symptoms include prolonged or worsening diarrhea, loose stools, cramping, nausea, low grade fever, anorexia, and onset of diarrhea more than 3 days after hospitalization.[3,8,12]

■ In the absence of diarrhea, the only indication for *C. diff* testing would be if an ileus is suspected.[13]

Monitoring

■ Monitoring is not recommended.

INTERPRETATION

■ Results are reported as positive or negative.[5]

Box 47.1: Risk Factors for *Clostridioides difficile* Infection

- Three or more watery stools in 24 hours
- Advanced age
- Cirrhosis
- Current/recent hospitalization
- Enteral feeding
- Gastric acid suppression medications
- Gastrointestinal surgery
- Immunocompromise
- Inflammatory bowel disease
- Obesity
- Recent antibiotic use
- Severe comorbid illness

Sources: Data from Zacharioudakis IM, Zervou FN, Pliakos EE, Ziakas PD, Mylonakis E. Colonization with toxinogenic *C. difficile* upon hospital admission, and risk of infection: a systematic review and meta-analysis. *Am J Gastroenterol.* 2015;110(3):381–390. doi:10.1038/ajg.2015.22; McDonald LC, Gerding DN, Johnson S, et al. Clinical practice guidelines for *Clostridium difficile* infection in adults and children: 2017 update by the Infectious Diseases Society of America (IDSA) and Society for Healthcare Epidemiology of America (SHEA). *Clin Infect Dis.* 2018;66(7):987–994. doi:10.1093/cid/ciy149.

FOLLOW-UP

- Test of cure not recommended since patients can remain colonized for up to 6 weeks.[2,6,7]
- Follow-up testing may be needed to evaluate for the differential diagnosis of CDI-like symptoms which includes Shigella, Salmonella, Campylobacter, or inflammatory bowel disease.

PEARLS & PITFALLS

- Do not test patients if there has previously been a negative test in the last 7 days or a positive test in last 14 days.[8,14]
- Do not test neonates or infants 12 months of age or younger with diarrhea.[8,12]
- Do not test children aged 1 to 2 years with diarrhea, unless all other causes of diarrhea have been ruled out.[8,12]
- In one study, approximately 77% of asymptomatic carriers had detectable toxin in their stool.[2]
- Watery diarrhea is the cardinal symptom in CDI, but other symptoms such as cramping, nausea, low grade fever, and anorexia do occur.
- The establishment of a best practice/test for CDI detection remains controversial because of the wide variation in testing with limited standardazation[15] It is important to remember that testing should be done only if the patient is symptomatic for CDI since *C. diff* colonization does not require treatment.
- *C. diff* toxin quickly degrades after 2 hours at room temperature. Therefore, samples must be refrigerated or tested immediately after collection.[1]
- In one study, up to 25% of patients experienced a CDI reinfection within 30 days of treatment.[16]

- Have high suspicion for CDI in hospitalized patients on acid-suppressing medication (ASM). Compared to patients not on ASM, any ASM confers a 64% increased risk of recurrent CDI, and PPI specifically confers an 84% increased risk of CDI.[17]
- Asymptomatic carriers can progress to CDI, so monitoring for symptom development is warranted.[18]
- Avoid testing patients with diarrhea due to laxative use.[8]
- In patients with inflammatory bowel disease, false-negative tests are more common for unclear reasons.[19]

PATIENT EDUCATION

- https://cdifffoundation.org
- https://medlineplus.gov/cdiffinfections.html

RELATED DIAGNOSES AND ICD-10 CODES

Diarrhea, unspecified	R19.7
Enterocolitis due to recurrent *Clostridium difficile*	A04.71
Enterocolitis due to *Clostridium difficile*	A04.72

REFERENCES

Full list of references can be accessed through Springer Publishing Company Connect™ at the following link: http://connect.springerpub.com/content/reference-book/978-0-8261 -8843-4/part/part03/toc-part/ch047

48. COLD AGGLUTININS

Beth Faiman and Mailey Wilks

PHYSIOLOGY REVIEW

The cold agglutinin titer (CAT) test is to be used as a laboratory test in the evaluation of suspected cold agglutinin syndrome (CAS) or cold agglutinin disease (CAD).[1] Cold agglutinins are IgM-agglutinating antibodies that, at a temperature of 3 °C to 4 °C, cause agglutination in cooler, usually distal, parts of the body.[2,3] Primary CAD is a distinct lymphoproliferative entity which occurs in approximately 15% of all patients with autoimmune hemolytic anemia (AIHA). Antibodies in the cooler parts of one's body recognize antigens on red blood cells (RBCs) and tag these for destruction. Immune hemolysis occurs and is entirely complement-dependent through the activation of the classical complement pathway. Cold agglutinins, usually IgM, attach to the patient's erythrocytes causing anemia. Symptoms other than anemia may include numbness and tingling of fingers and/or toes, or blood stasis in the skin capillaries.[4,5] Secondary CAS is often related to infection (viral or bacterial) or inflammatory disorders that can affect the complement system; this essential part of the innate immune system is associated with increased susceptibility to infections, inflammation, or disease, and termed "complementopathies." Genetic or acquired abnormalities can be seen in rheumatologic and hematologic disorders that affect the complement system.[2,6]

OVERVIEW OF LABORATORY TESTS

- There are two cold agglutinin serum tests available, the cold agglutinin screen (CPT code 86156) and the cold agglutinin titer (CPT code 86157).
- The cold agglutinin screening test is rarely used.
- The quantitative cold agglutinin titer (CPT code 86157) uses hemagglutination methodology that tests the patient's serum against type O blood cells at 2 °C and 8 °C.

INDICATIONS

Screening

- Universal and targeted screenings are not recommended.

Diagnosis and Evaluation

The CAT test is not diagnostic and should be used in conjunction with other parameters (e.g., evidence of hemolysis, positive direct Coombs' test for C3d) and the overall clinical picture to make the diagnosis of CAD.

Consider diagnostic testing with a CAT in individuals with:

- Cold-induced symptoms of pain or discomfort in an extremity upon exposure to cold
- Pain and/or discomfort on swallowing cold liquids or foods
- Unexplained hemolytic anemia despite an initial evaluation that fails to identify the cause of anemia from sources such as gastrointestinal bleeding, vitamin malabsorption, thyroid abnormalities, or other causes of decreased bone marrow production
- High mean corpuscle volume (MCV) secondary to RBC agglutination
  - Other common findings with CAD include RBC agglutination on blood smear, elevated or normal reticulocyte count, and increased serum lactate dehydrogenase and bilirubin. In hemolysis, the haptoglobin is often decreased or absent.

Monitoring

- Monitoring of cold agglutinin levels depends on the diagnosis.

INTERPRETATION

- Cold agglutinin test results are reported as a titer.
- A higher titer result represents the strength of the antibody and means that there are more autoantibodies present. A reference value is less than 1:64.
- Patients with CAD or CAS typically have a titer greater than 1:512. Rarely, CAD/CAS is seen in a patient with a titer of 1:64. In many instances, the titer is greater than 1:2048.

- An analysis of blood smear can reveal RBC clumping, especially under cold conditions.
- The degree of RBC hemolysis and hemolytic anemia can vary from person to person, and with each cold exposure.
- Not all individuals with cold agglutinin will present with anemia.
- Other conditions can cause an increase in cold agglutinins, such as mycoplasma pneumonia infections, cryoglobulinemia, mononucleosis, and viral infections such as human immunodeficiency virus (HIV), cytomegalovirus, and hepatitis.

FOLLOW-UP

- More than 70% of CAD cases can be attributed to infections, underlying malignancies, and autoimmune diseases. A thorough workup looking for these conditions should be considered.
- There is no recommended interval for follow-up testing on secondary CAS.
- The monitoring and treatment of patients with CAD secondary to a lymphoproliferative disorder is generally managed by hematology.
- If a patient has a high titer and significant anemia, a thorough evaluation by hematology for an underlying bone marrow disorder is warranted.

PEARLS & PITFALLS

- Not all individuals with cold agglutinins will exhibit symptoms. Cold avoidance in individuals without an underlying clonal bone marrow disorder, anemia, or viral/underlying disorder is still recommended.
- The importance of diagnosing cold agglutinin before cardiac surgery has been suggested to minimize the risk of agglutination during surgery. The incidence of asymptomatic cold agglutinins is low (less than 0.3%). Currently, a hematologist's opinion should be sought in patients with a significant antibody titer. Hemolysis is rarely seen if the titer is below 1:1000.[7]
- In patients with symptoms of cold or tingling feet, elevated cold agglutinin titers may be observed, but they may not exhibit anemia.
- CAD primarily affects women, and the median age of onset is 67.[7]

PATIENT EDUCATION

- https://rarediseases.info.nih.gov/diseases/6130/cold-agglutinin-disease

RELATED DIAGNOSES AND ICD-10 CODES

Chronic cold hemagglutinin disease	D59.12
Cold agglutinin disease	
Cold agglutinin hemoglobinuria	
Cold type (primary) (secondary) (symptomatic) autoimmune hemolytic anemia	
Cold type autoimmune hemolytic disease	

REFERENCES

Full list of references can be accessed through Springer Publishing Company Connect™ at the following link: http://connect.springerpub.com/content/reference-book/978-0-8261 -8843-4/part/part03/toc-part/ch048

49. COMPLEMENT STUDIES

Penelope Callaway

PHYSIOLOGY REVIEW

The complement system derives its name from its function; it "complements" the immune system.[1] The complement system consists of at least 60 proteins (and subcomponents) that promote immune and inflammatory responses.[1,2] Although the complement system is one of the first lines of defense of the innate immune system, it also contributes to the adaptive immune system by modulating the intensity of the immune response.[2,3] The complement system aids in identifying, destroying, and removing foreign pathogens, such as bacteria, fungi, parasites, and viruses. Additionally, this system assists in removing damaged or dead self-cells.[2,4-6] The complement cascade is the sequential activation of proteins in the complement system. Nine complement proteins (designated C1–C9) are key steps in the complement cascade.[1,2,4-6] Activation of the complement system begins when the body synthesizes antibodies either against its own tissues (as in autoimmune disease) or against foreign pathogens. Then, it takes one of three pathways (classical, alternative, or lectin) that converge with the same end-product, the membrane attack complex (MAC).[1,2] Congenital deficiencies and/or acquired dysregulation of the complement system are prominent aspects of many disorders and autoimmune diseases.[2,4-6]

Individual complement component levels vary with age. There is high variability of complement levels in infants.[2] Preterm infants display low C3 and C4, when compared with term infants.[2] These complement levels increase after birth but do not reach peak adult levels until about 18 months of age.[2] Total complement takes several years to match adult levels.[2] There is no evidence to indicate that complement levels decrease with age.[2]

Although initial identification of the complement system occurred over 100 years ago and the central role of this system is now much better understood, a thorough knowledge of its components and its many biologic effects is still emerging.[2,5]

OVERVIEW OF LABORATORY TESTS

Complement studies measure the amount of or activity level of complement proteins in the blood in order to diagnose or monitor autoimmune or immune complex-related diseases.[1,2,7-9] Disorders of the complement system can be congenital or acquired. Rare deficiencies of specific complement proteins can cause susceptibility to recurrent infections or autoimmune disorders.[2,8,9] When the complement system is activated, complement proteins are consumed, and complement levels fall. Specific complement components can be measured to determine if abnormalities of the complement system are related to a particular condition. For example, while total complement, C50 (CPT code 86162), is used to gain an overview of the entire classical complement pathway, C3 (CPT code 86160) and C4 (CPT code 86160) are commonly ordered as individual complement tests.[1,2,8] Both C3 and C4 levels are typically low in active systemic lupus erythematosus (SLE). In acute infections, however, it is common that only C3 is low.[1,2,8,9] Complement levels generally return to normal once the acute or chronic condition is resolved.[1,9]

INDICATIONS
Screening
■ Complement studies are not recommended for universal screening.[8]
■ The total complement assay (C50) should be used to screen for suspected complement-related disorders prior to measuring specific complement components. Consider screening with a total complement assay when:
  ● There are recurrent infections, or there is an unusual or persistent infection that does not respond to treatment;
  ● What is usually a mild childhood disease suddenly worsens or becomes life-threatening despite treatment; or
  ● The presence of abnormal results of complete blood cell counts (CBCs) is persistent and significant.[1,7,8]

Diagnosis and Evaluation
Abnormal complement levels are not diagnostic. An elevated or decreased complement level does not definitively rule in or rule out a particular condition. Instead, a complement level outside of the normal interval simply indicates that a specific part of the immune system is likely involved.[1,10] Complement studies provide additional information that can contribute to the overall clinical picture.

Following screening with a total complement assay (C50), measurement of specific complement components can contribute to diagnosing the following conditions:

■ Suspected autoimmune diseases
  ● Such as C3 and C4 for SLE or rheumatoid arthritis (RA);
■ Reasons for recurrent/persistent microbial (bacterial, fungal, parasitic, or viral) infections,
  ● Such as C1, C2, C4, C5, C6, C7, C8, and C9 for recurrent *Streptococcus pneumoniae*, *Neisseria meningitides*, or *Neisseria gonorrhea*; and
■ Causes of chronic conditions,
  ● Such as C1 and C4 for hereditary angioedema, or C1, C2, C3, and C4 for genetic complement deficiencies.[1,7-9,10]

Monitoring
Tracking levels of specific complement components can be used to:

■ Monitor the activity of acute and chronic autoimmune disorders, immune complex-related diseases, and certain inflammatory diseases.[1,7-9]
■ Help determine the effectiveness of treatment for acute and chronic autoimmune disorders, immune complex-related diseases, and certain inflammatory diseases.[1,5,7-9]

During acute phase exacerbations or prior to stabilization of an existing condition:

- Low levels of evidence (expert opinion) indicate complement levels should be repeated every 2 to 4 weeks.[11]

Complement components used to monitor treatment efficacy:

- Will need to be repeated in 2- to-6-month intervals, once the condition has stabilized.[11]

INTERPRETATION

A wide variety of conditions can lead to high or low levels of individual components of complement. Interpretation for each condition is unique and often requires results of other laboratory tests and findings from a clinical examination.

For example, utilizing complement levels for a diagnosis of SLE, with corroboration of clinical examination findings, yields a:

- C3 sensitivity of 87.11% and specificity of 82.74%,
- C4 sensitivity of 88.66% and specificity of 77.43%, and
- A combined C3 and C4 sensitivity of 92.78% and specificity of 79.20%.[12]

Neither C3 nor C4 alone is sufficient to meet immunologic criterion. When combined with an antinuclear antibody (ANA) and an anti-double-stranded DNA (anti-dsDNA) antibody, the sensitivity and specificity of all four indicators rise to 97.42 and 80.97%, respectively.[12]

For SLE, there is high diagnostic value in testing ANA, anti-dsDNA antibody along with complements C3 and C4.

A comprehensive analysis of the reciprocal relationships between individual complement components and each disorder is extensive. See Table 49.1. for disorders associated with general complement trends.

Although normal test value ranges vary among different laboratories, Table 49.2. is provided as a reference for the most commonly ordered complement protein levels. Of note, there is significant variability in the units of measurement between laboratories; U/mL = units per milliliter; mg/dL = milligrams per deciliter.

FOLLOW-UP

As the complement system is only one component of the innate immune system, abnormal results of complement testing warrant correlation and/or follow-up testing of other parts of the innate immune system. Often, laboratories will offer reflex testing, the process of proceeding on to subsequent related tests if initial tests' results are outside of the normal ranges.

Depending on the purpose of the testing and the differential diagnoses, ensuing or frequently accompanying tests may include:

- CBC with differential, complete metabolic panel (CMP), creatine kinase (CK), erythrocyte sedimentation rate (ESR), C-reactive protein (CRP), rheumatoid factor (RF) (IgA, IgG, and IgM), ANA, serum protein electrophoresis, UA,

TABLE 49.1: CONDITIONS ASSOCIATED WITH A DECREASE OR INCREASE IN COMPLEMENT ACTIVITY

↓ DECREASED COMPLEMENT ACTIVITY	↑ INCREASED COMPLEMENT ACTIVITY
• Recurrent microbial infections (usually bacterial) • Autoimmune diseases: systemic lupus erythematosus, rheumatoid arthritis, Sjögren syndrome, myasthenia gravis, and Henoch-Schonlein purpura • Hereditary or acquired angioedema • Various types of kidney disease, including glomerulonephritis, lupus nephritis, membranous nephritis, and IgA nephropathy, as well as kidney transplant rejection • Cirrhosis • Hepatitis • Malnutrition • Septicemia, shock • Serum sickness (immune complex disease) • Rare inherited complement deficiencies • Antiphospholipid syndrome • Mixed cryoglobulinemia • Malaria • Infective endocarditis • Congenital complement deficiencies • Inflammatory myopathies	• Cancer (leukemia, Hodgkin's lymphoma, sarcoma) • Ulcerative colitis • Thyroiditis • Acute myocardial infarction • Sarcoidosis • Active juvenile rheumatoid arthritis • Acute or chronic inflammation • Certain acute infections (usually viral) • Non-alcoholic fatty liver disease (NAFLD) • Metabolic syndrome • Obesity • Diabetes • Heart disease

Sources: Pagana K, Pagana T, Pagana T. *Mosby's® Diagnostic and Laboratory Test Reference.* 15th ed. Elsevier Health Sciences; 2021; Liszewski MK, Atkinson JP. Acquired disorders of the complement system. In: Feldweg A, Marsh R, Schur P, Post T, eds. *UpToDate.* UpToDate; 2021. www.uptodate.com; Ferri F. *Ferri's Best Test: A Practical Guide to Clinical Laboratory Medicine and Diagnostic Imaging.* 4th ed. Elsevier Health Sciences; 2019; Frazer-Abel A, Sepiashvili L, Mbughuni MM, Willrich MA. Overview of laboratory testing and clinical presentations of complement deficiencies and dysregulation. *Adv Clin Chem.* 2016;77:1–75. doi:10.1016/bs.acc.2016.06.001.

TABLE 49.2: COMPLEMENT LEVEL TESTS: REFERENCE INTERVALS

COMPLEMENT COMPONENT	LOW	NORMAL	HIGH
*Complement C1Q (CPT code 86160)	11.9 mg/dL or less	12–22 mg/dL	22.1 mg/dL or greater
Complement C2 (CPT code 86160)	24.9 U/mL or less	25–47 U/mL	47.1 U/mL or greater
Complement C3 (CPT code 86160)	74.9 mg/dL or less	75–175 mg/dL	175.9 mg/dL or greater
Complement C4 (CPT code 86160)	13.9 mg/dL or less	14–40 mg/dL	40.1 mg/dL or greater
Total complement (CH50) (CPT code 86162)	29.9 U/mL or less	30–75 U/mL	75.1 U/mL or greater

* The measurement of C1q is an indicator of the amount of C1 present, a different assay than C1q binding, which is an assay for circulating immune complexes.

Source: Frazer-Abel A, Sepiashvili L, Mbughuni MM, Willrich MA. Overview of laboratory testing and clinical presentations of complement deficiencies and dysregulation. *Adv Clin Chem.* 2016;77:1–75. doi:10.1016/bs.acc.2016.06.001.

urine protein-to-creatinine ratio, quantitative serum immunoglobulin (IgG, IgA, IgM, and IgE) levels, antibody titers to protein and polysaccharide vaccines; isohemagglutinins; and/or serology for viral infections.[1,2,7–10]

Other autoantibody tests are often needed to monitor specific disease activity or treatment efficacy, or to further guide the diagnostic reasoning process. These tests may include, but are not limited to:

- Anti-dsDNA, anti-Sm, lupus anticoagulant, anti-Ro/SSA, anti-La/SSB, anticardiolipin antibodies, anti-beta2-glycoprotein 1, anti-cyclic citrullinated peptide, mitochondrial antibodies, smooth muscle antibodies, RNP antibodies, and antineutrophil cytoplasmic antibodies.[1,2,7–10]

PEARLS & PITFALLS

- In addition to plasma, complement can be measured in other body fluids, such as pleural, pericardial, and synovial fluids. The complement levels in different body fluids vary and do not always positively correlate with the serum complement levels. For example, in people with RA, the serum complement levels can be low, normal, or high, depending on the phase of the condition; however, complement levels in synovial fluid may be very low.[1,8]
- A deficiency in any one of the individual complement components will result in a low or even undetectable total complement level.[1,2,10]
- Initial complement testing should be completed prior to any treatment and should not be repeated if treatment involves complement inhibitors, such as eculizumab or ravulizumab, as complement inhibitor therapies will affect the accuracy of the complement assays.[10]
- Phases of the same immune disorder may affect complement levels differently. For example, the acute phase of an immune disorder may cause a rise in complement levels, while a chronic phase may display low levels of complement components. It is important to establish the pattern that is unique to the individual.[1,10]
- Correct specimen handling (collection, processing, and storage) is essential for accurate results, as many of the complement components are highly unstable and can be activated prior to the clinical testing procedure. It is best to assay the serum sample on the day of collection. Always repeat an undetectable or very low CH50 with a separate sample.[1,2]
- Evaluate infants who present with recurrent, persistent, or severe infections (bacterial, viral, fungal, or parasitic) or failure to thrive for severe combined immunodeficiency (SCID), as this is a pediatric emergency.[8]
- Given the recognized role of complement in immune activation and promoting inflammation and the deleterious effect in autoimmune disease, research is focusing on the development of complement-inhibiting therapies.[13–15]

PATIENT EDUCATION

- https://medlineplus.gov/lab-tests/complement-blood-test

RELATED DIAGNOSES AND ICD-10 CODES

Defect in the complement system	D84.1
Other related diagnoses using the same ICD-10 code: angioedema, hereditary; circulating enzyme deficiency; complement deficiency disease; deficiency of circulating enzyme; heriditary angioneurotic edema; and hypocomplementemia, Bannister's disease, hereditary; giant urticaria, hereditary; Quincke's disease, hereditary; alternative pathways deficiency[8]	
Other specified disorders involving the immune mechanism, not elsewhere classified[8]	D89.9
Systemic involvement of connective tissue, unspecified	M35.9

Autoimmune, infectious, or other disorders involving the complement system will require additional ICD-10 codes specific to the condition.

REFERENCES

Full list of references can be accessed through Springer Publishing Company Connect™ at the following link: http://connect.springerpub.com/content/reference-book/978-0-8261 -8843-4/part/part03/toc-part/ch049

---

50. COOMBS' DIRECT AND INDIRECT ANTIBODY TESTS

Elizabeth Sharpe

PHYSIOLOGY REVIEW

There are four major blood group types: A, B, AB, and O. Each of these blood group types is characterized by the presence or absence of A and/or B antigens and the presence or absence of specific antibodies (see Chapter 31, Figure 31.1).

■ Individuals with type A blood have the A antigen and their sera contains IgM antibodies against the B antigen.
■ Individuals with type B blood have the B antigen and their sera contains IgM antibodies against the A antigen.
■ Individuals with type AB blood have the A and B antigens and their sera contains no A or B antibodies, making them the universal recipient.
■ Individuals with type O blood have no blood group antigens and their sera contains antibodies against both the A and B antigen, making them the universal donor.

In addition to the A and B antigens that are found on the surface of the red blood cells (RBCs), there is a protein called the Rh factor. The Rh factor is either present (+) or absent (-), thus forming the eight most common blood types (A+, A–, B+, B–, AB+, AB–, O+, and O–).

Infants are at risk for hemolytic disease of the newborn when the Rh (D) antigen status differs from the maternal Rh (d) antigen status (e.g., when an Rh-positive (+) infant is born to an Rh-negative (–) mother, or an Rh-negative (–) infant is born to a Rh-positive (+) mother). During pregnancy, an Rh-negative mother carrying a fetus conceived with an Rh-positive father is at risk for maternal-fetal mixing of blood causing maternal sensitization and formation of antibodies. When these antibodies transfer into the fetus, the antibodies attach to fetal blood cells, causing hemolytic disease of the newborn (also known as erythroblastosis fetalis). While this occurs rarely during the first pregnancy, the maternal response and risk to the fetus increases with subsequent pregnancies. Rh immune-globulin (RhoGAM) is administered to Rh-negative mothers at 28 weeks gestation and following delivery to prevent maternal recognition of any fetal D antigen and formation of antibodies that would cause hemolysis.[1] Patients across the life span are at risk for hemolytic transfusion reaction if they receive transfused blood with incompatible blood type or group. The patient's existing antibodies would attach to the incompatible erythrocytes leading to alloimmune hemolytic anemia. Pre-transfusion screening aims to detect existing antibodies to prevent erythrocyte destruction.

OVERVIEW OF LABORATORY TESTS

The direct Coombs' test (CPT code 86880), also called the direct antiglobulin test, detects antibodies on the surface of the RBC. When the antibody on the surface of the RBCs reacts with the anti-human globulin reagent producing a visible agglutination reaction, this is a positive result. The direct Coombs test is performed to identify antibodies coating the erythrocyte surface, such as the blood grouping antigens, ABO and Rh, and evaluate suspected transfusion reactions when anticipating hyperbilirubinemia. The direct Coombs' test is used to investigate suspected hemolytic transfusion reactions, diagnose and classify autoimmune hemolytic anemia, and assess for hemolytic disease of the fetus and newborn. The indirect Coombs' or indirect antiglobulin test (CPT code 86850) detects antibodies circulating in serum. It detects minor antibodies that are present and not attached to the erythrocyte surface. The indirect Coombs' is a two-stage test where the patient's serum is added to donor RBCs with known antigens, then the anti-human globulin reagent is added. Agglutination reaction indicates a positive result. Both the direct and indirect Coombs' tests are useful across the life span.[2]

INDICATIONS

Screening
Universal screening is not recommended.

Targeted screening using the direct Coombs' test should be obtained in the following:

- Infants of Rh-negative mothers
- Where the maternal antibody screen is negative and active hemolysis is suspected.[3]

Targeted screening using the indirect Coombs' test should be obtained in the following:

- For patients in advance of a blood transfusion[3]
- For each pregnancy at the first visit (at 12 weeks gestation)[4]

Diagnosis and Evaluation

Coombs' (Direct Antiglobulin Test)
- Suspected alloimmune-mediated hemolytic transfusion reactions
- Evaluation of hemolytic disease of the fetus and newborn
- Investigation of autoimmune-mediated hemolytic anemia[2]
- Assessment for drug-induced immune hemolytic anemia[5]

Coombs' (Indirect Antiglobulin Test)
- Maternal development of antibodies to common antigens to identify risk for hemolytic disease of the fetus and newborn[6]

Monitoring
- No routine monitoring of the Coombs' tests is recommended.

INTERPRETATION
- The strength of an antibody agglutination reaction is graded from 1+ (weak reaction) to 4+ (strong reaction) and a positive result.[2]
- No agglutination is a negative or normal result.

FOLLOW-UP
- No ongoing follow-up of the Coombs' tests are recommended.
- A positive direct Coombs' test with climbing bilirubin levels may require more frequent bilirubin monitoring and indicate the need for hematocrit and reticulocyte count evaluation.

PEARLS & PITFALLS
- Potential causes of false-positive results include:
  - Clotted or inadequate specimen
  - Intravenous immune globulin administration
  - Antiphospholipid syndrome
  - Human immunodeficiency virus (HIV), malaria
  - Wharton jelly
- Potential causes of false-negative results include:
  - Hemolysis
  - Inadequate specimen[2]
- Recent evidence demonstrated that 46% of COVID-19 patients had a positive direct antiglobulin test result and this was associated with increased incidence of anemia and transfusion requirements.[7,8]
- A positive direct Coombs' test in the absence of hemolytic anemia may be correlated with high acuity and poor renal response in systemic lupus erythematosus.[9]

PATIENT EDUCATION

■ https://med.stanford.edu/newborns/professional-education/jaundice
-and-phototherapy/the-coombs--test.html

RELATED DIAGNOSES AND ICD-10 CODES

Autoimmune hemolytic anemia	D59.10, D59.11, D59.12, D59.13, D59.19
Hemolytic transfusion reaction	T80.919A
ABO incompatibility with hemolytic transfusion reaction	T80.31
Non-ABO incompatibility with hemolytic transfusion reaction	T80.A1
Rh incompatibility with hemolytic transfusion reaction	T80.41
Rh isoimmunization of newborn	P55.0

REFERENCES

Full list of references can be accessed through Springer Publishing Company Connect™ at the following link: http://connect.springerpub.com/content/reference-book/978-0-8261
-8843-4/part/part03/toc-part/ch050

51. COPPER

Kelly Small Casler

PATHOPHYSIOLOGY REVIEW

Copper is one of the essential nutrients. It is absorbed by the enterocytes and transported to the liver where some copper is used for metabolism and the rest is attached to ceruloplasmin, the main transporter of copper.[1,2] Copper is excreted in bile. Excretion of copper and the ability to attach it to ceruloplasmin is impaired in Wilson's disease (WD).[1] Without copper attachment, ceruloplasmin is quickly degraded by the body.

OVERVIEW OF LABORATORY TESTS

Copper can be measured in serum as total copper.[3] Total copper includes copper that is both bound to protein (ceruloplasmin, albumin, and other proteins) and not bound to protein. Free copper (the amount of copper that is not attached to ceruloplasmin) can be estimated by tripling the serum ceruloplasmin level and subtracting that number from the total copper level.[4,5] Copper can also be measured in urine (usually 24-hour collection)[6,7] and tissue obtained during liver biopsy.[7]

INDICATIONS

Screening
■ Not used

Diagnosis and Evaluation
■ Serum copper testing is indicated with signs or symptoms of copper deficiency or excess.
  ● Signs/symptoms of deficiency:[6,8] anemia, leukopenia, myeloneuropathy (presents similarly to neuropathy seen in vitamin B12 deficiency)
  ● Signs/symptoms of excess:[9,10] nausea, vomiting, headache, diarrhea, liver failure, kidney failure, gastrointestinal (GI) hemorrhage, hemolytic anemia, methemoglobinemia
■ Urine copper and hepatic copper testing are used to evaluate for WD.

Monitoring
■ Urine and serum copper are used to monitor treatment response in WD. Usually serum copper is performed every 6 months.[11]
■ Free copper may also be used to monitor and guide WD treatment response with a goal of less than 10 µg/dL.[5]

INTERPRETATION

■ Reference interval for serum total copper (adults): 70–155 µg/dL[12]
■ Reference interval for serum total copper (children, older than 6 months): 90 to 190 µg/dL
■ Reference interval for free copper (adults): 8 to 12 µg/dl[4]
■ Reference interval for 24-hour urine copper (adults): 40.6 to 101.6 µg/24 hr[7]
■ Reference limit for 24-hour urine copper (children): 40.6 µg/24 hr or less[11]
■ Reference limit for hepatic copper: less than 50.8 µg/g[7]
■ Interpretation of copper levels is most often completed using ceruloplasmin, other laboratory tests, and other signs/symptoms to determine likelihood of WD. A calculator is available (sometimes called Leipzig criteria).
  ● https://gastroliver.medicine.ufl.edu/hepatology/for-physicians/wilsons-disease-scoring-system/#gf_8
■ For diagnosis of WD, elevated 24-urine copper had sensitivity of 50.0% to 80.0%, and specificity of 75.6% to 98.3%.[7]
■ For WD, hepatic copper greater than 254.1 µg/g had a sensitivity of 65.7% to 94.4%, and a specificity of 52.2% to 98.6%.[7]
■ In WD, serum copper will be decreased, but free copper will be elevated.[4]

FOLLOW-UP

■ If serum total copper is low, evaluate for causes of copper deficiency:[8] WD, celiac disease, gastric bypass and other malabsorption syndromes,[13–15] Menkes disease,[16] cholestasis,[17] eating disorders, prematurity, malnutrition, burns, and renal replacement therapy.

- If serum total copper is high, evaluate for causes of excess: thyrotoxicosis, biliary disease, accidental (excess copper in drinking water, for example) or intentional ingestion.[9,10]
- Mutation/genetic analysis (ATB7B) is used if confirmation of WD diagnosis is needed.[11]

PEARLS & PITFALLS

- Zinc excess can impair copper absorption and lead to deficiency.[18]
- Elevated hepatic copper levels can be seen in chronic obstructive/cholestatic liver diseases like primary biliary cirrhosis.[11,19]
- Mean values of serum copper are higher in females, especially those taking estrogens, and during pregnancy.[6]

PATIENT EDUCATION

- https://ods.od.nih.gov/factsheets/Copper-HealthProfessional

RELATED DIAGNOSES AND ICD-10 CODES

Elevated liver transaminases	R94.5
Disorder of copper metabolism	E83.00

REFERENCES

Full list of references can be accessed through Springer Publishing Company Connect™ at the following link: http://connect.springerpub.com/content/reference-book/978-0-8261-8843-4/part/part03/toc-part/ch051

---

52. CORONAVIRUSES (SARS-COV-2, MERS, SARS)

Heidi He

PHYSIOLOGY REVIEW

Coronaviruses, whose name derived from their characteristic crown-like appearance in electron micrographs, are divided into four genera: alpha, beta, gamma, and delta coronaviruses. Human coronaviruses (HCoVs) are in two of these genera: alpha and beta. Prior to 2019, six coronavirus serotypes have been associated with disease in humans: four common cold human coronaviruses (HCoV-229E, HCoV-NL63, HCoV-OC43, and HCoV-HKU1), Middle East Respiratory Syndrome coronavirus (MERS-CoV), and severe acute respiratory syndrome coronavirus (SARS-CoV). At the end of 2019, a novel coronavirus

(SARS-CoV-2) was identified as the cause of a cluster of pneumonia cases in Wuhan, China. It subsequently has spread throughout the world, becoming the unprecedented coronavirus disease 2019 (COVID-19) global pandemic. Of these viruses, only HCoV-229E and HCoV-NL63 are alpha coronaviruses; the rest are beta coronaviruses.[1-3] In this chapter, laboratory tests for diagnosing COVID-19, MERS, and SARS will be discussed.

SARS-COV-2

The disease caused by SARS-CoV-2 virus was designated as coronavirus disease 2019 (COVID-19) by the World Health Organization (WHO) in February 2020 to prevent the use of other names that can be inaccurate or stigmatizing.[4] At the time of this article, over 150 million confirmed cases of COVID-19 have been reported globally.[5] Updated case counts can be found on the WHO website.

The clinical symptoms of COVID-19 vary significantly and can range from asymptomatic to fatal. The understanding of COVID-19 continues to evolve, as is the guidance for diagnosing and managing COVID disease. While the exact mechanisms of COVID-19 pathophysiologic progression remain unclear, several key mechanisms have been proposed as contributing to the progression of COVID-19 disease.[2]

Coronaviruses consist of four main structural glycoproteins: spike (S), membrane (M), envelope (E), and nucleocapsid (N). Spike protein is responsible for viral binding and entry into host cells. Human angiotensin converting enzyme 2 (ACE2) has been identified as the entry receptor for both SARS-CoV and SARS-CoV-2. However, SARS-CoV-2 has been reported to have a higher affinity for the ACE2 receptor. Furthermore, the unique characteristic of SARS-CoV-2 virus spike makes the virus very pathogenic.[2]

ACE2 expression is high in the lungs, particularly on epithelial cells. SARS-CoV-2 is mostly transmissible through large respiratory droplets, directly infecting cells of the upper and lower respiratory tract, especially nasal ciliated and alveolar epithelial cells. When viremia is present, SARS-CoV-2 may also directly infect cells of other organ systems, because ACE2 is also expressed in the small intestine, kidneys, heart, thyroid, testis, and adipose tissue.[2]

SARC-CoV-2 can also be transmitted through the airborne route, but the extent to which this mode of transmission contributed to the pandemic is controversial. Similarly, SARC-CoV-2 has been detected in nonrespiratory specimens, including stool, blood, ocular secretions, and semen, but the role of these sites in transmission is unclear.[3,6]

In some COVID-19 patients, the combined immune response of initial cytokine release and activation of antiviral interferon response, followed by immune cell recruitment, is enough for successful SARS-CoV-2 clearance. However, in other patients, viral infection can progress to severe disease due to a dysregulated immune response.[6] Maladaptive release of post inflammatory cytokines and chemokines significantly correlate to disease severity and mortality. Many believe that extrapulmonary involvement in COVID-19 is a direct result of unrestrained inflammation. However, other contributing mechanisms, such as direct viral infection, have also been proposed. This is understandable, because ACE2 is expressed in multiple organ systems, although the expression is highest in the lungs. The high incidence of thrombotic events in COVID-19 patients can also be strongly linked to inflammation and cytokine release. One of the key hallmarks of COVID-19 severity is the progression to multisystem organ damage or failure.[2,3,6]

OVERVIEW OF LABORATORY TESTS

SARS-CoV-2 testing is essential in slowing and stopping the spread of the virus. The Centers for Disease Control and Prevention (CDC) recommends that the selection and interpretation of SARS-CoV-2 tests should be based on the context in which they are being used.[7] Types of tests that can be used for SARS-CoV-2 testing are detailed in Table 52.1.

INDICATIONS

Screening

Individuals who are asymptomatic or pre-symptomatic can transmit SARS-CoV-2 and contribute to the occurrence of COVID-19 infection in the community. Screening tests are an extremely important disease prevention strategy.

TABLE 52.1: TYPES OF SARS-COV-2 TESTS		
TESTING PURPOSE	**TEST NAME**	**COMMENTS**[3,7,9]
Tests for Current Infection (Viral Tests)	SARS-CoV-2 nucleic acid amplification tests (NAATs)	• Highly specific • Preferred initial test for COVID-19 • Most commonly with a reverse – transcription polymerase chain reaction (RT-PRC) assay, to detect RNA from the upper respiratory tract • Could be impacted by the SARS-CoV-2 variants with mutations in the spike protein • Rapid RT-PRC tests: appear to be comparable to laboratory-based NAAT • Rapid isothermal tests: less sensitive compared to laboratory based NAAT • Can be done at a testing facility or at home with an at home collection kit or an at home test
	Antigen tests	• Less sensitive than that of NAAT • Negative antigen tests should usually be confirmed with NAAT if clinically indicated • Most sensitive in the early stages of the infection • Would not be impacted by the SARS-CoV-2 variants with mutations in the spike protein • Can be done at a testing facility or at home with an at home collection kit or an at home test
Tests for Prior Infection (serologic tests/antibodies tests)	SARS-CoV-2 IgG or total antibody	• Should be performed 3 to 4 weeks after the onset of symptoms to optimize testing accuracy • The sensitivity of IgG or total antibody at 4 weeks was 88% and 95%, respectively • Sensitivity and specificity are highly variable • Cross reactivity with another coronavirus has been reported

It allows early identification and isolation of asymptomatic, pre-symptomatic, or mildly symptomatic individuals; and effectively decreases the spread of infection. Screening is particularly helpful in COVID-19 outbreaks or in communities with a high level of transmission.[7] As the vaccination rate for COVID-19 continues to increase, the screening priorities for SARS-CoV-2 continue to evolve.[7]

Diagnosis and Evaluation

While there are no specific clinical features that can reliably distinguish COVID-19 from other viral respiratory infections, the CDC recommends COVID testing in the following circumstances:[7]

1. People who have symptoms regardless of vaccination status or prior infection. Symptoms may appear 2 to 14 days after exposure to the virus and may be mild to severe. The following list includes common symptoms but does not include all possible symptoms.[7]
   - Fever or chills
   - Cough
   - Short of breath or difficulty breathing
   - Fatigue
   - Muscle or body aches
   - Headache
   - New loss of taste or smell
   - Sore throat
   - Congestion or running nose
   - Nausea or vomiting
   - Diarrhea
2. People who have had close contact (within 6 feet for a total of 15 minutes or more over a 24-hour period) with someone with confirmed COVID-19,[7] with **exceptions** for:
   - Fully vaccinated people (2 weeks after their second dose in a two-dose vaccine series or 2 weeks after a single dose vaccine) with no COVID-19 symptoms
   - People who have tested positive for COVID-19 within the past 3 months and have recovered, and do not have new symptoms
3. People who have participated in activities that put them at higher risk for COVID -19, such as travel, attending a large social or mass gathering, or being in a crowded or poorly ventilated indoor setting, because they cannot physically distance as needed to avoid exposure[7]

Monitoring

Antibody or serology tests that look for antibodies should not be used to diagnose a current infection. A positive antibody test can help support the diagnosis of COVID-19 illness or complications of COVID-19 in the following situations:[7]

1. When patients present with complications of COVID-19 illness, such as multisystem inflammatory syndrome and other post-acute sequalae of COVID-19

2. At least 7 days following acute illness onset in person with a previous negative antibody test (seroconversion) and who did not receive a positive viral test

INTERPRETATION

SARS-CoV-2 Nucleic Acid Amplification Tests

A summary of SARS-CoV-2 nucleic acid amplification test (NAATs) results and their interpretation, including clinical implications, is provided in Table 52.2.

SARS-CoV-2 IgG or Total Antibody Tests

A summary of SARS-CoV-2 IgG or total antibody test results and their interpretation, including clinical implications, is provided in Table 52.3.[8-10]

The spectrum of symptomatic COVID-19 infection ranges from mild to fatal. While severe illness can occur in otherwise healthy individuals of any age, older age is associated with increased mortality. Other comorbidities that have been associated with severe illness and mortality include cardiovascular disease, diabetes mellitus, lung diseases such as chronic obstructive pulmonary disease, cancer, chronic kidney disease, solid organ or hematopoietic stem cell transplantation, obesity, and smoking. Furthermore, certain demographic features have also been associated with more severe illness, such as male sex, Black, Hispanic, and south Asian ethnicities.[11]

TABLE 52.2: NAATS TEST RESULTS AND INTERPRETATION	
TEST RESULT	**INTERPRETATION AND CLINICAL IMPLICATIONS[7,10]**
Positive SARS-CoV-2 NAATs	• Confirm the diagnosis of COVID-19, no additional testing needed. • SARS-CoV-2 RNA can be detected for weeks after the onset of symptoms. • Highly specific tests; however, the accuracy and predictive values have not been systematically evaluated.

Persistent or recurrent positive SARS-CoV-2 NAATs	• Prolonged viral RNA does not necessarily indicate ongoing infectiousness.
	• The possibility of reinfection should be investigated in patients who:
	  ○ Have a repeat positive NAAT more than 90 days after the initial infection, regardless of symptoms, or
	  ○ Have a repeat positive NAAT 45 to 89 days after initial infection and have symptoms consistent with COVID-19 in the setting of recent exposure or with no alternative explanation.
	• Asymptomatic individuals who were previously diagnosed with SARS-CoV-2 in the prior 3 months should not be retested.[7,10]
	  ○ The likelihood that a repeat positive test during this interval represents an active infection is very low.
	  ○ Infectious virus from upper respiratory specimens is rarely isolated 10 days after illness onset.

Negative SARS-CoV-2 NAATs	• Generally, this excludes the diagnosis of COVID-19 in many individuals.
	• However, false-negative NAAT tests have been well documented.
	• May need to repeat the test if clinical suspicion for COVID-19 remains.
	  ○ Repeat testing is generally recommended to be performed 24 to 48 hours after the initial test.
	  ○ Repeat testing within 24 hours is not recommended.
	  ○ However, the optimal timing for repeat testing is not known.

The severity of COVID-19 infection is largely due to dysregulated immune response. Cytokine storm is strongly associated with COVID-19 severity and suggested as the predominant cause of the progression to multisystem organ damage or failure, the hypercoagulation state, and mortality in COVID-19 infection.[6]

A summary of laboratory features that have been associated with worse outcomes due to multisystem involvement[6,11] is detailed in Table 52.4.

TABLE 52.3: SARS-COV-2 IGG OR TOTAL ANTIBODY TEST RESULTS AND INTERPRETATION

TEST RESULT	INTERPRETATION AND CLINICAL IMPLICATIONS[7,9,10]
Positive SARS-CoV-2 IgG or total antibody[7,9,10]	• Previously had SARS-CoV-2 infection, or current infection who have had symptoms for 3 to 4 weeks • SARS-CoV-2 antibody, particularly IgG, may persist for months and possibly years • Cross reactivity with another coronavirus has been reported • Asymptomatic unvaccinated persons who test positive for SARS-CoV-2 antibody without recent history of COVID-19 have a low likelihood of active infection and do not need to be isolated
Negative SARS-CoV-2 IgG or total antibody[7,9,10]	• In the first several days of infection, or • No SARS-CoV-2 infection • A negative serologic test does not preclude previous infection

TABLE 52.4: LABORATORY FEATURES ASSOCIATED WITH WORSE COVID DISEASE OUTCOMES

SYSTEM INVOLVEMENT	LABORATORY PROFILE[6,11]
Systemic inflammatory	• Elevated inflammatory markers (e.g., C-reactive protein [CRP] and ferritin) • Elevated inflammatory cytokines (e.g., interleukin 6 [IL-6]) • Elevated tumor necrosis factor (TNF)-alpha
Hematologic	• Lymphopenia, thrombocytopenia • Elevated D-dimer • Elevated prothrombin time • Elevated activated partial thromboplastin time (aPTT)
Cardiac	• Elevated cardiac troponin • Elevated creatine phosphokinase (CPK) • Elevated brain natriuretic peptides (BNP)
Hepatic	• Elevated liver enzymes, including alanine aminotransferase (ALT), aspartate aminotransferase (AST), and albumin • Elevated lipase • Elevated amylase • Elevated lactate dehydrogenase (LDH)
Renal	• Elevated serum creatinine • Elevated urea • Proteinuria

FOLLOW-UP

The CDC does not recommend using COVID testing to determine when infection has resolved, when to end home isolation, or whether to discontinue precautions in a healthcare setting.[7] In some people, NAATs can remain positive months after they have recovered from COVID-19 infection. In individuals who are not severely immunocompromised, a symptoms-based strategy should be used to determine when to discontinue home isolation or precautions.[7]

PEARLS & PITFALLS

- COVID-19 vaccination does not influence the results of viral tests (NAAT or antigen tests).
- COVID-19 vaccination should lead to a positive result on a serologic test that detects on spike (S) protein.
- COVID-19 vaccine would not lead to a positive result on a serologic test that detects on nucleocapsid (N) protein.[7,9,10]
- Unvaccinated individuals who have had known SARS-CoV-2 exposure, even with a negative SARS-CoV-2 NAAT test result, should be quarantined for 14 days, or for the duration recommended by local public authorities.[7]
- Fully vaccinated individuals who have had known SARS-CoV-2 exposure, but have no COVID-like symptoms, do not need to be quarantined or be tested.[7]

SEVERE ACUTE RESPIRATORY SYNDROME

First reported in February 2003 in Guangdong Province of China, SARS is a rapidly progressive respiratory illness caused by SARS-CoV virus. By the end of the worldwide outbreak in July 2003, a total of 8,096 cases worldwide with a case fatality rate of 9.6% was reported. No case has been reported since mid-2004.[12,13]

The prodromal phase of SARS is often somewhat prolonged, lasting for 3 to 7 days. Most patients have no upper respiratory symptoms during this stage. However, at the end of the prodromal phase, the respiratory phase begins with a nonproductive cough, and progresses to dyspnea and respiratory failure with progressive pulmonary infiltrates on chest radiograph, necessitating ventilation. The lung injury resulting from severe disease of SARS is thought to reflect an excessive host response with production of large quantities of proinflammatory cytokines (cytokine storm).[12,14]

OVERVIEW OF LABORATORY TESTS

Reverse-Transcriptase Polymerase Chain Reaction (RT-PCR) Assays
When SARS is suspected, specimens for PCR testing should be obtained from at least two sites, such as the respiratory tract, stool, and serum or plasma.[12]

Serum Antibody Testing
Serum antibody tests, measured by enzyme-linked immunosorbent assay, are the most sensitive of the tests that are available.[12] They are less useful during the acute phase because antibodies typically develop several weeks into the illness.

In addition, cross reactivity with another coronavirus can occur resulting in a false-positive result, due to the antigenic similarity among coronaviruses.

INTERPRETATION

Unfortunately, no systematic study has been performed to determine the relative value of each type of specimen at various stages of illness.[12] Clinical observations found:

Reverse–Transcriptase Polymerase Chain Reaction (RT-PCR)

- Assays performed on samples obtained early in the illness had sensitivities as low as 50%.
- Nasopharyngeal aspiration appears to be most sensitive at the time of peak respiratory symptoms.[12]

Serum Antibody Testing

- Serum antibody testing has the greatest sensitivity early in the illness and diminishes greatly with time.[12]

Both higher serum and respiratory real time RT-PCR titers have been correlated with worse prognosis.[12]

MIDDLE EAST RESPIRATORY SYNDROME

First identified in 2012 in Saudi Arabia, MERS-CoV is different from the other human beta coronaviruses, such as SARS-CoV and SARS-CoV-2, but closely related to several bat coronaviruses. It is believed that the virus may have originated in bats and later transmitted to camels in the distant past.[15] Since 2013, 27 countries have reported cases, leading to 858 known deaths due to the infection and related complications.[15] The latest MERS large outbreak occurred in South Korea in 2015, which was associated with a traveler returning from the Arabian Peninsula.[16,17]

The spectrum of illness of MERS-CoV infection is not well defined. Most reported MERS-CoV patients were adults with severe pneumonia and acute respiratory distress syndrome, and some had acute kidney injury. Gastrointestinal symptoms, pericarditis, and disseminated intravascular coagulation have been reported as well.[16] Some infected people had no symptoms or mild cold-like symptoms.[17] While the exact mode of transmission is not fully understood, MERS-CoV likely is transmitted by large respiratory droplets. Only two cases were reported in the United States, both in 2014, and these were among healthcare providers who lived and worked in Saudi Arabia.[17] Although there has been no reported case of MERS in the United States since 2014, and the last large outbreak of MERS occurred in 2015, public health officials continue to monitor the incidence of MERS closely.

In the United States, patients who meet the following criteria are defined as Persons Under Investigation (PUI) by CDC and are recommended to be evaluated for MERS-CoV infection.[17,18]

1. Fever and pneumonia, or acute respiratory distress syndrome, and with either:
   - A history of travel from countries in or near the Arabian Peninsula within 14 days before symptoms onset; or,
   - Close contact with a symptomatic traveler who developed fever and acute respiratory illness within 14 days after traveling from countries in or near the Arabian Peninsula; or,
   - A history of being in a healthcare facility in South Korea within 14 days before symptoms onset; or,
   - Is a member of a cluster of patients with severe acute respiratory illness (e.g., fever and pneumonia requiring hospitalization) of unknown etiology in which MERS-CoV is being evaluated in consultation with state and local health departments.[17]
2. Fever and symptoms of respiratory illness (i.e., cough, shortness of breath) and being in a healthcare facility within 14 days before symptom onset in a country in or near the Arabian Peninsula in which recent healthcare-associated cases of MERS-CoV have been identified.[17]
3. Fever or symptoms of respiratory illness (i.e., cough, shortness of breath) and had close contact with a confirmed MERS-CoV case while the affected person was ill[17]

OVERVIEW OF LABORATORY TESTS

Real Time Reverse Transcriptase Polymerase Chain Reaction (rRT-PCR) Testing

- Used to detect active infection.[18]
- Multiple specimens should be collected from different sites and at different times to increase the likelihood of detecting MERS-CoV.[16,17,19]
- Testing of lower respiratory specimens should be the priority. It is more sensitive for detection of MERS-CoV than testing of upper respiratory specimens.[16–18]
- Lower respiratory tract (bronchalveolar lavage, sputum, and tracheal aspiration), upper respiratory tract (nasopharyngeal and oropharyngeal swabs), stool, and serum samples should be collected.[16–18]

Serology Tests

- Used to detect previous infection.[18]
- The CDC has developed a two-stage approach.[18]
  1. An enzyme-linked immunosorbent assay (ELISA) for screening to detect the antibodies against two different MERS-CoV proteins, the nucleocapsid (N) and spike (S).
  2. If positive by either ELISA, the test is followed by an indirect immunofluorescence test or microneutralization test for confirmation. The microneutralization test:
     - Is the gold standard for detection of specific antibodies in serum samples.
     - Requires at least 5 days before results are available.[18]

■ Any positive test by a single serologic assay should be confirmed with a microneutralization assay.

● A positive serology test in the absence of PCR testing or sequencing is considered a probable case if they meet other elements (e.g., a febrile acute respiratory illness with evidence of pulmonary parenchymal disease and a direct epidemic link with a laboratory confirmed MERS-CoV case).[18]

● There is limited data on the sensitivity and specificity of antibody tests for MERS-CoV.[18]

INTERPRETATION

Real Time Reverse Transcriptase Polymerase Chain Reaction (rRT-PCR) Testing

A summary of rRT-PCR test results and their interpretation is provided in Table 52.5.

MERS Serology Tests

A summary of MERS serology test results and their interpretation is provided in Table 52.6.

TABLE 52.5: rRT-PCR TEST RESULTS AND INTERPRETATION

TEST RESULT	INTERPRETATION[18]
Confirmed Case for Active MERS-CoV Infection	Laboratory confirmation of MERS-CoV infection: ● Positive PCR on at least two specific genomic targets, or ● A single positive target with sequencing on a second[18]
Probable Case for Active MERS-CoV Infection	A person under investigation (PUI) with absent or inconclusive laboratory results for MERS-CoV infection who is a close contact of a laboratory confirmed MERS-CoV case.[18] Examples of inconclusive laboratory results include: ● A positive serology test in the absence of rRT-PCR testing ● A positive test with an assay that has limited performance data available ● A negative test on an inadequate specimen[18]
Negative Case for Active MERS-CoV Infection	● A person under investigation (PUI) with one negative rRT-PCR test on the recommended specimens ● MERS patient with two consecutive negative rRT-PCR tests on all specimens[16-18]

TABLE 52.6: MERS SEROLOGY TEST RESULTS AND INTERPRETATION

TEST RESULT	INTERPRETATION[16,17,19]
Confirmed positive	● Positive by either ELISA, **and** ● Positive by microneutralization[16-18]
Indeterminate	● Positive by both ELISA, **and** ● Negative by microneutralization[16-18]
Negative	● Positive by only one ELISA and negative by microneutralization ● Negative by both ELISA[16-18]

Reporting of MERS Test Results

The CDC (2021) requires state and local health department to

- Report any MERS case and any PUI with equivocal or positive MERS test results immediately; and,
- Submit all MERS-CoV rRT-PCR assay test results, regardless of the findings.[16–18]

PATIENT EDUCATION

COVID-19

- www.cdc.coronavirus/2019-ncov/communication/print-resources .html?Sort=Date%3A%3Adesc

SARS

- www.cdc.gov/sars/about/fs-sars.html

MERS

- www.cdc.gov/coronavirus/mers/

RELATED DIAGNOSES AND ICD-10 CODES

Coronavirus Disease 2019 (COVID-19)[19]

Encounter for screening for COVID-19	Z11.52
Contact with and (suspected) exposure to COVID-19	Z20.822
Personal history of COVID-19	Z86.16
Multisystem inflammatory syndrome (MIS)	M35.81
Other specified systemic involvement of connective tissue	M35.89
Pneumonia due to coronavirus disease 2019	J12.82

Severe Acute Respiratory Syndrome (SARS)

Pneumonia due to SARS-associated coronavirus[20]	J12.82
Severe acute respiratory syndrome[20]	J12.81
Encounter for screening for respiratory disorder[20]	Z13.83
Coronavirus infection SARS associated[20]	B97.21

Middle East Respiratory Syndrome (MERS)

Coronavirus infection, unspecified	B34.2
Encounter for screening for respiratory disorder[20]	Z13.83
Viral infection, unspecified	B34.9

REFERENCES

Full list of references can be accessed through Springer Publishing Company Connect™ at the following link: http://connect.springerpub.com/content/reference-book/978-0-8261 -8843-4/part/part03/toc-part/ch052

53. CORRECTED THROMBIN TIME
AND MIXING STUDIES

Kathleen O'Neill

PHYSIOLOGY REVIEW

The coagulation pathway is a cascade of events that leads to hemostasis. There are two paths, intrinsic and extrinsic, which originate separately but meet at a specific point to form the common pathway, leading to fibrin activation. The purpose is to ultimately stabilize the platelet plug with a fibrin mesh.[1,2] When platelets and clotting factors circulate in an inactive form, blood flows freely through the vascular system. When there is injury to the vascular system and disruption to the endothelium, a complex hemostatic response is initiated.[3]

There are two types of hemostasis: primary and secondary. Primary hemostasis is an aggregation of platelets forming a plug at the damaged site of the exposed endothelial cells. Secondary hemostasis uses the intrinsic, extrinsic, and common pathways to activate fibrinogen to fibrin.[2] Fibrin is insoluble and forms a mesh around the platelet plug, strengthening and stabilizing the clot. These two processes happen simultaneously.

The thrombin time (TT) measures this final step of coagulation, the conversion of fibrinogen to fibrin. The TT is commonly used in clinical laboratories to detect the function of coagulation, anticoagulation, and fibrinolysis. Both the intrinsic and extrinsic coagulation cascades cumulate in the activation of prothrombin to thrombin and subsequently form a fibrin clot. Simultaneously, the fibrinolysis system is activated, and fibrinogen is lysed.[4]

Thrombin leads to the formation of fibrin. The prolongation of the thrombin time decreases the level of fibrinogen or alters its structure and results in overactive fibrinolysis in some conditions such as disseminated intravascular coagulation (DIC), heparin anticoagulant therapy, liver disease, amyloidosis, and malignancy.[4]

If the thrombin time is normal, then the problem is likely due to abnormalities in thrombin, and/or factors V or X. This may be seen in the setting of decreased production of one or more of these factors (e.g., DIC or vitamin K deficiency). Less commonly, an inherited factor deficiency or acquired factor inhibitor may be responsible. Mixing studies can be used to distinguish these possibilities.[5] If the thrombin time is abnormal, then a fibrinogen disorder is suspected. Liver disease and DIC can cause hypofibrinogenemia if severe.

OVERVIEW OF LABORATORY TESTS

The TT test (CPT code 85670) is a simple and inexpensive blood test performed by incubating citrated plasma in the presence of dilute thrombin (bovine [cow] or human) and measuring how much time it takes for clot formation to occur.[5]

The normal range for the TT varies by laboratory and reagent instrument combination, and is typically between 14 to 19 seconds. The thrombin time is prolonged if fibrinogen levels are low or if an anticoagulant that inhibits thrombin is present in the sample.[6]

The reptilase time (RT) test (CPT code 85635) is like the thrombin time in measuring the conversion of fibrinogen to fibrin. However, unlike the TT, the RT is insensitive to the effects of heparin because reptilase is an enzyme derived from the venom of Bothdrops snakes and is not inhibited by antithrombin or the antithrombin-heparin complex. The test is performed similarly to the TT, with the exception that reptilase is used instead of thrombin.[6]

Mixing studies (CPT codes 85610 and 85611) are performed by measuring the clotting time of the patient's plasma diluted serially with normal plasma. The clotting time of a 1:1 mixture of patient plasma and normal plasma can be measured immediately upon incubation, and after incubation at body temperature (typically 2 hours). The degree of "correction" of the coagulation time at both time points is reported.

INDICATIONS

Screening
Universal and targeted screenings for TT and mixing studies are not recommended. Screening is typically done with the prothrombin time (PT) and activated partial thromboplastin time (aPTT). The PT and aPTT will provide an overall assessment of clot formation; however, they do not provide information about fibrin or clot dissolution and will be insensitive to abnormalities of factor XIII function or abnormal fibrinolysis.[6] Refer to Chapter 133 for more information.

Diagnosis and Evaluation
If both the aPTT and PT (INR) are prolonged, the problem is likely to be in the final common pathway, which includes factor X, V, and prothrombin (factor II).

Common acquired conditions giving a prolonged PT and aPTT are:

- Liver disease,
- DIC, and
- Over-anticoagulation with warfarin or other vitamin K antagonists.[6]

TT is used to diagnose coagulation disorders within the blood. It is also used to test the effectiveness of fibrinolytic therapy. When the cause of bleeding is not obvious from the patient evaluation, the TT can be used to distinguish abnormalities of the common pathway from disorders affecting fibrinogen. The TT test, by itself, has little diagnostic value and should be interpreted within the context of additional coagulation assays (e.g., PT, aPTT, and reptilase time). This test may be done if an anticoagulation or fibrinogen disorder is suspected.[7]

Indications for testing TT include:

1. Excessive bleeding or thrombotic episodes,
2. Recurrent miscarriages,

3. When a PT and/or aPTT test is prolonged (especially if abnormal fibrinogen level or function is considered), and
4. When heparin contamination is suspected.

Mixing studies are appropriate in a patient with an unexplained prolonged clotting test. This study is useful because it can distinguish between an abnormally prolonged clotting time due to a factor deficiency versus a factor inhibitor. Inhibitors are autoantibodies that interfere with coagulation factor function in the patient or in the laboratory test (e.g., lupus anticoagulant; refer to Chapter 110). Other interfering substances that can act as inhibitors include heparins, fondaparinux, direct oral anticoagulants (DOACs), and elevated C-reactive protein.[6]

Monitoring

TT can be used in monitoring levels of dabigatran (Pradaxa). Dabigatran is an oral direct anticoagulant and a direct thrombin inhibitor. Dabigatran has a wide therapeutic window and does not necessarily require routine monitoring. However, in some cases, it may be valuable to determine the level of anticoagulation, such as in patients with massive hemorrhage or thrombosis, or excessive anticoagulation treatment. It is also reasonable to monitor TT to ensure blood concentration levels of dabigatran are within the normal range in patients with renal insufficiency.[8]

INTERPRETATION

The PT and aPTT are the most frequently ordered tests for initial evaluation of coagulation. If prolonged, further testing can be done, including TT (Tables 53.1, 53.2, and 53.3).

FOLLOW-UP

When TT is abnormal, DIC, the presence of plasma heparin, or a hepatopathy should be suspected.[7] Additional testing will likely be needed including fibrinogen and liver function tests in order to make a final diagnosis.

Most factor inhibitors will not correct in a mixing study. If the 1:1 dilution does not correct, further evaluation is needed on the suspected cause of the inhibitor and the patient's clinical status. Early involvement of the consulting

TABLE 53.1: NORMAL REFERENCE INTERVAL OF THROMBIN TIME AND MIXING STUDIES

	NORMAL
Thrombin time	14–19 seconds
Mixing studies (10)	APTT screen: <33.2 seconds
	APTT immediate mix: <33.2 seconds
	APTT incubated mix: <36 seconds

Notes: APTT immediate mix—performed immediately.

APTT incubated mix—performed after 1 hour incubation.

Reference intervals: May vary slightly based on lab and reagent instrument combination.

APTT, activated partial thromboplastin time.

TABLE 53.2: COMMON CAUSES OF PROLONGED THROMBIN TIME

CAUSE	RATIONALE
Anticoagulants	Heparin, LMWH, and direct thrombin inhibitors (bivalirudin or argatroban)[5]
Acquired fibrinogen disorders	Hypofibrinogenemia is fibrinogen level <100 Dysfibrinogenemia[5]
DIC (disseminated intravascular coagulation)	Coagulation factors become consumed and depleted and fibrinolysis is increased TT is prolonged both from depletion of fibrinogen and from the effects of fibrin degradation products, both from inhibiting thrombin and in interfering with fibrin polymerization[5]
Liver disease	Associated with decreased production of fibrinogen[5] Also associated with decreased production of anticoagulant factors
Hypoalbuminemia	Decreases coagulation competence and may cause prolonged TT[5]
Paraproteinemias	High concentrations of serum proteins (seen in multiple myeloma and amyloidosis) can prolong TT via interface with fibrin polymerization[5] LMWH, low molecular weight heparin; TT, thrombin time.

TABLE 53.3: COMMON CAUSES OF ABNORMAL CLOTTING TIMES—USES OF A MIXING STUDY

Pure factor deficiency	Normal pooled plasma (NPP) adds enough clotting factors to overcome the deficiency and correct the clotting time.[10]
Inhibitors	If an inhibitor is present, it typically inhibits the clotting factors in patient plasma and NPP so the clotting time remains prolonged.[10] • Specific inhibitors: antibodies directed against a specific coagulation factor • Nonspecific Inhibitors: lupus anticoagulant • Medications: heparin, direct thrombin inhibitors, or direct Xa inhibitors

hematologist and/or appropriate laboratory personnel is advised as some conditions can cause potentially life-threatening bleeding (acquired factor inhibitors), thrombosis (antiphospholipid antibodies), or both (DIC).[6]

PEARLS & PITFALLS

- To begin screening for a bleeding disorder, it is important to obtain a detailed personal and family history as well as physical examination. Spontaneous or unexpected bleeding after a procedure or surgery makes it more likely that the patient has a bleeding disorder.[3]
- Early involvement of a hematologist should be considered for those with evidence of bleeding disorder, both to assist with the evaluation and determination of likely causes as well as to help with obtaining and dosing hemostatic products if needed.[5]
- Coagulation tests must be performed on plasma rather than serum, because clotting factors are removed during serum preparation along with the clotted cellular elements.[6]

- Low molecular weight heparin (LWMH) inhibits thrombin-generating factor X; without factor X, thrombin is unable to turn fibrinogen into fibrin.[9]
- TT should not be used for monitoring anticoagulation therapy as it is too sensitive and not standardized for this purpose.[1]
- Ideally, the patient should be off anticoagulation at the time of testing. Avoid warfarin therapy for 2 weeks prior to the test and heparin, direct Xa, and thrombin inhibitor therapies for about 3 days prior to testing. It should not be drawn from an arm with a heparin lock or heparinized catheter.

PATIENT EDUCATION

- https://labtestsonline.org/tests/thrombin-time

RELATED DIAGNOSES AND ICD-10 CODES

Disseminated intravascular coagulation	D65
Adverse effect of antithrombotic drugs	T45.515A
Long-term use of anticoagulants	Z79.01

REFERENCES

Full list of references can be accessed through Springer Publishing Company Connect™ at the following link: http://connect.springerpub.com/content/reference-book/978-0-8261-8843-4/part/part03/toc-part/ch053

54. CORTISOL, SERUM

Lisa Ward

PATHOPHYSIOLOGY REVIEW

Serum cortisol is the main glucocorticoid produced in the adrenal glands. Ninety-five percent of cortisol is bound to corticosteroid-binding globulin (CBG) and albumin; and 5% of circulating cortisol is free (unbound).[1-5] The free cortisol is the active form that plays a critical role in the glucose metabolism and in the body's response to stress.[3,4] Cortisol levels are regulated by adreno-corticotropic hormone (ACTH) and the hypothalamus-pituitary-adrenal axis in a negative feedback loop (Figure 54.1). ACTH is released in a cyclical fashion with diurnal peaks in the morning (6 to 8 a.m.) and troughs in the evening (11 p.m.).[3] This circadian rhythm occurs in normal healthy adults. Infants do not develop this circadian rhythm or adult pattern of ACTH and cortisol secretion until at least 1 year of life.[6] Disruption of this rhythm, in cases such as hyper- and hypo-cortisolism, can lead to disease. Cortisol levels can increase with pregnancy, exogenous estrogen, and with age.[3,4,6,7]

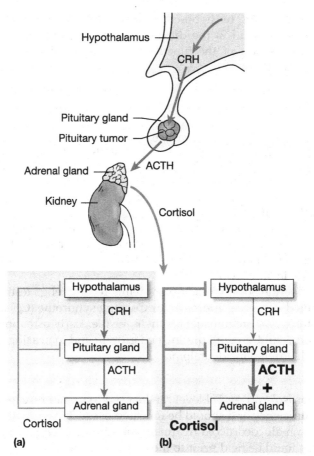

FIGURE 54.1. Hypothalamic-pituitary-adrenal axis. ACTH-stimulated cortisol production: the HPA axis and negative feedback. (a) In the normal HPA axis, hypothalamic CRH stimulates pituitary release of ACTH, resulting in stimulation of cortisol synthesis and secretion, and growth promotion of all of the adrenal gland layers. Cortisol also provides negative feedback to the pituitary and hypothalamus, inhibiting excessive ACTH and CRH secretion. (b) In Cushing disease, an ACTH-secreting pituitary adenoma continuously secretes supranormal amounts of ACTH, driving adrenal gland hyperplasia and excessive cortisol secretion. Negative feedback via increased cortisol inhibits hypothalamic CRH secretion, but is ineffective at reducing ACTH secretion from the autonomously activated tumor cells. ACTH, adrenal corticotropic hormone; CRH, corticotropin releasing hormone; HPA, hypothalamic-pituitary-adrenal. *Source*: Yedinak C, Hurtado CR, Leung AM, et al. Endocrine system. In: Tkacs NC, Hermann LL, Johnson RL, eds. *Advanced Physiology and Pathophysiology: Essentials for Clinical Practice*. Springer Publishing; 2020. Figure 17.13.

OVERVIEW OF LABORATORY TESTS

Serum cortisol levels (CPT code 004051) are often evaluated simultaneously with a serum ACTH level (CPT code 82024). Cortisol is normally secreted in a circadian rhythm with highest levels in the morning.[8] Therefore, timing of the blood draw is essential for best accuracy of results. Because of the episodic secretion of cortisol, interpreting a single value of cortisol is not recommended and further stimulation or suppression testing should be performed when hyper- or hypo-cortisolism is suspected.[4,6] Measurement of serum cortisol is useful in the diagnosis of hypercortisolism and adrenal insufficiency and as part of the functional evaluation of the hypothalamic-pituitary-adrenal (HPA) axis.[4]

INDICATIONS

Screening

■ The Endocrine Society clinical practice guideline recommends against universal screening of cortisol[9] because it is neither efficient nor indicated.[10]
■ The Endocrine Society recommends against screening serum cortisol levels.[4,9]

Diagnosis and Evaluation

■ The Endocrine Society recommends acutely ill patients with unexplained symptoms undergo diagnostic testing to rule out adrenal insufficiency.[11]
■ Consider testing in patients with the following symptoms consistent with cortisol excess in Table 54.1.[3,12]
■ The U.S. Endocrine Society practice guideline recommends testing cortisol with a targeted screening approach for Cushing syndrome (CS) in patients with symptoms that are unusual for their age (i.e., early osteoporosis, hypertension), children with diminished growth and increasing weight, and patients with adrenal incidentaloma.[9]

Monitoring

■ An 8 a.m. cortisol and ACTH level can be used to monitor treatment for adrenal insufficiency and should be repeated every 3 to 6 months.[13]
■ For patients on glucocorticoid treatment for adrenal insufficiency, medication should be held prior to the early morning laboratory test for the most accurate result.

INTERPRETATION

■ Reference intervals vary with different assays.[6]
■ Cortisol secretion is episodic; normal ranges are broad and vary by age.
■ Normal serum cortisol results are listed in Table 54.2.

TABLE 54.1: SIGNS AND SYMPTOMS OF CORTISOL EXCESS

COMMON	LESS COMMON
Obesity/weight gain	Dorsal fat pad
Round face	Edema
Menstrual changes	Abnormal glucose tolerance
Lethargy, depression	Recurrent infections
Striae/Plethora/thinning skin	Acne
Proximal muscle weakness	Female balding

- In adults, an early morning serum cortisol level of less than 3 mcg/dL is suggestive of adrenal insufficiency, whereas a level greater than10 mcg/dL makes adrenal insufficiency unlikely.[4]
- Further interpretation of abnormal cortisol levels is described in Table 54.3.

FOLLOW-UP

- The American Endocrine Society clinical guidelines recommend one of the four following tests for confirmation of Cushing syndrome following an abnormal morning cortisol level: two measurements of urinary-free cortisol, two measurements of late-night salivary cortisol, 1 mg dexamethasone stress test (DST), or a longer low-dose DST with 2 mg/day in divided doses for 48 hours.[9,14]
- Low morning serum cortisol levels specifically create suspicion for adrenal insufficiency and need to be followed up with an ACTH stimulation test.[4,15]

TABLE 54.2: CORTISOL REFERENCE INTERVALS

AGE	8 A.M. (5–11 A.M. ACCEPTABLE)	4 P.M.	8 P.M. (5–11 P.M. ACCEPTABLE)	MIDNIGHT
0–24 months	1–34 mcg/dL		1–30 mcg/dL	
2–10 years	1–33 mcg/dL		1–24 mcg/dL	
11–18 years	1–28 mcg/dL		1–22 mcg/dL	
Adult	5–25 mcg/dL	3–16 mcg/dL	50% of 8 a.m. value	<5 mcg/dL

Source: Lexicomp Online, Lab Tests and Diagnostic Procedures. UpToDate, Inc.; 2019.

TABLE 54.3: DIFFERENTIAL DIAGNOSES OF ABNORMAL CORTISOL LEVELS

POSSIBLE CAUSES OF ↑ CORTISOL LEVELS	POSSIBLE CAUSES OF ↓ CORTISOL LEVELS
• Excess pituitary production of ACTH (i.e., Cushing disease) • Adrenal gland overproduction (e.g., nodular hyperplasia, adrenal cancer) • Ectopic ACTH-secreting tumor (e.g., lung, thymic tumors, or neuroendocrine/carcinoid tumors) • Concurrent trauma, surgery, sepsis • Depression • Alcoholism • Obesity • Pregnancy or estrogen medication • Recent glucocortoid use • Nonpathologic physiologic hypercortisolism • Iatrogenic adrenal insufficiency	• Hypothalamic insufficiency • Pituitary insufficiency • Adrenal dysfunction (e.g., Addison disease) • Hypothyroidism • Corticosteroid long-term use • Medications (e.g., androgens, phenytoin) • Sepsis

Source: Lexicomp Online, Lab Tests and Diagnostic Procedures. UpToDate, Inc.; 2019.

PEARLS & PITFALLS

- Mitotane, a treatment for adrenal cancer, increases cortisol-binding globulin and cortisol levels; therefore, serum cortisol measurement is not an effective means to monitor therapeutic response to treatment.[3]
- Cortisol levels can be elevated in normal physiologic conditions (i.e., obesity, insulin resistance, alcoholism, neuropsychiatric disorders).[4,6,16] In patients with these conditions, a midnight serum cortisol level of less than 7.5 mg/dL is strongly suggestive of physiologic hypercortisolism and rules out Cushing syndrome.[17]
- Chronic opioid use can cause HPA suppression, thus causing false abnormal results.[15]
- Most patients with Cushing syndrome have early morning serum cortisol levels within or slightly above normal range; however, late evening levels are almost always high due to their abnormal or absent circadian rhythm.[4,6]
- Severe malnutrition can cause slight increases of serum cortisol levels.[6]
- Synthetic glucocorticoids can cause either falsely elevated cortisol or, if they suppress the HPA axis, falsely low levels of cortisol.[4,6] Because of these possible outcomes, exogenous glucocorticoid medications should be tapered or stopped if able prior to testing.
- Alcohol abuse can cause high serum cortisol levels or pseudo-Cushing syndrome.[6]
- Night-shift workers may have altered normal diurnal patterns of cortisol secretion and must be taken into consideration when interpreting test results.[4,18]
- Hypothyroidism may cause decreased levels of cortisol.[12]
- Iatrogenic hypercortisolism is the most common cause of Cushing syndrome. Patients should discontinue (if possible) all prescribed steroid dosages prior to further cortisol testing (DST, salivary cortisol, or 24-hour urine cortisol).[19]
- In critically ill patients, both ACTH and cortisol rise in response to illness.[20] After the initial phase, CBG and albumin levels start to decrease, causing lower serum cortisol levels.[3,5,6]
- Single random cortisol values drawn under uncontrolled conditions have no diagnostic value.[4]

PATIENT EDUCATION

- http://oregon-ent.com/patient-education/hw-view.php?DOCHWID=hw71646
- http://oregon-ent.com/patient-education/hw-view.php?DOCHWID=hw65865

RELATED DIAGNOSES AND ICD-10 CODES

Cushing disease	E24.9	Personal history of systemic steroid therapy	Z92.241
Cushing syndrome	E24.0	Ectopic ACTH	E24.3
Pseudo-Cushing	E24.4	Iatrogenic Cushing syndrome	E24.2
Abnormal cortisol level	E27.8	Hypercortisolism	E27.0

REFERENCES

Full list of references can be accessed through Springer Publishing Company Connect™ at the following link: http://connect.springerpub.com/content/reference-book/978-0-8261 -8843-4/part/part03/toc-part/ch054

---

55. CORTISOL (SALIVARY AND URINE)

Lisa Ward

PHYSIOLOGY/PATHOPHYSIOLOGY REVIEW

Cortisol is a steroid hormone produced in the adrenal glands and is the main glucocorticoid in humans. Cortisol plays a critical role in glucose metabolism, immune response regulation, and stress response.[1] Cortisol production is regulated by the hypothalamus-pituitary-adrenal axis (HPA) in a negative feedback loop (see Chapter 54, Figure 54.1)[2]. Adrenocorticotropic hormone (ACTH) is secreted in cyclic fashion with peak levels in the morning and trough levels in the evening.

Only about 5% of circulating cortisol is biologically active (free).[3] When plasma cortisol values increase, free cortisol increases and is filtered through the kidneys into the urine. Therefore, urinary free cortisol (UFC) in the urine correlates well with the plasma cortisol concentration[4,5] and provides an estimate of the circulating biologically active cortisol.[5,6] A 24-hour UFC is not affected by diurnal variation and is, therefore, a good initial test for hypercortisolism.

In Cushing syndrome (CS), the diurnal pattern of cortisol secretion is disrupted, causing elevated cortisol levels in the evening.[7,8] Subtle increases in midnight salivary cortisol are among the earliest abnormalities in CS. Therefore, the measurement of late-night salivary cortisol (LNSC) is useful to evaluate for CS.[8] Blood cortisol diffuses freely into the saliva and is independent on the rate and quantity of saliva production.[3,7,9] An increase in serum cortisol is reflected in a change in the late-night salivary cortisol levels within a few minutes.[9,10]

OVERVIEW OF LABORATORY TESTS

A 24-hour urine free cortisol (UFC) (CPT code 82530) and late night salivary cortisol (LNSC) (CPT code 500179) are common confirmatory tests for hypercortisolism.[8,9,] Salivary cortisol concentration is about less than one-tenth of that in serum cortisol.[4] Salivary samples are stable at room temperature; therefore, patients can delay returning specimens until multiple night collections are completed.[1,3] Eating, smoking, or teeth brushing should be avoided for 2 hours before collection[4,9] At least two samples of salivary cortisol on separate nights collected between 11 p.m. and midnight should be completed.[7,8,10] Patients should be instructed to stay awake until the sample is collected. The patient should

NOT fall asleep prior to testing, since the stress associated with awakening suddenly to an alarm is strong enough to result in cortisol secretion.[3] Additionally, patients should be instructed to avoid any activity or excitement just prior to and at the time the sample is collected to avoid any misleading high values.[3]

A 24-hour UFC is considered by some to be the gold standard for diagnosing CS because it provides an estimate of cortisol production.[3,6] However, the advantage of doing LNSC testing as opposed to 24-hour UFC is the option of an easy, non-invasive sample collection that can be done at home under stress-free conditions.[1,3,7,4,9] With 24-hour UFC, adequate urine excretion of creatinine appropriate for age and sex is assessed simultaneously through a 24-hour urine creatinine level (CPT code 82570) to confirm that enough urine was obtained for an accurate result.[3,6] Failure to adhere to the strict timing of collection can lead to an inadequate urine sample.[11] Accuracy of 24-hour UFC testing can be influenced by several factors summarized in Table 55.1.[3]

INDICATIONS

Screening

- Universal screening is discouraged due to overlap of symptoms from more common comorbidities (e.g., metabolic syndrome) and high rate of false positives. The Endocrine Society Clinical Practice Guideline Task Force recommends against widespread screening[10] as it is neither efficient nor indicated.[3]
- As a general rule, biochemical screening should only be performed if the pretest probability for CS is reasonably high.[3]

TABLE 55.1: POSSIBLE CAUSES OF ABNORMAL 24-HOUR URINE FREE CORTISOL (UFC) RESULTS

DRUG/CONDITION	ADVERSE EFFECT ON 24-HOUR UFC
Exercise/stress	Can cause false-positive results
Proteinuria	May effect cortisol binding in urine
Carbamazepine/ Fenofibrate	Can cause interference in the measurement of UFC
Licorice	Has steroid like chemical that can raise urine cortisol excretion
Polyuria	May abnormally increase urine amount in 24-hour period
Urinary tract infection	May lead to decreased UFC due to metabolism by urine bacteria
Low glomerular filtration rate <30 mL/min	Can lead to decrease UFC amount
Conditions that decrease 24-hour excretion	May cause abnormally decreased 24-hour urine amount
High fluid intake >3.5 liters/24 period	Can lead to abnormally high urine volume (and decreased UFC)

Sources: Bansal V, Elasmar N, Ausan WR, Arafah BM. Pitfalls in the diagnosis and management of Cushing's syndrome. *Neurosurg Focus.* 2015;38(2):E4. doi:10.3171/2014.11.FOCUS14704; Nieman LK. Diagnosis of Cushing's syndrome in the modern era. *Endocrinol Metab Clin North Am.* 2018;47(2):259–273. doi:10.1016/j.ecl.2018.02.001.

Diagnosis and Evaluation

- The 24-hour UFC and two-night LNSC are two of the three tests recommended by American Endocrine Society clinical guidelines as an initial test if CS/hypercortisolism is suspected (Table 55.2).[7,10]
- Consider testing with UFC or LNSC in patients with symptoms suggestive of hypercortisolism (Table 55.2):[7,9]
- Testing with LNSC and 24-hour UFC is also indicated in:[3,10]
  - Patients with multiple and progressive features, particularly those that are more predictive of Cushing syndrome
  - Patients with symptoms that are unusual for their age (e.g., early osteoporosis, hypertension)
  - Children with diminished growth and increasing weight
  - Patients with an adrenal incidentaloma

Monitoring

- A 24-hour UFC is not used to monitor most treatments, since it is a poor indicator of the adequacy of glucocorticoid replacement therapy.[6] However, it can be used to monitor efficacy of treatment with steroid inhibitors (metyrapone and osilodrostat).[6]
- LNSC can be used to monitor glucocorticoid treatment in patients with congenital adrenal hyperplasia and may be useful in monitoring hydrocortisone replacement therapy.[4]

INTERPRETATION

- Diagnosis of hypercortisolism requires that two different confirmatory tests are unequivocally abnormal and physiologic hypercortisolism has been excluded.[3,9,10]
- Differential diagnosis for abnormally elevated 24-hour UFC or LNSC includes iatrogenic Cushing syndrome, pseudo-Cushing syndrome, and nonpathologic physiologic hypercortisolism (NPPH).

TABLE 55.2: POSSIBLE SYMPTOMS OF HYPERCORTISOLISM	
COMMON	**LESS COMMON**
Obesity/weight gain	Dorsal fat pad
Round face	Edema
Menstrual changes	Abnormal glucose tolerance
Lethargy, depression	Recurrent infections
Striae/Plethora/thinning skin	Acne
Proximal muscle weakness	Female balding

Sources: Pappachan JM, Hariman C, Edavalath M, Waldron J, Hanna FW. Cushing's syndrome: a practical approach to diagnosis and differential diagnoses. *J Clin Pathol.* 2017;70(4):350–359. doi:10.1136/jclinpath-2016-203933; Urinary cortisol. Mayo Clinical Laboratories website. https://www.mayocliniclabs.com/test-catalog/Specimen/8546.

- Nonpathologic physiologic hypercortisolism (NPPH) should be considered during evaluation for mild abnormal results in patients since both clinical and/or biochemical features of CS can occur without the condition.[3] Examples of NPPH not associated with CS can be seen in Box 55.1. [3,10] In patients with NPPH, hypercortisolism self-resolves with triggers and avoided or underlying conditions are corrected.[6] Patients with NPPH tend to have urine cortisol excretion less than 3 times normal.

A 24-Hour Urine Free Cortisol

- A three- to four-fold increase over 24-hour UFC reference intervals is diagnostic of CS.[3,9]
- Reference interval 24-hour UFC values are listed in Table 55.3.[5,9]
- Interpretation/differential diagnosis of abnormal 24 UFC cortisol levels is listed in Table 55.4.[9]
- When interpreting 24-hour UFC results, be aware of the most common causes of false-positive, false-negative, or false-normal results listed in Table 55.5.[9]

Box 55.1: Causes of Nonpathologic Physiologic Hypercortisolism (NPPH)

- Pregnancy
- Uncontrolled diabetes
- Sleep apnea
- Uncontrolled pain
- Alcoholism, especially withdrawal
- Psychiatric disorders
- Physical or emotional stress
- Extreme obesity
- Glucocorticoid resistance syndromes

Sources: Bansal V, Elasmar N, Ausan WR, Arafah BM. Pitfalls in the diagnosis and management of Cushing's syndrome. *Neurosurg Focus*. 2015;38(2):E4. doi:10.3171/2014.11.FOCUS14704; Nieman LK, Biller BM, Findling JW, et al. The diagnosis of Cushing's syndrome: an Endocrine Society clinical practice guideline. *J Clin Endocrinol Metab*. 2008;93(5):1526–1540. doi:10.1210/jc.2008-0125.

TABLE 55.3: 24-HOUR URINE FREE CORTISOL (UFC) VALUES REFERENCE INTERVALS

AGE	mcg/24 HOURS
0–2 years	Not established
3–8 years	1.4–20 mcg/24 hours
9–12 years	2.6–37 mcg/24 hours
13–17 years	4.0–56 mcg/24 hours
>18 years	3.5–45 mcg/24 hours

*For pediatric patients >45 kg, adult normal intervals may be used.[13]

Sources: Lexicomp Online, Lab Tests and Diagnostic Procedures. UpToDate Inc.; 2019, October 27, 2020; Urinary cortisol. Mayo Clinical Laboratories website. https://www.mayocliniclabs.com/test-catalog/Specimen/8546.

TABLE 55.4: CAUSES FOR ABNORMAL CORTISOL LEVELS FOR 24-HOUR URINE FREE CORTISOL (UFC)

↓ LEVELS OF CORTISOL	↑ LEVELS OF CORTISOL
• Decreased production of cortisol due to adrenal, pituitary, or hypothalamic insufficiency* • Insufficient collection of urine during collection time	• Cushing disease (pituitary source) • Ectopic ACTH syndrome • Adrenal gland excess cortisol secretion (due to adrenal cancer or benign adrenal hyperplasia) • Pseudo-Cushing (e.g., severe depression, alcoholism, uncontrolled DM)

*UFC cannot be relied upon to diagnose hypocortisolism.

ACTH, adrenocorticotropic hormone; DM, diabetes mellitus.

Source: Lexicomp Online, Lab Tests and Diagnostic Procedures. UpToDate Inc.; 2019, October 27, 2020.

TABLE 55.5: CAUSES OF FALSE RESULTS FOR 24-HOUR URINE FREE CORTISOL (UFC)

FALSE POSITIVES	FALSE NEGATIVES	FALSE NORMAL
• High fluid intake (>3.5 L/day) • Conditions that increase cortisol production (i.e., pregnancy, depression, morbid obesity) • Intervals of acute physical or emotional stress (e.g., surgery, acute illness) • > 24-hour collection	• Moderate to severe renal insufficiency • Incomplete urine collection (<24 hour)	• Cyclic disease when the condition is inactive • Mild CS • Incomplete urine collection (<24 hour)

Source: Lexicomp Online, Lab Tests and Diagnostic Procedures. UpToDate Inc.; 2019, October 27, 2020.

TABLE 55.6: REFERENCE INTERVALS FOR LATE-NIGHT SALIVARY CORTISOL (LNSC)

TIME OF COLLECTION	NORMAL SALIVARY CORTISOL LEVEL
7 a.m.–9 a.m.	100–750 ng/dL
3 p.m.–5 p.m.	<401 ng/dL
11 p.m.–midnight	<100 ng/dL

Sources: Lexicomp Online, Lab Tests and Diagnostic Procedures. UpToDate Inc.; 2019, October 27, 2020; Nieman LK, Biller BM, Findling JW, et al. the diagnosis of Cushing's syndrome: an Endocrine Society clinical practice guideline. *J Clin Endocrinol Metab.* 2008;93(5):1526–1540. doi:10.1210/jc.2008-0125; Salivary cortisol, Free Serum. Mayo Clinical Laboratories website. https://www.mayocliniclabs.com/test-catalog/Clinical+and+Interpretive/84225.

Late Night Salivary Cortisol

■ Reference intervals for LNSC are dependent on time of collection (Table 55.6)[8–10]

FOLLOW-UP

■ Patients with concordant normal results (e.g., two normal confirmatory tests) generally do not require further assessment for hypercortisolism.[9,10,12,13]
■ A three- to four-fold increase over 24-hour UFC reference intervals is diagnostic of CS and no additional testing is required to confirm the diagnosis.[3,9] If there is less than a three-fold increase in 24-hour UFC, another diagnostic test is needed to confirm diagnosis and rule out a false positive.[3,13]

- Once confirmation of abnormally elevated cortisol is established, the cause of the hypercortisolism (adrenal vs. pituitary vs. ectopic ACTH production) must be established.[3,5,14] This process is typically complex and requires a referral to an endocrinologist.
- If clinical suspicion for CS persists despite multiple normal UFC or LNSC tests, repeat testing in 6 months and referral to an endocrinologist should be considered[9,10]

PEARLS & PITFALLS

- Pregnancy, exogenous estrogen use, and aging can all increase cortisol levels.[5,9,10,15]
- Urine cortisol excretion is reduced in moderate and severe chronic kidney disease (CrCl less than 50 mL/min).[5,11] Therefore, 24-hour UFC is not recommended in this patient population.[9]
- 24-hour UFC and LNSC are not used to evaluate for hypercortisolism or Addison disease. Serum cortisol and ACTH are used instead.[5,6,8,9]
- 24-hour UFC is not affected by the use of estrogen; therefore, patients do not need to discontinue therapy prior to collection.[3,6]
- Acute physical or emotional stress, alcoholism, depression, and drugs (e.g., exogenous glucocorticoids, anticonvulsants) can alter normal diurnal variation of cortisol and will cause elevated cortisol levels.[5,14] Use of UFC or LNSC is not recommended under these scenarios.
- Salivary cortisol collection may be difficult in patients with oral diseases (e.g., bleeding gingivitis or Sjogren's syndrome).[4]
- Direct contamination of saliva sample with acidic or high sugar foods can cause false-positive LNSC results.[3,9]
- Night-shift workers may have altered normal diurnal patterns of cortisol.[3,9,16] Salivary cortisol testing might not be the most appropriate test for this population, unless the shift worker has the same bedtime every day.[10,11]
- Chronic kidney disease (CrCl greater than 20 mL/min) is associated with increased salivary cortisol levels.[11]
- Hypothyroidism may cause decreased levels of salivary and/or 24-hour UFC cortisol.[17]
- If unable to obtain an LNSC or 24-hour UFC, a dexamethasone suppression test can also be used for evaluation of hypercortisolism.[9,12]
- In patients with nonpathologic physiologic hypercortisolism (NPPH) who need repeat testing, clinicians should first assure treatment/control of the underlying condition.[11]
- Salivary cortisol results correspond with blood cortisol values since levels equilibrate within minutes and are not affected by serum-binding proteins or by the rate of saliva production.[3,8,9]
- Iatrogenic hypercortisolism is the most common cause of CS.[14] Patients should discontinue (if possible) all prescribed oral, inhaled, or topical steroid dosages prior to further cortisol testing.[9]

- Urinary cortisol levels are disproportionately high after ACTH stimulation testing. Therefore, UFC measurement should be avoided after stimulation testing.[6]
- Ingestion of licorice 24 hours prior to specimen collection may result in falsely elevated salivary and urine cortisol level.[3,9]

PATIENT EDUCATION

- http://www.dmcul.org/upload/docs/Patient%20instructions%20for%20 24%20hr%20urine.pdf
- https://www.mayocliniclabs.com/it-mmfiles/Cortisol_-_Saliva_Collection_ Instructions.pdf

RELATED DIAGNOSES AND ICD-10 CODES

Cushing disease	E24.9
Cushing syndrome	E24.0
Pseudo-Cushing	E24.4
Abnormal cortisol level	E27.8
Personal history of systemic steroid therapy	Z92.241
Ectopic ACTH	E24.3
Iatrogenic Cushing syndrome	E24.2
Hypercortisolism	E27.0

REFERENCES

Full list of references can be accessed through Springer Publishing Company Connect™ at the following link: http://connect.springerpub.com/content/reference-book/978-0-8261 -8843-4/part/part03/toc-part/ch055

56. CREATININE KINASE

LouAnn B. Bailey and Kelly Small Casler

PHYSIOLOGY REVIEW

Creatinine kinase (CK), formally called creatine phosphokinase (CPK), is an enzyme composed of two subunits, M (muscle) and B (brain), that is configured in one of three combinations: MM, MB, and BB.[1] CK-MM is present in the skeletal muscle, CK-MB in the myocardium, and CK-BB in neuronal/brain tissue.[1] Small amounts of CK are also found in the colon, lung, and bladder.[1] CK is important for cellular energy storage and transfer and is released into circulation with muscular injury. Normal skeletal muscle CK is more than 99% MM with a small amount of MB.[2]

OVERVIEW OF LABORATORY TESTS

CK can be assessed by a total CK level (CPT code 82550) or total CK with isoenzymes (CPT code 82552), which separates out levels by combination (CK-MB, CK-MM, and CK-BB). There is limited data to support the need for separating CK by levels, however. CK is predominantly used to evaluate neuromuscular disease and is the most sensitive indicator of muscle injury available.[3] It has also historically been used to diagnosis acute myocardial infarction; however, total CK levels lack specificity for this indication. Specificity improves if only the CK-MB combination is measured, but skeletal muscle breakdown can also lead to elevations in CK-MB.[4] Therefore, its use in the evaluation for myocardial injury/infarction has been replaced by cardiac troponin.[4-8] Normal reference intervals for CK can vary depending on age, sex, race, muscle mass, and activity level.[9,10]

INDICATIONS

Screening

- There is disagreement in the literature about whether patients should be screened for CK elevations prior to statin initiation and if routine screening/monitoring should be done. Canadian guidelines and an older U.S. guideline support screening,[11,12] while newer guidelines and findings from a 2003 study argue against this practice.[13,14]
- There is some consideration being given to adding CK measurement to newborn screening panels in an effort to screen for Duchenne muscular dystrophy.[15]

Diagnosis and Evaluation

- CK is used to evaluate for muscle damage in the setting of persistent myalgia, myopathy (subjective or objective muscle weakness), or generalized muscle tenderness.[14] It is also used to evaluate for suspected rhabdomyolysis.[16]

Monitoring

- CK levels may be monitored during rhabdomyolysis. In general, levels rise within 12 hours of symptom onset and peak on day two to three before returning to baseline.[16]
- CK may be one of several parameters used to monitor severity of COVID-19 infection.[17]
- CK levels may be monitored during statin therapy, though evidence to support this practice is conflicting and generally lacking.

INTERPRETATION

- Reference intervals are highly variable based on age, sex, race, and performing laboratory.

- Generally, levels below the 97.5th percentile are considered normal. One reference suggests the following reference limits as the cutoff for normal, also called the upper limit of normal (ULN):[18]
  - Black males less than 520 U/L
  - Black females; nonblack males less than 345 U/L
  - Nonblack females less than 145 U/L
- Interpretation of abnormalities is usually stratified into mild, moderate, and severe elevations of CK. Elevations greater than 3 x the ULN are considered mild, 10 x ULN or more are considered moderate, and 50 x ULN or more are considered severe.[19]
- Multiple conditions and situations are associated with elevated CK levels (Table 56.1).[19–24]

FOLLOW-UP

- Women with persistent CK elevations can be offered DNA testing for Duchenne muscular dystrophy carrier status.[25]
- If exercise is suspected as the cause of elevation, repeat CK after 7 days of rest.[26]
- In patients with elevated CK (especially those greater than 5–10x ULN) and persistent muscle weakness or muscle tenderness, consider the possibility of autoimmune or myopathic muscle disorders.[19,27] These patients may benefit from referral for electromyogram, nerve conduction study, or muscle biopsy.[26] Patients with persistent elevations greater than 10x ULN should especially be evaluated.[27]
- Hypothyroidism is a common cause of myalgia. Evaluate thyroid-stimulating hormone if this is suspected. [19,22,26]
- For persistent elevations, consider evaluating parathyroid hormone (to evaluate for hypoparathyroidism), vitamin D levels (to evaluate for vitamin D deficiency), and phosphorus (to evaluate for hypophosphatemia).[19,22]
- If rhabdomyolysis cannot be ruled out based on history/physical examination, evaluate estimated glomerular filtration rate, creatinine, and urine myoglobin along with CK.[19,23] Liver transaminases may also be evaluated.

TABLE 56.1: CONDITIONS AND SITUATIONS ASSOCIATED WITH ELEVATED CREATINE KINASE LEVELS	
NEUROLOGIC CONDITIONS	**OTHER CONDITIONS**
CNS injury: stroke, brain cancer, brain bleed, seizures, shock	Adenocarcinoma especially of the breast and lung
Electroconvulsive therapy	Pulmonary infarction
	Hypothyroidism
	Hypoparathyroidism
	Chronic kidney disease/AKI
	Alcohol abuse
	Vitamin D deficiency
	Hypophosphatemia

(continued)

TABLE 56.1: CONDITIONS AND SITUATIONS ASSOCIATED WITH ELEVATED CREATINE KINASE LEVELS (continued)

CARDIAC CONDITIONS	MUSCULOSKELETAL CONDITIONS
Acute myocardial infarction	Rhabdomyolysis
Cardiac aneurysm surgery	Inflammatory/infectious myopathies
Cardiac defibrillation	Sex-linked muscular dystrophies
Myocarditis	Myositis
Ventricular arrhythmias	Metabolic myopathies
Cardiac ischemia	Recent surgery
	Trauma
	Crush injuries
	Delirium tremens
	Malignant hyperthermia
	Recent seizures
	Electrolyte disorders/derangements
	Thyroid/parathyroid disease
	Dermatomyositis/polymyositis
	Periodic paralyses
	Malignant hyperthermia
	Neuroleptic malignant syndrome

NO DISEASE	MEDICATIONS
Exercise	HMG-CoA reductase inhibitors
Needle electromyography	Hydroxychloroquine
IM injections	Isotretinoin
	Colchicine
	Corticosteroids
	Rheumatologic agents
	Antiretrovirals/HIV therapy
	Cocaine

AKI, acute kidney injury; CNS, central nervous system; HIV, human immunodeficiency virus; IM, intramuscular.

Sources: Rosenson RS, Baker SK, Jacobson TA, Kopecky SL, Parker BA, The National Lipid Association's Muscle Safety Expert Panel null. An assessment by the Statin Muscle Safety Task Force: 2014 update. *J Clin Lipidol.* 2014;8(3 Suppl):S58–71. doi:10.1016/j.jacl.2014.03.004; Miller M. Muscle enzymes in the evaluation of neuromuscular disease. In: *Up To Date.* Wolters Kluwer; 2020; Valiyil R, Christopher-Stine L. Drug-related myopathies of which the clinician should be aware. *Curr Rheumatol Rep.* 2010;12(3):213–220. doi:10.1007/s11926-010-0104-3; Lacomis D. Electrodiagnostic approach to the patient with suspected myopathy. *Neurol Clin.* 2012;30(2):641–660. doi:10.1016/j.ncl.2011.12.007; Stroes ES, Thompson PD, Corsini A, et al. Statin-associated muscle symptoms: impact on statin therapy-European Atherosclerosis Society Consensus Panel Statement on assessment, aetiology and management. *Eur Heart J.* 2015;36(17):1012–1022. doi:10.1093/eurheartj/ehv043; Zuckner J. Drug-related myopathies. *Rheum Dis Clin North Am.* 1994;20(4):1017–1032. doi:10.1016/S0889-857X(21)00078-8

PEARLS & PITFALLS

■ Serum CK is the most sensitive marker available for muscle damage/injury, though it lacks specificity for any one condition.[3,9]

■ Serum CK and CK-MB are not recommended to be used to assess acute myocardial ischemia or injury and should not take the place of cardiac troponin.[4]

- Serum CK greater than 5 to 10 times the ULN or greater than 1,000 U/L is seen with rhabdomyolysis.[28] However, CK is not highly specific or sensitive for the condition.[28]
- In studies of asymptomatic and well individuals where CK was assessed at regular intervals, CK has been found to rise incidentally (always less than 10x ULN) without signaling any underlying problem.[23]
- Elevations in CK often occur from hypothyroidism or exercise.[23]
- Persistent CK elevations present concern for neuromuscular disorders.[18]
- The prevalence of statin-associated muscle symptoms (SAMS) is 7% to 29%. Muscle symptoms are mild with mild to no elevations in CK.[23] On rare occasions, the CK may be 4 to 10x the ULN.[29] However, SAMS is primarily a clinical diagnosis, and there is no range of CK elevation that provides high specificity for SAMS.
- It is safe to use/continue statins in patients with CK levels up to 5 times the ULN. Levels greater than 10 x ULN argue against SAMS and clinicians should evaluate for other disorders that cause elevated CK levels.[30]
- When assistance is needed in assessing for SAMS, the American College of Cardiology offers a decision aide tool at https://tools.acc.org/statinintolerance/#!/

PATIENT EDUCATION

- https://medlineplus.gov/lab-tests/creatine-kinase/

RELATED DIAGNOSES AND ICD-10 CODES

Myocardial ischemia	I24.8
Myocardial injury	I21.9
Rhabdomyolysis	M62.82
Acute kidney injury	S37.0
Myalgia	M79.1
Myositis	M60
Electrolyte derangements	T50.3X5
Thyroid derangements	E07.89
Myocarditis	I51.4
Stroke	I69.30
Critical illness myopathy	G72.81

List is not all inclusive.[5]

REFERENCES

Full list of references can be accessed through Springer Publishing Company Connect™ at the following link: http://connect.springerpub.com/content/reference-book/978-0-8261-8843-4/part/part03/toc-part/ch056

57. CYCLIC CITRULLINATED PEPTIDE ANTIBODY AND RHEUMATOID FACTOR

Elizabeth Kirchner

PHYSIOLOGY REVIEW

Autoimmune disease arises when the body loses immunologic tolerance and attacks self-molecules.[1] For this to occur, the immune system must not only mistake "self" for "non-self" but must also identify self-molecules as a danger or threat.[2] When it does so, the immune system may create antibodies (in this case autoantibodies) to attack the "threat." Two autoantibodies that are most commonly (but not exclusively) associated with rheumatoid arthritis (RA) are rheumatoid factor (RF) and cyclic citrullinated peptide (ACPA, CPT code 86200).

RF is a single antibody directed against the Fc portion of immunoglobulin G.[3] In contrast, the ACPA test refers to a group of autoantibodies directed against "citrullinated" peptides and proteins. During inflammation, arginine amino acid residues can be converted into citrulline, a process called citrullination. If their shapes are significantly altered, the proteins (e.g., keratin, filaggrin, vimentin) may be seen as antigens by the immune system, thereby generating an immune response.[4]

OVERVIEW OF LABORATORY TESTS

RF (CPT code 86431) testing measures the amount of rheumatoid factor that is present in the blood. A titer value can also be provided to quantify how much rheumatoid factor is in the blood. Immunoturbidimetric is the methodology utilized to conduct the test. The specificity of RF for RA in adults ranges from 72%[5] to 85%.[6] Other connective tissue diseases, infections, malignancies (especially after radiation or chemotherapy), and primary biliary cirrhosis may all cause RF to be positive.[7] In addition, between 1% and 5% of healthy individuals may have positive RF.[7] Typically, false positives are low-level; a strongly positive RF along with a history and physical examination consistent with RA would signify that the RF is indeed diagnostic for RA. RF is elevated in (i.e., has a sensitivity of) 60% to 80% in adult patients with RA at some point during their disease course;[8] however, the sensitivity for early RA is less than 40% so it is not as useful a test for patients with recent onset of symptoms.[7] Levels of RF can fluctuate somewhat with disease activity, though titers generally remain high even in patients with drug-induced remission.[7]

ACPA (CPT code 11173) is elevated early in the course of adult RA (often before symptoms are present), which allows the diagnosis of RA to be made at a very early stage.[9] Early tests detected only cyclic citrullinated proteins and were therefore called anti-CCP (the term "ACPA" includes both cyclic and noncyclic and is therefore more inclusive). The sensitivity of the first generation anti-CCP test (used from 2000 to 2001) was 53%, with 96% specificity.[10] Second- and third-generation anti-CCP testing has been used since 2001 with a sensitivity for RA between 50% and 75% and a specificity of 90%.[9] ACPA sensitivity is 72% (20% to 25% in early RA); specificity is 96%–98% (95% in early RA).[10]

Both RF and ACPA testing are typically performed during the initial adult patient evaluation when RA is suspected. If both tests are positive, this increases diagnostic specificity. Approximately 50% of RA patients will test negative on both tests at presentation; however, close to 75% of RA patients will eventually test positive for ACPA. About 20% of patients diagnosed with RA will continue to test negative for both throughout their disease; this is called "seronegative RA".[9]

Importantly, neither RF nor ACPA are included in the American College of Rheumatology recommendations for disease activity measurement tools.[11] Levels of RF can fluctuate somewhat with disease activity, though titers generally remain high even in patients with drug-induced remission.[7] However, these fluctuations are not reliable enough to guide treatment decisions.

Missing from the previous discussion are the roles of RF and ACPA in screening for juvenile idiopathic arthritis (JIA). This is because only 4% to 30% of children with JIA have a positive RF,[12,13] and ACPA is even less commonly seen.[14] These tests are not widely used in the pediatric population; the American Academy of Pediatrics and the Choosing Wisely® initiative recommend against their use in pediatric patients with musculoskeletal concerns.[12]

INDICATIONS

Screening
- Universal and targeted screenings are not recommended.

Diagnosis and Evaluation
History and symptoms of RA include:

- Tender, warm, and swollen joints (typically symmetrical and affects the small joints first then spread to the larger joints)
- Joint pain that is worse in the morning or after inactivity
- Fatigue
- Fever
- Anorexia
- Symptoms that can come and go
- 40% of people experience symptoms that do not involve the joints but involve other organs including the eyes, skin, lungs, heart, kidneys, salivary glands, nerve tissues, bone marrow, and blood vessels
- Familial history of RA or other autoimmune conditions

Diagnostic criteria from the 2010 American College of Rheumatology (ACR)/ European League Against Rheumatism (EULAR) guidelines require the patient have at least one joint with definite clinical synovitis and with the synovitis that is not better explained by another disease. In addition, the patient must have a score of 6/10 or greater (Table 57.1).

TABLE 57.1: CRITERIA FOR NEWLY DIAGNOSED RA DIAGNOSIS

CLINICAL CRITERIA	SCORE
A. Joint involvement	
(defined as any swollen or tender joint)	
1 large joint*	0
2–10 large joints*	1
1–3 small joints** (+/– large joints)	2
4–10 small joints** (+/–large joints)	3
>10 joints (at least 1 small joint)	5
B. Serology	0
Negative RF and negative ACPA	
Low-positive RF or low-positive ACPA	2
High-positive RF or high-positive ACPA	3
C. Acute phase reactants	0
Normal C-reactive protein (CRP) and normal erythrocyte sedimentation rate (ESR)	
Abnormal CRP or abnormal ESR	1
D. Duration of symptoms	0
<6 weeks	
≥ 6 weeks	1

*Large joints include shoulder, elbows, hips, knees, and ankles.

**Small joints include metacarpophalangeal joints, proximal interphalangeal joints, 2nd-5th metatarsophalangeal joints.

Source: Aletaha D, Neogi T, Silman AJ, et al. 2010 Rheumatoid arthritis classification criteria: an American College of Rheumatology/European League Against Rheumatism collaborative initiative. *Arthritis Rheum.* 2010;62:2569–2581. doi:10.1002/art.27584.

Monitoring

■ Repeat RF/ACPA is not indicated for those who test positive.
■ Repeat testing several months/years after an initial negative test may be indicated if the clinical picture is strongly suggestive of RA.
■ Seropositivity in both pediatric and adult populations is associated with a higher incidence of erosive disease and a worse prognosis than seronegative RA.

INTERPRETATION

■ RF
  • Less than 20 IU/mL is negative.
  • Greater than 20 IU/mL is positive; typically 20 to 50 is considered "weakly positive."

- A weakly positive RF may indicate any of the following:
  - Infection (especially hepatitis C)
  - Other autoimmune disease (Hashimoto's thyroiditis, multiple sclerosis)
  - Overlap rheumatic disease (e.g., lupus)
  - Malignancy
- ACPA
  - Less than 20 units: negative
  - 20 to 39 units: weak positive
  - 40 to 59 units: moderate positive
  - 60 units or more: strong positive

FOLLOW-UP

- A strongly positive RF and/or ACPA with correlating clinical presentation does not typically require any follow-up testing in order to secure the diagnosis of RA.
- A weakly positive RF, especially in the setting of an atypical clinical presentation, should be a clue to the clinician that further testing may be warranted. This should be guided by signs and symptoms and may include testing for infectious hepatitis, thyroid disease, malignancies, inflammatory lung disease, mixed connective tissue disease, or Sjögren's syndrome.

PEARLS & PITFALLS

- A positive RF or ACPA is not enough to secure a diagnosis of rheumatoid arthritis! The clinical picture must also support the diagnosis (synovitis of at least one joint, symptoms for at least six weeks, and a certain number/size of joints involved – see the 2010 EULAR/ACR Criteria Classification for RA[15]).
- Conversely, a negative RF/ACPA does not rule out RA, especially in a patient with a clinical presentation strongly suggestive of RA.
- The older a patient is, the more likely they are to have a false-positive RF.
- Patients can (and frequently do) have more than one type of arthritis. Radiographs are helpful in distinguishing which symptoms are from RA and which are from osteoarthritis, old damage, or possibly gout.

PATIENT EDUCATION

- https://www.rheumatology.org
- https://eular.org
- https://www.arthritis.org
- https://creakyjoints.org

RELATED DIAGNOSES AND ICD-10 CODES

Rheumatoid arthritis, seropositive	M05.79
Rheumatoid arthritis, seronegative	M06.09

REFERENCES

Full list of references can be accessed through Springer Publishing Company Connect™ at the following link: http://connect.springerpub.com/content/reference-book/978-0-8261 -8843-4/part/part03/toc-part/ch057

58. CYSTATIN

M. Danielle Atchley

PHYSIOLOGY REVIEW

Cystatin C (CysC) is a renal biomarker and small protein produced throughout the body and found in an array of body fluids including blood.[1] Production and filtration of cystatin C occurs via the kidneys at a constant rate, and the concentration found within the serum is inversely correlated with glomerular filtration rate (GFR).[2]

OVERVIEW OF LABORATORY TESTS

Cystatin C (CPT code 82610) is evaluated via a serum or plasma sample.[3,4] Unlike creatinine, cystatin C is not affected by nutrition, body mass, inflammation, infection, or medications. Therefore, it may be a more reliable indicator of overall kidney function.[1,2,5,6] Additionally, estimated glomerular filtration rate (eGFR) calculations based on cystatin C have greater accuracy for the assessment of chronic kidney disease (CKD) especially in patients with eGFR less than 60 mL/min/1.73.[5,7]

INDICATIONS

Screening
- In general, cystatin C is not used for universal screening for CKD,[8] but is used for targeted screening when eGFR based on serum creatinine could be inaccurate (alterations in muscle mass, malnutrition, use of medications that block creatinine secretion, and eGFR 45 to 59 mL/min/1.73 m²).[6,9–11,15] It is also listed as an alternative CKD screening method in patients with diabetes mellitus.[12]
- Cystatin C should not be used to screen for cardiovascular risk.[9]
- Cystatin C may be used in addition to creatinine for CKD screening in situations where confirmation of adequate kidney function is imperative.
- Examples include high-risk renally excreted pharmacotherapy or evaluation for kidney donation.[5,9]

Diagnosis and Evaluation
- Cystatin C is used to confirm declines in creatinine-based eGFR.[6,10,12]

Monitoring

- Serum cystatin C may be used in monitoring when creatinine-based methods are inaccurate.[6,10,13,15]

INTERPRETATION

- In general, the reference interval for cystatin C is 0.63 to 1.21. Cystatin C reference intervals vary based on age range and laboratory equipment used and there is lack of consensus for appropriate reference intervals for individuals younger than 22 years of age.[2] Therefore, it is recommended that clinicians utilize reference intervals provided by the referring laboratory.[2,3]
- In addition to decreased renal function, increased cystatin C levels can be seen in hyperthyroidism, hyperhomocysteinemia, malignant and rheumatic diseases, obesity, steroid use, alcohol consumption, tobacco use, hypoglycemia, hyperglycemia, human immunodeficiency virus, and acquired immunodeficiency syndrome. These conditions may influence the accuracy of cystatin C for estimating GFR.[6,17]

FOLLOW-UP

- Abnormal cystatin C levels or cystatin-based eGFR warrants follow-up testing for the underlying cause of renal dysfunction and evaluation for proteinuria.

PEARLS & PITFALLS

- When monitoring eGFR, it is important to not just compare creatinine and eGFR but also cystatin C-based eGFR due to the fact it is a more active marker and true reflection of GFR[16]
- Sex-specific and age-specific references for cystatin C should be used when evaluating kidney function.[17]
- Compared to measurement of creatinine, cystatin C is more costly and less convenient.[5,17]
- Cystatin C is not considerably affected by muscle mass.[6,18-20]
- There have been more recent studies which have indicated that increased levels of cystatin C may be indicative of a higher risk of heart failure and heart disease leading to mortality.[6]
- Similar to creatinine, cystatin C is more useful when used as part of a calculation for eGFR, rather than interpreting cystatin C concentrations alone.[14]
- When estimating GFR, cystatin C-based CKD-epidemiology calculations have more accuracy and present less bias than observing the estimate of the measured GFR alone.[21]
- In diabetic mellitus patients, observing cystatin C equations either alone or combined in as a reflection of creatinine to estimate GFR provides a reliable indicator of what the overall status is of the eGFR.[22]

PATIENT EDUCATION

■ https://www.kidney.org/atoz/content/cystatinC

RELATED DIAGNOSES AND ICD-10 CODES

Chronic kidney disease, stage 1	N18.1
Chronic kidney disease, stage 2 (mild)	N18.2
Chronic kidney disease, stage 3 (moderate)	N18.3
Chronic kidney disease, stage 4 (severe)	N18.4
Chronic kidney disease, stage 5	N18.5
End-stage renal disease	N18.6
Chronic kidney disease, unspecified	N18.9

REFERENCES

Full list of references can be accessed through Springer Publishing Company Connect™ at the following link: http://connect.springerpub.com/content/reference-book/978-0-8261 -8843-4/part/part03/toc-part/ch058

59. CYTOMEGALOVIRUS

Stephanie C. Evans and Kate Sustersic Gawlik

PHYSIOLOGY REVIEW

Cytomegalovirus (CMV) is a human viral pathogen classified as a ubiquitous double-stranded DNA prototypical β-herpesvirus. The virus infects epithelial cells, macrophages, and T lymphocytes. The virus establishes a lifelong latent infection in myeloid progenitor cells, and possibly other cells as well. Epithelial cells, endothelial cells, fibroblasts, and smooth muscle cells are the predominant targets for virus replication.[1] It is transmitted by sexual contact or direct contact with infected blood, urine, or saliva. There is an incubation period of 28 to 60 days with a mean of 40 days. CMV infection is a concern for immunocompromised individuals and for women of childbearing age. Immunocompetent individuals, on the other hand, show mild or no symptoms despite periodic reactivation of the virus during myeloid cell differentiation. In individuals who have weakened immune systems, such as individuals with human immunodeficiency virus (HIV) and transplant recipients, an active CMV infection could lead to considerable morbidity and mortality. Both initial infection as well as reactivation of latent CMV infection can cause serious complications.[2]

CMV infection in a pregnant woman can lead to a possible congenital CMV infection in the fetus/infant and result in birth defects. About one out of every 200 infants is born with a congenital CMV infection. The role of gestational age at the time of maternal infection is an important determinant of both transmission and infant outcome. Transmission to the fetus is greatly reduced (only about 20%) when contracted in the first trimester but rises to 75% transmission if infection occurs during the third trimester. Maternal immunity from past CMV infection decreases the risk of fetal infection by around 70%.[3] Among those born with congenital CMV, one in five will have long-term health problems that may include hearing loss, vision loss, developmental delay, microcephaly, and seizure disorder.[4]

OVERVIEW OF LABORATORY TESTS

Cytomegalovirus may be detected by viral culture or polymerase chain reaction (PCR) of infected blood, urine, saliva, cervical secretions, amniotic fluid, or breast milk, although diagnosis of CMV infection in adults usually is established by serologic testing.[5] Testing for adults or children over the age of 1 uses a serologic test (blood/plasma) to detect CMV antibodies (IgM and IgG) (CPT codes 86644 and 86645) for determination of possible past or present infections. CMV infection induces immunoglobulin M (IgM) antibody production followed by an immunoglobulin G (IgG) antibody response. Viremia can be detected for 2 to 3 weeks after primary infection.[6] The IgG avidity enzyme-linked immunosorbent assay (ELISA) test (CPT code 86644) is a titer.

Congenital CMV infection is not diagnosed by antibody testing. Testing for congenital CMV in children under the age of 1 year is completed with use of the CMV, PCR test (CPT code 87496) and may use whole blood, plasma, cerebrospinal fluid, or urine. Congenital CMV also can be detected in the amniotic fluid of infected fetuses by either culture or PCR. Sensitivity of CMV amniotic fluid culture is 70% to 80% and the PCR test has a higher sensitivity of 78% to 98% and a specificity of 92% to 98%. The sensitivity of amniotic fluid testing for prenatal diagnosis of congenital CMV infection is markedly improved if performed after 21 weeks of gestation.[6]

INDICATIONS

Screening

Universal screening for CMV infections in healthy individuals is not recommended. Targeted screening is recommended for the following individuals:

- Donors and transplant candidates should be screened before transplant for serum anti-CMV IgG to determine their risk for primary and re-activated CMV infection.
  - Allogeneic hematopoietic stem cell transplantation[7]
  - Solid organ transplant[8]
- Patients with HIV who are at low risk for latent CMV[9]
- Certain states in the United States are performing targeted CMV testing on infants who fail hearing screening after birth.[10]

Choosing Wisely® guidelines advise against targeted screening for the following populations:[9,11]

■ Routine maternal CMV testing as part of prenatal screening
■ Routine screening for CMV IgG in HIV patients who have a high likelihood of being infected with CMV

Diagnosis and Evaluation

CMV testing should be completed on the following:

Individuals with signs/symptoms of CMV infection:[6]

■ Mononucleosis-like syndrome, with fever, chills, myalgias, malaise, leukocytosis, abnormal liver function tests, and lymphadenopathy (also termed heterophile-negative mononucleosis syndrome)
■ Negative monospot test and/or negative Epstein-Barr virus (EBV) titers with previous symptoms
■ Lymphocytosis with atypical presentation
■ Unexplained jaundice and/or anemia
■ Immune system compromise and for
■ Infants who have signs of congenital CMV at birth. suspected of congenital CMV

Infants who have signs/symptoms of congenital CMV at birth:[6]

■ Petechiae/purpura
■ Jaundice
■ Microcephaly
■ Intrauterine growth restriction
■ Hepatosplenomegaly
■ Seizures
■ Retinitis
■ Thrombocytopenia
■ Myocarditis
■ Failed hearing screening
■ Developmental problems
  • Congenital CMV infection is diagnosed by detection of CMV DNA in the urine, saliva (preferred specimens), or blood. It must be diagnosed within 3 weeks after birth. Any testing after this cannot distinguish between congenital infection and an infection acquired during or after delivery.[5] CMV can also be diagnosed in vitro using amniotic fluid.[6]

Pregnant individuals with signs/symptoms of CMV infection:

■ Pregnant individuals should have IgG, IgM titers with avidity testing 3 to 4 weeks apart. IgG avidity assays measure the maturity of the IgG antibody and provide greater sensitivity and specificity for diagnosing recent primary CMV infection.

Monitoring

Serum samples should be collected 3 to 4 weeks apart and monitored for either seroconversion from negative to positive or a significant increase (greater than fourfold [e.g., from 1:4 to 1:16]) in CMV IgG titers.

Any infant diagnosed with congenital CMV infection needs routine hearing and vision screening. This should be completed annually and more frequently if needed as hearing loss can present later in children and may progress with age.[12]

In stem and solid-organ transplant patients, CMV immune monitoring and current clinical and DNA-based monitoring for CMV should be considered. This type of routine monitoring has the potential to be incorporated into clinical care to better improve CMV management of these populations.[13]

INTERPRETATION

PCR viral detection test interpretation (Table 59.1):

- A positive CMV test may mean CMV is present and there is an active infection.
- A negative CMV test may mean there is no active infection or a very low viral load present on sample tested.

IgG avidity testing:

- Seroconversion from negative to positive or a significant increase (greater than fourfold [e.g., from 1:4 to 1:16]) in CMV IgG titers indicates evidence of a current CMV infection. This in combination with IgM titers increases sensitivity to 92%. For pregnant individuals, CMV IgM should not be used in isolation. CMV-specific IgM, which have a reported sensitivity of 50% to 90%, may not be positive during an acute infection, may persist for many months after the primary infection, may be present during reactivation or reinfection, or may be present in the absence of infection[6,14]

TABLE 59.1: SEROLOGIC CMV IgG AND IgM TEST INTERPRETATION	
RESULT	**INTERPRETATION**
IgG Negative IgM Negative	Not previously CMV infected
IgG Positive IgM Positive	Recent CMV infection
IgG Positive IgM Negative	Past CMV infection that is not recent

Source: Cytomegalovirus (CMV) and Congenital CMV Infection—Interpretation of laboratory tests. Centers for Disease Control and Prevention. https://www.cdc.gov/cmv/clinical/lab-tests.html.

FOLLOW-UP

■ Follow-up testing is not typically indicated unless there is a question regarding response to treatment.
■ The clinician may repeat levels for PCR labs to determine the effectiveness of treatment. Decreasing levels indicate positive response to antiviral treatments.

PEARLS & PITFALLS

■ If the patient is a female of childbearing age and has a recent CMV infection, it is recommended to delay conception for 6 to 12 months or until antibody levels represent a past infection.[6]
■ CMV is one of the tests included on the TORCH testing panel. This is a panel often completed on pregnant individuals for diseases which are known to cause birth defects. TORCH is for Toxoplasmosis, Rubella, Cytomegalovirus, and Herpes simplex virus.[6]
■ Cytomegalovirus infection is associated with a significantly increased relative risk of CVD.[15]
■ In immunocompromised patients, CMV infection surveillance by quantitative CMV DNA PCR may be useful during the maintenance phase.[16]
■ CMV infection can present with signs and symptoms similar to the common cold.
■ There should be a high suspicious index for CMV in a patient who presents with mononucleosis type symptoms who lives in communal settings, such as college-age students in dorms.

PATIENT EDUCATION

■ https://www.cdc.gov/cmv/fact-sheets/parents-pregnant-women.html
■ https://www.cdc.gov/cmv/index.html

RELATED DIAGNOSES AND ICD-10 CODES

Viral illness	B34.09
Mononucleosis	B27.9
Hearing loss, unspecified	H91.93
Congenital hearing loss	H91.90
Visual loss, unspecified	H54.7

REFERENCES

Full list of references can be accessed through Springer Publishing Company Connect™ at the following link: http://connect.springerpub.com/content/reference-book/978-0-8261-8843-4/part/part03/toc-part/ch059

60. D-DIMER

Dayna Jaynstein

PATHOPHYSIOLOGY REVIEW

D-dimer is a small protein fragment, referred to as a fibrin degradation product (FDP), released into the bloodstream after fibrinolysis, or clot degradation.[1] During hemostasis (Figure 60.1), the coagulation cascade converts fibrinogen to fibrin, leading to the formation of thrombus.[2] During fibrinolysis, plasmin cleaves the thrombus into multiple fibrin degradation products, one of which is D-dimer. D-dimer measurements, therefore, serve as a marker of fibrin turnover and provide an indication of fibrinolytic activity.[3] Hemostasis and fibrinolysis are physiologically normal processes the body is always balancing. Not all thrombus formation leads to venous thromboembolism (VTE) or other acute pathology; therefore, slightly elevated levels of D-dimer can be a normal finding. Thus, the finding of an elevated D-dimer could be normal or indicative of acute pathology. Additional evaluation is therefore necessary in patients with elevated levels in whom a thrombotic disorder is suspected.

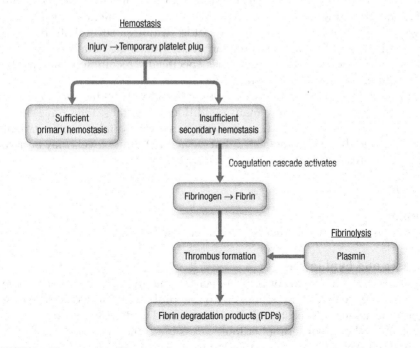

FIGURE 60.1. The process of hemostasis.

OVERVIEW OF LABORATORY TESTS

D-dimer assays can be obtained from whole blood or plasma.[4] Currently available assays include manual immunoagglutination assays, manual immunochromatographic assays, immunofiltration assays, microtiter plate enzyme-linked immunosorbent assay [ELISA]) systems, automated ELISA systems, and latex-enhanced photometric immunoassays.[3] Each test uses a specific monoclonal antibody to quantify D-dimer levels and result times also vary.[3,4] Sensitivity and specificity of the different tests can vary widely; therefore, it is important that clinicians are aware of the limitations associated with specific tests they obtain. In general, however, D-dimer assays are considered to have good sensitivity and poor specificity. The D-dimer test is, therefore, most helpful in ruling out VTE than ruling in. Depending on the D-dimer assay, the overall sensitivity can near 100% while specificity can range from 58% to 94%.[3]

D-dimer testing is useful in the evaluation of multiple thrombotic disorders such as VTE, deep vein thrombosis (DVT), pulmonary embolism (PE), disseminated intravascular coagulation (DIC), assessment of anticoagulation treatment, and, more recently, as a prognostic indicator.[4,5]

Recent research in D-dimer testing has included expanded use of highly sensitive assays, age-adjusted analysis, and D-dimer assessment in pregnant individuals. When used within clinical practice, the D-dimer test should be employed to exclude the probability of VTE; therefore, highly sensitive D-dimers are preferred. D-dimer levels are age dependent and often patients over the age of 60 years old have nonclinically significant elevations.[5] Current recommendations encourage using an age-adjusted cutoff (patient's age in years × 10 mcg/L) for patients above 50 years old.[6] Although several studies have evaluated the use of D-dimers in pregnant individuals, the data is unclear and the American Thoracic Society guidelines specifically recommend against the use of D-dimer to exclude PE in pregnancy.[7]

In addition to the ability to assess fibrinolytic activity, D-dimers can also be used as a prognostic indicator in many conditions.[3] Several studies have shown that levels greater than 4 mcg/dL portray an increased mortality rate in patients with PE.[8] Studies have also suggested that elevated D-dimer levels may be associated with increased mortality in COVID-19 patients.[9]

INDICATIONS

Screening

■ D-dimer is not used for universal or targeted screening.

Diagnosis and Evaluation

■ D-dimers are used as part of clinical decision-making pathways to evaluate for the presence of VTE in patients with low probability/low risk. Multiple clinical decision tools exist, and clinicians should understand pretest probabilities before ordering D-dimers. Possible clinical decision tools include the Wells' Criteria for DVT, Wells' Criteria for PE, Geneva Score for PE, Pulmonary Embolism Rule-Out Criteria (PERC) Rule for PE, and the Age-Adjusted D-Dimer for VTE.[10-14]

- The American College of Physicians recommends that in patients with a low pretest probability of VTE, a highly sensitive D-dimer assay should be the initial diagnostic test.[15]
- American Thoracic Society guidelines specifically recommend against the use of D-dimer to exclude PE in pregnancy.[7]

Monitoring

- D-dimer levels may be monitored to assess progression of malignancy and mortality rate in cancer patients.[16]
- D-dimer elevations are monitored for disease severity and mortality risk determination in patients with COVID-19.[9]
- D-dimer levels can be trended to monitor response to anticoagulation therapy. Decreasing levels can provide assurance that a patient is adequately anticoagulated.[5] There are no formal guidelines for this use, however.

INTERPRETATION

- Reference intervals are established by each manufacturer. Typically, the reference cutoff is considered less than 250 ng/mL, or less than 0.4 mcg/mL,[17] and a D-dimer level less than 500 ng/mL reasonably excludes VTE.[3,5]
- There is little data correlating the level of D-dimer elevation with likelihood of VTE. All D-dimers over 500 ng/mL should be considered abnormal.
- D-dimer analysis in patients over the age of 50 should be adjusted with the following calculation:[6,18]
  - Patient's age in years × 10 mcg/L
- Multiple patient factors and comorbidities aside from acute VTE can cause an elevated D-dimer (Table 60.1).

FOLLOW-UP

- An elevated D-dimer only indicates the possibility of VTE. Therefore, additional diagnostic workup is warranted, which often includes imaging studies to evaluate for DVT or PE.

PEARLS & PITFALLS

- Because D-dimer tests have poor specificity, correlation with a clinical pretest probability score can increase the test's ability to help rule out VTE.[5]
- D-dimer is considered the most sensible blood test to evaluate hypercoagulability. It is positive in more than 90% of cases of VTE.[4]
- D-dimer levels less than 500 ng/mL reasonably exclude the possibility of VTE.
- D-dimers should be age-adjusted for interpretation in patients over the age of 50.
- D-dimers should not be used in the evaluation of VTE in pregnancy until expert consensus is obtained.
- D-dimers should not be used in patients with high likelihood of VTE by clinical prediction rules. These patients should proceed straight to diagnostic imaging to evaluate for VTE.

TABLE 60.1: FACTORS OTHER THAN ACUTE VENOUS THROMBOEMBOLISM THAT CAN CAUSE AN ELEVATED D-DIMER

PATIENT FACTORS	COMORBIDITIES
Age (levels increase above 60 yo)	Acute limb ischemia
Cigarette use	Acute and chronic renal failure
Pregnancy	Atrial fibrillation
African American or Black	Cerebral vascular accident
Hospitalization	Congestive heart failure
	Inflammatory processes
	Liver disease (severe)
	Malignancy
	Myocardial infarction
	Preeclampsia and eclampsia
	Sepsis/SIRS
	Sickle cell disease
	Surgery
	Trauma
	Upper gastrointestinal bleed

SIRS, systemic inflammatory response syndrome.

Sources: Data from Wakai A, Gleeson A, Winter D. Role of fibrin D-dimer testing in emergency medicine. *Emerg Med J.* 2003;20:319–325. doi:10.1136/emj.20.4.319; Greenberg CS. The role of D-dimer testing in clinical hematology and oncology. *Clin Adv Hematol Oncol.* 2017;15(8):580–583. https://www.hematologyandoncology.net/archives/august-2017/the-role-of-d-dimer-testing-in-clinical-hematology-and-oncology/

■ The age-adjusted D-dimer cutoff levels to rule out pulmonary embolism (ADJUST PE) study evaluated age-adjusted cutoff values for patients over the age of 50.[18] The European Society of Cardiology and American College of Physicians have both adopted age-adjustment analysis into their VTE guidelines.[19,20]

PATIENT EDUCATION

■ https://medlineplus.gov/lab-tests/d-dimer-test/

RELATED DIAGNOSES AND ICD-10 CODES

Abnormal coagulation profile	R79.1

REFERENCES

Full list of references can be accessed through Springer Publishing Company Connect™ at the following link: http://connect.springerpub.com/content/reference-book/978-0-8261-8843-4/part/part03/toc-part/ch060

61. DEHYDROEPIANDROSTERONE

Lisa Ward

PHYSIOLOGY REVIEW

Dehydroepiandrosterone (DHEA) and its conjugated sulfate metabolite, DHEA-S, are weak androgen steroid hormone precursors that are made in and secreted by the adrenal gland. The pituitary gland releases adrenocorticotropic hormone (ACTH), which stimulates the adrenal gland to secrete DHEA-S via a negative feedback loop (Figure 61.1). DHEA-S is further converted into androstenedione and then to testosterone or estrogen (Figure 61.2). During pregnancy, the fetal adrenal gland secretes large amounts of DHEA-S until birth; however, these levels fall shortly after birth and remain low until adrenarche.[1,2] Adrenarche, an adrenal maturational event associated with increase in DHEA-S, causes the appearance of pubic hair, axillary hair, body odor, and acne.[3] DHEA-S levels gradually decrease after age 30, and fall to about 10% to 24% of their peak levels by the seventh decade of life.[1,2]

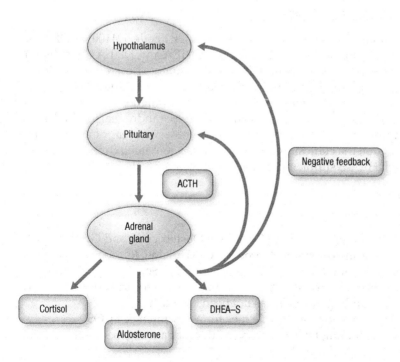

FIGURE 61.1. Dehydroepiandrosterone secretion. ACTH, adrenocorticotropic hormone; DHEA-S, dehydroepiandrosterone sulfate.

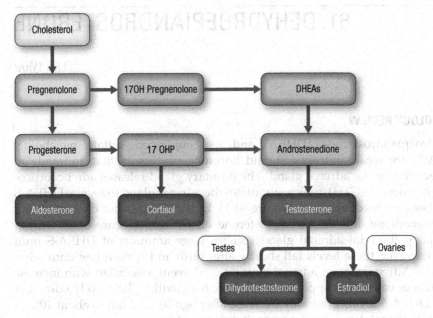

FIGURE 61.2. Steroid pathway. DHEA, dehydroepiandrosterone.

OVERVIEW OF LABORATORY TESTS

Laboratory evaluation can be assessed by DHEA (CPT code 004100) or DHEA-S (CPT code 004020). In most clinical situations, DHEA and DHEA-S results can be used interchangeably; however, DHEA-S is usually chosen because it has minimal diurnal variation, minimal variation during menstrual cycles, a longer half-life, and circulating concentrations are much higher (greater than 100 fold).[3,4] Elevated DHEA-S in females can cause hyperandrogenism. Males are usually asymptomatic. DHEA-S levels decline with every year of age after the age of 20;[5] however, the clinical significance of this age-related drop is unknown and generally DHEA-S supplementation is not recommended.[4,6-8]

INDICATIONS

Screening

- The Endocrine Society, American College of Obstetricians and Gynecologists (ACOG), American Society for Reproductive Medicine, European Society of Endocrinology, and the International Menopause Society recommend against universal DHEA/DHEA-S screening because a correlation between symptoms and androgen levels has not been established.[5]
- International evidence-based guidelines for assessment of PCOS recommend evaluating DHEA-S along with other androgens if total or free testosterone are not elevated.[9]
- ACOG recommends evaluating female adolescents with hirsutism and acne with lab testing serum androgens, including DHEA-S.[10]
- In a polycystic ovary syndrome (PCOS) workup, ACOG recommends evaluating DHEA-S levels in females with rapid virilization.[11]

Diagnosis and Evaluation

- The Endocrine Society recommends evaluating androgen levels, including DHEA-S, in all women with hirsutism and suspected PCOS.[12,13]
- Used to help determine adrenal cause of androgen excess.
- Typically done in conjunction with other steroid hormone levels (i.e., testosterone, 17 OHP, androstenedione).[2,14] Rarely is DHEA-S diagnostic of any condition alone.[2,14]
- Aids in the diagnosis of:
  - Congenital adrenal hyperplasia (CAH)
  - Hyperandrogenism and virilization
  - Virilizing adrenal tumor
  - Premature adrenarche
  - Evaluation of adrenal insufficiency or hypopituitarism
- Differential diagnosis:
  - The differential diagnosis of elevated DHEA-S includes PCOS, CAH, adrenal gland tumor, normal aging, premature adrenarche, and Cushing disease.[2]
  - The differential diagnosis of decreased DHEA-S includes normal aging; pre-pubertal, adrenal insufficiency; hypopituitarism; corticosteroid therapy; and chronic illness.[2]

Monitoring

- In adolescents with hirsutism and chronic acne related to PCOS, DHEA-S may be monitored every 3 to 6 months to assess response to treatment. Once the condition is stable, it may be monitored annually.[10]
- DHEA-S and other androgen levels may be done 3 to 6 weeks after initiation of androgen deficiency therapy and every 6 months thereafter to assess androgen excess.[5,14]

INTERPRETATION

- Normal values are based off sex and age (Table 61.1)[2] Normal values can also be determined based off Tanner staging (Table 61.2)[2]
- Mild elevations in adults are usually idiopathic.[14]
- An increased DHEA-S level is not diagnostic to a specific condition;[14] rather, it usually indicates further testing is needed to determine the cause of hormonal imbalance.
- DHEA-S values of greater than 600 to 700 mcg/dL may be indicative of an androgen-secreting adrenal tumor.[2,14] Elevated levels may also indicate premature adrenarche, PCOS,[9] Cushing disease, smoking, or ectopic ACTH-secreting tumor.
- DHEA-S levels that are increased for age suggest precocious puberty.[3]
- Decreased levels can be seen in adrenal insufficiency (AI),[14] cortisol-secreting adrenal nodule, hypopituitarism,[14] corticosteroid therapy, or chronic illness.

FOLLOW-UP

- High DHEA-S level in an infant or child with signs and symptoms of CAH should prompt additional hormonal testing,[6] including laboratory evaluation of 17 hydroxyprogesterone (17OHP), androstenedione (AE), testosterone, ACTH, and cortisol.

TABLE 61.1: DHEA-S NORMAL RANGES (mcg/dL)

AGE	MALE	FEMALE
1–5 day	12–254	10–248
1 month–5 y/o	1–41	5–55
6–9 y/o	2.5–145	2.5–140
10–11 y/o	15–115	15–260
12–17 y/o	20–555	20–535
18–30 y/o	125–619	45–380
31–50 y/o	59–452	29–379
51–60 y/o	20–413	29–379
61–83 y/o	13–285	
Postmenopausal female		30–260

DHEA-S, dehydroepiandrosterone sulfate.

Source: Data from Lexicomp Online, Lab Tests and Diagnostic Procedures. UpToDate, Inc; 2019, October 27, 2020.

TABLE 61.2: DHEA-S NORMAL RANGES (mcg/dL)

TANNER STAGE	MALE	FEMALE
1	5–265	5–125
2	15–380	15–150
3	60–505	20–535
4	65–560	35–785
5	165–500	75–530

DHEA-S, dehydroepiandrosterone sulfate.

Source: Data from Lexicomp Online, Lab Tests and Diagnostic Procedures. UpToDate, Inc; 2019, October 27, 2020.

- In adults with significantly high levels of DHEA-S (greater than 600 to 700 mcg/dL), further testing with androgen laboratory tests (androstenedione and testosterone) and abdominal imaging is needed to exclude adrenal tumors.
- In adults with high levels of DHEA-S, additional adrenal steroid laboratory testing (AE, 17OHP, testosterone, ACTH, cortisol) should be done to evaluate for nonclassic CAH.[6]
- In female patients with symptoms of PCOS, simultaneous measurement of AE along with testosterone and DHEA-S leads to more accurate diagnosis of PCOS.[15]

■ Low DHEA-S levels can indicate adrenal insufficiency (AI). In patients with concerning clinical symptoms of AI (hypotension, fatigue, weight loss), further testing should be conducted to look for adrenal or pituitary causes of the AI. These follow-up laboratory results should include adrenocorticotropic hormone (ACTH), cortisol, luteinizing hormone (LH), follicle-stimulating hormone (FSH), thyroid-stimulating hormone (TSH), free thyroxine (T4), total triiodothyronine (T3), testosterone, growth hormone (GH), and insulin-like growth factor 1 (IGF1).

PEARLS & PITFALLS

■ DHEA-S levels are decreased in obesity and aging.[4,16] There is no current correlation for DHEA-S level with human well-being established. In addition, there are no established guidelines for DHEA-s preplacement or supplementation therapy.[6] In most settings, the value of DHEA-S therapy is doubtful.[6]

■ DHEA-S levels are typically significantly increased in persistent acne in adults and in PCOS.[17]

■ High DHEA-S levels in infant females can cause ambiguous genitalia.[14]

■ DHEA-S can be normal, elevated, or decreased in CAH patients depending on the enzyme deficiency.[2]

■ 30% to 50% of PCOS patients have elevated DHEA-S,[15,18] which is indicative of adrenal androgen excess.

■ Elevated DHEA-S levels can lead to amenorrhea in females.

■ DHEA-S, along with other hormones (FSH, LH, prolactin, estrogen, and testosterone) can be evaluated to help diagnose the cause of infertility.[14]

■ Certain drugs can cause elevated blood levels (Table 61.3). These drug-induced changes, besides DHEA-S supplements, likely are not significant enough to cause diagnostic confusion. If clinically concerned, the patient should stop all interacting medications for 4 weeks, and testing should be repeated.

TABLE 61.3: MEDICATIONS THAT CAN AFFECT DHEA-S LEVELS

CAUSE ↑DHEA-S	CAUSE ↓ DHEA-S
DHEA-S supplements	Insulin
Metformin	Oral contraceptives
Troglitazone	Corticosteroids
Calcium channel blockers	Dopamine
Nicotine	Carbamzaepine/imipramine/phenytoin
Danazol	Herbal supplements (fish oil, vitamin E)

DHEA-S, dehydroepiandrosterone sulfate.

Source: Data from DHEA-S, Serum. Mayo Clinical Laboratories website. https://endocrinology.testcatalog.org/show/ANST.

PATIENT EDUCATION

- https://healthy.kaiserpermanente.org/health-wellness/health-encyclopedia/he.dhea-s-test.abp5017

RELATED DIAGNOSES AND ICD-10 CODES

Androgen excess	E28.1
Congenital adrenal hyperplasia	E25.0
Ambiguous genitalia	Q56.4
Hirsutism	L68.0
PCOS	E28.2
Adrenal nodule	E27.9
Premature adrenarche	E30.1

REFERENCES

Full list of references can be accessed through Springer Publishing Company Connect™ at the following link: http://connect.springerpub.com/content/reference-book/978-0-8261 -8843-4/part/part03/toc-part/ch061

---

62. DEXAMETHASONE SUPPRESSION TEST

Lisa Ward

PATHOPHYSIOLOGY REVIEW

The dexamethasone suppression test (DST) is used to test patients for excess cortisol production. The DST assesses the lack of suppression of the hypothalamic-pituitary-adrenal (HPA) axis by exogenous corticosteroids. When the HPA axis is intact, any supraphysiologic dose of dexamethasone will suppress pituitary adrenocorticotrophic hormone (ACTH) secretion, thus reducing cortisol production (Figure 62.1).[1] Dexamethasone is a potent synthetic corticosteroid with minimal mineralocorticoid activity. It does not interfere with cortisol measurement in the plasma, urine, or saliva.

OVERVIEW OF LABORATORY TESTS

Laboratory evaluation of each DST can be assessed by cortisol (CPT code 004051) and dexamethasone level (CPT code 500118). Measuring serum dexamethasone provides verification that the drug was taken appropriately.[2] Cortisol is normally secreted in a circadian rhythm with highest levels in the morning.[3] Therefore;

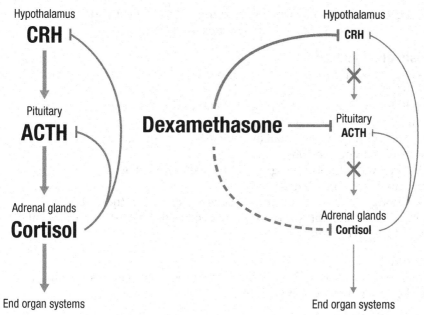

FIGURE 62.1. Normal cortisol HPA axis (left) and HPA axis reaction to dexamethasone (right).
ACTH is produced in the pituitary, and when released will stimulate the adrenal glands to produce cortisol. During a DST, the supraphysiologic dose of dexamethasone suppresses the pituitary secretion of ACTH, thus reducing cortisol production. If cortisol fails to decrease after dexamethasone administration, further evaluation for hypercortisolism should be completed. ACTH, adrenocorticotropic hormone; CRH, corticotropin-releasing hormone.

timing of the blood draw is essential for best accuracy of results. There are two types of DST: low dose (LDDST) and high dose (HDDST).

1. LDDST is used as a screening or confirmatory test in the initial diagnosis of excess cortisol.
   - Patient takes 1 mg dexamethasone tablet orally between 11 p.m. and midnight. Serum cortisol and dexamethasone levels are drawn the next morning at 8 a.m.
2. HDDST is used to determine if excess cortisol is from a pituitary source or from a nonpituitary ACTH secreting source.
   - Patient takes 8 mg dexamethasone tablet orally between 11 p.m. and midnight. Serum cortisol level and dexamethasone levels are drawn at 8 a.m. the next morning.

INDICATIONS

Screening
■ Universal screening is discouraged due to overlap of symptoms from more common comorbidities (e.g., metabolic syndrome) and high rate of false positives.
   - The Endocrine Society Clinical Practice Guideline Task Force recommends against widespread screening.[4]

● As a general rule, endocrinologists recommend against widespread screening because it is neither efficient nor indicated.[5]

Diagnosis and Evaluation

■ Consider testing patients with the symptoms suggestive of excess cortisol (Table 62.1).
■ The U.S. Endocrine Society Practice also notes the following situations are indications for testing for Cushing syndrome with DST:[4]
   ● Patients with symptoms that are unusual for their age (e.g., early osteoporosis, hypertension)
   ● Children with diminished growth and increasing weight
   ● Patients with adrenal incidentaloma
■ In the setting of suspected hypercortisolism, begin with the LDDST.
■ If LDDST does not suppress cortisol, proceed with HDDST to differentiate source of hypercortisolism.[2,4,6–12]

Monitoring

■ Normal DST result should be repeated in 6 months in patients with high clinical suspicion of Cushing syndrome.[7,9]

INTERPRETATION

■ LDDST interpretation guidelines are listed in Table 62.2.[2,13]
■ HDDST interpretation guidelines are listed in Table 62.3.[2,13]

TABLE 62.1: SYMPTOMS OF EXCESS CORTISOL PRODUCTION

COMMON	LESS COMMON
Obesity/weight gain	Dorsal fat pad
Round face	Edema
Menstrual changes	Abnormal glucose tolerance
Lethargy, depression	Recurrent infections
Striae/plethora/thinning skin	Acne
Proximal muscle weakness	Female balding

TABLE 62.2: LDDST INTERPRETATION GUIDELINES

TEST	NORMAL	INTERPRETATION
Cortisol	<1.8 mcg/dL	No hypercortisolism
Cortisol	>1.8 to <5 mcg/dL	Indeterminate, more testing may be needed if clinically indicated
Cortisol	>5 mcg/dL	Possible hypercortisolism, more testing needed
Dexamethasone	140–295 ng/dL	Patient took dexamethasone appropriately

TABLE 62.3: HDDST INTERPRETATION GUIDELINES		
TEST	**RESULT**	**INTERPRETATION**
Cortisol	Suppresses by 50%	Normal finding, Cushing disease is unlikely
Cortisol	Not suppressed	Cushing syndrome is likely
Dexamethasone	1,600–2,850 ng/dL	Patient took dexamethasone appropriately

HDDST, high-dose dexamethasone suppression test.

FOLLOW-UP

- If LDDST is indeterminate, proceed to the HDDST.[2,11]
- If LDDST is abnormal, further testing is needed (i.e., salivary cortisol, urinary free cortisol) to confirm diagnosis of Cushing syndrome.[2,5] Referral to an endocrinologist may be needed.[3]
- Simultaneous measure of serum dexamethasone level is useful to ensure the dexamethasone tablet was taken, absorbed, and reached sufficient blood levels to exert proper HPA feedback.[2,6,12,13]

PEARLS & PITFALLS

- Exogenous corticosteroids (inhaled/topical/parenteral/intraarticular) can cause inaccurate results. If Cushing syndrome is clinically suspected, exogenous corticosteroids should be stopped or tapered to the lowest dose possible before testing.[2]
- Any acute illness (emotional or physical) can falsely elevate cortisol levels.[6] DST should not be done until at least 1 week after resolution of acute stress.
- Oral contraceptives and estrogen therapy can cause falsely elevated DST.[6,10] Patients on these medications should stop the medication for 6 weeks before DST.
- Cortisol levels can be elevated in normal physiologic conditions (i.e., obesity, insulin resistance, alcoholism, neuropsychiatric disorders).[2,10] In patients with these conditions, a midnight serum cortisol level of less than 7.5 mg/dL excludes Cushing syndrome and suggests physiologic hypercortisolism.[9]
- If patient compliance is a concern, dexamethasone level can be used to verify the patient took the medication at 11 p.m. the night before the DST.[12]
- A low clinical suspicion of Cushing syndrome and a negative DST makes the diagnosis of Cushing syndrome very unlikely.[8]
- Cortisol levels can increase with age.[14]
- Poor absorption of dexamethasone, as would occur in patients with malabsorption or celiac disease, will result in a lower concentration of dexamethasone level and subsequently lower degrees of cortisol suppression.[6]
- As a general rule, DST should only be performed if the pretest probability for Cushing syndrome is reasonably high.[5]
- The DST should not be used to evaluate Cushing syndrome in pregnancy, epilepsy, and renal failure due to high false-positive results.[4]

■ Iatrogenic hypercortisolism is the most common cause of Cushing syndrome. Patients should discontinue (if possible) all prescribed steroid medications prior to completing DST.[7]

PATIENT EDUCATION

■ https://www.mountsinai.org/health-library/tests/dexamethasone -suppression-test
■ https://www.labcorp.com/resource/dexamethasone-suppression -screening-for-cushing-disease-syndrome

RELATED DIAGNOSES AND ICD-10 CODES

Cushing syndrome	E24.9
Cushing disease	E24.0
Pseudo-Cushing	E24.4
Abnormal cortisol level	E27.8
Personal history of systemic steroid therapy	Z92.241

REFERENCES

Full list of references can be accessed through Springer Publishing Company Connect™ at the following link: http://connect.springerpub.com/content/reference-book/978-0-8261 -8843-4/part/part03/toc-part/ch062

---

63. DIVALPROEX SODIUM/VALPROIC ACID

Shannon L. Linder

PHYSIOLOGY REVIEW

Valproic acid (VPA), most commonly otherwise known as valproate, is a simple-chain branch of the carboxylic acid family and is converted rapidly to the acid form in the stomach.[1] There are numerous preparations available and all of them are therapeutically equivalent medications due to the dissociation of valproic acid into valproate ion at physiologic pH levels.[1] It was first approved for epilepsy, then manic episodes, bipolar disorder, and migraine prophylaxis.[2]

Valproic acid is in the medication class of anticonvulsants, in which the exact mechanism of action is unknown. Valproic acid has positive effects of mood stabilization and anti-migraine, in addition to the anticonvulsant actions. Of the proposed theories of mechanism of action, valproic acid may lower excessive transmission of ions through voltage-sensitive sodium channels by changing the sensitivity by altering their phosphorylation, thus enhancing mood stabilization antimanic effects.[3] The theory presents as less sodium being available, less release of glutamate, and less excitatory neurotransmission, thus stabilizing mood.[3] In terms of antimanic effects, valproic acid may also enhance GABA actions by increasing its release, decreasing its reuptake, or slowing its metabolic inactivation, causing more inhibitory neurotransmission.[3] The downstream actions on complex signal transduction cascades include more recent theories of mechanism of action which are less understood.

Valproic acid Food and Drug Administration (FDA) indications include proven effectiveness for the acute manic phase of bipolar disorder, mixed episodes of bipolar disorder, complex partial seizures, simple and complex absence seizures, multiple seizure types for adjunctive treatment, and migraine prophylaxis.[4] Off-label indications for use include prevention of reoccurrence of mania, bipolar depression, rapid cycling of bipolar disorder, agitation associated with dementia, personality disorders and brain injury, and adjunctive treatment of psychosis and schizophrenia.[4] Less common uses for valproic acid include intermittent explosive disorder, kleptomania (case reports), posttraumatic stress disorder (PTSD), alcohol withdrawal and relapse prevention, panic disorder, borderline personality disorder, behavioral agitation, dementia, and obsessive compulsive disorder (OCD).[1] Remission of symptoms is the goal of treatment; thus, treatment can be indefinite. The side effect profile of VPA is extensive with some significant warnings and considerations. Side effects can occur with use of valproic acid and may increase with dosage (Table 63.1).[4-7]

OVERVIEW OF LABORATORY TESTS

Laboratory evaluation of VPA level status can be assessed by VPA serum level (CPT code 80165). VPA level should be ordered as a trough, 12 hours post-dose of medication. For example, if a patient takes their last dose of VPA in the evening around 8 p.m., they should skip their morning VPA dosage if they take one and have the laboratory level drawn at 8 a.m..

INDICATIONS

Screening
- Universal and targeted screenings are not applicable.

TABLE 63.1: SIDE EFFECTS WITH VALPROIC ACID	
Black box warnings	Fetal congenital malformations, pancreatitis, and hepatotoxicity
Common side effects	Sedation, tremor, dizziness, ataxia, asthenia, headache, abdominal pain, nausea, vomiting, diarrhea, decreased appetite, constipation, dyspepsia, weight gain, metabolic changes, and alopecia
Potential side effects*	Polycystic ovary syndrome (PCOS), hyperandrogenism, hyperinsulinemia, dyslipidemia, decreased bone mineral density, and amenorrhea

*These side effects are considered controversial due to inconsistent evidence demonstrating direct correlation.

Sources: Data from Stahl SM, Grady MM. *Stahl's Essential Psychopharmacology: Prescriber's Guide.* 6th ed. Cambridge University Press; 2017; Kee JL. *Laboratory & Diagnostic Tests With Nursing Implications.* Prentice Hall; 2002; Jacobson SA. *Laboratory Medicine in Psychiatry and Behavioral Science.* American Psychiatric Pub; 2012; Padder TAM. *Practical Guide to Psychiatric Medications: Simple, Concise, & Up-To-Date.* CreateSpace; 2015.

Diagnosis and Evaluation

Consider evaluation of VPA level for the following:

- Routine monitoring of pharmacotherapy
- Failure to respond to treatment
- Presence of side effects
- Signs and symptoms of serious adverse effects including tachycardia, bradycardia, hepatotoxicity with liver failure, pancreatitis, drug reaction with eosinophilia (DRESS), and rare activation of suicidal ideation or suicidal behavior[4]
- Overdose is suspected such as central nervous system (CNS) depression, coma, miotic pupils, tachycardia, hypotension, QTc prolongation, and respiratory depression, restlessness, hallucinations, or heart block.[4,7]

Monitoring

- VPA serum concentration levels are monitored for patients receiving VPA medication pharmacotherapy to ensure VPA levels are in the therapeutic dosage range.[5]
- Monitoring plasma drug levels may assist with efficacy, side effects, and compliance in patients treated with VPA.[4]
- Evaluate VPA serum level as needed to check noncompliance or toxicity with both mood and seizure disorders.[6] It may also be useful to check serum levels in patients who are on VPA and other medications with pharmacokinetic interactions or other clinical conditions that may present a concern to the clinician.[8]
- When treating seizure disorders, the VPA serum monitoring has been controversial. Repetitive serum monitoring is not recommended once dosage of VPA and seizures have stabilized.[9]
- The National Institute for Health Care and Excellence (NICE) recommends not routinely measuring VPA levels in adults and children unless there is a clinical indication such as suspicion of ineffectiveness, poor compliance, or toxicity.[8,10] The correlation between serum drug concentration with clinical response may be more accurate, however, than with the actual dosage.[9]
- VPA levels should be monitored regularly, at suggested intervals, for acute mania at 5 days after starting or adjusting the dosage.[11] The level should then be repeated once, and then maintenance monitoring every 3 to 6 months.[11] According to the Canadian Network for Mood and Anxiety Treatments (CANMAT) and the International Society for Bipolar Disorders (ISBP), there has been some evidence supporting a linear relationship between improvement of mania and VPA levels; however, this has not been proven with the maintenance phase.[11] The patient's mood symptoms should be monitored closely. Other guidelines such as the Royal Australian and New Zealand College of Psychiatrists (RANZCP) state that serum levels and clinical efficacy are not closely correlated in the treatment of mania.[12]
- Monitoring of various labs and other screenings should take place before the start of and during VPA treatment (Table 63.2).

TABLE 63.2: MONITORING CONSIDERATIONS DURING VALPROIC ACID TREATMENT	
Before starting treatment with VPA	• Prior to starting VPA, patients should have the following laboratory tests: thyroid function starting with thyroid-stimulating hormone (TSH), complete blood count (CBC) with platelets, coagulation tests, fasting lipid profile, liver function tests (LFTs), fasting glucose, and a human chorionic gonadotropin (HCG) in childbearing women.[1,4,6] • Metabolic screening should be completed prior to initiating VPA treatment: weight, height, body mass index (BMI), waist circumference, blood pressure, fasting glucose, and fasting lipid profile.[4,6]
During VPA	• During initial titration: CBC with platelets and LFTs weekly[6] for the first few months of treatment, followed bi-annually or annually following the initiation period[4] • CBC with platelets, LFTs, serum ammonia, TSH, amylase and lipase every 6 months[6] • Metabolic screening should also be completed at regular intervals throughout treatment: weight, height, body mass index (BMI), waist circumference, blood pressure, fasting glucose, and fasting lipid profile.[4,6] • Frequently monitor for pregnancy in individuals of childbearing age.[4,10]
Special considerations	• Monitor coagulation tests prior to a planned surgery or if there is a bleeding history.[4] • Monitor for signs and symptoms of thrombocytopenia and instruct patients to report any signs or symptoms of easily bruising or bleeding.[4] • The older adult population may experience more side effects of VPA; therefore, monitor for increased somnolence, dehydration, reduced nutritional intake, and weight loss, and start with lower doses and increase slowly.[4] The older adult population is also at increased risk for developing thrombocytopenia, particularly those in long-term care facilities.[4] Monitor gait disturbances and tremor in this population as well.[10]

INTERPRETATION

▪ There can be slight variations of normal reference intervals; however, VPA has a relatively wide therapeutic index. Table 63.3 summarizes current interpretation guidelines.

▪ Serum concentrations shown to be effective for mania associated with bipolar disorder are greater than 45 to 50 µg/mL.[1,4] The maintenance range is usually 50 to 125 µg/mL.[13] Despite these recommendations, it is imperative to treat the patient, not the laboratory value.

▪ Free VPA levels range from 6 to 22 µg/mL and % free VPA ranges from 5% to 18% (calculated).[6]

FOLLOW-UP

▪ The recommendation from the NICE guidelines for adjunctive monitoring includes BMI, weight, LFTs, and CBC at 6 months after initiating VPA treatment and then subsequent annual testing.[10] The RANZCP guidelines for BMI, waist circumference, LFTs, and CBC are at initiation of treatment, 6 months, 12 months and 24 months, respectively.[12] Refer to Table 63.2.

TABLE 63.3: INTERPRETATION VALPROIC ACID DRUG LEVEL		
	NORMAL	**HIGH**
Sadock, Sadock, & Ruiz[1]	>50 µg/mL for antimanic effects	
Jacobson[6]	50–125 µg/mL	>150 µg/mL
Stahl[4]	>45 µg/mL for antimanic and/or anticonvulsant effects	
	Up to 100 µg/mL well tolerated	
	Up to 125 µg/mL may be needed for some acute manic patients	
Hirschfeld RMA, Bowden CL, Gitlin MJ, et al. [14]	50–125 µg/mL	

PEARLS & PITFALLS

- VPA does not interfere with other laboratory tests; however, it is important to consider the drug interaction effects on VPA levels such as carbamazepine, lamotrigine, and fluoxetine, to name the most common interactions.[6]
- Although the risks for pancreatitis and hepatotoxicity are rare, they can be fatal.[4] Inform patients of early symptoms of liver disease and pancreatitis. Idiosyncratic hepatic failure is not dose dependent and is rare. Hemorrhagic pancreatitis is typically seen in the first 3 months of treatment.[15]
- The use of VPA is never recommended in females of childbearing age unless there are no other options, pregnancy prevention measures are in place, and risks are reviewed in depth.[8] VPA has the highest incidence of teratogenic effects on fetuses (between 6.2% and 16%) and has been shown to have lasting developmental delays.[15]
- There were not any studies found suggesting cultural variances should change treatment or monitoring of VPA. However, VPA is contraindicated in patients with any known or suspected mitochondrial disorders, fatty acid metabolism disorders, and in women with X-linked hyperammonemia.[16]
- Drug–drug interactions are plentiful and can affect serum concentrations.
- Hyperammonemia has been reported in patients taking topirimate combined with VPA; therefore, ammonia levels should be measured in patients who develop unexplained lethargy, vomiting, or change in mental status.[4]
- VPA administration is contraindicated for the following reasons: thrombocytopenia; urea cycle disorders due to the potential for hyperammonemic encephalopathy; pregnancy; known severe liver disease; children under 10, particularly under 2 years of age; known pancreatitis; or proven allergy to VPA or any of the components.[4] Urea cycle disorders may be associated with unexplained encephalopathy, mental retardation,

elevated plasma ammonia, cyclical vomiting, and lethargy.[4] Any patient who develops a new onset neurologic symptom may be at risk for hyperammonemic encephalopathy and should be evaluated for such.[11] VPA- induced encephalopathy has also been documented in the treatment of seizure disorders.[15]

- With the treatment of seizure disorders, it is not recommended to switch manufacturers of VPA due to changes in serum concentrations.[8]
- In patients with alopecia-related side effects, multivitamins with zinc and selenium may help.[4]

PATIENT EDUCATION

- https://nami.org/About-Mental-Illness/Treatments/Mental-Health -Medications/Types-of-Medication/Valproate-(Depakote)

RELATED DIAGNOSES AND ICD-10 CODES

Bipolar and other bipolar spectrum	F31
Cyclothymia	F34.0
Schizophrenia	F20
Monitoring for therapeutic medication levels	Z51.81
Epilepsy and recurrent seizures	G40
Migraine	G43

REFERENCES

Full list of references can be accessed through Springer Publishing Company Connect™ at the following link: http://connect.springerpub.com/content/reference-book/978-0-8261 -8843-4/part/part03/toc-part/ch063

---

64. ELECTROLYTES (BASIC METABOLIC PANEL)

Kelly Small Casler and Kristopher R. Maday

Electrolytes are positive or negative charged ions that constitute the various body fluid compartments. Maintenance of normal levels of electrolytes is essential to muscle, nerve, and other physiologic processes.[1,2] Laboratory evaluation of electrolytes provides information regarding the body's acid-base balance and also reflects kidney function. In serum and plasma samples, electrodes specific to each electrolyte are used to capture and quantify the amount of electrolytes in a sample.[3]

SODIUM

PHYSIOLOGY REVIEW

Sodium is a positive charged electrolyte (cation) that is obtained through the diet and is greatly affected by water homeostasis. Normal sodium levels are important to neuron physiology and neuroelectrical transmission. Normal sodium levels are regulated by the renin-angiotensin-aldosterone system (RAAS) and by the secretion of antidiuretic hormone (vasopressin) from the posterior pituitary gland.[2] Patients with abnormalities in these systems are, therefore, at risk for alterations of sodium balance.[4]

OVERVIEW OF LABORATORY TESTS

Sodium can be measured in serum, plasma, or whole blood. It also can be measured indirectly or directly. Whole blood is commonly used for tests performed on arterial blood gas analyzers or point-of-care machines and provides direct measurements, whereas samples analyzed in the central laboratory use indirect methods to measure sodium in the serum or plasma.[5] Indirect methods rely heavily on normal water content (93%) in the serum or plasma, something that is often abnormal in critically ill patients.[5]

INDICATIONS

Screening
■ Not typically used.

Diagnosis and Evaluation
■ Used in the differential diagnosis of signs/symptoms that may be related to sodium imbalances, such as cardiac arrhythmias, heart failure, liver failure, renal failure, myalgias, mental status changes, muscle weakness, and dehydration.

Monitoring
■ Used in the monitoring of electrolyte disturbances and replacement therapies. Exact monitoring intervals will vary.

INTERPRETATION
■ **Reference interval:** 135 to 145 mEq/L[6,7]
■ **Critical values:** less than 121 mEq/L or greater than 158 mEq/L[6]

FOLLOW-UP

Hyponatremia
■ The first step in the differential diagnosis of hyponatremia is to obtain a plasma or serum osmolality and classify the hyponatremia as hypotonic, isotonic, or hypertonic (Table 64.1).[8] In complex cases of hyponatremia, urine osmolality and urine sodium are also used (Table 64.2).[8–10]
■ If hypotonic hyponatremia (most common type of hyponatremia) is suspected, the differential diagnoses can be categorized further by determining volume status (Table 64.2).

TABLE 64.1: CLASSIFICATION OF HYPONATREMIA USING SERUM/PLASMA OSMOLALITY

OSMOLALITY IN mOSm/kg	CLASSIFICATION	DIFFERENTIAL DIAGNOSIS FOR CAUSE OF ABNORMAL SODIUM
<280 (low)	Hypotonic hyponatremia	Large differential (see Table 64.2) including SIADH, cirrhosis, heart failure
280–295 (normal)	Isotonic hyponatremia	Hyperglycemia, pseudohyponatremia
>295 (high)	Hypertonic hyponatremia	Severe hyperglycemia with dehydration, mannitol adverse effects, pseudohyponatremia from hyperglycemia

SIADH, syndrome of inappropriate antidiuretic hormone.

Source: Verbalis JG, Goldsmith SR, Greenberg A, et al. Diagnosis, evaluation, and treatment of hyponatremia: expert panel recommendations. *Am J Med.* 2013;126(10):S1–S42. doi:10.1016/j.amjmed.2013.07.006

TABLE 64.2: DIFFERENTIAL DIAGNOSIS AND CATEGORIZATION OF HYPOTONIC HYPONATREMIAS

CATEGORIZATION BASED ON VOLUME STATUS	OTHER POTENTIAL ASSOCIATED LABORATORY CHANGES	PEARLS	DIFFERENTIAL DIAGNOSES
Hypovolemic	Elevated BUN and Cr or uric acid.	Serum Na should improve with fluid resuscitation. If it does not, consider SIADH.	**If urine sodium <20–30 mEq/L:** excessive vomiting/diarrhea, burns, third spacing **If urine sodium >30 mEq/L:** side effects of diuretics, head injury (cerebral salt wasting), primary adrenal insufficiency
Euvolemic	Normal/low uric acid, or BUN and Cr. Urine sodium ≥ 20–30 mEq/L	Urine sodium might be elevated due to diuretics A urine osmolality >100 mOsm/kg suggests SIADH.	SIADH, secondary adrenal insufficiency, hypothyroidism, excessive exercise, polydipsia, beer potomania, diuretic use
Hypervolemic	Elevated BNP if heart failure Elevated BUN and Cr if AKI or CKD	Can also be caused by severe hyperglycemia with dehydration or use of potent diuretics (mannitol)	**If urine sodium is <20–30 mEq/L:** heart failure, cirrhosis **If urine sodium >30 mEq/L:** AKI, CKD

AKI, acute kidney injury; BNP, brain natriuretic peptide; BUN, blood urea nitrogen; CKD, chronic kidney disease; Cr, creatinine; Na, sodium; SIADH, syndrome of inappropriate antidiuretic hormone.

Sources: Verbalis JG, Goldsmith SR, Greenberg A, et al. Diagnosis, evaluation, and treatment of hyponatremia: expert panel recommendations. *Am J Med.* 2013;126(10):S1–S42. doi:10.1016/j.amjmed.2013.07.006; Spasovski G, Vanholder R, Allolio B, et al. Clinical practice guideline on diagnosis and treatment of hyponatraemia. *Eur J Endocrinol.* 2014;170(3):G1–47. doi:10.1530/EJE-13-1020; Seay NW, Lehrich RW, Greenberg A. Diagnosis and management of disorders of body tonicity—hyponatremia and hypernatremia: core curriculum 2020. *Am J Kidney Dis.* 2020;75(2):272–286. doi:10.1053/j.ajkd.2019.07.014

Hypernatremia

■ To follow-up hypernatremia, first determine fluid status. Urine sodium and urine osmolality can then be used to assist in the differential diagnosis (Table 64.3).

PEARLS & PITFALLS

■ Hyperglycemia causes pseudohyponatremia, so for every 100 mg/dL rise in glucose above 100 mg/dL, sodium should be corrected by 1.6 to 2.4 mEq/L.[11] For example, in a patient with a glucose of 700 mg/dL and sodium of 122 mg/dL, the corrected sodium for glucose would be 132 to 136 mEq/L. A calculator is available for this conversion at https://www.mdcalc.com/sodium-correction-hyperglycemia
■ Hyperlipidemia or hyperproteinemia can also cause a pseudohyponatremia.[8]
■ Serum sodium concentration of 105 mEq/L or less combined with hypokalemia should alert the clinician to a risk of osmotic demyelination syndrome.
■ Sodium may need to be corrected for abnormalities in albumin. For every 1 gm/dL that albumin rises/falls, sodium can be corrected by 0.7 mEq/L in the same direction.[5]
■ Hyponatremia is more common in geriatrics, probably partially related to polypharmacy.[12]
■ Much work is being done to exactly characterize the role that sodium plays in predicting mortality in hospitalized patients.[13–16]

TABLE 64.3: DIFFERENTIAL DIAGNOSIS OF HYPERNATREMIA BASED ON FLUID STATUS

FLUID STATUS	URINE TEST	DIFFERENTIAL DIAGNOSIS	OTHER LABORATORY FINDINGS OR FOLLOW-UP TESTS
Hypovolemia	Urine sodium >20 mEq/L	Diuretic use Renal disease	
	Urine sodium <20 mEq/L	Heat exhaustion, burns, diarrhea	
Euvolemia	Urine osmol >600 mOsm/kg	Fluid loss, inadequate water intake	Elevated lithium level, hypercalcemia, hypokalemia
	Urine osmol <300 mOsm/kg	DI	Hypokalemia and hypercalcemia may be seen with nephrogenic diabetes insipidus. Water deprivation test can be used to confirm suspected DI
Hypervolemia	Urine osmol >600 mOsm/kg	Excessive salt intake, Cushing syndrome, primary hyperaldosteronism	Urine Na >100 mEq/L

DI, diabetes insipidus.

Source: Data from Seay NW, Lehrich RW, Greenberg A. Diagnosis and management of disorders of body tonicity—hyponatremia and hypernatremia: core curriculum 2020. *Am J Kidney Dis.* 2020;75(2):272–286. doi:10.1053/j.ajkd.2019.07.014

- Hyponatremia is the most common electrolyte abnormality in inpatients and outpatients and is associated with increased fracture risk as well as morbidity and mortality.[4,8,17–19]
- Some medications can cause hyponatremia, especially benzodiazepines, antiepileptics, and diuretics.[4]

POTASSIUM

PHYSIOLOGY REVIEW

Potassium is the most abundant intracellular cation (only 2% is found extracellularly) and is important for cardiac, skeletal, and neuromuscular electrical transmission and contractility.[2] Excessive potassium is excreted by the kidneys.[1] In acidemic states, serum potassium may rise due to potassium moving out of the cell; the opposite is true of alkalemic conditions.[6]

OVERVIEW OF LABORATORY TESTS

Potassium can be measured in either serum or plasma. Plasma usually allows faster analysis (since plasma must first clot to produce serum), but serum is more commonly used.[3,20,21] Whole blood samples are also sometimes used, mainly in emergencies where point-of-care potassium can be performed along with arterial blood gases.[22] Samples must be collected and handled with care since things like excessive use of tourniquets, pneumatic tube transport, and hand pumping can distort values, causing pseudohyperkalemia.[3,22,23] Under- or overactivity of the RAAS is a common cause of abnormal potassium levels.[4]

INDICATIONS

Screening
- Patients with poor nutrition or gastrointestinal (GI) illness are especially at risk for hypokalemia and may warrant screening for abnormalities.[4]

Diagnosis and Evaluation
- Used in the differential diagnosis of signs/symptoms that may be related to potassium imbalances, such as cardiac arrythmias, renal failure, myalgias, mental status changes, muscle weakness, constipation, fatigue, muscle cramping, and paresthesia.
- Used to evaluate for dyskalemia as a cause of electrocardiogram abnormalities:
  - Hypokalemia will cause flat T-waves, ST-segment depression, and U-wave development.
  - Hyperkalemia will cause peaked T-waves, PR prolongation, widened QRS, and loss of P-wave.

Monitoring
- Used in the monitoring of electrolyte disturbances and replacement therapies.
- Used to monitor patients with risk factors for dyskalemias. Optimal frequency of monitoring is unknown.[4]

■ Used to monitor for side effects of antimineralcorticoid pharmacotherapy in patients with heart failure.[24]
■ May be used to routinely monitor patients on antimineralcorticoid pharmacotherapy for acne, though one study suggests this is not evidence-based.[25]
■ Used in monitoring for hyperkalemic side effects of angiotensin-converting enzyme inhibitor (ACE-I) or angiotensin-receptor blocker (ARB) pharmacotherapy.

INTERPRETATION

Reference interval for ages 1 year and older: 3.5 to 5.3 mEq/L[6]
Critical values for ages 1 year and older: less than 2.6mEq/L or greater than 7.5 mEq/L[6]
Hyperkalemia emergencies (Note: Individuals with renal failure may be allowed higher thresholds before considering it an emergency.):[26]

■ ANY patients with signs or symptoms of hyperkalemia
■ Potassium greater than 6.0 mEq/L (and pseudohyperkalemia is ruled out)
■ A 24-hour increase in potassium greater than 1.0 mEq/L that is associated with neuromuscular weakness or critical illness

FOLLOW-UP

■ Magnesium levels should be assessed in hypokalemia, especially when patients fail to respond to replacement therapies.[27]
■ Follow-up of abnormal potassium levels is guided based on differential diagnoses (Table 64.4)[28,29]

TABLE 64.4: DIFFERENTIAL DIAGNOSIS OF HYPERKALEMIA AND HYPOKALEMIA

HYPERKALEMIA CAUSE	FOLLOW-UP	HYPOKALEMIA CAUSE	FOLLOW-UP
Hypoaldosteronism	Plasma renin activity, aldosterone, cortisol	Hyperaldosteronism	Aldosterone/renin ratio
Pseudohyperkalemia	Repeat potassium level	Excessive catecholamines as seen in ACLS	None, monitor patient
Diabetic ketoacidosis	Gluose, beta hydroxybutyrate	Diuretics, especially loop diuretics	Other electrolytes
Metabolic acidosis	Other electrolytes, arterial blood gas	Vomiting/diarrhea	Other electrolytes
Renal disease or dysfunction	BUN/Cr/GFR		

ABG, arterial blood gas; ACLS, advanced cardiac life support; BUN, blood urea nitrogen; Cr, creatinine; GFR, glomerular filtration rate.

Sources: Data from Funder JW, Carey RM, Mantero F, et al. The management of primary aldosteronism: case detection, diagnosis, and treatment: an Endocrine Society clinical practice guideline. *J Clin Endocrinol Metab.* 2016;101(5):1889–1916. doi:10.1210/jc.2015-4061; Rodan AR. Potassium: friend or foe? *Pediatr Nephrol.* 2017;32(7):1109–1121. doi:10.1007/s00467-016-3411-8

PEARLS & PITFALLS

- Many patients on ACE-I/ARB therapy are not monitored for hyperkalemia, even though routine monitoring has been shown to reduce chances of hyperkalemic events.[30,31]
- If hypokalemia is identified in the presence of hypertension, look for secondary causes of hypertension, such as Conns syndrome and other primary aldosteronism states.[28,32]
- Medications that are associated with hyperkalemia include ARBs, ACE-Is, spironolactone, drospirenone, amiloride, triamterene, trimethoprim, heparin, ketoconazole, nonsteroidal anti-inflammatory drugs, and beta blockers.[29,33]
- Potassium determined through whole blood samples may be more accurate in cases of severe leukocytosis and either whole blood or plasma samples may be more accurate if platelets are greater than 500,000.[21,34]
- Conditions that cause delay in clotting such as anticoagulant therapy or liver disease can cause pseudohyperkalemia in serum samples.[35]
- Point-of-care devices (whole blood) are more prone to result in pseudohyperkalemia in the presence of hemolysis, thrombocytosis, or leukocytosis.[33]
- Diabetes limits renal potassium excretion, increasing blood potassium and urinary potassium levels.[33]
- Medications that increase urinary potassium excretion and cause hypokalemia include thiazide and loop diuretics.[33]
- Patients are at most risk of hyperkalemia from ACE-I/ARB therapy when glomerular filtration rate (GFR) is 60 mL/min per 1.73 m^2 or less.[36,37]
- For every 10 mEq of oral potassium chloride replacement, potassium is predicted to rise by 0.1 mEq/L.[38,39]

CALCIUM

Physiology Review

Calcium is considered both an electrolyte and mineral and is important for the functions of action potentials, nerve conduction, and blood coagulation.[2] Most of the body's calcium is found in bone; along with phosphorus and vitamin D, calcium is important in bone homeostasis. Calcium homeostasis in the body is regulated through parathyroid hormone, calcitonin (thyroid), and calcitriol (kidneys).[40]

OVERVIEW OF LABORATORY TESTS

Serum calcium measures total calcium, calcium that is either bound to proteins or unbound (free).[6]

INDICATIONS

Screening

- Screening of total calcium levels is indicated in individuals with chronic kidney disease (CKD) and GFR lower than 45 mL/min/1.73 m^2 at least once to evaluate for metabolic bone disease.

Diagnosis and Evaluation

■ Used in the differential diagnosis of signs/symptoms that may be related to calcium imbalances, such as cardiac arrythmias, bone pain, abdominal pain, depression/confusion, renal failure, myalgias, fatigue, lethargy, urolithiasis, tetany, or muscle weakness.

Monitoring

■ This is used to monitor electrolyte disturbances.
■ Although an uncommon complication, calcium may be used to monitor for hypoparathyroidism after thyroidectomy.[41,42]

INTERPRETATION

■ Reference interval: 8.7 to 10.7 mg/dL
■ Critical: less than 6.6 or greater than 12.9 mg/dL
■ Malnourished patients with hypoalbuminemia may have a pseudo-hypocalcemia. The calcium level can be corrected through the following calculation: 0.8 x (normal lab albumin – patient's albumin) + serum calcium. Alternatively, ionized calcium can be evaluated, which will not be influenced by albumin levels.[40]

FOLLOW-UP

■ If hypocalcemia is noted, follow-up evaluation includes parathyroid hormone (to assess for hypoparathyrodism), magnesium (to assess for hypomagnesemia), vitamin D levels (to assess for vitamin D deficiency), serum phosphorus, and urine calcium/phosphate.[40]
■ If hypercalcemia is noted, evaluate parathyroid hormone (to assess for hyperparathyroidism), thyroid-stimulating hormone (TSH) and free T4 (to assess for thyrotoxicosis), and blood urea nitrogen (BUN)/creatinine/GFR (to assess for renal dysfunction). Also consider the possibility of malignancy.[40]

PEARLS & PITFALLS

■ In the setting of primary hyperparathyroidism, total serum calcium is a more reliable reflection of calcium status compared to ionized calcium.[43]

CHLORIDE

PHYSIOLOGY REVIEW

Chloride is an anion that often moves with sodium; likewise, low sodium states will also be accompanied by low chloride. Chloride is the most abundant anion in serum and it is key to regulating body fluids.[44] In conjunction with bicarbonate, chloride helps maintain acid-base relationships in the body. Too little chloride is termed "hypochloremia," while too much is termed "hyperchloremia."

OVERVIEW OF LABORATORY TESTS

Chloride can be tested in sweat, serum, urine, and feces.[44] This section focuses on serum testing.

INDICATIONS

Screening
■ Not used.

Diagnosis and Evaluation
■ Used in the differential diagnosis of electrolyte abnormalities and to evaluate metabolic acidosis.

Monitoring
■ Used along with sodium, potassium, and bicarbonate levels to monitor electrolyte disturbances and acidosis/alkalosis.

INTERPRETATION
■ Reference interval: 97 to 110 mEq/L[6]

FOLLOW-UP

■ Follow-up testing should be guided based on the suspected differential diagnoses (Table 64.5).[44,45]

PEARLS & PITFALLS
■ Chloride levels rise and fall in an inverse relationship with bicarbonate.[44]

CARBON DIOXIDE

PHYSIOLOGY REVIEW

Carbon dioxide is a gas produced as a product of cellular metabolism. It is carried in the blood to the lungs for excretion during respiration.

OVERVIEW OF LABORATORY TESTS

Total carbon dioxide is measured in the serum. Three components make up the total carbon dioxide: bicarbonate (HCO3-), dissolved carbon dioxide (dCO_2), and carbonic acid (H_2CO_3)[46]; however, 95% of total carbon dioxide is actually in the form of bicarbonate, and so when interpreting carbon dioxide levels, it is

TABLE 64.5: DIFFERENTIAL DIAGNOSIS OF ALTERATIONS OF CHLORIDE LEVELS	
CAUSES OF HYPOCHLOREMIA[44,45]	**CAUSES OF HYPERCHLOREMIA**[44,45]
Excessive GI losses (severe diarrhea or vomiting very common), compensation for metabolic acidosis, adrenal insufficiency, burns, alkalosis, loop diuretics, sodium bicarbonate infusion, SIADH, excessive hypotonic solutions, CHF, hyponatremia	Metabolic acidosis, renal disease, salicylate intoxication, excessive intravenous saline, diabetes insipidus, dehydration, diarrhea, renal tubular acidosis, renal failure, diabetes insipidus, diuretics, hypermetabolic states, hypernatremia, carbonic anhydrase inhibitors

CHF, congestive heart failure; GI, gastrointestinal; IV, intravenous; SIADH, syndrome of inappropriate diuretic hormone.

often used to approximate bicarbonate levels in the absence of an arterial blood gas.[47] It seems to perform quite well in this role, only overestimating plasma bicarbonate levels by 1 to 1.5 mEq/L.[48,49]

INDICATIONS

Screening
- Not used.

Diagnosis and Evaluation
- Used in the differential diagnosis of electrolyte abnormalities and to evaluate acidosis/alkalosis.

Monitoring
- Used along with other parameters of the basic metabolic panel (BMP) to monitor electrolyte disturbances and acidosis/alkalosis.

INTERPRETATION
- Reference interval: 24–32 mEq/L[6]

FOLLOW-UP
- Most acid–base disorders are initially recognized because of abnormalities in CO_2.[48] In critically ill states or those with persistent abnormalities, measuring true bicarbonate levels and other elements of the arterial blood gas help to clarify the clinical picture.[48]

PEARLS & PITFALLS
- Do not use CO_2 as a proxy for HCO_3 when the patient has severe hyperlipidemia as it will not be accurate.[47]

ANION GAP AND CHLORIDE/SODIUM RATIO

PHYSIOLOGY REVIEW
The anion gap reflects the amount of acid present in serum and helps to clarify acidosis/alkalosis since increased acid reduces serum bicarbonate levels.[50]

OVERVIEW OF LABORATORY TESTS
Over the years, the anion gap has had varying definitions but is most often calculated by subtracting serum sodium from the sum of chloride and bicarbonate (carbon dioxide is used in place of bicarbonate, if bicarbonate levels are not available). Historically, serum potassium was included in the calculation, but most clinicians exclude this information since the changes in potassium are so small, they do not seem to influence results. However, this decision would cause an inaccurate anion gap in the setting of elevated potassium levels.[51] The chloride/sodium ratio is sometimes used as an alternative to the anion gap.[52,53] A ratio of less than 0.75 is used as a predictor of a high anion gap and greater than 0.79 predicts a normal anion gap.

INDICATIONS

Screening
■ Not used.

Diagnosis and Evaluation
■ Used in the differential diagnosis of electrolyte abnormalities and to evaluate acidosis/alkalosis.

Monitoring
■ Used along with other parameters of the BMP to monitor electrolyte disturbances and acidosis/alkalosis.

INTERPRETATION

■ Serum anion gap helps in the differential diagnosis of metabolic acidosis as either a high anion gap metabolic acidosis or a normal anion gap acidosis. Causes of a metabolic acidosis with high anion gap associations are recalled through the mnemonic "GOLD MARK": Glycols (ethylene and propylene), Oxoproline, L-lactate, D-lactate, Methanol, Aspirin, Renal failure, and Ketoacidosis.[54] Metabolic acidosis with a normal anion gap can result from diarrhea, vomiting, renal tubular acidosis, excess saline infusion, ingestion of salt water, chronic kidney disease, d-lactic acidosis, and diabetic ketoacidosis.[55]

■ Anion gap greater than 10 is often seen in diabetic ketoacidosis.[56]

FOLLOW-UP

■ Other components of the BMP help differentiate between the causes of metabolic acidosis.[55]
■ Serum lactate levels or beta hydroxybutarate may be used if sepsis or diabetic ketoacidosis are suspected.

PEARLS & PITFALLS

■ Metabolic acidosis can still be present in the setting of a normal anion gap.
■ Serum albumin can influence anion gap interpretation.[57] For every 1 gram decrease in albumin, the anion gap is reduced by up to 2.5 mEq/L.[51] Because of this, anion gap calculation may need correction factors if albumin is abnormal—for every 1 g/dL decrease in albumin, add 2.5 mEq/L to the anion gap.[44,49] However, these correction factors are fraught with error and have not been shown to ease clinical decision-making.[58] The following link offers an anion gap calculation that takes into account the albumin level: https://www.mdcalc.com/anion-gap

PATIENT EDUCATION

■ https://medlineplus.gov/lab-tests/comprehensive-metabolic-panel-cmp/

RELATED DIAGNOSES AND ICD-10 CODES

Hypokalemia/hyperkalemia	E87.6 / E87.5
Hyponatremia/hypernatremia	E87.0 / E87.1
Acidosis	E87.2
Dehydration	E86.0

REFERENCES

Full list of references can be accessed through Springer Publishing Company Connect™ at the following link: http://connect.springerpub.com/content/reference-book/978-0-8261-8843-4/part/part03/toc-part/ch064

65. EPSTEIN-BARR VIRUS TESTING

Kelly Small Casler

PHYSIOLOGY/PATHOPHYSIOLOGY REVIEW

Epstein-Barr virus (EBV) is a herpes DNA virus that infects B lymphocytes. Exposure to the virus produces a humoral and cell-mediated inflammatory response where B-cells proliferate and T-cells produce atypical (morphologically abnormal) lymphocytes. In an immunocompetent patient, these responses are regulated by apoptosis and cytokine activation. In immunocompromised individuals, however, these responses can be dysregulated and there is excessive, disordered lymphocyte proliferation in response to EBV. Examples include post-transplant lymphoproliferative disease (PTLD) in patients with stem cell or solid organ transplant[1] and X-linked lymphoproliferative disease, a genetic immune system abnormaility.[2]

Primary EBV infection occurs in a previously non-infected person and causes infectious mononucleosis (IM), although some patients have asymptomatic disease.[3] Recurrent EBV infection occurs when the virus is reactivated, usually as a result of an immunocompromised state. EBV-DNAemia refers to the detection of DNA in the blood from molecular tests.[4]

OVERVIEW OF LABORATORY TESTS

There are several laboratory tests that are used in the evaluation of patients with EBV infection symptoms.

Complete Blood Count, Differential, and Peripheral Smear

These laboratory tests may be used individually or as a group with the focus looking for elevations in (a) white blood cells (leukocytes), (b) atypical lymphocytes, and/or (c) total lymphocytes. Elevations in monocyte counts may also occur. Peripheral smear is rarely needed for evaluation of EBV but if completed may provide clues to the diagnosis.

Heterophile Antibody Test

Heterophile antigens are antigens that are shared among different species. Heterophile antibodies refer to the antibodies that bind with these types of antigens. The heterophile antibody test (CPT code 86308) is most often performed using bovine antigens and latex agglutination. In this process, patient capillary or venous whole blood is mixed with a solution containing latex beads coated with small amounts of bovine antigen that mimic EBV antigens. If the patient's blood contains EBV antibodies, agglutination will occur, causing a positive test. This test can be performed as a point-of-care test or laboratory test. There are 44 different point-of-care test options which result in significant variability in accuracy depending on the product used.[5]

Direct Molecular Test and Epstein-Barr Virus Viral Load

Direct molecular tests (CPT code 87799) and tests that report viral loads (CPT code 87799) for EBV DNA can be performed on serum, whole blood, and cerebrospinal fluid specimens.[6,7] Direct molecular tests are reported as positive or negative and viral load will report a numerical value reflecting the amount of DNA detected.

Liver Transaminases

Alanine aminotransferase (ALT) and aspartate amino transferase (AST) can be elevated in up to 50% of individuals with infectious mononucleosis.[8–10] However, there are many causes of liver transaminase elevations so this finding is very nonspecific.

Epstein–Barr Virus Antibodies

Epstein-Barr Nuclear Antigen (EBNA) Antibodies (CPT Code 86664)

EBNA are protein components of EBV particles. Antibodies to EBNA are produced when an individual is exposed to the virus. Primarily measured as EBNA IgG, this antibody is seen 6 to 12 weeks after primary infection with EBV. When produced, EBNA antibodies remain detectable for the rest of a patient's life span, but up to 10% of people may never develop EBNA antibodies in response to EBV infection.[6]

Viral Capsid Antigen (VCA) Antibodies (CPT Code 86665)

VCAs are antigens present on the virus wall or capsule, hence their name. Laboratory tests are available to look for antibodies to VCA in the form of IgG and IgM.[6,11]

Early Antigen (EA) Antibody (CPT Code 86663)

Antibodies to EA detect antigens produced in the early stages of IM. Their role in detection of nasopharyngeal cancer is a topic of ongoing research.[12]

INDICATIONS

Screening

■ Screening EBV antibody or direct molecular tests may be used for organ and stem cell donors and recipients to assess and mitigate EBV transmission risk prior to and after the procedures/surgeries.

■ Direct molecular tests may be used to screen individuals at risk for certain cancers. Research is ongoing regarding this purpose, although a recent Cochrane review did not find evidence to support nasopharyngeal cancer screening with molecular tests.[13,14]

Diagnosis and Evaluation

■ Testing may be warranted in the presence of fever, pharyngitis, lymphadenopathy, and a negative streptococcal pharyngitis test (most common symptoms suggestive of IM). However, remember the diagnosis of IM can be made clinically (Figure 65.1).[6,15]

  ● If laboratory testing is desired for confirmation of IM, the complete blood count and differential along with heterophile antibodies are usual first-line diagnostic tests. Antibody tests can be used if further clarification is needed.

  ● Although the Centers for Disease Control and Prevention recommends against using the heterophile antibody test, several other sources support its use due to low cost, ability to be performed at the point of care, and quick turnaround time.[6,16–18]

■ Direct molecular tests for EBV may be used if PTLD is suspected. Biopsy is used to confirm all positive tests.

Monitoring

■ Monitoring immunocompetent patients with IM is not needed.

■ Molecular tests are used to monitor patients with immunocompromise (especially stem-cell transplants) as frequently as twice a week.[1,6,7]

■ EBV viral load may be monitored in those with HIV or other immunodeficiencies (especially X-linked immunodeficiency). A difference in viral load of $0.5 \log^{10}$ or more between samples is considered a significant change.[6] Caution should be used when comparing viral load trends performed at different laboratories as there is a lack of agreement.[19]

INTERPRETATION

Complete Blood Count and Differential

CBC and differential findings suggestive of IM (Table 65.1):

■ Absolute lymphocyte count greater than 4×10^9

■ Lymphocytosis to 50% or greater

■ Monocytes greater than 1×10^9

■ Leukocytosis greater than 10×10^9/L

■ Atypical lymphocytes 10% or greater

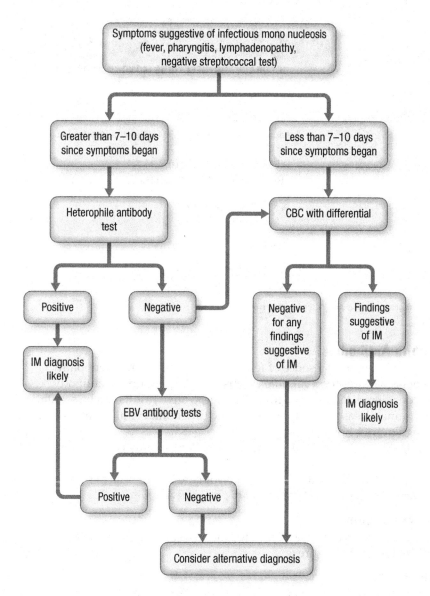

FIGURE 65.1. Algorithm for testing. CBC, complete blood count; EBV, Epstein-Barr virus; IM, infectious mononucleosis.

Peripheral Smear

Peripheral smear findings suggestive of IM:

- Smudge cells or cloverleaf lymphocyte nuclei (high specificity but low sensitivity).[20]
- Smudge/smear/basket cells are also seen in chronic lymphocytic leukemia (CLL) and cloverleaf nuclei are also seen in T-cell leukemia and human immunodeficiency virus (HIV). Therefore, history, physical, and follow-up are imperative with these findings.[20]

TABLE 65.1: INTERPRETATION OF COMPLETE BLOOD COUNT AND DIFFERENTIAL FINDINGS IN INFECTIOUS MONONUCLEOSIS

	ACCURACY FOR INFECTIOUS MONONUCLEOSIS[20,24–26]
Leukocytosis > 10 x 10^9 L	Specificity 87% Sensitivity 40%
Absolute lymphocyte count > 4x 10^9 L	Specificity = 96.8% Sensitivity = 61.8% Positive predictive value (PPV) = 95% Negative predictive value (NPV) =71.7%–99% +LR 26 (adults) -LR 0.04 (adults) +LR 5.6 (pediatrics) -LR0.49 (pediatrics)
Atypical lymphocytes ≥ 10%*	Specificity 92% Sensitivity 66% +LR of 11 - LR 0.37
Lymphocytosis ≥ to 50%*	Specificity 84.5% Sensitivity 66.3%
Monocytes > 1 x 10^9	Specificity 95%–98% Sensitivity 33% +LR 2.9–14 -LR.69–.90

*If both are present, the specificity is 95% and the sensitivity is 61.3%.

LR, likelihood ratio.

Heterophile Antibodies

- When positive in the presence of fever, pharyngitis, lymphadenopathy, and a negative streptococcal pharyngitis test, the heterophile antibody test is considered consistent with IM. False-positive results can be seen in autoimmune disease, leukemia, pancreatic carcinoma, viral hepatitis, and cytomegalovirus, however.[6]
- False-negative tests are common with this test, especially early in the process of IM.
- Sensitivities and specificities of the point-of-care heterophile antibody tests vary from 63% to 84% and 84% to 100%, respectively.[21]

Antigen Antibodies

- Results reported as a titer level that is graded as positive, equivocal, or negative (Table 65.2; Figure 65.2).

Molecular Tests

- Reported as positive or negative. Test offers 77% sensitivity and 98% specificity for EBV.[22]

FOLLOW-UP

- Cytomegalovirus (CMV) infection, human herpes virus 6, human immunodeficiency virus, toxoplasmosis, adenovirus, and acute leukemia all cause similar symptoms to IM. Follow-up testing may be needed if symptoms persist and these diagnoses cannot be excluded[6,18,23,24]

PEARLS & PITFALLS

- Up to 10% of individuals with mononucleosis may have a falsely negative heterophile antibody.[6,20]

- Heterophile antibodies are generally not produced by the body or detectable until day 6 to 10 of illness; lymphocyte production is seen earlier.[6,20]
- The heterophile antibody test is not accurate in patients younger than the age of 4.[3,17]
- CMV is a strong differential diagnosis for IM, especially if EBV serology is negative.[30]

TABLE 65.2: INTERPRETATION OF EPSTEIN-BARR VIRUS ANTIBODY TESTING			
	POSITIVE IN	**ACCURACY FOR IM**[27–29]	**NOTES**
Early Antigen IgG	Early and active disease		
VCA IgM	Early disease	98% specificity 89% sensitivity	
VCA IgG	Recent or past infection	98.1% sensitivity 97.4% specificity	
EBNA IgG	Past infection at least 2–3 months ago	92.2% sensitive and 84.6%–90% specific	May be negative early in disease. Lasts for lifetime

EBNA, Epstein–Barr nuclear antigen; IgG, immunoglobulin G; IgM, immunoglobulin M; VCA, viral capsid antigen.

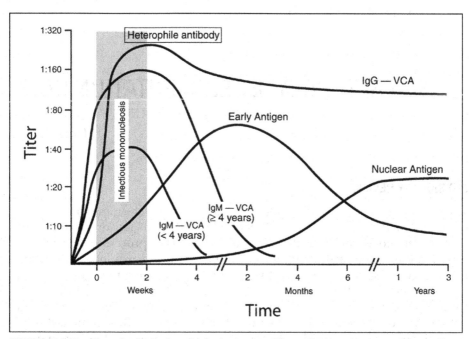

FIGURE 65.2. Timeline of expected positivity for heterophile antibody and common Epstein-Barr virus antibody tests. *Source:* Reproduced with permission from Detrick B, Schmitz JL, Hamilton RG. *Manual of Molecular and Clinical Laboratory Immunology.* ASM Press; 2016:637–647.

- Ninety percent of adults have been infected with EBV.[3]
- CMV, toxoplasmosis, rubella, tick borne illness, and rheumatoid arthritis can all cause false-positive results on VCA IgM.[19,31]
- Molecular testing and viral load testing are more accurate than antibody testing, but also more expensive.[32]

PATIENT EDUCATION

- https://www.ucsfhealth.org/medical-tests/003513

RELATED DIAGNOSES AND ICD-10 CODES

Fever	R50.9
Acute pharyngitis, unspecified	J02.9
Enlarged lymph nodes	R59.9
Post-transplant lymphoproliferative disorder (PTLD)	D47.Z
Infectious mononucleosis, unspecified	B27.9

REFERENCES

Full list of references can be accessed through Springer Publishing Company Connect™ at the following link: http://connect.springerpub.com/content/reference-book/978-0-8261-8843-4/part/part03/toc-part/ch065

66. ERYTHROCYTE SEDIMENTATION RATE

Darla Gowan

PHYSIOLOGY REVIEW

The erythrocyte sedimentation rate (ESR) is a test that determines the amount of time that it takes for the red blood cells (RBCs) to fall or separate out from other blood components in the test tube. This process of the rate of separation is called "sedimentation."[1] The faster the sedimentation, the more inflammation is present. This test is an indirect assessment of inflammation and/or necrosis. When inflammation or damage is present, the RBCs tend to clump together, get heavier, and settle more quickly in the test tube.[1] In a patient without inflammation, the rate of separation of RBCs in the test tube is relatively slow. The ESR level shows a slower increase with inflammation usually rising about 24 to 49 hours after the onset of inflammation and takes more time to return to normal.[2] An ESR is not indicative of a specific disease;

however, it is often the first indicator that inflammation is present. The ESR should not be used as a disease marker on its own as it is not specific for any one disease. It should be used with other tests to evaluate for the presence of inflammation and add additional information to the overall clinical picture.[3] Life span, sex, and pregnancy differences in ESR have been noted in some studies.[3-5]

OVERVIEW OF LABORATORY TESTS

Laboratory evaluation of the ESR can be done by ordering a sedimentation rate, modified westergren (CPT code 85652). Turnaround time is usually within 24 hours. It should be collected as whole blood in a lavender tube, requiring 2 to 4 mL of blood to complete the test.[6,7]

INDICATIONS

Screening

- There is currently no recommendation for universal screening using ESR.
- The Choosing Wisely recommendations from the American Society for Clinical Pathology recommend using a C-reactive protein (CRP) test to determine inflammation, in lieu of the ESR test.[8-10] The CRP is stated to be more sensitive and specific to acute inflammation; rising faster in the face of inflammation and falling more quickly once the inflammation is resolved.[10]
- Despite the concerns that the ESR is not the first-line test to perform, it is often ordered along with a CRP for added data collection. In patients where an ESR and CRP were both assessed, the results was statistically more specific than either alone. The ESR and CRP together were statistically superior in sensitivity to the ESR alone, and at least comparable to the CRP alone.[11]

Diagnosis and Evaluation

As previously noted, the ESR test is not diagnostic to any condition and using both the ESR and CRP gave superior results overall.[12] ESR is often tested with the following conditions:

- *Rheumatoid arthritis (RA):* Some evidence does not show a significant correlation between ESR and RA, whereas other evidence shows that the ESR may remain normal in these patients.[13]
- *Vasculitis, temporal arteritis:* Lower ESR levels do not completely rule out these diagnoses, but a high ESR will mean that a vasculitis is most likely the diagnosis.[14,15]
- *Autoimmune disease (e.g., systemic lupus erythematosus, psoriatic arthritis):* May be helpful in monitoring the disease process as well as treatment response.[16]

- *Malignancies:* Associated with more advanced stage and poor performance in patients with large B-cell lymphoma;[17] associated with worse survival in patients with cutaneous malignant melanoma.[18]
- *Kidney disease:* The ESR is almost always elevated to a degree (>25 mm/hr) in most patients with end-stage renal disease (ESRD). Higher levels (>60 mm/hr) are noted in more than 50% of patients with ESRD, so an elevated ESR does not necessarily indicate that there is infection present or a change in disease activity.[19]
- *Inflammatory bowel disease (IBD):* A pilot study showed that patients with a higher ESR (greater than 25 mm/hr) also expressed lower disease-specific quality of life.[20]
- *Ankylosing spondylitis (AS):* An ESR and CRP are often used as part of the diagnosis of AS but it is only seen to be elevated in 40% to 50% of patients. Due to this, a normal level cannot rule out AS.[21]
- *Medications:* In giant cell arteritis (GSA), studies have shown that the ESR tends to be lower in patients who are also taking nonsteroidal anti-inflammatory drugs (NSAIDs) or statins. However, the CRP does not seem to be lower.[22]
- *Osteomyelitis in adults:* The ESR may not be as useful in diagnosis but may play a role in monitoring resolution or relapse.[23]
- *Invasive bacterial infections in children:* Increased sensitivity of ESR at the level of 20 mm/h has been noted in helping to identify bone/joint infections in children. However, the best indication was the use of both ESR and CRP in the evaluation.[24] Another meta-analysis looking at pyelonephritis in children showed that an ESR alone is not helpful in differentiating between pyelonephritis and cystitis in children.[25]
- *Technical* (e.g., dilution, increased temperature of blood, tilted ESR tube).[26]
- *COVID:* Meta-analysis suggests that a highly elevated ESR (along with other nonspecific markers) may suggest disease in those suspected of COVID and suggest more severe disease in those diagnosed with COVID.[27,28]

If a low ESR result is found in a patient who is known to have an acute or chronic inflammatory process, then the following need to be considered:

- An abnormality in the red blood cell
- Heart failure
- Cachexia
- High levels of bile salt related to liver or gallbladder disease
- Significant leukocytosis
- Technical issues with the lab draw (delay in testing, low room temperature, short ESR tube)[19]

Monitoring
Monitoring of the ESR is not well delineated in the research. For a disease process where you are worried about relapse (temporal arteritis or polymyalgia rheumatic), the ESR can help to establish relapse.[29]

INTERPRETATION

Normal reference intervals vary between labs, but generally are:

- Male: less than 50 years of age 0 to 15 mm/hour; greater than 50 years of age 0 to 20 mm/hour
- Female: less than 50 years of age 0 to 20 mm/hour; greater than 50 years of age 0 to 30mm/hour
- Child: 10 mm/hour or less
- Newborn: 0 to 2 mm/hour[14,19]

An increased result can be affected by increased age, pregnancy, anemia, any process that causes an increase in fibrinogen levels, obesity, and technical issues (room temperature, delay in testing blood, amount of blood collected).[14,19] A decreased result can also occur with technical issues (time from collection to resulting, direct sunlight, icteric samples, hemolysis).[3]

If the ESR is greater than 100 mm/hr, it is more likely to be associated with the following conditions:

- Giant cell arteritis, vasculitis/arteritis, metastatic cancer, chronic infection, hyperfibrinogenemia, Waldenström macroglobulinemia, or polymyalgia rheumatic[7]
- A systematic review of several studies was done looking at the sensitivity and specificity of the ESR in several different diagnoses (periprosthetic infections, pediatric orthopedic infections, inflammatory bowel disease (IBS), and two different major studies on giant cell arteritis). The sensitivity of the ESR ranged from 0.79 to 0.97 and the specificity ranged from 0.3 to 0.7.[11]
- Other tests may be ordered at the same time to also look for inflammatory processes in the body including antinuclear antibody (ANA), C-reactive protein (CRP), complete blood count (CBC), complete metabolic panel (CMP), rheumatoid factor (RF), and serum fibrinogen.[1,30,31]

FOLLOW-UP

- Follow-up testing is not usually required unless the patient has a mild/moderate elevation in the ESR. In that case, a repeat ESR in a patient with no known etiology would be a more cost-effective way to assess the patient status.[14]
- If a significant level (greater than 100 mm/hour) is discovered in a patient who is asymptomatic, then other testing may be warranted. Chest x-ray, tuberculosis (TB) testing, liver function tests, kidney function tests, a hematology profile, urinalysis, and stool for occult blood should be considered.[14]

PEARLS & PITFALLS

- There are some medications/supplements that can interfere with the test results including aspirin, contraceptives, steroids, echinacea, or vitamin A.

- ESR should not be used as a screening tool for malignancies or systemic diseases as it has limited value as a single data point.[2,14]
- ESR may be useful for assessment of specific infectious processes, especially when paired with a CRP level.[11]

PATIENT EDUCATION

- https://medlineplus.gov/lab-tests/erythrocyte-sedimentation-rate-esr/
- https://www.mayoclinic.org/tests-procedures/sed-rate/about/pac-20384797

RELATED DIAGNOSES AND ICD-10 CODES[32]

Giant cell arteritis	M31.6
Vasculitis/arteritis	I77.6
Large B cell lymphoma	C83.3
Cutaneous malignant melanoma	C3
Chronic infection–osteomyelitis	M86.9
Hyperfibrinogenemia	D68.8
Waldenström macroglobulinemia	C88.0
Polymyalgia rheumatic	N35.3
Ankylosing spondylitis	M45.9
Rheumatoid arthritis	M06.9
Inflammatory bowel disease	K51.90
COVID[33]	U07.1
Encounter for screening for COVID-19	Z11.52
Contact with and (suspected) exposure to COVID-19	Z20.822
Personal history of COVID-19	Z86.16
Multisystem inflammatory syndrome (MIS)	M35.81
Other specified systemic involvement of connective tissue	M35.89
Pneumonia due to coronavirus disease 2019	J12.82

REFERENCES

Full list of references can be accessed through Springer Publishing Company Connect™ at the following link: http://connect.springerpub.com/content/reference-book/978-0-8261 -8843-4/part/part03/toc-part/ch066

67. ESTROGEN: ESTRONE, ESTRADIOL, AND ESTRIOL

Emily Neiman

PHYSIOLOGY REVIEW

Estrogen is a steroid sex hormone present in both males and females. There are three main forms of estrogen: estrone (E1) and estradiol (E2) are the most active. Estriol (E3) is the dominant estrogen during pregnancy; it does not play much of a role outside of this.

In both males and females, E1 is synthesized primarily from the adrenals and is converted from the steroid hormone androstenedione. In contrast, E2 is synthesized primarily from the gonads. In males, estradiol is synthesized in the testes from aromatization of testosterone and is primarily responsible for regulating follicle-stimulating hormone (FSH) secretion. Estradiol is not stored in males. In females, estradiol is also aromatized from testosterone and primarily stored in body fat. E2 is secreted by the ovaries in response to FSH and luteinizing hormone (LH). E3 is mainly converted from E1 but is also converted from dehydroepiandrosterone-sulfate (DHEA-S) in the placenta during pregnancy and diffuses into the maternal circulation.[1-5]

Estradiol plays a large role in female reproductive and gynecologic function and is primarily responsible for the development of secondary sex characteristics. Estradiol, FSH, and LH work on a feedback loop in the hypothalamic-pituitary-gonadal (HPG) axis. Estrogen has also been shown to have effects on a multitude of other body organs and systems, such as the nervous system, body fat distribution, bone, muscle, and skin, among others (Box 67.1).[1-2] It has even been studied as a marker for female psychologic health.[6] Additionally, risk for coronary artery disease, thromboembolic events such as stroke and clots, and breast cancer are all linked to estrogen levels.[3,7]

In males, estrogen levels normally remain low throughout the life span. For females, estrogen levels begin to increase as they near puberty. Levels of estradiol vary widely during the menstrual cycle, rising from a nadir at the beginning of the cycle. Estradiol continues to rise through the follicular phase to a pre-ovulatory peak, then decreases throughout the luteal phase. Estrogen levels begin an overall decline throughout perimenopause and menopause, leading to the hypoestrogenic state found in postmenopausal females.[1-3,8] Low or fluctuating levels of estrogen are thought to contribute to the mood changes, sleep disturbances, and increased headaches that are frequently reported by peri- and postmenopausal females.[8]

OVERVIEW OF LABORATORY TESTS

Estradiol (E2) is the most common form of estrogen to be tested by laboratory methods in clinical practice. Estrone (E1) is occasionally evaluated, usually in

---

Box 67.1: Selected Functions of Estradiol in Females

- Puberty, including thelarche, pubarche, and menarche
- Stimulation of ovulation
- Rebuilding of endometrium after menses (proliferative phase)
- Stimulation of mammary glands/ducts during pregnancy
- Cervical changes around ovulation (softening of the cervix, thinning of cervical mucus)
- Supports movement of the ovum through fallopian tubes
- Vaginal lubrication

Sources: Data from Schuiling KD, Likis FE. *Gynecologic Health Care: With an Introduction to Prenatal and Postpartum Care.* 4th ed. Jones and Bartlett; 2020; Carcio HA, Secor RM. *Advanced Health Assessment of Women: Clinical Skills and Procedures.* Springer Publishing; 2018; Rieder JK, Darabos K, Weierich MR. Estradiol and women's health: considering the role of estradiol as a marker in behavioral medicine. *Int J Behav Med.* 2020;27(3):294–304. doi:10.1007/s12529-019-09820-4; Allshouse A, Pavlovic J, Santoro N. Menstrual cycle hormone changes associated with reproductive aging and how they may relate to symptoms. *Obstet Gynecol Clin North Am.* 2018;45(4):613–628. doi:10.1016/j.ogc.2018.07.004; Kumar V, Abbas AK, Aster JC. *Robbins Basic Pathology* Elsevieron Vitalsource. 10th ed. Elsevier; 2017.

---

combination with estradiol or as part of the total estrogen level (estrone plus estradiol), while estriol is primarily used as part of screening for genetic anomalies in pregnancy.[1,2] E1 may be individually evaluated by ordering estrone, serum (CPT code 82679). E2 can be measured individually by ordering serum estrogen (estradiol; E2; CPT code 82670). Additionally, it is possible to order E2 and E1 together for a measure of total estrogen by ordering fractionated estrogens (CPT code 82671).[3-5]

When elevated levels of estrogen are suspected, testing may be performed through an immunoassay (or "direct assay") test on a serum sample. When levels are anticipated to be low (men, postmenopausal women, women treated with aromatase inhibitors, and children), immunoassays have poor sensitivity and specificity so liquid chromatography-tandem mass spectrometry (LC/MS) is used.[7,9-11]

INDICATIONS

Screening

- There is no current evidence that supports universal testing of estrogen.

Diagnosis and Evaluation

- Consider evaluation of estrogen levels for the clinical presentations and scenarios noted in Table 67.1.[12-17]
- The American Academy of Pediatrics (AAP) recommends against drawing estradiol levels for children with pubic hair and/or body odor but no other signs of puberty.[18]

Monitoring

- Ongoing monitoring of E2 may be performed for:[4,12,16-17,19]
  - Patients with breast cancer being treated with aromatase inhibitors
  - Patients undergoing ovulation induction/assisted reproduction
  - Screening for ovarian hyperstimulation with ovulation induction

TABLE 67.1: INDICATIONS FOR ESTROGEN TESTING BASED ON SIGNS/SYMPTOMS/TREATMENT

FEMALE PATIENTS	MALE PATIENTS
Menstrual irregularities	Infertility
Amenorrhea (primary or secondary)	Early/delayed puberty
Infertility	Feminization, including gynecomastia
Early/delayed puberty	Fracture risk assessment
Virilization	
Ovarian status in assisted reproduction patients	
Use of ovulation induction medications	
Use of hormone replacement therapy	
Use of gender-affirming therapy	
Use of aromatase inhibitors	
Fracture risk assessment	

Sources: Data from Schuiling KD, Likis FE. *Gynecologic Health Care: With an Introduction to Prenatal and Postpartum Care.* 4th ed. Jones and Bartlett; 2020; Carcio HA, Secor RM. *Advanced Health Assessment of Women: Clinical Skills and Procedures.* Springer Publishing; 2018; EEST – Clinical: Estradiol, Serum. Mayocliniclabs.com. https://www.mayocliniclabs.com/test-catalog/Clinical+and+Interpretive/81816; ESTF – Fees: Estrogens, Estrone (E1) and Estradiol (E2), Fractionated, Serum. Mayocliniclabs.com. https://www.mayocliniclabs.com/test-catalog/Fees+and+Codes/84230; UE3 – Clinical: Estriol, Unconjugated, Serum. Mayocliniclabs.com. https://www.mayocliniclabs.com/test-catalog/Clinical+and+Interpretive/81711; Kumar V, Abbas AK, Aster JC. *Robbins Basic Pathology Elsevieron Vitalsource.* 10th ed. Elsevier; 2017; Thurston L, Abbara A, Dhillo WS. Investigation and management of subfertility. *J Clin Pathol.* 2019;72(9):579–587; American Association of Clinical Chemistry. Estradiol Testing in Men. Aacc.org. Published June 2020. https://www.aacc.org/advocacy-and-outreach/optimal-testing-guide-to-lab-test-utilization/a-f/estradiol-testing-in-men; Teede HJ, Misso ML, Costello MF, et al. Recommendations from the international evidence-based guideline for the assessment and management of polycystic ovary syndrome. *Clin Endocrinol (Oxf).* Published online 2018. doi:10.1111/cen.13795; Klein DA, Emerick JE, Sylvester JE, Vogt KS. Disorders of puberty: an approach to diagnosis and management. *Am Fam Physician.* 2017;96(9):590–599; Hamidi O, Davidge-Pitts CJ. Transfeminine hormone therapy. *Endocrinol Metab Clin North Am.* 2019;48(2):341–355. doi:10.1016/j.ecl.2019.02.001

- Transfeminine individuals receiving gender-affirming hormone therapy (levels kept under 200 pg/mL)
- Assessment of ovarian reserve
- Timing of ovulation (may be drawn with E1)
- National Institute for Health Care and Excellence (NICE) guidelines recommend against using E2 to predict the outcome of fertility treatments.[17]

INTERPRETATION

- Reference intervals for estrogen vary based on age, sex, stage of puberty, and the menstrual cycle in females. Table 67.2 provides commonly used reference ranges for E1 and E2 but it should be noted that best practice is to follow the reference ranges provided by the laboratory.[3–4]
- Estradiol levels vary widely throughout the menstrual cycle and with body fat.[3,7,10,11]

TABLE 67.2: ESTRONE (E1) AND ESTRADIOL (E2) REFERENCE RANGES		
	E1	**E2**
Female (prepubertal)	Undetectable–29 pg/mL	Undetectable–10 pg/mL
Female (premenopausal)	17–200 pg/mL	15–350 pg/mL
Follicular phase		10–180 pg/mL
Midcycle peak		100–300 pg/mL
Luteal phase		40–200 pg/mL
Female (postmenopausal)	7–40 pg/mL	<10 pg/mL
Male (prepubertal)	Undetectable–16 pg/mL	Undetectable–5 pg/mL
Male (>18 years)	10–60 pg/mL	10–40 pg/mL

Sources: Data from EEST – Clinical: Estradiol, Serum. Mayocliniclabs.com. https://www.mayocliniclabs.com/test-catalog/Clinical+and+Interpretive/81816; ESTF – Fees: Estrogens, Estrone (E1) and Estradiol (E2), Fractionated, Serum. Mayocliniclabs.com. https://www.mayocliniclabs.com/test-catalog/Fees+and+Codes/84230; American Board of Internal Medicine. ABIM laboratory test reference ranges. Abim.org. Published January 2021. https://www.abim.org/Media/bfijryql/laboratory-reference-ranges.pdf

- Reference intervals for men, children, women taking aromatase inhibitors, and postmenopausal women are based on very scant evidence.[7,11,20] Results should be interpreted with caution.
- Results of immunoassay tests for E2 levels may be affected by the use of exogenous substances. Examples of these substances are medications such as fulvestrant, birth control pills, and hormone replacement therapy.[3,7,10–11]
- Table 67.3 summarizes common reasons for elevated or decreased estrogen levels.

FOLLOW-UP

- Follow-up testing will depend on the original indication for testing.
- Consider FSH for patients undergoing ovulation induction treatments or E1 for determining when ovulation is taking place.[4,12]
- To further assess infertility concerns, FSH and anti-Müllerian hormone (AMH) may be ordered, and an antral follicle count may be performed via transvaginal ultrasound.[1,2,12,17]
- In cases of precocious puberty, FSH, LH, TSH, and a brain MRI should be considered. Testosterone should be drawn instead of estrogen for male patients with possible precocious puberty.[15]
- In cases of delayed puberty, FSH, LH, and bone age radiography should be obtained. Testosterone should be drawn instead of estrogen for male patients with delayed puberty.[15]
- Other serum tests that may be ordered depending on clinical presentation are total and free testosterone, prolactin, thyroid-stimulating hormone (TSH), fasting blood glucose, or hemoglobin a1c.[1,2,6,8,13,14,17]

TABLE 67.3: DIFFERENTIAL DIAGNOSIS OF ABNORMAL E2 LEVELS

FEMALE

DECREASED E2	INCREASED E2
Menopause	Infertility
Premature ovarian failure	Precocious puberty
Delayed puberty	Pseudo precocious puberty
Estrogen deficiency	Decreased estrogen clearance in liver
Disorder of sex steroid metabolism	Estrogen-producing tumor
Anovulatory cycles	Estrogen ingestion
Polycystic ovarian syndrome (PCOS)	Anovulatory cycles
Premenstrual syndrome (PMS)/premenstrual dysphoric disorder (PMDD)	Polycystic ovarian syndrome (PCOS)
	Endometrial hyperplasia
Hypopituitarism	Hyperthyroidism
Hypogonadism	Obesity
Low body fat	
Turner syndrome	

MALE

DECREASED E2	INCREASED E2
Estrogen deficiency	Infertility
Disorder of sex steroid metabolism	Androgen-producing tumor
Hypopituitarism	Androgen therapy
Hypogonadism	Decreased estrogen clearance in liver
	Estrogen-producing tumor
	Estrogen ingestion
	Hyperthryoidism

Sources: EEST – Clinical: Estradiol, Serum. Mayocliniclabs.com. https://www.mayocliniclabs.com/test-catalog/Clinical+and+Interpretive/81816; ESTF – Fees: Estrogens, Estrone (E1) and Estradiol (E2), Fractionated, Serum. Mayocliniclabs.com. https://www.mayocliniclabs.com/test-catalog/Fees+and+Codes/84230; UE3 – Clinical: Estriol, Unconjugated, Serum. Mayocliniclabs.com. https://www.mayocliniclabs.com/test-catalog/Clinical+and+Interpretive/81711; Rieder JK, Darabos K, Weierich MR. Estradiol and women's health: considering the role of estradiol as a marker in behavioral medicine. *Int J Behav Med.* 2020;27(3):294–304. doi:10.1007/s12529-019-09820-4; Allshouse A, Pavlovic J, Santoro N. Menstrual cycle hormone changes associated with reproductive aging and how they may relate to symptoms. *Obstet Gynecol Clin North Am.* 2018;45(4):613–628. doi:10.1016/j.ogc.2018.07.004; Kumar V, Abbas AK, Aster JC. *Robbins Basic Pathology Elsevieron Vitalsource.* 10th ed. Elsevier; 2017; Thurston L, Abbara A, Dhillo WS. Investigation and management of subfertility. *J Clin Pathol.* 2019;72(9):579–587; American Association of Clinical Chemistry. Estradiol Testing in Men. Aacc.org. Published June 2020. https://www.aacc.org/advocacy-and-outreach/optimal-testing-guide-to-lab-test-utilization/a-f/estradiol-testing-in-men; Teede HJ, Misso ML, Costello MF, et al. Recommendations from the international evidence-based guideline for the assessment and management of polycystic ovary syndrome. *Clin Endocrinol (Oxf).* Published online 2018. doi:10.1111/cen.13795; Klein DA, Emerick JE, Sylvester JE, Vogt KS. Disorders of puberty: an approach to diagnosis and management. *Am Fam Physician.* 2017;96(9):590–599.

PEARLS & PITFALLS

- Estrone and estradiol levels are elevated at birth but fall to prepubertal levels within a few days.[4]
- Estrone levels may rise in obese children after adrenarche.[4]
- If E2 levels are elevated in cases of suspected precocious puberty, E1 levels should also be measured. If both are elevated, this suggests true precocious puberty. If only one is elevated, this is likely to be pseudo precocious puberty.[4,15]

- Anovulatory cycles may be caused by either increases or decreases in baseline levels of E2. The baseline level may be decreased and remain low throughout the cycle, but it is also possible that baseline levels may be elevated without a midcycle peak to trigger ovulation.[4,12,14,17]
- Estriol (E3) is part of a genetic screening test, typically known as the "quad screen," that is offered to pregnant people during their second trimester of pregnancy to evaluate risk for trisomy 18 and Down syndrome.[5]
- Estradiol can also be measured by commercially available saliva testing kits.[7]
- If performing estradiol testing on any female who is having ovulatory menstrual cycles, it is key to note where the patient is in their menstrual cycle, as the levels normally vary throughout the cycle.[3,8]
- If prepubertal, anovulatory, menopausal, or male, estradiol may be tested at a random time.
- Pregnancy should always be ruled out first for a complaint of amenorrhea.
- Interpreting the results in the context of other laboratory results may be helpful in confirming a diagnosis.

PATIENT EDUCATION

- https://labtestsonline.org/tests/estrogens
- https://www.aacc.org/cln/articles/2012/november/fertility-testing

RELATED DIAGNOSES AND ICD-10 CODES

Hypogonadism, male	E29.1
Hypogonadism, female	E28.39
Delayed puberty	E30.0
Precocious puberty	E30.1
Polycystic ovarian syndrome (PCOS)	E28.2
Primary ovarian failure	E28.3
Menopausal and female climacteric states	N95.1
Primary amenorrhea	N91.0
Secondary amenorrhea	N91.1
Female infertility associated with anovulation	N97.0
Encounter for procreative investigation and testing	Z31.4
Hypopituitarism	E23.0
Testicular hypofunction	E29.1
Estrogen excess	E28.0
Androgen excess	E28.1
Hypertrophy of breast (gynecomastia)	N62

Other long-term (current) drug therapy	Z79.8
Obesity, unspecified	E66.9
Underweight	R63.6
Premenstrual syndrome (PMS)	N94.3
Premenstrual dysphoric disorder (PMDD)	F32.81

REFERENCES

Full list of references can be accessed through Springer Publishing Company Connect™ at the following link: http://connect.springerpub.com/content/reference-book/978-0-8261-8843-4/part/part03/toc-part/ch067

68. ETHANOL/ALCOHOL LEVELS

Tammy L. Tyree

PHYSIOLOGY REVIEW

Alcohol is typically ingested by humans in the form of ethyl alcohol or ethanol. Alcohol is a molecule that is both water- and lipid-soluble and therefore is quickly and easily absorbed into the bloodstream from the gastrointestinal tract via the stomach, small intestine, or large intestine.[1-3] When alcohol reaches systemic circulation, it is distributed throughout the body, crosses the blood-brain barrier, and ultimately affects most organs.[2] Alcohol penetrates tissue and body fluids, depending on water concentration, resulting in a difference between serum alcohol levels and whole blood alcohol levels.[2] The rate of absorption depends on the ethanol concentration, the presence of food in the stomach, and the patient's gastric emptying time.[1,2,4]

Ethanol is rapidly absorbed following ingestion with approximately 85% being absorbed within 1 hour under optimal conditions.[3] Alcohol switches from first order (steady percentage/time) to zero order (steady amount/time) kinetics at low concentrations. At low concentrations, metabolism occurs at a steady rate. The average rate of metabolism of ethanol is about 20 mg/dL/hour in serum.[3] There is a difference when comparing ethanol concentrations measured for legal purposes in the form of blood alcohol concentration (BAC; reported as grams/100 mL) and medical testing in serum. Serum (or plasma) ethanol concentrations are about 18% higher than whole blood. Related to this, the average rate of ethanol metabolism in whole blood is about 0.017 g% per hour. Ethanol metabolism, however, can increase with prolonged exposure resulting in tolerance.[3,5] Most alcohol is metabolized by alcohol dehydrogenase (ADH) and CYP450 2E1 but a small amount (approximately 5%)

is exhaled/excreted unchanged by the lungs, kidney, and skin.[1-3] Alcohol is oxidized by ADH into acetaldehyde.[3] Acetaldehyde is then oxidized by ADH into acetate, which is secreted in the urine.[3]

Alcohol elimination is affected by several factors including the amount of alcohol ingested, sex, age, body size (fat content), amount and rate of ingestion, use of other medications, tolerance, environmental influences, and genetic and induced metabolic capacities.[2] Due to these multiple variables, laboratory-determined ethanol concentrations (or levels calculated indirectly) do not correlate well with objective clinical effects.[6] In fact, there are no scientific data to prove that observers, including trained professionals, can reliably determine the degree of ethanol intoxication in others.[7]

OVERVIEW OF LABORATORY TESTS

The accurate measurement of alcohol levels has implications not only medically, but also legally. Consumption of alcohol impairs motor and cognitive skills and can impair one's ability to operate motor vehicles and heavy machinery, which can result in legal issues for the consumer. Alcohol can be measured in whole blood, serum, breath, saliva, urine, and vitreous fluid of the eye.[2] In addition, post-mortem, ethanol levels can be measured in gastric contents, liver tissue, and cerebrospinal fluid.[8] However, these levels can be affected by the time interval between death and the fluid sample collection, how long the sample was stored, how the fluid was obtained, varying temperatures of the body, the additives in the tubes that store the sample, the cap that seals the specimen, and the quality of air within the sample, among other things.[8]

The most common laboratory tests for alcohol are whole blood and serum ethanol concentration levels (CPT code 80320) and the method of laboratory analysis is gas chromatography.[8,9] As mentioned previously, there is a difference between serum and whole blood ethanol concentrations because of the varying water contents between these two fluids. Urine ethyl alcohol levels (CPT code 80307) can also be ordered and are analyzed via immunoassay/chromatography. Breath ethanol levels can be ordered (CPT code 82075); however, these not frequently used. They may not be available at most institutions.

INDICATIONS

Screening
There are no universal screening recommendations for checking alcohol levels. Targeted screenings using serum ethanol levels should be considered in the following patients:

- Occupational drivers
  - A systematic review of literature performed to determine whether mandatory drug and alcohol screening among occupational drivers contributed to prevention of injury.[10] There were two studies included in the review. Authors determined that mandatory alcohol testing showed some reduction in immediate workplace injury but did not affect the long-term downward trend of alcohol-related injuries compared to no mandatory testing.[10]

- Court-ordered (most often breath or urine screenings are ordered)
  - Child custody cases
  - Probation testing
- Parents/guardians can request alcohol level in a minor; however, clinicians are typically not obligated to test unless clinically indicated. These laws can vary by state and policies can vary by institution. Clinicians should check local laws and organization's policy.

Diagnosis and Evaluation

Whole blood and serum ethanol concentration levels are used to determine whether a patient has been consuming alcohol, how much they have consumed, and whether intoxication and alcohol poisoning should be considered as diagnoses. Ethanol level should be considered in the following patients:

- With unexplained altered mental status[11]
- With signs and symptoms that suggest intoxication or alcohol poisoning including difficulty with balance and coordination, slurred speech, slowed reflexes, nausea and vomiting, mood changes, poor judgment, confusion, irregular breathing, seizures, and low body temperature[11]
- With concern that alcohol ingestion will interfere with other illicit substances, drugs, or medications[11]
- With concern about the ability of the patient to make decisions or give consent for procedures
- With drug overdose
- With cases of encephalopathy, head injury, trauma, or infection
- For legal implications
  - Does impaired driver have BAC over the legal limit?[11]
  - Has a minor been drinking?[11]
  - Has alcohol contributed to an accident?[11]
  - Is it following the healthcare institution's policies and procedures for alcohol testing?[12]
  - Is it adhering to the state and federal regulations regarding legal compliance and alcohol testing?[12]
- Serum ethanol levels are usually not required for isolated mild intoxication.
- Consider complete metabolic panel in patients with alcohol intoxication and chronic alcohol use. Common metabolic abnormalities in alcoholic and intoxicated patients include:[13]
  - Acid–base disorders
  - Hypomagnesemia
  - Hypocalcemia
  - Hypokalemia
  - Hypophosphatemia
  - Hyponatremia

Monitoring

- Monitoring alcohol level and repeat testing for serial alcohol concentrations is not indicated for medical purposes or ordered on a routine basis.
- Do not repeat blood tests to "medically clear" intoxicated patients in the emergency department; use clinical examination findings.

■ Patient disposition should be based on clinical signs/symptoms. Alcohol positive patients are "medically stable" (in terms of ethanol effects) when they are no longer clinically intoxicated (i.e., they no longer exhibit slurred speech, nystagmus, or ataxia).

INTERPRETATION

■ Be certain to check the sample source (plasma/serum or whole blood) and units.
■ Medical units: mg/dL (in serum or plasma)
■ Legal (forensic) units: mg% (100 mg/dL = 1 g/L = 100 mg% = 0.100%) in whole blood
■ See Table 68.1 for a point of reference; however, it is important to remember that signs/symptoms of clinical intoxication cannot be accurately predicted from an ethanol concentration.

FOLLOW-UP

Serum ethanol levels are ordered specifically to measure acute ingestion and have little, if any, bearing on chronic diseases or sequelae of long-term alcohol use. Chronic diseases, adverse sequelae, and disorders that have been associated with excessive and long-term alcohol use and abuse include fatty liver, hepatitis, cirrhosis, cardiomyopathy, sexual dysfunction, cancers (e.g., mouth, tongue, esophagus, liver, pancreas, pharynx, larynx, stomach, lung, colon, rectal, and breast), as well as fetal alcohol syndrome, and Wernicke-Korsakoff syndrome.[3] There are direct and indirect biomarkers of alcohol use that can be used to guide clinicians in screening for, diagnosing, prognosticating, and monitoring patients with these alcohol-related disorders.[2] These biomarkers include but are not limited to:

■ Common indirect biomarkers
  ● Liver enzymes (hepatic function panel; CPT code 80076)
  ● Mean corpuscular volume (reported in complete blood count [CBC]; CPT code 85027)

TABLE 68.1: CLINICAL EFFECTS OF BLOOD ALCOHOL CONCENTRATION

BLOOD ALCOHOL CONCENTRATION	CLINICAL EFFECTS
20–50 mg/dL (4.4–11 mmol/L)	Diminished fine motor coordination
50–100 mg/dL (11–22 mmol/L)	Impaired judgment; impaired coordination
100–150 mg/dL (22–33 mmol/L)	Difficulty with gait and balance
150–250 mg/dL (33–55 mmol/L)	Lethargy; difficulty sitting upright without assistance
300 mg/dL (66 mmol/L)	Coma in the non-habituated drinker
400 mg/dL (88 mmol/L)	Respiratory depression

Source: Adapted from: Marx JA. *Rosen's Emergency Medicine: Concepts and Clinical Practice.* 5th ed. Mosby, Inc.; 2002:2513. Copyright © 2002 Elsevier.

- Lipid function panel (CPT code 80061)
- Carbohydrate-deficient transferrin (CPT code 82373)
- common direct biomarkers
  - Ethyl glucuronide (urine; CPT code 80307 or 80321)
  - Ethyl sulfate (urine; CPT code 80321)
  - Fatty acid ethyl esters (serum; CPT code 80322)

PEARLS & PITFALLS

- Understand units/sample source.
  - Serum/plasma versus whole blood's units will vary.
    - Medical units = mg/dL (in serum or plasma)
    - Legal or forensic units = mg% (in whole blood)
- Do not rely on ethanol levels to determine the degree of clinical intoxication.
- Measuring ethanol concentrations for medical purposes does not include chain-of-custody standard and cannot be used for legal purposes.
- Know the state laws and facility policies regarding requests from police for ethanol (and other) blood testing.

PATIENT EDUCATION

- https://www.niaaa.nih.gov/alcohols-effects-health/alcohol-basics
- https://www.niaaa.nih.gov/publications/brochures-and-fact-sheets/alcohol-facts-and-statistics

RELATED DIAGNOSES AND ICD-10 CODES

Trauma (injury, unspecified, initial encounter)	T14.90XA
Overdoses (poisoning by unspecified drugs, medicaments, and biologic substances, accidental)	T50.901A
Alcohol abuse with intoxication	F10.129
Alcohol dependence with withdrawal	F10.239
Alcoholic ketoacidosis	F10.988
Alcoholic hepatitis without ascites	K70.10
Alcoholic cirrhosis without ascites	K70.30
With ascites	K70.31
Alcoholic fatty liver	K70.0
Alcoholic gastritis with bleeding	K29.21

REFERENCES

Full list of references can be accessed through Springer Publishing Company Connect™ at the following link: http://connect.springerpub.com/content/reference-book/978-0-8261 -8843-4/part/part03/toc-part/ch068

69. EXTRACTABLE NUCLEAR ANTIGEN ANTIBODIES

Elizabeth Kirchner

PHYSIOLOGY REVIEW

Autoimmune disease arises when the body loses immunologic tolerance and attacks self-molecules.[1] These attacks may be in the form of autoantibodies. This chapter will discuss specific autoantibodies called extractable nuclear antigen antibodies (ENA), which are typically tested when there is a high index of suspicion for a rheumatologic illness. This test typically follows a positive antinuclear antibody (ANA) test, which indicates that a patient has antibodies against one or more nuclear proteins but does not tell us which protein(s). Since ENA testing is simply a more specific form of ANA testing, the same epidemiologic patterns hold true: autoimmunity can and does happen across the life span, but women are far more likely to have autoimmune disease than men.[2] The ENA panel takes the next step and reveals exactly which nuclear antigen the immune system is making antibodies against, if any.

OVERVIEW OF LABORATORY TESTS

The components of a typical ENA panel are included in Table 69.1.[3-7] The tests in the table are included in most ENA panels, but different laboratories and healthcare systems include different autoantibodies in their ENA panels. Also included in the table is double-stranded DNA antibody (dsDNA), which is an antinuclear antibody. The dsDNA test is typically not included in an ENA panel, but is often ordered when there is strong clinical suspicion for systemic lupus erythematosus (SLE). Sensitivities and specificities can vary depending on the type of test used (immunoelectrophoresis vs. enzyme-linked immunoabsorbent).[3] ENA tests have low sensitivity but are highly specific (see Table 69.1), making them useful for confirming diagnoses.

INDICATIONS

Screening
■ Universal and targeted screenings are not recommended.

Diagnosis and Evaluation
■ ENA is considered follow-up testing after a positive ANA is found in a patient with signs/symptoms highly suspicious for autoimmune rheumatic disease. It is recommended that ANA subserologies should *not* be tested without first having a positive ANA result and a high clinical suspicion of immune-mediated disease.[8]

TABLE 69.1: COMMON COMPONENTS OF THE EXTRACTABLE NUCLEAR ANTIGEN PANEL WITH ASSOCIATED DISEASE STATE, SENSITIVITY, AND SPECIFICITY

TEST NAME	CURRENT PROCEDURAL TERMINOLOGY (CPT) CODE	ASSOCIATED DISEASE	SENSITIVITY	SPECIFICITY
SSA/Ro Antibody	86235	Sjögren's syndrome	85%–97%[3]	50%–60%[3]
SSB/La Antibody	86235	Sjögren's syndrome	70%–85%[3]	50%–70%[3]
Sm Antibody	86235	SLE	35%–50%[3]	99%–100%[3]
RNP Antibody	86235	Mixed connective tissue disease (MCTD)	90%–98%[3]	50%–75%[3]
Scl-70/ Scleroderma Antibody	86235	Systemic sclerosis	25%–45%[3]	80%–99%[3]
Jo 1 Antibody	86235	Myositis	25%–45%[3]	90%–99%[3]
Centromere Antibody	86235	Systemic sclerosis/ CREST	36%[4]	97%[4]
Chromatin Antibody	86235	SLE (esp renal involvement or drug-induced lupus)	69%[5]	92%–100%[5]
Ribosome P Antibody (IgG)	83516	SLE (esp CNS involvement)	37%[6]	96%[6]
dsDNA Antibody	86225	SLE (esp renal involvement)	57%[7]	94%[7]

CNS, central nervous system; SLE, systemic lupus erythematosus.

Signs and symptoms of autoimmune diseases vary. Final diagnosis of autoimmune rheumatic disease is usually based on multiple criteria, which often includes, but is not solely based on, antibodies found in the ENA panel. Associated diagnoses are listed in Table 69.1.

Monitoring
- No monitoring is indicated once antibodies have been identified.

INTERPRETATION
- ENA results should not be interpreted in isolation—the entire clinical picture must be considered.
- Because assays vary between labs, results typically include the type of assay as well as a range to aid in interpretation.
- If a result that is just above the normal range is reported and the diagnosis remains in question, repeat testing may be helpful; ENA results are not a reliable measure of disease activity but may fluctuate over time.

FOLLOW-UP

■ A positive ANA and ENA in the setting of confirmed signs and symptoms of the suspected disease is typically enough to establish a diagnosis of an autoimmune rheumatic disease.

■ Follow-up testing is usually not indicated with the exception of patients diagnosed with scleroderma and systemic sclerosis (SSc), in whom a SCl-70 should be performed.[9] The SCl-70 can help identify SSc patients at risk for organ involvement and a worse prognosis.[9]

■ Monitoring of affected systems post-diagnosis may include renal function panel, complete blood count (CBC), renal biopsy for SLE, echocardiogram and pulmonary function tests for systemic sclerosis, creatine kinase (CK), and aldolase for myositis.

PEARLS & PITFALLS

■ ENA levels fluctuate over time but are not reliable measures of disease activity. The exception to this rule is the dsDNA, in which higher levels do correlate with increased disease activity.

■ dsDNA levels can be used to measure response to SLE therapy.[10]

PATIENT EDUCATION

■ https://rarediseases.info.nih.gov/diseases/diseases-by-category/27/connective-tissue-diseases

■ https://my.clevelandclinic.org/health/diseases/14803-connective-tissue-diseases

RELATED DIAGNOSES AND ICD-10 CODES

A chronic disorder, possibly autoimmune, marked by excessive production of collagen which results in hardening and thickening of body tissues	P83.8
Systemic lupus erythematosus, unspecified	M32.9
A disorder characterized by inflammation involving the skeletal muscles	G72.41
Sjögren syndrome	M35.0

REFERENCES

Full list of references can be accessed through Springer Publishing Company Connect™ at the following link: http://connect.springerpub.com/content/reference-book/978-0-8261-8843-4/part/part03/toc-part/ch069

70. FACTOR ASSAYS

Beth Faiman and Mailey Wilks

PHYSIOLOGY REVIEW

Coagulation factors are proteins and essential components of the coagulation system that lead to proper blood clot formation. This occurs through a complex interplay of actions that result in the conversion of soluble fibrin to insoluble fibrin strands. Primary hemostasis occurs when activated platelets and multiple clotting mediators become attached to damaged endothelium and form a clot. Secondary hemostasis changes soluble fibrinogen into fibrin strands via one of two clotting pathways: the intrinsic or the extrinsic pathway.[1] Figure 70.1 depicts the coagulation cascade.

OVERVIEW OF LABORATORY TESTS

Factor assays provide a quantitative determination of blood clotting activity. To test for clotting factor deficiencies or excess, a patient's blood sample is added to deficiency plasma of the factor of interest and run in a prothrombin time (PT)

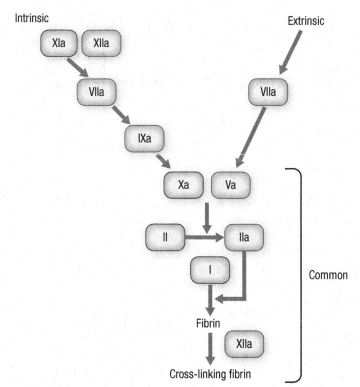

FIGURE 70.1. The coagulation cascade. Intrinsic, extrinsic, and common coagulation pathways.

to test for extrinsic and common pathway factors or activated partial thrombin time (aPTT) for intrinsic factors.[1,2]

■ PT: Value of 11–16 seconds indicates the extrinsic pathway is functioning normally.
■ aPTT: Value of 33 to 45 seconds indicates the intrinsic coagulation system is functioning normally.

Each blood clotting factor number, name, function, associated pathway, and chapter number of this book (if applicable) can be found in Table 70.1.

INDICATIONS

Coagulation factor assay testing is typically performed when someone has a prolonged PT and/or aPTT.

Patients should not be screened in the following situations: recent major surgery, trauma, immobilization, active malignancy, lupus, inflammatory bowel disease, myeloproliferative disorders, heparin-induced thrombocytopenia with thrombosis, preeclampsia at term, retinal vein thrombosis, or upper limb deep vein thrombosis.[2,3]

Screenings, diagnostic considerations, monitoring, interpretation, and follow-up testing can be found within the individual clotting factor chapter. Refer to Table 70.1.[4]

TABLE 70.1: NOMENCLATURE OF THE COAGULATION PROTEINS/CLOTTING FACTORS

CLOTTING FACTOR NUMBER	CLOTTING FACTOR NAME	FUNCTION	PATHWAY	ASSOCIATED CHAPTER OF THIS BOOK
I	Fibrinogen	Clot formation	Both	75
II	Prothrombin	Activation of I, V, VII, VII, VIII, XI, XIII, protein C, platelets	Both	133
III	Tissue factor	Cofactor of vilia	Extrinsic	
IV	Calcium	Facilitates coagulation factor binding to phospolipids	Both	36
V	Proacclerin, labile factor	Cofactor of prothrombinase complex	Both	104
VI (same as Va)	Accelerin		Both	
VII	Proconvertin, serum prothrombin conversion accelerator	Activates factors IX, X	Extrinsic	

(continued)

				ASSOCIATED
CLOTTING FACTOR NUMBER	**CLOTTING FACTOR NAME**	**FUNCTION**	**PATHWAY**	**CHAPTER OF THIS BOOK**

TABLE 70.1: NOMENCLATURE OF THE COAGULATION PROTEINS/CLOTTING FACTORS (*continued*)

CLOTTING FACTOR NUMBER	CLOTTING FACTOR NAME	FUNCTION	PATHWAY	ASSOCIATED CHAPTER OF THIS BOOK
VIII	Antihemophilic factor A	Cofactor of IX-tenase complex	Intrinsic	
IX	Antihemophilic factor B or Christmas factor	Activates factor X, forms tenase complex with factor VIII	Intrinsic	
X	Stuart-Prower factor	Prothrombinase complex with factor V: activates factor II	Both	
XI	Plasma thromboplastin antecedent	Activates factor IX	Intrinsic	
XII	Hageman factor	Activates factor XI, VII, and prekallikrein	Intrinsic	
XIII	Fibrin-stabilizing factor	Crosslinks fibrin	Both	
XIV	Prekallikrein (F Feletcher)	Serine protease zymogen	Intrinsic	
XV	High molecular weight kininogen (HMWK)	Cofactor	Intrinsic	
XVI	von Willebrand factor	Binds to VIII, mediates platelet adhesion	Intrinsic	164
XVII	Antithrombin III	Inhibits IIa, Xa, and other proteases	Intrinsic	25
XVIII	Heparin cofactor II	Inhibits IIa	Extrinsic	
XIX	Protein C	Inactivates Va and VIIIa	Intrinsic	129
XX	Protein S	Cofactor with activated protein C	Intrinsic	131

Source: Adapted from: Palta S, Saroa R, Palta A. Overview of the coagulation system. *Indian J Anaesth.* 2014;58(5):515–523. doi:10.4103/0019-5049.144643

RELATED DIAGNOSES AND ICD-10 CODES

Diseases of the blood and blood-forming organs and certain disorders involving the immune mechanism	D50–D89
Other coagulation defects	D68
Primary thrombophilia	D68.5

REFERENCES

Full list of references can be accessed through Springer Publishing Company Connect™ at the following link: http://connect.springerpub.com/content/reference-book/978-0-8261 -8843-4/part/part03/toc-part/ch070

---

71. FECAL ELASTASE

Jill S. Buterbaugh

PHYSIOLOGY REVIEW

Exocrine pancreatic insufficiency is defined as a lack of pancreatic enzyme production, inadequate enzyme activity, or early enzyme degradation resulting in fat malabsorption.[1-5] The most widely used test to diagnose exocrine pancreatic insufficiency is fecal elastase-1, also referred to as pancreatic elastase-1 or stool elastase-1.[1,6-8] The exocrine pancreas expresses and secretes 28 different proteases, including elastase, which contribute to the digestion of food proteins and are detectable in fecal samples.[9] Chymotrypsin-like elastases (CELA) are secreted by the pancreas and detectable in stool with minimal degradation, and are detectable by monoclonal or polyclonal enzyme-linked immunosorbent assay (ELISA) testing.[2,4-10] The fecal elastase-1 test is a misnomer because it actually tests for CELA3, as the human pancreas does not secrete CELA1.[6,9] Concentrations of pancreatic elastase found in stool samples have been found to correlate with levels in pancreatic fluid and accurately identifies exocrine pancreatic insufficiency when the exocrine function is impaired due to the stability of the enzyme as it passes through the gastrointestinal tract.[2,4-11]

OVERVIEW OF LABORATORY TESTS

- Fecal (pancreatic or stool) elastase-1 is the most widely accepted test due to its simplicity, availability, sensitivity, and specificity.[1,6-8] Sensitivity rates correlate with disease severity, increasing proportionately with more severe disease.[1,2-7] Fecal elastase-1 was found to be superior to other pancreatic testing in the pediatric population.[12] Depending on the laboratory and payer prior authorization, it may be coded as CPT code 83520 (most commonly), immunoassay for analyte other than infectious agent antibody, or CPT code 82656, pancreatic elastase (enzyme) measurement.
- The 72-hour quantitative fecal fat test (CPT code 82710) is considered to be the gold standard test for malabsorption but has poor patient tolerance and lacks standardization.[4,8,10,13,14]
- Qualitative fecal fat (CPT code 82705), which is a single fecal sample test, may increase the suspicion of malabsorption/maldigestion but has lower sensitivity (78%) and specificity (70%) than quantitative studies.[8,15]

- Fecal chymotrypsin (CPT code 84311) is another enzyme that may be used to detect pancreatic insufficiency, but it has much lower specificity and sensitivity (49% in mild and 85% in moderate disease) than fecal elastase-1.[3,7] Fecal chymotrypsin is degraded during intestinal transit, is sensitive to dilution in stool, and this test cannot differentiate exogenous chymotrypsin introduced through pancreatic enzyme supplementation.[5,9]
- Serum trypsinogen (CPT code 83519) might be of benefit in severe pancreatic insufficiency, but it is not sensitive for mild to moderate disease and may be elevated in acute pancreatitis or nonpancreatic abdominal pain conditions.[5,7,10]
- Secretin tests (CPT code 84311) are still considered the gold standard to diagnose pancreatic insufficiency but are invasive, no longer used routinely, and lack standardization. They may be useful if indirect testing is inconclusive but are unsuitable for use in the pediatric population.[1,3,6,7,10–12]
- Breath tests for 13C-marked substrates are nonspecific and inaccurate in mild exocrine pancreatic insufficiency, not routinely used, and are not approved for use to diagnose pancreatic insufficiency in the United States.[3,7,10]

INDICATIONS
Screening
Because pancreatic insufficiency can result from multiple disorders, there are no published recommendations for or against the universal screening for fecal elastase-1 in the general population in asymptomatic patients. Some research suggests the potential to use fecal elastase-1 testing to screen for cystic fibrosis in the newborn; however, a normal test in the first year of life was not found to exclude the diagnosis due to fluctuations in fecal elastase levels in that population.[16] Screening for fecal (pancreatic) elastase-1 should be considered in patients exhibiting symptoms suggestive for pancreatic insufficiency, including but not limited to:[2–5,7,11,17]

- Chronic diarrhea
- Steatorrhea
- Large, foul smelling stools
- Chronic abdominal pain
- Chronic nausea
- Malnutrition
- Unexplained weight loss
- Bloating/cramping/flatulence
- Anemia
- The American College of Gastroenterology recommends the use of fecal elastase to screen for suspected exocrine pancreatic insufficiency in those patients with the diagnosis of chronic pancreatits.[18]
- Screen the pediatric population with cystic fibrosis and intestinal manifestations who are demonstrating failure to thrive.[2]
- Consider screening in other conditions in symptomatic patients that may result in pancreatic insufficiency (see "Related Diagnoses and ICD-10 Codes").

Diagnosis and Evaluation

■ Fecal elastase-1 can be used to confirm the diagnosis of malabsorption based on the three most common symptoms of:
  ● Chronic diarrhea
  ● Unexplained weight loss
  ● Unexplained nutrient deficiencies
■ Fecal elastase-1 can be used for diagnosing pancreatic insufficiency in patients with the following conditions: [2–4,7,10–12,16]
  ● Chronic pancreatitis
  ● Cystic fibrosis
  ● Pancreatic resection

Monitoring

■ The European Society for Clinical Nutrition and Metabolism, the European Society for Paediatric Gastroenterology, Hepatology and Nutrition, and the European Cystic Fibrosis Society recommend that the fecal elastin-1 test be performed at early intervals in pancreatic-sufficient patients with cystic fibrosis to determine their need for pancreatic enzyme supplementation.[10] This recommendation has not been adopted in the United States.

INTERPRETATION

■ 200 µg/g stool or lower is positive for exocrine pancreatic insufficiency.
  ● Sensitivity and specificity vary with severity of symptoms and is reported to range from 93% to 100% sensitivity and 88% to 100% specificity in moderate to severe disease.[3,4,7,8,10,11,13,16]

FOLLOW-UP

■ There are no published recommendations for follow-up fecal elastase-1 testing in patients with levels greater than 200 µg/g stool once the diagnosis is confirmed.
■ Patient with levels of 200 µg/g stool and lower would require additional workup based on symptomology and correlation with other tests for definitive diagnosis of underlying pathology.[7]

PEARLS & PITFALLS

■ Consider quality of sample if results are 200 µg/g stool or lower and symptoms are consistent with pancreatic insufficiency. Watery stools may produce a false-negative result.[3,5,7,8,10]
■ Results may be falsely negative in patients with mild to moderate pancreatic insufficiency.[1,2,10]
■ Results are not affected by the use of pancreatic enzyme replacement therapy, which is extracted from porcine cells and is CELA1.[6,10]
■ Monitor lipid-soluble vitamins (A, D, E, & K) which are lost along with fecal fat and vitamin B12 levels, although that is rarer.[2,3,7,11,14]

- Patients with pancreatic exocrine deficiency are at higher risk for osteoporosis, visual impairment, neurologic difficulties, muscle wasting, and hemorrhagic disorders.[2,10]
- There are no reliable tests to definitively diagnose pancreatic insufficiency in mild to moderate disease.[1]

PATIENT EDUCATION

- https://gastro.org/news/aga-releases-new-epi-patient-education-page/
- https://medlineplus.gov/lab-tests/stool-elastase/
- https://labtestsonline.org/tests/stool-elastase

RELATED DIAGNOSES AND ICD-10 CODES

Chronic pancreatitis	K86.1
Pancreatic resection (acquired loss of pancreas)	Z90.411
Cystic fibrosis with intestinal manifestations	E84.19
Pancreatic cancer	C25.9
HIV/AIDS	B20
Diabetes mellitus	E00-E89
Inflammatory bowel disease	K51.90
Irritable bowel disease	K58.9
Celiac disease	K90
Small bowel intestinal bacterial overgrowth	K90.89
Alterations in the natural anatomy of the digestive tract (acquired absence of other specified parts of digestive tract)	Z90.49
Zollinger-Ellison syndrome	E16.4
Shwachman-Diamond syndrome (rare)	D61.0
Johanson-Blizzard syndrome (rare)	Q87.8
Giardiasis	A07.1

REFERENCES

Full list of references can be accessed through Springer Publishing Company Connect™ at the following link: http://connect.springerpub.com/content/reference-book/978-0-8261-8843-4/part/part03/toc-part/ch071

72. FECAL OCCULT BLOOD TEST, FECAL IMMUNOCHEMICAL TEST, AND MULTITARGET STOOL DNA TESTS

Christine Colella and Kelly Small Casler

PATHOPHYSIOLOGY REVIEW

Colorectal cancer (CRC) causes abnormal colonic cell growth in the colon and may also cause occult bleeding. Occult blood may also be seen with advanced adenomatous polyps, a pre-cancer growth.[1] When hemoglobin is passed in feces, detecting either heme or globin through laboratory methods allows screening for occult bleeding, and thus, CRC.[2] Identifying deoxyribonucleic acid (DNA) from cancer cells shed in the feces is another way to screen for CRC. Since CRC is the fourth most common cancer diagnosed among adults and the second-leading cause of death from cancer, screening for early detection can significantly improve morbidity and mortality.[3]

OVERVIEW OF LABORATORY TESTS

Both invasive and noninvasive methods can be used to screen for CRC. Colonoscopy and sigmoidoscopy are the two invasive methods available. This chapter will focus on noninvasive methods that use a patient's stool sample. Fecal occult blood tests (FOBT) examine the stool for small amounts of occult blood and can be guaiac-based tests (gFOBTs) or fecal immunochemical-based tests (FITs). Multitarget stool DNA (MT-sDNA) tests look for occult blood along with degraded, aberrant DNA shed in CRC or pre-cancerous adenomas.[4] These tests are described in detail in the text that follows and compared in Table 72.1[1-3,5-8].

gFOBT CPT CODE 82270

gFOBTs have been the traditional tool to screen for CRC and have been in use for almost 150 years.[1,7,9] gFOBTs rely on the chemical guaiac, a wood resin derived from the Guajacum tree, to detect blood in the feces. A series of three stool samples (from three different days) are collected, usually at home, by the patient and smeared onto guaiac-containing paper inside a card which is then returned to the clinician. The clinician then applies hydrogen peroxide to the guaiac paper/fecal sample. In the absence of heme, an oxidative reaction occurs, turning the guaiac paper blue slowly after several minutes. In the presence of heme or other peroxidase-containing substances (listed in Box 72.1), however, the process is catalyzed and the blue color appears over a few seconds, resulting in a positive test.[2] The interaction of peroxidase-containing substances in gFOBTs is a drawback as they can cause false-positive results. gFOBTs detect bleeding from anywhere in the gastrointestinal tract and not just the colon, which is another

TABLE 72.1: COMPARISON OF NONINVASIVE COLORECTAL SCREENING TESTS

	HS-GFOBTS	FIT	MT-SDNA
Diet restrictions	Avoid vitamins/red meat	No diet restrictions	No diet restrictions
Detection target	Heme	Globin	Globin and DNA biomarkers from cancer cells
Approximate cost	$20	$20	$500–$600
Recommended testing interval	Every 1–2 years	Every 1–2 years	Every 3 years
Sample collection	3 samples each on different days	1 spontaneous sample	1 spontaneous sample
Accuracy/performance	SN 62%–79% SP 87%–96%	SN 79%–99% SP 94%–99%	SN 92% SP 84%–89%

FIT, fecal immunochemical test; hs-gFOBTs, high-sensitivity fecal occult blood tests; MT-sDNA, multitarget stool DNA test; SN, sensitivity; SP, specificity.

Sources: Data from Daly JM, Xu Y, Levy BT. Which fecal immunochemical test should I choose? *J Prim Care Community Health.* 2017;8(4):264–277. doi:10.1177/2150131917705206; Lee JK, Liles EG, Bent S, Levin TR, Corley DA. Accuracy of fecal immunochemical tests for colorectal cancer: systematic review and meta-analysis. *Ann Intern Med.* 2014;160(3):171. doi:10.7326/M13-1484; Qaseem A, Alguire P, Dallas P, et al. Appropriate use of screening and diagnostic tests to foster high-value, cost-conscious care. *Ann Intern Med.* 2012;156(2):147. doi:10.7326/0003-4819-156-2-201201170-00011; Rex DK, Boland RC, Dominitz JA, et al. Colorectal cancer screening: recommendations for physicians and patients from the U.S. Multi-Society Task Force on Colorectal Cancer. *Am J Gastroenterol.* 2017;112(7):1016–1030. doi:10.1038/ajg.2017.174; Robertson DJ, Lee JK, Boland CR, et al. Recommendations on fecal immunochemical testing to screen for colorectal neoplasia: a consensus statement by the US Multi-Society Task Force on colorectal cancer. *Gastrointest Endosc.* 2017;85(1):2–21.e3. doi:10.1016/j.gie.2016.09.025; Wolf AMD, Fontham ETH, Church TR, et al. Colorectal cancer screening for average-risk adults: 2018 guideline update from the American Cancer Society. *CA Cancer J Clin.* 2018;68(4):250–281. doi:10.3322/caac.21457; Young GP. Fecal immunochemical tests (FIT) vs. office-based guaiac fecal occult blood test (FOBT). *Practical Gastroenterology.* Published online 2004. http://adphweb01.adph.org/colon/assets/FIT_vs_FOBT.pdf.

Box 72.1: Foods and Medicines That Contain Peroxidase

These substances can cause false-positive results and should be avoided 3 days prior to gFOBT testing, if possible:[2]

- Aspirin
- Beets
- Broccoli
- Cantaloupe
- Carrots
- Nonsteroidal anti-inflammatory drugs
- Red meat
- Turnips
- Vitamin C

drawback of this type of test.[4] Newer gFOBTs are referred to as high-sensitivity gFOBTs (hs-gFOBT; Brand name-Hemocult Sensa) and should be used over traditional gFOBTs due to 2- to 3-times higher sensitivity.[4,8]

FIT CPT Code 82274

FITs were invented over 50 years ago and there are over 25 different brands of FIT tests currently on the market.[1] FITs have gained international acceptance as being superior to the traditional gFOBT because they use antibodies specific for human hemoglobin.[10] This property results in fewer false positives compared to gFOBT because substances (Table 72.1) will not interfere with the results. Therefore, there are no dietary restrictions before gathering the sample as with FoBTs. FITs also tend to only identify occult bleeding from the lower part of the gastrointestinal tract. With FITs, monoclonal or polyclonal antibodies present in the test bind to the globin component of any hemoglobin from colonic bleeding that is present in the feces. This mechanism can detect smaller amounts of blood compared to gFOBT. FITs are performed one of two ways: through instrument-based immunoassays, which provide a quantitative result, or lateral flow immunoassays, which provide a qualitative result and can be used as a point-of-care test.[1,5,10] With quantitative assays, cutoff levels can be modified to a lower level if greater sensitivity is desired with the screening test.[6] Patients are able to complete a FIT test at home by collecting a sample of stool and then delivering or mailing in the sample to a laboratory or clinic. In general, patients prefer the easier and more agreeable collection method of FIT compared to gFOBT and clinicians and experts prefer the better performance.[1,11] The advantage of FITs are its noninvasiveness and one-time sensitivity for cancer of 79% to 99%.[1,6,7.] FIT is relatively inexpensive and is recommended annually in the United States.[3]

FIT-DNA/MT-sDNA Test (CPT Code 81528)

Approved by the Food and Drug Administration in 2014 and added to CRC cancer screening recommendations in 2016, FIT-DNA tests (also called mutitarget stool DNA tests, brand name Cologuard) combine the occult blood detection methods of FITs with additional mechanisms to detect degenerated DNA biomarkers from CRC and adenoma cells.[4,12] FIT-DNA tests are more sensitive for CRC and precancer lesions than FIT alone, but less specific than FIT.[12,13] In one study, the stool DNA test had a sensitivity rate of 92% for CRC and 69% for high-grade adenomas; its specificity was 86% to 89%.[13] MT-sDNA tests are approved for screening in patients age 45 and older and are performed once every 1 to 3 years.[14]

INDICATIONS

Screening

■ Patients at average risk of CRC, can be screened with hs-gFOBT, FIT, or MT-sDNA according to frequencies listed in Tables 72.1 and 72.2. Patients at high risk of CRC due to family history should have colonoscopy instead.

Diagnosis and Evaluation

■ Noninvasive tests are meant for screening only and are not used for diagnosis. Evaluation of bowel movement pattern changes, abdominal pain or trauma, anemia, bleeding, or signs/symptoms of inflammatory bowel disease requires colonoscopy.[9,15]

- Noninvasive tests are commonly misused for diagnostic purposes, especially for anemia. It is important to avoid this practice as the tests lack adequate sensitivity when used in this manner.[16,17]

Monitoring

- Not used.

INTERPRETATION

- gFOBTs and FITs are reported as positive or negative for hemoglobin.
- MT-sDNA tests are reported as positive or negative. Detection of either hemoglobin or DNA will result in a positive test.[18]
- Remember, the tests detect blood or DNA in the stool but do not identify any specific disease process.

FOLLOW-UP

- Colonoscopy is the recommended follow-up for a positive finding on FIT, gFOBT, or MT-sDNA tests.[5] If colonoscopy is negative, clinicians can consider esophagogastroduodenoscopy if there is suspicion for higher GI bleeding as a cause of the positive test.[19]

PEARLS & PITFALLS

- Performing a gFOBT with a stool sample obtained during a digital rectal examination lacks adequate accuracy for screening.[4,5]
- Do not use gFOBTs as a screening test for gastric cancer. Even though gFOBTs can detect upper gastrointestinal bleeding, the sensitivity is not high enough to be used in this manner.[19]
- In one study, yearly FIT had better accuracy and cost profile than MT-sDNA performed every 3 years.[7]
- Hemoglobin degrades more quickly in warm temperature, so FITs could have lower sensitivity in warm months if samples are exposed to the warm temperatures for too long.[1,5]
- In general, FITs are generally recommended over gFOBT due to patient preference. Patients feel they are less "disgusting" since (a) samples do not have to be kept in the residence, (b) fewer samples are required, and (c) the test tube for FIT is less messy and easier to use than gFOBT cards.[5,20]
- Educate patients to return FITs within 24 hours of collection, if possible.[5]
- Education is paramount since up to 40% of patients fail to turn-in FIT samples after dispensing the materials.[5] In addition to education, follow-up reminder phone calls can improve patient return of FIT samples.[21]
- It is important to remember that FITs do not replace colonoscopy. Although FITs are highly sensitive for CRC, they only have a sensitivity of 42% for other colon abnormalities like large polyps which, if missed, can advance to CRC.[13]

- The best role for noninvasive CRC screening tests seems to be in patients who decline or are uncomfortable with colonoscopy as a screening method or in those who prefer sigmoidoscopy to colonoscopy. For a comparison of common guidelines for CRC screening, see Table 72.2.[22]
- False negatives can also occur with gFOBTs and FITs if colonic abnormalities do not bleed.[23]
- MT-sDNA accuracy decreases with age older than 65.[7]
- If patients have had a normal colonoscopy in the last 10 years, CRC screening recommendations are met and noninvasive screening tests do not need to be performed.[5]
- Although generally recommended to occur yearly, one study showed no difference in mortality if gFOBT was performed every other year.[24]
- The FLU-FIT initiative pairs FIT testing kit handouts to encounters for influenza vaccination and increases CRC screening rates (Odds Ratio 2.75).[25,26]
- New research is looking at only screening patients with an elevated 15-year CRC cancer risk per the following calculator: https://qcancer.org/15yr/colorectal/[27] Further validation of the calculation is needed.

TABLE 72.2: SCREENING RECOMMENDATIONS FOR COLORECTAL CANCER

ORGANIZATION	START SCREENING	STOP SCREENING	SCREENING OPTIONS
American College of Physicians[8]	40 years old for Black/AA 50 years old for others	If >75 years old* or less than 10-year life expectancy	1. FIT or hs-gFOBT Q2Y 2. sigmoidoscopy Q10Y with FIT Q2Y 3. Colonoscopy Q10Y
USPSTF[28]	Age 50 (grade A) Age 45–49 (grade B)	At age 76–85* (grade C)	1. FIT or hs-gFOBT Q1Y 2. Sigmoidoscopy Q10Y with FIT Q2Y 3. MT-sDNA Q1–2Y 4. Colonoscopy Q10Y
American Cancer Society[3]	≥45 years old	>85 years old or less than 10-year life expectancy	1. FIT or hs-gFOBT Q1Y 2. MT-sDNA Q3Y 3. Colonoscopy Q10Y
U.S. Multi Society Task Force on CRC[7]	≥50 years ≥45 years old for Black/AA	Age >75 years old* or less than 10-year life expectancy	1. FIT Q1Y^ 2. MT-sDNA Q3Y 3. Colonoscopy Q10Y^

^ Preferred tests

*Most guidelines agree that individuals between 75 and 85 should undergo screening if they have never been screened before and prefer FIT over Cologuard.

AA, African American; FIT, fecal immunochemical test; hs-gFOBTs, high sensitivity fecal occult blood tests; MT-sDNA, multitarget stool DNA test; Q, every; USPSTF, United States Preventive Services Task Force; Y, years.

PATIENT EDUCATION

- https://www.cdc.gov/cancer/colorectal/basic_info/screening/index.htm
- https://www.cologuardtest.com/
- https://www.cdc.gov/cancer/colorectal/basic_info/screening/tests.htm#:~:text=The%20U.S.%20Preventive%20Services%20Task,if%20you%20should%20be%20screened
- https://medlineplus.gov/ency/patientinstructions/000704.htm

RELATED DIAGNOSES AND ICD-10 CODES

Guaiac positive, other fecal abnormalities, blood in feces	R19.5
Encounter for screening for malignant neoplasm of colon	Z12.11
Encounter for screening of malignant neoplasms of the rectum	Z12.12
Gastrointestinal hemorrhage unspecified	K92.2

REFERENCES

Full list of references can be accessed through Springer Publishing Company Connect™ at the following link: http://connect.springerpub.com/content/reference-book/978-0-8261-8843-4/part/part03/toc-part/ch072

---

73. FERRITIN AND IRON STUDIES

Samara Linnell and Kelly Small Casler

PHYSIOLOGY REVIEW

Iron is an essential element in the human body and low levels can result in iron deficiency anemia (IDA). Iron is the central component of heme, the molecule that binds and transports oxygen. About two-thirds of the body's iron is used for this function.[1,2] The rest of iron is used in adenosine triphosphate (ATP) formation, immune system function, connective tissue maintenance, and neurotransmitter formation.[3]

Iron levels are regulated through a complex interplay of hormones and proteins. Storage occurs mainly in the liver within iron's main storage protein, ferritin.[3] Ferritin is an acute phase reactant, meaning it is released into the bloodstream in response to inflammation, infection, or malignancy.[2,4] Ferritin is also elevated in iron overload states, such as hereditary hemochromatosis or transfusion hemosiderosis.[3] Iron is transported to the bone marrow by binding to transferrin, a protein produced in the liver. Transferrin delivers iron to cells by binding with transferrin receptors on the cell wall.[5] Transferrin levels decrease in malnourished states or in the presence of inflammation. The hepatic hormone hepcidin regulates iron levels by controlling its absorption and release; higher hepcidin levels limit iron release.[3] Hepcidin increases in response to inflammatory cytokines, which is often seen in anemia of chronic disease (ACD).[6]

OVERVIEW OF LABORATORY TESTS

There are several laboratory tests available to evaluate iron status and availability.

Ferritin

Ferritin (CPT code 82728) is a sensitive and specific test to reflect iron stores; low levels signal iron deficiency.[1,4,7] It is the laboratory test of choice to detect iron deficiency anemia unless there is inflammation, malignancy, or liver disease, in which case total iron binding capacity (TIBC) or transferrin saturation are used in addition to ferritin.[8] Ferritin is measured through the use of immunoassays using antibodies to ferritin and results from one laboratory to another are not interchangeable due to differences in immunoassay approach.[9] One of the biggest challenges with ferritin measurement is determining the most appropriate reference limit reflecting iron deficiency. Suggestions range from 15 to 45 ng/mL.[4] With the higher cutoff, the sensitivity rate nears 100%, but there is loss of specificity.[10] Lower cutoffs near 15 ng/mL result in less sensitivity, but improved specificity,[4] and a cutoff in the middle (30 ng/mL) provides 92% sensitivity and 98% specificity for IDA.[11] Because of these nuances, different clinical guidelines recommend different cutoff levels related to patient's history.[12] In most instances, however, levels 20 to 100 ng/mL are considered indeterminate. Results in this range require other laboratory tests, such as the tests described in the text that follows, to clarify the exact clinical picture.[7,13]

Iron Studies (Iron, Transferrin, Iron Binding Capacity, and Saturation)

Iron studies assess iron level (CPT code 83540), iron binding capacity (CPT code 83550), iron/transferrin saturation (CPT code 83550), and, sometimes, transferrin levels (CPT code 84466). These tests are summarized in Tables 73.1 and 73.2. Iron levels simply measure the amount of iron in a sample. Unsaturated iron binding capacity (UIBC) is determined by adding external iron to a serum sample to allow it to find and bind to all open binding sites on transferrin. Then, any of the unbound external iron leftover is measured and subtracted from the total external iron that was added to the sample.[9] TIBC refers to the total availability for iron and transferrin to bind. It reflects the amount of iron that is in the body and how much additional binding spots there are on transferrin (usually only about one-third of binding sites are ever used).[9] It is calculated by adding iron levels to UIBC. Transferrin saturation is reported as a percentage and reflects how many available iron binding sites on transferrin are currently occupied by iron. It is usually calculated (by dividing the serum iron concentration by the TIBC and multiplying by 100) rather than directly measured, although calculations can overestimate the result.[9] Transferrin can be measured directly but is often calculated by adding serum iron and UIBC.[8] TIBC and transferrin are

TABLE 73.1: OVERVIEW OF IRON STUDIES

	DEFINITION	CALCULATION	AUROC[8] FOR IDA
Iron	Element essential to oxygen delivery and body homeostasis	n/a	77% if low
Total iron binding capacity (TIBC)*	Maximum available capacity for iron binding (indirect measure of transferrin)	Serum iron + UIBC	94% if high
Unsaturated iron binding capacity (UIBC)	Amount of transferrin that is available for binding, but does not have iron bound to it	n/a	n/a
Transferrin	Transport protein for iron	*	n/a
Transferrin saturation (TSAT) (also called iron saturation)	% Occupied iron binding sites on transferrin^	(Serum iron/TIBC) × 100	87% if low

*Transferrin can be directly measured, but more commonly TIBC is used as an indirect measurement of transferrin.

^Normally only one-third of binding sites on transferrin are used.

AUROC, area under the receiver operating curve; IDA, iron deficiency anemia; n/a, not applicable.

sometimes used interchangeably though they are not determined in the same manner.[9]

Soluble Transferrin Receptor (sTfR) and Transferrin Receptor-Ferritin (sTfR-F) Index

Soluble transferrin receptors (sTfR) (CPT code 84238) are circulating protein remnants from the transferrin receptors on erythroblasts. They can be measured in the serum by immunoenzymatic assays.[9] sTfR is most often used to help distinguish between ACD and IDA when ferritin is in indeterminate ranges (20 to 100 ng/mL) since sTfR is less affected by inflammation than ferritin.[2,4,10] It is particularly helpful in chronic kidney disease (CKD).[14,15] Because sTfR is from erythroblasts, it reflects erythropoiesis, with high levels reflecting bone marrow response to iron deficiency, bleeding, hemolysis, or erythropoiesis-stimulating agents.[16] Decreased sTfR may be seen in conditions that impair erythropoiesis like chemotherapy. sTfR is not used as an initial test to differentiate causes of microcytotic anemia (especially iron deficiency anemia) due to its expense.[14] The transferrin receptor-ferritin index (sTfr-F index) (also called transferrin receptor-ferritin log ratio) expands on the use of sTfR by using it in combination with ferritin levels.[17,18] In patients with acute and chronic inflammation, a sTfR-ferritin index of 1.5 mg/L or more can detect IDA with a sensitivity of 88% to 100% and a specificity of 93% to 100%, which improves accuracy compared to use of sTfR alone.[2,17] In its original study with adults, the AUROC was 100% for distinguishing IDA from ACD[15] and in a study of its use in pediatrics for the same use, the AUROC was 97%.[18]

TABLE 73.2: FERRITIN AND IRON STUDIES INTERPRETATION

	REFERENCE INTERVALS*	INCREASED IN	DECREASED IN
Iron	28–147 µg/dL	Sideroblastic anemia	Iron deficiency, infection, inflammation
Ferritin	15–45 ng/mL	Inflammation, liver disease, hyperthyroidism, sideroblastic anemia	Iron deficiency anemia
TIBC (Serum iron + UIBC)	250–450 µg/dL	Iron deficiency	Inflammation, malnutrition, malignancy
Transferrin saturation (TSAT)	>16%–20% to <50%	Hemochromatosis, iron overload	Iron deficiency
Transferrin	200–400 mg/dL	IDA	Liver disease, malnutrition
Mean soluble transferrin receptor (sTfR)	Adults: 0.85–2.5 mg/L Children: 0.78–1.9 mg/L	IDA, sickle cell anemia, megaloblastic anemia, hemolytic anemias	Severe CKD, aplastic anemia, chemotherapy

*Values vary between laboratories, be sure to reference local reference intervals.

CKD, chronic kidney disease; IDA, iron deficiency anemia.

Sources: Data from Daru J, Colman K, Stanworth SJ, De La Salle B, Wood EM, Pasricha S-R. Serum ferritin as an indicator of iron status: what do we need to know? *Am J Clin Nutr.* 2017;106(suppl 6):1634S–1639S. doi:10.3945/ajcn.117.155960; De Franceschi L, Iolascon A, Taher A, Cappellini MD. Clinical management of iron deficiency anemia in adults: systemic review on advances in diagnosis and treatment. *Eur J Intern Med.* 2017;42:16–23. doi:10.1016/j.ejim.2017.04.018; Koulaouzidis A, Said E, Cottier R, Saeed AA. Soluble transferrin receptors and iron deficiency, a step beyond ferritin. A systematic review. *J Gastrointestin Liver Dis.* 2009;18(3):345–352; Kundrapu S, Noguez J. Laboratory assessment of anemia. In: Makowski GS, ed. *Advances in Clinical Chemistry.* Vol 83. Elsevier; 2018:197–225. doi:10.1016/bs.acc.2017.10.006; McPherson R. Specific proteins. In: McPherson RA, Pincus MR, eds. *Henry's Clinical Diagnosis and Management by Laboratory Methods.* 23rd ed. Elsevier:253–266; Vázquez-López MA, López-Ruzafa E, Ibáñez-Alcalde M, Martín-González M, Bonillo-Perales A, Lendínez-Molinos F. The usefulness of reticulocyte haemoglobin content, serum transferrin receptor and the sTfR-ferritin index to identify iron deficiency in healthy children aged 1–16 years. *Eur J Pediatr.* 2019;178(1):41–49. doi:10.1007/s00431-018-3257-0; Vázquez-López MA, López-Ruzafa E, Lendinez-Molinos F, Ortiz-Pérez M, Ruiz-Tudela L, Martín-González M. Reference values of serum transferrin receptor (sTfR) and sTfR/log ferritin index in healthy children. *Pediatr Hematol Oncol.* 2016;33(2):109–120. doi:10.3109/08880018.2015.1138007; World Health Organization. Iron deficiency anaemia. Assessment, prevention, and control. A guide for programme managers. Published 2001. https://www.who.int/nutrition/publications/en/ida_assessment_prevention_control.pdf

INDICATIONS

Screening

- When possible, use ferritin instead of hemoglobin (Hg) to screen patients at risk for iron deficiency or iron deficiency anemia.[11] Ferritin levels are much more accurate and pick up on iron deficiency much sooner compared to screening with Hg. For iron deficiency, ferritin has a sensitivity of 89%, while Hg has a sensitivity of 26%.[11]
- Consider using ferritin to screen populations at risk for iron deficiency (Table 73.3). Also consider screening patients at risk for iron excess related to past history of iron excess or frequent transfusion needs (sickle cell disease, leukemia, myelodysplastic syndrome, thalassemia, or aplastic anemia).

TABLE 73.3: POPULATIONS AT RISK FOR IRON DEFICIENCY	
Bleeding disorders	Von Willebrand disease, storage pool deficiency, hemophilia, heavy/abnormal uterine bleeding, endometrial hyperplasia
Chronic kidney failure/end-stage renal disease	Iron may be removed with dialysis
Malabsorptive states/ occult blood loss	Celiac disease, Chron's or ulcerative colitis, cystic fibrosis, history of gastric bypass surgery or bowel resection, lactose intolerance, irritable bowel disease or inflammatory bowel disease, thyroid disease, history of multiple GI surgeries, gastric or colorectal cancer, *Helicobacter pylori* or other infection of GI tract, esophagitis, autoimmune atrophic gastritis.
Metabolic derangements	Lack of iron-rich foods in diet. Uncontrolled diabetes mellitus.
Pregnant individuals	Increased demand for iron and fetal development considerations[3]
Children	During periods of rapid growth, breastfeeding
Use of certain medications	Proton pump inhibitors. Antipsychotics/antiepileptics

GI, gastrointestinal.

Sources: Data from Daru J, Colman K, Stanworth SJ, De La Salle B, Wood EM, Pasricha S-R. Serum ferritin as an indicator of iron status: what do we need to know? *Am J Clin Nutr.* 2017;106(suppl 6):1634S–1639S. doi:10.3945/ajcn.117.155960; Girelli D, Nemeth E, Swinkels DW. Hepcidin in the diagnosis of iron disorders. *Blood.* 2016;127(23):2809–2813. doi:10.1182/blood-2015-12-639112; Koch TA, Myers J, Goodnough LT. Intravenous iron therapy in patients with iron deficiency anemia: dosing considerations. *Anemia.* 2015;2015:763576. doi:10.1155/2015/763576; Trotti LM, Becker LA. Iron for the treatment of restless legs syndrome. *Cochrane Database Syst Rev.* 2019;1(1):CD007834. doi:10.1002/14651858.CD007834.pub3.

Diagnosis and Evaluation

- Ferritin and iron studies are most often ordered to differentiate between IDA and other causes of microcytic anemia and to further evaluate abnormalities of Hg, hematocrit, or other red blood cell abnormalities.[4,10,17] Ferritin is the usual first step, with iron studies being ordered if ferritin levels are in the indeterminate range.
- Ferritin and other iron studies are also used in the evaluation of signs and symptoms of iron excess such as abdominal discomfort or hyperpigmentation on the face or hands.[3,19]
- Ferritin and iron studies are used to evaluate signs and symptoms of iron deficiency (Box 73.1).

Monitoring

- In the setting of oral or intravenous iron repletion, monitor ferritin levels every 8 weeks.
- In the setting of chelation therapy, monitor iron levels every 1 to 3 months.
- In the setting of hereditary hemochromatosis, ferritin levels are used to monitor and guide the need for periodic phlebotomies. The target ferritin level is 50 to 100 ng/mL.[20]
- In the setting of IDA, ferritin is monitored monthly in children and every 2 months in adults.[21]

Box 73.1: Signs and Symptoms of Iron Deficiency

■ Cold intolerance
■ Drop in hemoglobin from baseline
■ Exercise intolerance
■ Fatigue
■ Hair loss
■ Heart murmurs
■ Low hemoglobin
■ Pale mucous membranes
■ Pica
■ Prior anemia history
■ Shortness of breath
■ Trouble concentrating/decreased cognitive function

Sources: Data from Berlin T, Meyer A, Rotman-Pikielny P, Natur A, Levy Y. Soluble transferrin receptor as a diagnostic laboratory test for detection of iron deficiency anemia in acute illness of hospitalized patients. *Isr Med Assoc J.* 2011;13(2):96–98; Infusino I, Braga F, Dolci A, Panteghini M. Soluble transferrin receptor (sTfR) and sTfR/log ferritin index for the diagnosis of iron-deficiency anemia a meta-analysis. *Am J Clin Pathol.* 2012;138(5):642–649. doi:10.1309/AJCP16NTXZLZFAIB; O'Brien KO, Ru Y. Iron status of North American pregnant women: an update on longitudinal data and gaps in knowledge from the United States and Canada. *Am J Clin Nutr.* 2017;106(suppl 6):1647S–1654S. doi:10.3945/ajcn.117.155986; Pettei MJ, AAP NY State Chapter 2 Nutrition Committee, Weinstein T, Eden A. Screening for iron deficiency. *Pediatrics.* 2016;137(6):e20160714A. doi:10.1542/peds.2016-0714A.

TABLE 73.4: CLUES TO DIFFERENTIATING IRON DEFICIENCY ANEMIA FROM ANEMIA OF CHRONIC DISEASE (INFLAMMATION)

	SERUM IRON LEVEL	FERRITIN LEVEL	TIBC LEVEL	TSAT LEVEL	sTfR LEVEL
IDA	Low	Low	High	Low	High
ACD	Low	Normal or high	Low	Normal	Normal

ACD, anemia of chronic disease (inflammation); IDA, iron deficiency anemia; sTfR, soluble transferrin receptor; TIBC, total iron binding capacity; TSAT, transferrin saturation.

Sources: Data from Berlin T, Meyer A, Rotman-Pikielny P, Natur A, Levy Y. Soluble transferrin receptor as a diagnostic laboratory test for detection of iron deficiency anemia in acute illness of hospitalized patients. *Isr Med Assoc J.* 2011;13(2):96–98; Hawkins RC. Total iron binding capacity or transferrin concentration alone outperforms iron and saturation indices in predicting iron deficiency. *Clin Chim Acta.* 2007;380(1–2):203–207. doi:10.1016/j.cca.2007.02.032; Kundrapu S, Noguez J. Laboratory assessment of anemia. In: Makowski GS, ed. *Advances in Clinical Chemistry.* Vol 83. Elsevier; 2018:197–225. doi:10.1016/bs.acc.2017.10.006.

■ In the setting of erythropoiesis-stimulating therapy, ferritin and TSAT are monitored every 3 months and more frequently during dose titration or initiation.[14]

INTERPRETATION

■ Interpretation of ferritin and iron studies is summarized in Tables 73.1 and 73.2. Specific considerations are discussed in the text that follows. Additionally, Table 73.4 summarizes the interpretation of iron studies, ferritin,

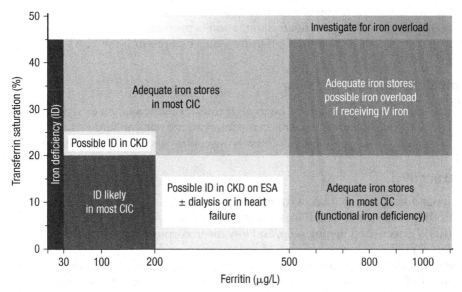

FIGURE 73.1. Assessment of iron stores in chronic inflammatory conditions (CIC). Ferritin is challenging to interpret in the setting of chronic inflammation. In these instances, using transferrin saturation in combination ferritin can assist in the interpretation of results. CKD, chronic kidney disease; ESA, erythropoiesis-stimulating agent. *Source:* Fertrin KY. Diagnosis and management of iron deficiency in chronic inflammatory conditions (CIC): is too little iron making your patient sick? *Hematology.* 2020;2020(1):478–486. doi:10.1182/hematology.2020000132.

and sTfR for differentiating IDA and ACD and Figure 73.1 summarizes the interpretation of ferritin and TSAT in chronic inflammatory states.

Ferritin

- Consider diagnosing IDA in premenopausal females with ferritin less than 50 ng/mL.[5,7]
- Consider diagnosing IDA in patients with inflammatory conditions with ferritin less than 70 ng/mL.[2,5,10]
- Consider diagnosing IDA in patient with heart failure when ferritin is less than 100 ng/mL with low transferrin levels.[17,19,22]
- Consider diagnosing IDA in patients who are athletes when ferritin levels are lower than 30 to 40 ng/mL.[23]
- Consider diagnosing IDA in patients with restless leg syndrome when ferritin levels are lower than 45 ng/mL.[24,25]

Iron and Iron Studies

- Serum iron levels are influenced by nutritional intake in the days preceding measurement.[10]

■ A transferrin saturation of less than 20% is considered diagnostic of IDA regardless of whether or not inflammation is present.[5]
■ In patients with CKD or ACD, IDA may also be present if the TSAT is between 20% and 25%.[10]

Soluble Transferrin Receptor

■ Use local laboratory reference intervals/limits for interpretation of sTfR and sTfR-ferritin index, since reference intervals are not standardized and agreements on appropriate cutoff levels are controversial and vary with age.[18,26]

FOLLOW-UP

■ If not done prior, evaluate a complete blood count (CBC) for the following findings associated with IDA: increased red blood cell distribution width (RDW), decreased hemoglobin, and low mean corpuscular volume (MCV).[2,5,17]
■ Zinc protoporphyrin (ZPP) is a low cost, rapid test that helps confirm iron deficiency if elevated. However, it may also be elevated in lead toxicity.[4,9]
■ If further clarity is needed, reticulocyte indices can assist in differentiating types of anemia.[4]
■ In the presence of indeterminate ferritin levels or iron studies and when trying to differentiate between IDA or ACD, C-reactive protein (CRP), erythrocyte sedimentation rate (ESR), hepcidin, and α1 acid glycoprotein (AGP) can be used to evaluate for inflammation.[2,10]
  ● Hepcidin levels are elevated in the presence of inflammation if iron deficiency is absent. If iron deficiency is present, hepcidin is usually not elevated even if there is inflammation.[2-4,10]
  ● Elevated CRP and AGP suggest inflammation and ACD, while low AGP suggests IDA.[2,10]
■ Always consider referral for evaluation of occult gastrointestinal bleeding, especially with no apparent/obvious reason for iron deficiency.[7,27] In one study, males and post-menopausal females with IDA had a 11% incidence of malignancy.[4]
■ In patients with IDA, consider the differential diagnoses of celiac disease[5,21] or *Helicobacter pylori* infection[5] especially if IDA recurs or is difficult to correct.
■ Consider referral and testing for HFE-associated hereditary hemochromatosis genotyping for C282Y and H63D in patients with iron excess and evidence of liver disease, elevated ferritin (greater than 300 ng/mL), transferrin saturation (greater than 45%), or a known family history of HFE-associated hereditary hemochromatosis.[4,19,28]
■ Consider referral for possible sideroblastic anemia in patients with elevated TSAT, iron, and ferritin. These patients may require bone marrow biopsy for diagnostic evaluation.

PEARLS & PITFALLS

■ Inflammatory conditions can increase the serum ferritin level by 30% to 90%.[5]

■ Black individuals have higher incidence of IDA during pregnancy. Prioritize these individuals for screening.[25]

■ Levels of hemoglobin do not begin to decline until a person has already been iron deficient for several months; ferritin will decline first in iron deficiency.[7]

■ If left undiagnosed, IDA can contribute to problems such as heart failure and chronic fatigue, poor work performance, poor fetal development, and depression.[3]

■ Patients can experience ACD and IDA simultaneously.[15]

■ Ferritin is not susceptible to short-term variations in iron intake.[26]

■ Ferritin lower than 200 mg/dL is consistent with iron deficiency in dialysis patients.[14]

■ In a review of international guidelines, ferritin was found to be the most favored test for IDA, followed by TSAT, then sTfR.[12]

■ Iron studies have lower cost compared to ferritin testing.[8]

■ sTfR rise is seen prior to the development of anemia and will be seen prior to a decline in the hemoglobin.[1]

PATIENT EDUCATION

■ https://www.cdc.gov/genomics/disease/hemochromatosis.htm

■ https://www.nhlbi.nih.gov/health-topics/iron-deficiency-anemia

RELATED DIAGNOSES AND ICD-10 CODES

Iron deficiency anemia related to chronic blood loss	D50.0
Elevated ferritin	R79.89
Hereditary hemochromatosis	E83.110
Iron deficiency anemia, unspecified	D50.9
Hemosiderosis	E83.19
Iron overload from blood transfusions	E83.111

REFERENCES

Full list of references can be accessed through Springer Publishing Company Connect™ at the following link: http://connect.springerpub.com/content/reference-book/978-0-8261-8843-4/part/part03/toc-part/ch073

74. FETAL FIBRONECTIN

Elizabeth Sharpe

PHYSIOLOGY REVIEW

Fetal fibronectin (fFN) is a glycoprotein produced by fetal cells and detectable in cervicovaginal fluid. It is found at the border where the placenta and membranes attach to the wall of the uterus.[1,2] Fetal fibronectin adheres the placenta and membranes to the uterine wall and facilitates physiologic separation after delivery.[3] fFN levels in cervicovaginal secretions are high early in gestation, usually absent between 16 and 22 weeks, and rise again just before delivery.[4] This rise and fall with subsequent elevation approaching term enables its use as one parameter, though not a sole predictor, for preterm labor.[5]

OVERVIEW OF LABORATORY TESTS

fFN is evaluated through sterile speculum-guided sampling of the cervicovaginal secretions. As fFN can be present in amniotic fluid, the sampling should be performed in advance of digital examination. Detection of fFN is performed using a monoclonal antibody-based immunoassay. Commercial assay tests produce rapid qualitative results providing visual interpretation as positive or negative. Quantitative testing expressing results at and above 50 ng/mL are interpreted as a positive test.[6] There is high positive predictive value for preterm birth associated with levels at or above 200 ng/mL demonstrating the superiority of the quantitative testing over qualitative assay.[7] fFN is associated with preterm birth but should not be considered as the primary driver to direct management due to lack of high-level evidence.[5] As a single determinant, it has only produced poor positive predictive value for impending labor.[8] It has greater value in combination with other clinical findings such as transvaginal ultrasound measurement of cervical length shortening.[9] In twin pregnancies, fFN measured between 22 and 27+6 weeks accurately predicted spontaneous preterm delivery at fewer than 30 weeks of gestation.[10] The United States Food and Drug Administration (FDA) approved use of fFN testing for assessing risk of preterm birth within 7 or 14 days following specimen collection.[11] Identification of mothers at increased risk for preterm labor enables avoidance of—as well as preparation for—prematurity and its comorbidities and appropriate utilization of high-level resources.[12]

INDICATIONS

Screening

■ Not recommended as a universal screening tool in asymptomatic females.[5,13]

Diagnosis and Evaluation

■ Used to identify patients at increased risk for preterm delivery. There is lack of universal agreement on specific indications for fFN testing, but in general[5,14]:
  ● It is not recommended to use fFN or cervical length shortening alone for decision making regarding patients with signs of preterm labor.[5]
  ● Utilization of fFN in conjunction with transvaginal ultrasound is most useful in patients with borderline cervical length of 20 to 29 mm.[14]

Monitoring

■ Not used for monitoring.

INTERPRETATION

■ Qualitative assay: positive or negative
■ Quantitative assay: 50 mg/mL or more is the usual cutoff for positive results. Table 74.1 reviews further interpretation of quantitative results.
■ A negative fFN is not adequately reassuring on its own to modify management.[14]

FOLLOW-UP

■ fFN should be used in conjunction with cervical length assessments.

PEARLS & PITFALLS

■ False-positive results can result from rupture of membranes, recent cervical disruption, digital examination, coitus within 24 to 48 hours, or presence of amniotic fluid or blood.
  Traditional contraindications to testing: cervical dilatation greater than 3 cm, ruptured membranes, cerclage, moderate or more vaginal bleeding, multiple gestations, placenta previa, or fewer than 22 weeks gestation.
■ Recent work found that cervical manipulation and cerclage did not alter fFN results.[16,17]
■ Results must be interpreted in clinical correlation with maternal history, gestational age, fetal ultrasound, and other findings.[5]
■ Clinicians should be alert to emerging research in ongoing pursuit of consensus for evidence-based indications for fFN testing and standardization in management of preterm labor.

TABLE 74.1: ODDS RATIO (OR) FOR OUTCOMES BASED ON QUANTITATIVE ASSAY RESULTS		
Quantitative Level	OR for Birth at Fewer Than 34 Weeks Gestaiton[15]	OR for Birth Within Next 7 Days[15]
≥50 ng/mL	7.11	10.5
≥200 ng/mL	12.5	32.7

PATIENT EDUCATION

■ https://www.acog.org/womens-health/faqs/preterm-labor-and-birth

RELATED DIAGNOSES AND ICD-10 CODES

Preterm labor, unspecified trimester	060.00

REFERENCES

Full list of references can be accessed through Springer Publishing Company Connect™ at the following link: http://connect.springerpub.com/content/reference-book/978-0-8261 -8843-4/part/part03/toc-part/ch074

---

75. FIBRINOGEN

Carolyn McClerking

PHYSIOLOGY REVIEW

Fibrinogen, a glycoprotein produced by the liver, represents the last step in the coagulation cascade.[1] As an acute phase reactant, fibrinogen can increase significantly in such conditions as inflammation, tissue damage, and infection. The half-life of fibrinogen is approximately 4 to 5 days. Both the extrinsic and intrinsic pathways permit the proteolytic conversion of fibrinogen to fibrin.[1]

There are three primary forms of congenital fibrinogen disorders: afibrinogenemia, hypofibrinogenemia, and dysfibrinogenemia. Congenital afibrinogenemia, which is a rare condition associated with total absence of fibrinogen, has only been documented in a minute number of cases in the literature.[2] Congenital afibrinogenemia affects males and females equally, and due to their inability to produce fibrin, individuals with this disorder have prolongation of protime (PT) and activated prothrombin time (aPTT) levels, putting them at risk for life-threatening bleeding or thrombotic events.[2] Acquired dysfibrinogenemia is associated with acquired conditions leading to an imbalance of fibrinogen mass to fibrinogen function.[3] Acquired dysfibrinogenemia can be seen in hepatic disease or in interference of autoantibodies of fibrinogen molecular polymerization such as with multiple myeloma, systemic lupus erythematosus, drugs, or possibly idiopathic issues.[3] In acquired dysfibrinogenemia, as opposed to patients with congenital forms of afibrinogenemia, bleeding can be more prominent.[3,4]

OVERVIEW OF LABORATORY TESTS

There are several methods in which fibrinogen can be directly analyzed. The different methods include clottable protein, nephelometric, clot based, and immunologic.[5] The most common technique used in the laboratory for measurement of fibrinogen is the Clauss assay (CPT code 85384).[5] The fibrinogen Clauss assay is a quantitative, clot-based functional assay that evaluates fibrinogen's ability to form fibrin clot after exposure to purified thrombin.[5]

INDICATIONS

Screening
- Universal screening for fibrinogen is not recommended.
- Target screening for fibrinogen is recommended for conditions that predispose individuals to hypo- and hyperfibrinogenemia (Table 75.1).

Diagnosis and Evaluation
- Fibrinogen levels should be evaluated in patients who have a bleeding history in the setting of a normal protime (PT) and activated partial thromboplastin time (aPTT). This is significant as PT and aPTT are usually unaffected by a fibrinogen deficiency unless levels fall below 100 mg/dL.[6]
- Fibrinogen is often used to diagnosis and evaluate the following:
  - Unexplained bleeding or thrombosis,
  - Pregnancy morbidity without a known cause,

TABLE 75.1: SIGNS AND SYMPTOMS OF HYPO- AND HYPERFIBRINOGENEMIA

HYPOFIBRINOGENEMIA	HYPERFIBRINOGENEMIA
Congenital fibrinogen disorders	Acute ischemic stroke
Hemarthrosis	Acute leukemia
Hemorrhage	Hemophagocytic lymphocytosis
Intracranial hemorrhage	Joint infection
Menorrhagia	Pulmonary embolism
Obstetric hemorrhage	
Interosseous hemorrhage	
Recurrent miscarriages	
Splenic rupture	

Sources: Data from Berger MD, Heini AD, Seipel K, Mueller B, Angelillo-Scherrer A, Pabst T. Increased fibrinogen levels at diagnosis are associated with adverse outcome in patients with acute myeloid leukemia. *Hematol Oncol.* 2017;35(4):789–796. doi:10.1002/hon.2307; Casini A, de Moerloose P. Fibrinogen concentrates in hereditary fibrinogen disorders: past, present and future. *Haemophilia.* 2020;26(1):25–32. doi:10.1111/hae.13876; Casini A, Undas A, Palla R, Thachil J, de Moerloose P. Diagnosis and classification of congenital fibrinogen disorders: communication from the SSC of the ISTH. *J Thromb Haemost.* 2018;16(9):1887–1890. doi:10.1111/jth.14216; Chen X, Li S, Chen W, et al. The potential value of D-dimer to fibrinogen ratio in diagnosis of acute ischemic stroke. *J Stroke Cerebrovasc Dis.* 2020;29(8):104918. doi:10.1016/j .jstrokecerebrovasdis.2020.104918; Matsunaga S, Takai Y, Seki H. Fibrinogen for the management of critical obstetric hemorrhage. *J Obstet Gynaecol Res.* 2019;45(1):13–21. doi:10.1111/jog.13788; McBride D, Tang J, Zhang JH. Maintaining plasma fibrinogen levels and fibrinogen replacement therapies for treatment of intracranial hemorrhage. *Curr Drug Targets.* 2017;18(12):1349–1357. doi:10.2174/1389450117666 151209123857; Wang XJ, Wang Z, Zhang ZT, Qiu XS, Chen M, Chen YX. Plasma fibrinogen as a diagnostic marker of infection in patients with nonunions. *Infect Drug Resist.* 2020;13:4003–4008. doi:10.2147/IDR.S269719; Wu H, Meng Z, Pan L, Liu H, Yang X, Yongping C. Plasma fibrinogen performs better than plasma D-dimer and fibrin degradation product in the diagnosis of periprosthetic joint infection and determination of reimplantation timing. *J Arthroplasty.* 2020;35(8):2230–2236. doi:10.1016/j.arth.2020.03.055; Yin G, Man C, Huang J, et al. The prognostic role of plasma fibrinogen in adult secondary hemophagocytic lymphohistiocytosis. *Orphanet J Rare Dis.* 2020;15(1):332. doi:10.1186/s13023-020-01622-2; Zhang Z, Zhang R, Qi J, et al. The prognostic value of plasma fibrinogen level in patients with acute myeloid leukemia: a systematic review and meta-analysis. *Leuk Lymphoma.* 2020;61(11):2682–2691. doi:10.1080/10428194.2020.1780587.

- Inflammation,[7]
- Progressive liver disease,[8]
- Individuals undergoing thrombolytic therapy,[9] and
- Other signs/symptoms that could be related to altered fibrinogen levels (Table 75.1)

Monitoring

Certain conditions may require periodic monitoring of fibrinogen levels:

■ Monitor fibrinogen for risk of bleeding during catheter-directed thrombolysis with tissue plasminogen activator (tPA).[10]
■ Monitor fibrinogen for patients with disseminated intravascular coagulopathy(DIC).[11]
■ Monitor fibrinogen for hospitalized patients with COVID-19 associated coagulopathy.[12]
■ Monitor fibrinogen in individuals with severe cytokine release syndrome (CRS) undergoing chimeric antigen receptor T- cell (CAR -T) therapy.[13]

INTERPRETATION

■ Normal reference interval: 200 to 400 mg/dL[14]
■ Newborn: 125 to 300 mg/dL
■ 7 months to 16 years: 180 to 383 mg/dL
■ 17 years or more: 193 to 507 mg/dL
■ Possible critical value: less than 100 mg/dL

Table 75.2 provides target fibrinogen replacement levels for bleeding and Table 75.3[15–18] provides differential diagnoses for elevated and decreased levels of fibrinogen.

FOLLOW-UP

■ Based on the determined diagnosis, additional testing may be indicated.
■ The following tests should be done to assist in confirming the diagnosis of DIC: prolonged thrombin time (PT); prolonged prothrombin time (aPTT), direct thrombin inhibitors (DTI), D-dimer, and platelet count.[19]

TABLE 75.2: CONDITIONS ASSOCIATED WITH ALTERED LEVELS OF FIBRINOGEN	
DECREASED FIBRINOGEN LEVELS	**ELEVATED FIBRINOGEN LEVELS**
DIC	Inflammation
Abnormal fibrinolysis	Tissue damage/trauma
Large-volume blood transfusions	Infection
Severe malnutrition	Cancer
End-stage liver disease	Acute coronary syndrome
Hypofibrinogenemia	Strokes
Afibrinogenemia	Inflammatory conditions

TABLE 75.3: TARGET FIBRINOGEN REPLACEMENT LEVELS FOR BLEEDING

Cardiovascular surgery	1.5 to 2.0 g/L
Obstetrics	<2.0 g/L
Trauma	1.5 to 2.0 g/L
Hematologic malignancies	<1 g/L

Sources: Data from Levy JH, Goodnough LT. How I use fibrinogen replacement therapy in acquired bleeding. *Blood.* 2015;125(9):1387–1393. doi:10.1182/blood-2014-08-552000; Levy JH, Welsby I, Goodnough LT. Fibrinogen as a therapeutic target for bleeding: a review of critical levels and replacement therapy. *Transfusion.* 2014;54(5):1389–1405; quiz 1388. doi:10.1111/trf.12431; Kozek-Langenecker SA, Afshari A, Albaladejo P, et al. Management of severe perioperative bleeding: guidelines from the European Society of Anaesthesiology. *Eur J Anaesthesiol.* 2013;30(6):270–382. doi:10.1097/EJA.0b013e32835f4d5b; Spahn DR, Bouillon B, Cerny V, et al. Management of bleeding and coagulopathy following major trauma: an updated European guideline. *Crit Care.* 2013;17(2):R76. doi:10.1186/cc12685.

Box 75.1: Disorders of Fibrinogen

- Disseminated intravascular coagulation (DIC); major hemorrhage
- Evaluation of the effectiveness of thrombolytic therapy
- Diagnose fibrinogen deficiency, homozygous and heterozygous
- Neurologic diseases
- Tissue damage
- Hemostasis and thrombosis
- Diagnosis of joint infection
- Determine risk of cardiovascular disease

Sources: Data from Bialkower M, McLiesh H, Manderson CA, Tabor RF, Garnier G. Rapid, hand-held paper diagnostic for measuring fibrinogen concentration in blood. *Anal Chim Acta.* 2020;1102:72–83. doi:10.1016/j.aca.2019.12.046; Kattula S, Byrnes JR, Wolberg AS. Fibrinogen and fibrin in hemostasis and thrombosis. *Arterioscler Thromb Vasc Biol.* 2017;37(3):e13-e21. doi:10.1161/ATVBAHA.117.308564; Petersen MA, Ryu JK, Akassoglou K. Fibrinogen in neurological diseases: mechanisms, imaging and therapeutics. *Nat Rev Neurosci.* 2018;19(5):283–301. doi:10.1038/nrn.2018.13.

PEARLS & PITFALLS

- Females with congenital fibrinogen disorders usually have issues of pre- and post-delivery hemorrhage, menorrhagia, spontaneous abortion, and infertility.[20]
- Evidence suggests plasma fibrinogen may have a major role as a biomarker in such conditions as peri-prosthetic joint infection as compared to circulating D-dimer.[21]
- A study suggests plasma fibrinogen is similarly beneficial in diagnosing polymyalgia rheumatica as the diagnostic markers C-reactive protein (CRP) and erythrocyte sedimentation rate (ESR).[22]
- A longitudinal observational study found a positive correlation between higher fibrinogen levels and end-stage peritoneal dialysis patients' increased risk for cardiovascular disease. The results were supported by prior studies linking high fibrinogen and heart disease.[23]
- Evidence suggests non-small cell lung cancer patients with elevated fibrinogen levels not only have an increased risk of disease progression,

but a higher chance of death than patients with normal fibrinogen levels.[24]

■ Persistent elevation of plasma fibrinogen in patients with acute ischemic stroke may be associated with less favorable outcomes.[25]

■ One study concluded that the impaired fibrinolysis and fibrinogen disulfide-linked albumin complexes likely contributed to a patient's multiple cerebral infarcts.[26]

■ Fibrinogen level may be a good diagnostic marker in determining the presence of acute appendicitis, thus providing useful data to prevent unnecessary surgical intervention.[27]

■ COVID-19 patients have significantly high fibrinogen levels, increasing their risk of developing venous pulmonary embolism.[14,28]

■ The prognostic significance of fibrinogen in acute myeloid leukemia patients was evaluated at initial diagnosis. Results suggest a negative correlation between higher fibrinogen levels and overall survival and progression-free survival.[29,30]

■ Serum fibrinogen plays a significant role in distinguishing between infection around the prosthetic joint and prosthesis aseptic loosening.[31]

■ There is evidence that a causal link exists between dysfibrinogenemia and multiple sclerosis; however, further research is needed to validate this theory.[32]

PATIENT EDUCATION

■ https://www.testing.com/fibrinogen-test/
■ https://www.labtestsonline.org.au/learning/test-index/fibrinogen

RELATED DIAGNOSES AND ICD-10 CODES

Other specified coagulation defects	D68.8
Other primary thrombophilia	D68.59

• Synonyms: Hypofibrinogenemia, acquired fibrinogen abnormality, afibrinogenemia, hyperfibrinogenemia, congenital hypofibrinogenemia

REFERENCES

Full list of references can be accessed through Springer Publishing Company Connect™ at the following link: http://connect.springerpub.com/content/reference-book/978-0-8261-8843-4/part/part03/toc-part/ch075

76. FIRST TRIMESTER SCREENING

Melissa Bogle

PHYSIOLOGY REVIEW

First trimester screening tests are performed via maternal serum sampling to screen for fetal abnormalities including aneuploidy, a condition in which a cell has an incorrect number of chromosomes.[1] In particular, this screening is used to identify possible signs of Down syndrome (trisomy 21), Edwards' syndrome (trisomy 18), or Patau's syndrome (trisomy 13).[2] It can also be used as a screening mechanism for anticipated pregnancy complications such as stillbirth, infant death, intrauterine growth restriction, preterm birth, and pre-eclampsia.[3] Two specific biomarkers which are produced by the placenta become detectable in the first trimester and fluctuate throughout the pregnancy.[1] The first biomarker, pregnancy-associated plasma protein-A (PAPP-A), increases insulin-like growth factor, thus regulating glucose and amino acid transport in the placenta.[1] The second biomarker, human chorionic gonadotropin, has multiple functions including endometrial growth and maternal immune system suppression.[1]

OVERVIEW OF LABORATORY TESTS

Laboratory evaluation of human chorionic gonadotropin (hCG) and pregnancy-associated plasma protein-A (PAPP-A) can be obtained through the first trimester screening test (CPT code 81508). This screening test includes PAPP-A levels, hCG levels, and a maternal risk calculation inclusive of nuchal translucency (NT) measures.[4] When results are determined to be low risk, they can be incorporated with the second trimester values as part of an integrated testing process or sequential integrated screen (CPT code 81508).[5] The initial sample is typically collected between 10.0 weeks to 13.9 weeks' gestation. Maternal pregnancy demographics such as estimated pregnancy gestation are used for interpretation.[5] A statistic called the multiple of the median (MoM) is often used to describe and standardize biomarker levels due to variations in maternal characteristics and gestational age.[6]

INDICATIONS

Screening

- The United States Preventive Services Task Force does not currently have recommendations regarding first trimester screening with biomarkers.[7]
- The American College of Obstetricians and Gynecologists (ACOG) recommends first trimester screening be offered to all patients early in pregnancy regardless of maternal age or baseline risk.[8]

■ While offering universal screening during the first trimester is preferred, the risk of aneuploidy conditions is often higher with increased maternal age. Counseling of risk level and screening options should include this information (Figure 76.1).

Diagnosis and Evaluation

■ Low maternal PAPP-A can be associated with stillbirth, infant death, intrauterine growth restriction, preterm birth, and preeclampsia when there are no chromosomal abnormalities present.[3]

■ Abnormal biomarker levels have also been indicated in gestational diabetes, preeclampsia, and preterm labor.[3]

■ In ectopic pregnancy, hCG levels increase at a slower-than-normal rate.[6]

Monitoring

■ Low-risk results of initial FTS are often incorporated with the second trimester values as part of an integrated testing process or sequential integrated screen.[5]

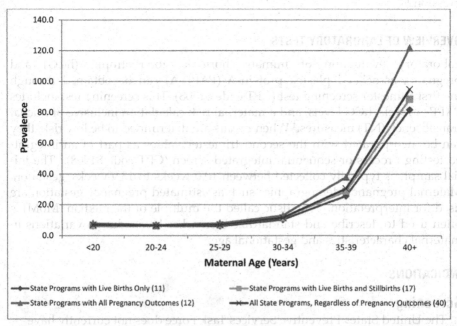

FIGURE 76.1. Pooled prevalence (per 10,000 live births) of Down syndrome by maternal age (years). *Source:* Mai CT, Kucik JE, Isenburg J, et al. Selected birth defects data from population-based birth defects surveillance programs in the United States, 2006 to 2010: Featuring trisomy conditions. *Birth Defects Res A Clin Mol Teratol.* 2013;97(11):709–725. doi:10.1002/bdra.23198.

INTERPRETATION

■ Abnormal maternal biomarkers are not diagnostic but used as a screening tool. Interpretation of results requires the combination of biomarkers along with gestational age and, ideally, a nuchal translucency ultrasound examination. Table 76.1 provides guidelines for interpretation.

FOLLOW-UP

■ For abnormal test results, diagnostic follow-up should be offered through chorionic villus sampling (CVS) or amniocentesis.

PEARLS & PITFALLS

■ Invasive diagnostic tests such as CVS and amniocentesis carry a procedure-related risk of miscarriage of about 0.3%.[9]
■ First-trimester ultrasound remains an important evaluation test with or without the serum biomarker screening.[6]
■ Levels of PAPP-A and hCG may be affected by maternal behaviors such as smoking, alcohol use, and drug use.[10]
■ Pregnant individuals with chinese genetic heritage may have a higher level of PAPP-A.[11]
■ First-trimester screening markers (hCG, PAPP-A) and nuchal translucency can vary depending on maternal weight and ethnicity.[12]
■ Some ovarian and testicular tumors can also release hCG.[6]

PATIENT EDUCATION

■ https://www.geneticsupport.org/genetics-pregnancy/prenatal-screening-tests/first-trimester-screening/?gclid=CjwKCAjwqcKF BhAhEiwAfEr7zXEJ6dvIeumvh-MMWBaAZXOa7GyeaEROEg_ mhvKxGDcEx2Fb0OxChRoC61IQAvD_BwE[13]
■ https://www.mayoclinic.org/tests-procedures/first-trimester-screening/ about/pac-20394169[14]

TABLE 76.1: MATERNAL BIOMARKERS BY TRISOMY CATEGORY		
	PAPP-A MEDIAN LEVEL	**HCG MEDIAN LEVEL**
Normal karyotype	Normal (1.0 MoM)	Normal (1.0 MoM)
Trisomy 21 (Down syndrome)	Low (0.5 MoM)	High (2.0 MoM)
Trisomy 18 (Edwards' syndrome)	Low (0.2 MoM)	Low (0.2 MoM)
Trisomy 13 (Patau's syndrome)	Low (0.3 MoM)	Low (0.5 MoM)

Source: Kagan KO, Wright D, Spencer K, Molina FS, Nicolaides KH. First-trimester screening for trisomy 21 by free beta-human chorionic gonadotropin and pregnancy-associated plasma protein-A: impact of maternal and pregnancy characteristics. *Ultrasound Obstet Gynecol.* 2008;31(5):493–502. doi:10.1002/uog.5332

RELATED DIAGNOSES AND ICD-10 CODES

Encounter for supervision of normal pregnancy, unspecified	Z34.9
Abnormal biochemical finding on antenatal screening of mother	O28.1
Supervision of high-risk pregnancy, unspecified, first trimester	O09.91

REFERENCES

Full list of references can be accessed through Springer Publishing Company Connect™ at the following link: http://connect.springerpub.com/content/reference-book/978-0-8261-8843-4/part/part03/toc-part/ch076

---

77. FOLATE

Elizabeth Wright and Kate Sustersic Gawlik

PHYSIOLOGY REVIEW

Folate is water soluble vitamin B9. The bioactive form of folate is tetrahydrofolic acid (THF). Naturally occurring folates are hydrolyzed in the intestine and converted to monoglutamates. Folic acid is a synthetic monoglutamide form of folate.[1] The monoglutamide combines with carbon fragments to convert to THF. "At least 85% of folic acid is estimated to be bioavailable when taken with food, whereas, only about 50% of folate naturally present in food is bioavailable."[1] Folates function as a coenzyme in the synthesis of DNA and RNA. It is necessary for metabolism of amino acids and biosynthesis of neurotransmitters and phospholipids. It also aids in the conversion of homocysteine to methionine. Thus, it is necessary for normal cell division and erythrocyte production. It is especially critical during early embryogenesis when rapid cell division is occurring. It is well established that a correlation exists between low folate levels and increased risk of neutral tube defects.[1]

Without folate, the body cannot form the red blood cells it needs in order to carry and deliver oxygen to all parts of the body. Without this oxygen, the body does not function as well, and anemia develops. Low levels of folate cause megaloblastic anemia, which is when the red blood cells are larger than normal, there are fewer in number, and they are oval shaped in appearance instead of round like typical erythrocytes.[1]

Folate is naturally occurring in foods such as

- Green leafy vegetables (especially spinach, Brussel sprouts, and asparagus)
- Fruits and fruit juices (bananas, oranges, peaches)
- Nuts (almonds, soya products)
- Dairy

■ Meat (especially liver, chicken, egg yolk)
■ Grains (whole wheat and enriched)

In addition, processed grains are fortified with folic acid in the United States and Canada, so folate deficiency is rare. It is seen more often in lower income countries.

OVERVIEW OF LABORATORY TESTS

Folate screening is done by examination of the serum folic acid level. Folate can be tested two ways; through the serum or within erythrocytes (red blood cell folate levels). Folates are most often tested by analysis of the serum folic acid level (CPT code 82746). There are some limitations to this testing. For example, the serum levels are influenced by food if consumed immediately prior to testing.[2]

Red blood cell folate tests (CPT code 82747) were used in the past, but now confirmatory testing is completed using other tests (typically MMA and homocysteine). The American Society for Clinical Pathology released a Choosing Wisely® guideline that recommends that clinicians do not order red blood cell folate levels at all. In lieu of testing, folate supplementation should be considered in patients with macrocytic anemia.[3]

INDICATIONS

Serum folate levels are used in the diagnosis of folate deficiency.

Screening

■ Universal screening is not recommended.

Targeted screenings are often used in the following individuals who are considered at risk for folate deficiency[4-9]:

● Patients with alcohol addiction
● Nutritional deficiency
● Malabsorptive disorders (celiac disease, inflammatory bowel disease, gastritis, gastric or bowel surgery)
● Exfoliative skin diseases
● Hemodialysis
● Pregnancy/breast feeding
● Adults older than 65 years old
● Medications (methotrexate, phenytoin)
● Patients with cancer
● Patients who have undergone bariatric surgery
● People with the MTHFR polymorphism

Diagnosis and Evaluation

Folate deficiency usually coexists with other nutrient deficiencies.
Signs and symptoms of folate deficiency anemia include[1,4]:

■ Megablastic anemia with a low reticulocyte count
■ Hypersegmented neutrophils
■ Fatigue
■ Weakness

- Headaches
- Dizziness
- Pale skin
- Decreased appetite
- Gastrointestinal signs (diarrhea, nausea, weight loss)
- Lack of energy
- Neurologic signs (tingling, burning, peripheral neuropathy)
- Psychologic signs (confusion, memory and judgment problems)
- Being irritable

Megaloblastic anemia without neuropathy is the most common clinical presentation of folate deficiency. The differential diagnoses for folate deficiency are broad and based on the initial presenting signs/symptoms. Since folate is water soluble, folate overdose/toxicity is rare.[10]

Monitoring

- Routine monitoring is recommended in patients who have undergone bariatric surgery.[9]
- There is currently no recommendation on monitoring folate serum levels following initial folate deficiency diagnosis.

INTERPRETATION

- In the clinical scenario where the patient has borderline folate deficiency results (Table 77.1), the clinician should order homocysteine and methylmalonic acid (MMA) testing. Homocysteine and MMA are both elevated in B12 deficiency, whereas only homocysteine, and not MMA, is elevated in folate deficiency.[10,11]
- An MCV value greater than 115 fL is more specific to vitamin B12 or folate deficiency than other conditions in the differential diagnosis such as hypothyroidism or myelodysplastic syndrome.
- When there is incongruence between the test result and clinical features of folate deficiency, folate treatment should not be delayed to ensure neurologic impairment is avoided.[4]

FOLLOW-UP

- Folate deficiency can occur with vitamin B12 deficiency, so these tests are often ordered together.[4]
- As previously noted, homocysteine and MMA can provide more information for diagnosis.
- Once the diagnosis of vitamin B12 and/or folate deficiency is made, additional historical information and/or testing should be used to determine the underlying cause.

TABLE 77.1: ADULT PLASMA FOLATE REFERENCE INTERVAL		
NORMAL	**BORDERLINE**	**DEFICIENT**
>4 ng/mL	2 to 4 ng/mL	<2 ng/mL

Note: Will vary by laboratory, source, and patient age.

PEARLS & PITFALLS

- All individuals who are planning on, or are capable of, pregnancy should take 0.4 to 0.8 mg of folic acid to prevent congenital neural tube defects.[12]
- Folate deficiency can be implicated with an increased risk of atherosclerosis due to high homocysteine levels.[10]
- There is some evidence that suggests that folate could be used as a supplement to augment other treatment for depression.[13]
- In older adults with or without dementia, there is no evidence that supports the role of folic acid (with or without vitamin B12) for improving cognitive function. Those older adults with high homocysteine levels do benefit from long-term folic acid supplementation.[14]

PATIENT EDUCATION

- https://www.womenshealth.gov/a-z-topics/folic-acid

RELATED DIAGNOSES AND ICD-10 CODES

Megablastic anemia	D52.1
Neural tube defects	Q05.9
Alcoholism	F10.20

REFERENCES

Full list of references can be accessed through Springer Publishing Company Connect™ at the following link: http://connect.springerpub.com/content/reference-book/978-0-8261-8843-4/part/part03/toc-part/ch077

78. GAMMA-GLUTAMYL TRANSFERASE

Pam Kibbe and Kelly Small Casler

PHYSIOLOGY REVIEW

Gamma(γ)-glutamyl transferase (GGT) is an enzyme that is present in the kidney, pancreas, liver, brain, and prostate.[1,2] It has several functions, including counteraction of oxidative stress and the production of glutamate.[3,4] GGT is activated in the presence of alcohol when the liver microsomes oxidize ethanol.[5] It has a half-life of 14 to 26 days.[4]

OVERVIEW OF LABORATORY TESTS

Although GGT is present in many tissues, laboratory evaluation methods for GGT (CPT code 82977) are structured to primarily detect GGT levels in the liver.[4]

It is often used to evaluate for cholestatic liver disease, but elevation in serum levels of GGT can also be seen in diseases of the biliary tract and pancreas. GGT is also used to assess alcohol use. Daily consumption of moderate levels of alcohol for several weeks are known to increase GGT levels, and levels can decrease after 2 weeks of abstinence.[4] The test is generally considered sensitive but not specific for both uses.[3]

GGT levels fluctuate with age and sex. GGT levels in full-term infants are six to seven times the upper limit of the normal adult range. The level declines and will plateau to low levels at 5 to 7 months of age after which there is a gradual increase through adolescence.[1,6] Males generally have higher levels of GGT.[3]

INDICATIONS

Screening

■ GGT is not used as a screening test.[7]

Diagnosis and Evaluation

■ GGT is used to assist in evaluation of elevated alkaline phosphatase (ALP) levels. An elevation of both GGT and ALP indicates liver dysfunction, namely cholestatic liver disease. However, if ALP is elevated and GGT is not, non-liver causes of ALP elevations should be considered.[8]

■ GGT is used in the evaluation of jaundice in a newborn/infant since ALP levels are less reliable in a newborn (normal levels of ALP vary in growing infants).[9]

Monitoring

■ In some instances, GGT may be used to monitor alcohol consumption in those with chronic alcoholic liver disease, but this use is not supported by the evidence. It lacks specificity for alcohol abuse, but does remain the best predictor out of all liver enzymes to detect moderate or heavy use.[10] However, when compared to self-report, GGT still misses several patients with alcohol use disorder.[11-14]

INTERPRETATION

■ Reference intervals:
  ● 16 years and older: 7 to 50 IU/L[15]
  ● Younger than 3 months of age: 4 to 120 IU/L[15]
  ● 3 months of age to 16 years old: 2 to 35 IU/L[15]
■ Increased in cholestasis, pancreas/kidney damage, obesity, alcohol abuse, diabetes, hypertriglyceridemia, or cardiovascular disease.[4,8,16]
■ Increased with medications such as phenytoin or barbiturates, carbamazepine, some antiretroviral drugs, and warfarin.[3,4,8,16,17]
■ Decreased in pregnancy.[15]

FOLLOW-UP

- If not already performed, ALP, ALT, AST, and bilirubin should be evaluated so levels can be correlated with GGT level. All are usually elevated in cholestatic liver disease.
- Alcohol consumption history should be collected if not previously, to evaluate for alcohol misuse as a cause of elevation.
- If cholestasis is suspected, imaging and other diagnostic testing for cause of cholestasis will need to be performed.

PEARLS & PITFALLS

- Elevations of GGT have been noted in COVID-19.[18]
- GGT elevations are seen in patients with cardiovascular disease[19] and may be a predictor of prognosis in genitourinary cancer.[20]
- Research is ongoing regarding the use of GGT combined with other clinical indicators to detect non-alcoholic fatty liver disease (NAFLD).[21]
- Although there is much interest in using GGT to screen for alcohol use disorders, be sure to consider the limitations of this role. One study showed it was only positive in 59% to 67% of individuals admitted to an alcohol rehabilitation program.[11] In a Finish study, it was elevated in less than 60% of heavy drinkers.[12] Its performance for pregnant patients was even worse, with a sensitivity of 26%.[13] However, it is able to differentiate between chronic rather than episodic heavy alcohol use.[16]
- Age, sex, BMI, and puberty all influence ALT, ALP, and GGT. Therefore, research is underway to see if percentiles similar to growth charts are needed for normal ranges in children.[6,22]
- If GGT is elevated in isolation of ALT, AST, and bilirubin, and if AST/ALT ratio is greater than 2, GGT elevations are more likely to be from alcohol abuse than cholestatic disease.[17]

PATIENT EDUCATION

- https://medlineplus.gov/lab-tests/gamma-glutamyl-transferase-ggt-test/

RELATED DIAGNOSES AND ICD-10 CODES

Elevated serum GGT level or abnormal GGT test	R74.8
Elevation of liver transaminase levels	R74.01

REFERENCES

Full list of references can be accessed through Springer Publishing Company Connect™ at the following link: http://connect.springerpub.com/content/reference-book/978-0-8261-8843-4/part/part03/toc-part/ch078

79. GASTRIN AND PEPSINOGEN

Kelly Small Casler

PHYSIOLOGY REVIEW

Gastrinomas are neuroendocrine tumors that arise from the duodenum or pancreas; they secrete gastrin and lead to hypergastrinemic states.[1] Gastrin, a hormone normally released by gastric cells, acts on enterochromaffin-like cells (ECL), chief cells, and parietal cells, resulting in gastric motility and gastric acid secretion.[1] Hypergastrinemia can result in a triad of symptoms (hyperchlorhydria, peptic ulcerations, and gastrinoma) known as Zollinger Ellison syndrome (ZES).[2] ZES and other hypergastrinemic states increase the risk of gastric tumors.[3]

Pepsinogen (PG) is a gastric cell enzyme used in protein digestion. PG is secreted by the chief cells of the stomach and is converted to pepsin by gastric acid. PG can be further differentiated into PG I, which is secreted by gastric fundal mucosa, and PGII, which is secreted by both fundal and other gastric mucosa.[4]

OVERVIEW OF LABORATORY TESTS

Serum gastrin and PG testing are conducted through immunoassays and are usually ordered as individual tests, though in some countries they are performed together as a gastric panel.[5,6] Both tests require fasting states.[7,8] Proton pump inhibitors (PPI) can increase gastrin levels and should be held for 1 week prior to gastrin testing[9] and for 48 hours prior to pepsinogen testing.[7] Accuracy of gastrin immunoassays is influenced by the type of gastrin tested for since there are multiple circulating forms of gastrin.[5,6,10]

INDICATIONS

Screening

- Not currently recommended. PG use in gastric cancer screening and surveillance is being researched in Asian populations at high risk of gastric cancer.[11–17]

Diagnosis and Evaluation

- Gastrin is used in combination with a measurement of gastric pH to evaluate for gastrinoma as part of the differential diagnosis for peptic ulcer disease combined with chronic diarrhea when symptoms are refractory to treatment and *Helicobacter pylori* infection has been ruled out.[1,8,9]
- Gastrin is also measured as part of a secretin stimulation test (used for gastrinoma diagnosis) and measured at 2, 5, and 10 minutes after secretin injection.[9]

Monitoring

■ Can be used to monitor for successful gastrinoma resection and gastrinoma recurrence after treatment.[2]

INTERPRETATION

■ Gastrin reference intervals vary by age but the usual reference limit is less than 100 pg/mL.[2]

■ A gastrin level greater than 1,000 pg/mL with a gastric pH lower than 2 is diagnostic of ZES.[8,9] If gastric pH is 2 or more, look for other differentials of hypergastrinemic conditions like *Helicobacter pylori*, atrophic gastritis, PPI use, vagotomy, or renal failure.[8,10,18–21]

■ If gastrin is used as part of a secretin stimulation test, a greater than 50% increase in baseline gastrin levels or level of 120 to 200 ng/mL or more within 15 minutes of secretin administration diagnoses ZES.[2,8,9]

FOLLOW-UP

■ With suspected gastrinoma, diagnostic imaging is usually performed by a specialist to determine tumor location.[9]

■ Over 60% of patients with ZES have gastrin levels below 1,000 pg/mL.[8,9] In these cases, the secretin stimulation test is the follow-up test to confirm diagnostic suspicion.

■ ZES may be a sign of multiple endocrine neoplasia (MEN)-1 syndrome. ZES in the presence of an elevated calcium is especially suspicious for MEN-1 syndrome. Laboratory evaluation of prolactin and parathyroid hormone as well as genetic testing for MEN-1 may be warranted to evaluate for MEN-1.[9]

PEARLS & PITFALLS

■ PG levels and PGI/II ratios in combination with gastrin levels are current research foci for gastrinoma screening in patients with chronic autoimmune atrophic gastritis[22] and to identify atrophic gastritis, a precursor to gastric cancer.[23–31]

■ Weaning off PPIs in suspected ZES to allow accurate testing is challenging; histamine-2 receptor antagonists can be substituted for PPIs without test interference, but are not always strong enough to control symptoms.[32,33]

■ Females have lower levels of gastrin than males.[23]

■ Gastrin levels should not be used alone to diagnose ZES; diagnostic testing should be paired with pH testing.[21]

RELATED DIAGNOSES AND ICD-10 CODES

Gastrinoma	D37.9
Gastritis, unspecified without bleeding	K29.70

REFERENCES

Full list of references can be accessed through Springer Publishing Company Connect™ at the following link: http://connect.springerpub.com/content/reference-book/978-0-8261 -8843-4/part/part03/toc-part/ch079

80. GLUCOSE (WHOLE BLOOD, SERUM, OR PLASMA)

Kelly Small Casler

PHYSIOLOGY REVIEW

Glucose is a monosaccharide and an important mediator in bodily functions. Glucose is absorbed into the body through the intestines and is also produced by the liver during gluconeogenesis (production of glucose by the liver when fasting) and glycogenolysis (breakdown of glycogen into glucose). Glucose is found in blood and interstitial space and cells. The amount of glucose in plasma is related to a balance between glucose entering circulation and being removed from circulation. There are multiple hormones that regulate glucose levels in circulation and keep it in range through activation of glycogenolysis and gluconeogenesis.[1]

OVERVIEW OF LABORATORY TESTS

Glucose can be measured in plasma or serum. Serum samples are used more often, since plasma samples must be analyzed within an hour of collection to avoid false low levels due to red blood cell glycolysis.[2] Serum samples are also preferred since they can be included as part of a basic or complete metabolic panel. Whole blood samples from arterial, venous, or capillary sources are also used to measure glucose, with capillary being the most frequently used.[3,4] Glucose can also be measured in interstitial fluid as is the case for continuous glucose monitoring.[3] It is also possible to measure glucose in pleural fluid, cerebrospinal fluid, and urine.[3]

Glucose is the most commonly used point-of-care (POC) test.[4] Measurements can be obtained from capillary whole blood[3] or in arterial blood while also performing an arterial blood gas.[5] Whole blood samples tend to read 10% to 15% lower than plasma/serum, but this can vary based on the timing of the sample (fasting vs. nonfasting) or hematocrit level.[3]

INDICATIONS

Screening

Hypoglycemia

■ Point-of-care tests are used to screen neonates at 1 to 2 hours of age for hypoglycemia of the newborn and at regular intervals up to 48 hours of age if symptoms of hypoglycemia, small for gestational age, large for gestational age, perinatal stress, premature or post-term delivery, infant of a mother with diabetes, family history of genetic hypoglycemia, and presence of congenital syndromes/abnormal physical features.[6–8]

Hyperglycemia

- Fasting plasma glucose or plasma glucose after a glucose loading dose are two of three methods recommended by the American Diabetic Association (ADA) to screen for diabetes mellitus or prediabetes.[9] Start screening at age 45 or younger if risk factors, and repeat at 3-year intervals if normal.[9] Screen people with history of prediabetes yearly due to higher risk for transition to type 2 diabetes mellitus (T2DM).[10] Note that these guidelines recommend plasma, not serum glucose, be used to screen.[9,11]
  - Screen for prediabetes and/or T2DM if body mass index (BMI) is 25 kg/ m^2 or greater, especially in patients planning pregnancy or with one or more risk factors (Boxes 80.1 and 80.2). Patients with Asian genetic heritage should be considered for screening at a BMI of 23 kg/m^2 or more.[9]
  - Screen children ages 11 and older if BMI is at the 85th percentile or higher.[9]
  - The United States Preventive Services Task Force recommends screening individuals at age 40 to 70 years with BMI at 25.0 or higher at 3-year intervals.[12]

Box 80.1: Risk Factors for Type 2 Diabetes Mellitus in Adults

- First-degree relative
- Polycystic ovarian syndrome
- HDL less than 35 mg/dL or TG greater than 250 mg/dL
- Blood pressure 140/90 or higher or on medication
- Genetic heritage of African American, Latinx, Native American, Asian American, or Pacific Islander
- Physical inactivity
- History of gestational diabetes mellitus
- Cardiovascular disease
- Acanthosis nigricans
- Human immunodeficiency virus

HDL, high density lipoprotein; TG, triglycerides.

Source: Adapted from American Diabetes Association. 2. Classification and diagnosis of diabetes: standards of medical care in diabetes-2021. *Diabetes Care.* 2021;44(suppl 1):S15–S33. doi:10.2337/dc21-S002.

Box 80.2: Risk Factors for Diabetes in Children

- First-degree or second-degree relative
- Polycystic ovarian syndrome in history
- Dyslipidemia
- Genetic heritage of African American, Latinx, Native American, Asian American, or Pacific Islander
- Physical inactivity
- Maternal history of diabetes or gestational diabetes mellitus (GDM)
- Small for gestational age birth weight
- Acanthosis nigricans

Source: Adapted from American Diabetes Association. 2. Classification and diagnosis of diabetes: standards of medical care in diabetes-2021. *Diabetes Care.* 2021;44(suppl 1):S15–S33. doi:10.2337/dc21-S002.

Diagnosis and Evaluation

■ Used to evaluate neonates, pediatric patients, and adult patients with signs/symptoms of hypoglycemia.[6,7]

■ Used to diagnose T2DM, type 1 diabetes, or prediabetes. Two different abnormal test results should be received before diagnosing. The tests could be completed with two different test types (fasting plasma glucose, glucose tolerance test, or hemoglobin A1C) on the same or additional days or using the same test type with two different samples from two different days. The latter is recommended most often.[9,12–14]

■ If there are symptoms of diabetes (hyperglycemia crisis or classic hyperglycemia symptoms) and a random plasma glucose of 200 mg/dL or more, two abnormal results are not needed.[9]

Monitoring

■ May be used for monitoring of hypoglycemic and hyperglycemic states and for response to pharmacologic therapies.

■ Patients on intensive insulin regimens should monitor glucose before meals/snacks, after meals/snacks as needed, at bedtime, during symptoms or treatment of hypoglycemia, before exercise, and before driving.[15,16]

■ Patients on basal insulin or oral medication regimens should monitor a fasting morning glucose and other times as needed.[15,16]

■ Continuous glucose monitoring is used for patients requiring insulin more than once per day.[15,16]

INTERPRETATION

■ Normal reference interval is between 70 and 110 mg/dL, but experts are considering changing the upper limit to 100 mg/dL.[13]

■ Hypoglycemia definition[13,17]:
  ● Glucose lower than 50 mg/dL in 0 to 12 months of age. Critical values are lower than 35 mg/dL.
  ● Glucose less than 70 mg/dL for ages 1 year and older. Critical values are less than 45 mg/dL.
  ● The most common differential diagnosis of hypoglycemia is an adverse reaction to diabetic medications.

■ Hyperglycemia definition[13,17]:
  ● Glucose greater than 110 mg/dL.
  ● Critical values: greater than 500 mg/dL for ages 1 year or older and greater than 325 mg/dL for ages 0 to 1 year.[17]
  ● The most-common differential diagnoses for hyperglycemia are prediabetes, diabetes, diabetic ketoacidosis, hyperglycemic hyperosmolar state (HHS), and sepsis.

■ Table 80.1 provides a summary of interpretation related to diabetes diagnosis.

■ Table 80.2[9,15,19] provides a summary of interpretation related to diabetes control.

TABLE 80.1: INTERPRETATION OF GLUCOSE FOR DIAGNOSIS OF DIABETES

	PREDIABETES (ADA)	DIABETES	ADVANTAGES[10]	DISADVANTAGES[10]
Fasting plasma glucose (FPG)	100–125 mg/dL	≥125 mg/dL	More convenient than post prandial. More sensitive than A1C.	Fasting state needed.
2 hour 75 OGTT	140–199 mg/dL	≥200 mg/DL	More sensitive than A1C and FPG	Time intensive
HgB A1C	ADA 5.7%–6.4%[10] WHO 6.0%–6.4%[18]	≥6.5%	Convenience (no fasting, less disturbance by day-to-day fluctuations in glucose from illness/stress/diet, fewer preanalytical errors	Greater cost, limited availability, less sensitivity

FPG, fasting plasma glucose.

TABLE 80.2: TARGET REFERENCE INTERVAL FOR PATENTS WITH DIABETES

	AACE (PREGNANT)	ADA (NONPREGNANT)	ADA (PREGNANT)
Postprandial 2 hours	<140 mg/dL	<180	<120
Postprandial 1 hour			<140 mg/dL
Fasting plasma glucose	<110 mg/dL	70–130	<95

Guidelines recommend individualization of treatment goals based on age and other factors.

Note: The goal for nonpregnant individuals is that they should spend 70% or more of their time in the target range (70–180 mg/dL) and less than 4% of their time should be under 70 mg/dL.

AACE, American Academy of Clinical Endocrinologists; ADA, American Diabetic Association.

Sources: Data from American Association of Clinical Endocrinology. *Type 2 Diabetes Glucose Management Goals.* 2020. https://pro .aace.com/disease-state-resources/diabetes/depth-information/type-2-diabetes-glucose-management-goals; American Diabetes Association. 2. Classification and diagnosis of diabetes: standards of medical care in diabetes-2021. Diabetes Care. 2021;44(suppl 1):S15–S33. doi:10.2337/dc21-S002; American Diabetes Association. 6. Glycemic targets: standards of medical care in diabetes-2021. *Diabetes Care.* 2021;44(suppl 1):S 73–S84. doi:10.2337/dc21-S006

FOLLOW-UP

- Follow-up testing for underlying conditions is needed for those infants who cannot maintain blood glucose concentrations greater than 50 mg/dL in the first 48 hours of life or greater than 60 mg/dL after 48 hours of life.[6]
- Follow-up testing may be needed to differentiate between type 1 diabetes and T2DM in patients with rapid appearance of hyperglycemic states.

PEARLS & PITFALLS

- Whole blood glucose concentrations can differ by 10% to 15% from serum and plasma levels so they cannot be used interchangeably.[8] Venous and whole blood should also not be used interchangeably since venous whole blood glucose levels read around 10 mg/dL higher than capillary whole blood glucose levels.[20]

- POC glucose tests are only approved for monitoring and should not be used for diagnosis or screening of diabetes; use plasma glucose or hemoglobin A1C for these indications.[3,20]
- Humidity, extremes of temperature, milking of the finger, and expired test strips can all give inaccurate readings on POC glucometers.[4]
- POC glucose testing was originally designed for home use where they have shown reduction of complications, morbidity, and mortality.[4]
- Not all glucometers have FDA approval for POC testing in critically ill patients.[4]
- Capillary glucose reading may not be accurate in critically ill patients, especially in those with anemia where there is up to 30% difference compared to laboratory received value.[5,21] Their use in this setting continues to be debated.[22]
- Although previous guidelines have included random plasma glucose (RPG) level in diagnosis of diabetes, RPG is not included in current USPSTF or ADA guidelines although a RPG of 100 mg/dL or greater was associated with an odds ratio of 20.4 for diabetes.[23]
- RPG should not be used for gestational diabetes screening.[24]
- Older glucometers use GDH-PQQ technology; non-glucose sugars can interact with these glucometers, causing false readings. Although these are no longer being manufactured, some patients may still own these glucometers.[25–27]
- Interestingly, a systematic review and Cochrane review recently noted that screening for diabetes did not reduce mortality rates, but it did help delay progression to diabetes.[28,29] Another systematic review confirmed that screening was cost-effective and saved healthcare costs related to prevention of diabetes complications.[30]
- A recent metanalysis showed that for screening, HgB A1C may lack sensitivity and specificity and fasting glucose may lack sensitivity. Additionally, screening may not have as large of an effect on the diabetes epidemic as once thought.[18]
- Patients who self-monitor blood glucose have a better chance of achieving treatment goals.[9]

PATIENT EDUCATION

- https://www.diabetes.org/risk-test

RELATED DIAGNOSES AND ICD-10 CODES

Hypoglycemia	E16.2
Hyperglycemia	R73.9

REFERENCES

Full list of references can be accessed through Springer Publishing Company Connect™ at the following link: http://connect.springerpub.com/content/reference-book/978-0-8261 -8843-4/part/part03/toc-part/ch080

81. GLUCOSE TOLERANCE TEST

Lucia M. Jenkusky and Kate Sustersic Gawlik

PHYSIOLOGY REVIEW

Gestational diabetes mellitus (GDM) is a common pregnancy complication. GDM is defined as diabetes diagnosed in the second or third trimester of pregnancy in patients who have not previously been diagnosed with diabetes prior to gestation.[1] The physiologic changes in pregnancy include a metabolic adaptation of insulin sensitivity. This sensitivity changes based on the requirements of the pregnancy. In early gestation, insulin sensitivity increases, promoting uptake of glucose into adipose stores in preparation for the energy demands of late pregnancy.[1] There is a progressive increase in postprandial glucose levels that is the result of impaired glucose tolerance due to pancreatic B-cell dysfunction.[2-4]

According to the International Diabetes Federation (IDF), in 2019, one in six births was affected by gestational diabetes with the vast majority of cases occurring in low to middle income countries where there is limited access to maternal healthcare.[5] Twenty million (16%) of all live births had some form of hyperglycemia in pregnancy with an estimated 84% due to gestational diabetes.[5] The American Diabetes Association estimates that nearly 10% of all pregnancies in the United States are affected by gestational diabetes every year.[1] Risk factors for GDM include overweight/obesity, advanced maternal age, and a family history of insulin resistance and/or diabetes. Patients who have GDM are at an increased risk for cardiovascular disease, type 2 diabetes, macrosomia and complications at birth such as instrumental delivery, increased risk for cesarean delivery, and shoulder dystocia. Infants born to individuals with preexisting diabetes or GDM are heavier at birth and have an increased risk of obesity and type 2 diabetes.[2-4] Patients who had GDM have a long-term risk of obesity and type 2 diabetes.[2-4]

OVERVIEW OF LABORATORY TESTS

The oral glucose challenge test (OGCT) (CPT code 82950) is where a blood specimen is drawn 1 hour post administration of an oral glucose solution. If this test shows elevated glucose, it is typically followed by an oral glucose tolerance test (OGTT).

The OGTT (CPT codes 82951 and 82952) is where three to four serum glucose specimens are drawn over the course of 2 to 3 hours. The first is drawn while fasting, then at specific times after the patient consumes the oral glucose solution (typically at 1-hour, 2-hour +/− 3-hour intervals).

INDICATIONS

Screening

- The American College of Obstetricians and Gynecologists (ACOG) and the United States Preventive Services Task Force recommend screening all pregnant individuals for gestational diabetes between 24 and 28 weeks gestation.[6,7] Screening is recommended only for pregnant individuals not previously found to have diabetes.[6,7] There are two options for screening and diagnosis of gestational diabetes.
  1. The "one-step" approach (2-hour glucose tolerance test): Obtain a fasting blood sample then have the patient consume 75 grams(g) of glucose as quickly as possible. A blood glucose level should then be drawn at 1 and 2 hours.
  2. The "two-step" approach: The patient consumes a 50-g (non-fasting) oral glucose solution; then, after 1 hour, the patient has their blood drawn and their glucose is tested. If this test is determined to be positive (a level of 130 to 140 mg/dL or higher depending on the institution), the patient returns at a later date for the second test. The second test is a 100-g OGTT, 3-hour diagnostic test.
- Screening for undiagnosed prediabetes and diabetes at the first prenatal visit should be completed in those with risk factors using standard diagnostic criteria. Risk factors include physical inactivity, first-degree relative with diabetes, high risk race/ethnicity (Black, Latino, Native American, Asian, Pacific Islander), prior birth of an infant weighing 4,000 g or more, previous GDM, chronic hypertension, polycystic ovary syndrome (PCOS), history of impaired glucose tolerance, insulin resistance, or history of cardiovascular disease.[6,7]

Diagnosis and Evaluation

Many individuals are asymptomatic. Signs and symptoms of gestational diabetes include:

- Polyuria
- Polyphagia
- Polydipsia
- Overweight/obesity
- Fatigue
- Diaphoresis

Differential diagnoses include:

- Type 1 diabetes mellitus
- Type 2 diabetes mellitus
- Prediabetes mellitus

Monitoring

If the diagnosis of gestational diabetes is confirmed, the patient will need to monitor their glucose levels throughout the duration of the pregnancy. According to the Choosing Wisely initiative, it is not necessary to perform antenatal testing (e.g., biophysical profile [BPP]) or nonstress test (NST) on individuals who are well controlled by diet alone and who have no other indications for testing.[8]

INTERPRETATION

The "One-Step" 75-g 2-Hour Oral Glucose Tolerance Test

The International Association of Diabetes and Pregnancy Study Group (IADPSG) and the American Diabetes Association (ADA) recommend that the following criteria establish a diagnosis of GDM for the 75-g, 2-hour OGTT:

- Fasting value, 92 mg/dL;
- 1-hour value, 180 mg/dL; or
- 2-hour value, 153 mg/dL

The diagnosis of GDM should be established when any single threshold value was met or exceeded.

The "Two-Step" Approach

For the 50-g (nonfasting) screen: Cutoff values of 130 to 140 mg/dL are used to initiate a 3-hour 100-g OGTT diagnostic test.

Of the four blood draws during the test, two or more criteria must either meet or exceed the reference levels as indicated in Table 81.1 for the diagnosis of GDM although even one abnormal value on the two-step test is associated with a significantly increased risk of adverse perinatal outcomes compared to patients without GDM and is supported by ACOG as sufficient for diagnosis.[1,6]

FOLLOW-UP

- Postpartum: Test individuals who had gestational diabetes mellitus for prediabetes or diabetes at the 4 to 12 weeks postpartum visit, using the 75-g OGTT and clinically appropriate nonpregnancy diagnostic criteria.[6]
- Health maintenance: Individuals with a history of gestational diabetes mellitus should have lifelong screening for the development of diabetes or prediabetes at least every 1 to 3 years.[6]

PEARLS & PITFALLS

- Individuals with a history of gestational diabetes mellitus found to have prediabetes should receive intensive lifestyle interventions and/or metformin to prevent diabetes.[6]

TABLE 81.1: TWO-STEP APPROACH DIAGNOSTIC CRITERIA FOR GESTATIONAL DIABETES MELLITUS	
TIME POINT	**PLASMA GLUCOSE LEVEL**
Fasting	≥ 95 mg/dL (5.1 mmol/L)
1 hour	≥ 180 mg/dL (10.0 mmol/L)
2 hours	≥ 155 mg/dL (8.5 mmol/L)
3 hours	≥ 140 mg/dL (7.8 mmol/L)

Note: The American Diabetes Association states there must be two or more abnormal values on the 3-hour oral glucose tolerance test for diagnosis; however, the American College of Obstetricians and Gynecologists states that one abnormal value meets criteria for diagnosis.

- Individuals with a history of depression or vitamin D insufficiency may be at an increased risk of gestational diabetes.[9–10]
- When a patient has the diagnosis of GDM, they have a twofold higher risk of cardiovascular events postpartum compared with their peers.[10]
- There is a significant but not strong association between thyroid antibodies and the risk of GDM.[10]

PATIENT EDUCATION

- https://www.acog.org/womens-health/faqs/gestational-diabetes
- https://www.cdc.gov/reproductivehealth/maternalinfanthealth/diabetes -during-pregnancy.htm
- https://www.diabetes.org/diabetes/gestational-diabetes

RELATED DIAGNOSES AND ICD-10 CODES

Gestational diabetes mellitus in pregnancy, unspecified control	O24.419
Preexisting type 2 diabetes mellitus in pregnancy, unspecified trimester	O24.119
Preexisting type 1 diabetes mellitus in pregnancy, unspecified trimester	O24.019

REFERENCES

Full list of references can be accessed through Springer Publishing Company Connect™ at the following link: http://connect.springerpub.com/content/reference-book/978-0-8261 -8843-4/part/part03/toc-part/ch081

---

82. GONORRHEA AND CHLAMYDIA

Deanna Hunt and Courtney DuBois Shihabuddin

PHYSIOLOGY REVIEW

Gonorrhea and chlamydia are two of the most common sexually transmitted infections, both transmitted almost exclusively through sexual contact. Coinfection with both gonorrhea and chlamydia is common and both are reported communicable diseases within the United States. Chlamydia is caused by the bacteria *Chlamydia trachomatis* and gonorrhea is caused by the bacteria *Neisseria gonorrhoeae*.[1] Gonorrhea and chlamydia are most common in younger people, aged 15 to 24 years.[1,2] Gonorrhea can infect the cervix, uterus, fallopian tubes, mouth, throat, eyes, and rectum.[2] Chlamydia and gonorrhea, if left untreated, can lead to serious consequences including pelvic inflammatory disease (PID), infertility, ectopic pregnancy, and chronic pelvic pain.[1]

OVERVIEW OF LABORATORY TESTS

Molecular tests, specifically nucleic acid amplification tests (NAATs), are the most used tests for gonorrhea and chlamydia testing.[3] These tests are highly sensitive and as a result are considered the standard of care. The optimal urogenital specimen types when using NAATs include the first-catch urine in patients with a penis and vaginal swabs in patients with a vagina.[1,2,4] However, laboratory evaluation of chlamydia and gonorrhea in patients with a vagina can be assessed by testing first-catch urine (CPT codes 87491 and 87591) or by the collection of vaginal or endocervical cells (CPT codes 87491, 87563, 87591, 87798). Another option for NAAT testing in patients with a vagina is with a brush, spatula, or broom during a liquid-based Pap test. While this is an acceptable method and convenient for patients who are already undergoing a Pap test, the test sensitivity might be lower compared with cervical or vaginal swabs.[5] In patients with a penis, laboratory evaluation can be assessed through a urethral swab (CPT codes 87491, 87563, 87591, 87798) or first-catch urine (CPT codes 87491 and 87591). NAAT testing can now also be completed with anal and oropharyngeal swabs (extragenital sites) in those patients with receptive anal intercourse or receptive oral intercourse history.[6,7]

An alternative laboratory evaluation for gonorrhea and chlamydia is a cell culture (Chlamydia CPT codes 87110 and 87140). The culture differs from an NAAT test because with a culture, an endocervical or urethral swab specimen is required. A cell culture and detection of the chlamydia or gonorrhea is completed using fluorescent antibody staining.[4] A notable difference in the testing of gonorrhea and chlamydia is the use of Gram staining. Gram staining is less commonly used when testing for gonorrhea despite the benefits in certain situations. A Gram stain of urethral secretions has a high specificity and sensitivity if it demonstrates polymorphonuclear leukocytes with intracellular Gram-negative diplococci.[5]

Self-collection kits and point-of-care (POC) tests are available for the testing of gonorrhea and chlamydia, providing the patient with comfort, ease, and autonomy. Based on high levels of evidence (systematic review, large cross-sectional study), there is sufficient evidence to support not only self-obtained vaginal swab samples, but POC tests for gonorrhea and chlamydia testing as well.[6,8-10] Currently, POC tests are available, and many more options for POC tests are slated to launch, pending improvement of current suboptimal sensitivity.[11] Rapid POC tests are available that use either antibody or NAAT methods. In a systematic review of the listed assays, it was found that while chlamydia antigen detection rapid POC tests demonstrated high specificity (97% to 100%), their sensitivity was much lower.[12] Antibody tests are also available for detection of gonorrhea. Just as the POC chlamydia test demonstrated, POC gonorrheal tests also have high specificity, but lower sensitivity. Due to the sensitivities, antibody tests for chlamydia and gonorrhea are not recommended. Currently, there are three NAAT-based options for the POC diagnosis of chlamydia and gonorrhea; however, only one is available in the United States, the GeneXpert system (Cepheid).[13] Self-collection NAAT kits are a valuable method for testing and are equivalent in sensitivity and specificity compared with clinician-collected samples.[1,14] When using both self-collection kits and POC tests, a patient can receive results quicker than the standard sample taken in a clinic setting.

INDICATIONS

Screening

Of Extragenital Sites

■ Men who have sex with men (MSM) should be screened at the anatomical site (rectal, pharyngeal, or urethral) most likely to have been exposed for proper disease identification and treatment.[15,16] Extragenital sites, specifically the oropharynx and rectum, are more likely to test positive for gonorrhea and/or chlamydia in asymptomatic MSM. The urogenital tract will only test positive for insertive MSM and women who have vaginal intercourse.[17–19]

■ Some studies have shown there may be a benefit to begin screening sexually active adolescents (14 to 17+) for extragenital gonorrhea and chlamydia.[20]

■ There are no recommendations to routinely screen for rectal chlamydia infections in patients with a vagina, including in those who report anal sex.[21] This is because the adverse consequences of undetected, untreated infection at this site are not known.[22] These patients, however, should be educated about the risk of extragenital infection and may be offered screening.[23,24]

Of Urogenital Tract

■ The United States Preventive Services Task Force (USPSTF) recommends annual screening for sexually active patients with a vagina aged 24 years or younger, and those older who are at increased risk of infection (Box 82.1).[25]

■ The Centers for Disease and Control and Prevention (CDC) recommend annual screening for
  ● Sexually active patients with a vagina under 25 years of age and those 25 years and older who are at increased risk (Box 82.1).[26]
  ● Sexually active men who have sex with men (MSM)[26]
  ● All pregnant patients under 25 years of age[26]
  ● Pregnant patients, aged 25 years and older who are at increased risk[26]

Diagnosis and Evaluation

■ Testing is indicated in the presence of signs and symptoms suggestive of gonorrhea/chlamydia infection.

Box 82.1: Factors Placing Patients at Increased Risk of Gonorrhea/Chlamydia

■ New or multiple sex partners[25]
■ Aged 20 to 24 years[25]
■ Sex partner with concurrent partners[25]
■ Those in high-risk fields (exchanging sex for money or drugs)[25,26]
■ History of STIs[25]
■ Those who are not in a mutually monogamous relationship[25]
■ Inconsistent condom use[25]

- Dysuria
- Urethral discharge
- Vaginal discharge
- Pelvic inflammatory disease
- Post-coital vaginal bleeding
- Dyspareunia

Monitoring

- A test-of-cure for chlamydia can occur as late as 3 months after but no earlier than 3 weeks after treatment in patients with[23,26]:
  - Persistent symptoms
  - Pregnancy
  - Previous treatment with suboptimal regimen, such as azithromycin, doxycycline, levofloxacin, or ofloxacin
- A test-of-cure for treatment of uncomplicated gonorrhea is not necessary, assuming the patient received treatment with ceftriaxone and is having no additional symptoms.[27]
- If performing a test-of-cure for gonorrhea, perform it at least 7 days following therapy if using a culture or at least 14 days if using NAATs.[27]

INTERPRETATION

- NAATs will return as either positive or negative.
- A Gram stain is suggestive of gonorrhea if staining demonstrates polymorphonuclear leukocytes with intracellular Gram-negative diplococci.[5]

FOLLOW-UP

- In cases of gonorrheal treatment failure, a culture and antimicrobial susceptibility test should be ordered (nonculture tests including NAAT cannot provide susceptibility).[28]

PEARLS & PITFALLS

- Sex partners should be tested and considered for presumptive treatment if they have had sexual contact with the partner within the last 60 days.[26]
- Asymptomatic presentation of gonorrhea and chlamydia is common, which is why screening is important.[29,30]
- Gonorrhea and chlamydia are reportable diseases in all states.[31]
- Gonorrhea and chlamydia can facilitate the transmission of HIV infection.[32]
- Pregnant individuals infected with chlamydia can pass the infection to their infants during delivery, potentially resulting in ophthalmia neonatorum, which can lead to blindness, and pneumonia.[33]
- Self-collected vaginal swabs appear to be more sensitive for diagnosing gonorrhea and chlamydia than health-professional-collected swabs and/or first catch urine samples. When a pelvic examination is not required, self-collected vaginal swabs are recommended.[8]

PATIENT EDUCATION

- https://www.cdc.gov/std/
- https://www.cdc.gov/std/healthcomm/fact_sheets.htm (STD Fact Sheets)
- https://www.cdc.gov/std/prevention/NextSteps-GonorrheaOrChlamydia.htm (Next Steps)

RELATED DIAGNOSES AND ICD-10 CODES

Gonorrhea (acute, chronic)	A54.9	Gonococcal pharyngitis	A54.5
Screening for gonorrhea	Z11.3	Gonococcal infection of anus and rectum	A54.6
Chlamydia	A74.9	Chlamydial infection of pharynx	A56.4
Screening for chlamydia	Z13.8	Chlamydial infection of anus and rectum	A56.3

REFERENCES

Full list of references can be accessed through Springer Publishing Company Connect™ at the following link: http://connect.springerpub.com/content/reference-book/978-0-8261-8843-4/part/part03/toc-part/ch082

83. GRAM STAIN, CULTURE, AND SENSITIVITIES

Kelly Small Casler

PHYSIOLOGY REVIEW

Bacteria, viruses, and fungi may exist as normal flora or, in other instances, may cause infectious diseases. Bacteria are single-celled organisms without a nucleus and are usually categorized as either aerobic or anaerobic. Aerobic bacteria can only survive in the presence of oxygen, although some, called facultative aerobes, can shift their metabolism to survive if oxygen is absent. Anaerobic bacteria do not require oxygen for survival and, in fact, may die when exposed to it. However, facultative anaerobes do not die in the presence of oxygen but may not be able to replicate when exposed. Some bacteria, called fastidious bacteria, have complex growth requirements, and replicate slowly. These bacteria may not grow readily in usual culture mediums. Other bacteria can produce spores (e.g., Bacillus or clostridium) allowing them to survive in dormant states and hostile environments.[1] Viruses are infectious microbes that, unlike bacteria, require a host cell to replicate and contain their own genetic material. Fungi also contain their own genetic material and reproduce by forming spores.

OVERVIEW OF LABORATORY TESTS

Gram stain, culture, and sensitivities can be performed on a variety of specimens (Table 83.1) and are useful in the differential diagnosis of suspected infections. They have been the traditional gold standard laboratory test to diagnose significant infections and guide antimicrobial therapy. Over time, however, molecular testing has replaced culture for some common complaints like pharyngitis. This trend may continue to reduce the need for Gram stain, culture, and sensitivities.[2] Gram stains (CPT code 87205) can be performed relatively quickly (within 15 minutes) after obtaining a sample, but are usually performed after sample incubation for 24 hours at 35 °C. Gram stain provides a general categorization of bacterium as either gram positive or gram negative based on

TABLE 83.1: SPECIMEN COLLECTION SITES FOR GRAM STAIN, CULTURE, AND SENSITIVITY

SPECIMEN SITE	INDICATIONS	COLLECTED THROUGH
Joint/synovial fluid	Swollen, fluid-filled joint and signs/symptoms of infection	Arthrocentesis
Peritoneal fluid	Spontaneous bacterial peritonitis	Pericentesis
Pleural fluid	Pleural effusion and signs/symptoms of infection	Pleurocentesis
Pericardial fluid	Pericardial effusion	Pericardiocentesis
Sputum	Cough, suspicion of tuberculosis	Bronchoscopy or induced sputum sample
Throat*	Pharyngitis when suspected to be due to streptococcus or gonorrhea	Posterior oropharynx swab
CSF	Fever, headache, nuchal rigidity	Lumbar puncture
Eye	Purulent drainage	Swab of conjunctiva or cornea
Vaginal/cervical*	Purulent vaginal/cervical drainage	Swab to collect secretions
Urine	Pyelonephritis or complicated cystitis	Clean catch, suprapubic or catheter aspiration
Wound/tissues	Nonhealing wound, signs/symptoms of infection	Incision and drainage, aspiration, or swab
		Surgical irrigation or debridement
Nail	Thickened hypertrophic nails suspicious for onychomycosis	Nail clipping
Stool	Severe diarrhea/dysentery	Stool sample
Blood	Sepsis/signs or symptoms of bacteremia	Venous or arterial blood draw
Bone	Suspected osteomyelitis (nonhealing fracture, pain)	

*Denotes specimens where Gram stain, culture, and sensitivities have mostly been replaced with molecular tests.

CSF, cerebrospinal fluid; TB, tuberculosis.

whether they retain the Gram stain dye.[3] They are also categorized as rods or cocci, based on morphology. This preliminary information along with knowledge of bacteria associated with the site of infection (Table 83.2) allows the clinician to begin treatment for the most likely cause. Gram stain interpretation may be complicated in the presence of anaerobic bacteria given that gram-positive anaerobic bacteria may not retain the dye (e.g., Clostridium).[4] After Gram stain, specimens are allowed to incubate for 48 to 120 hours post-collection, depending on the growth rate of the suspected microbe.[1,3,5] Some cultures, such as blood cultures, may be separated into different mediums so that testing can

TABLE 83.2: SUSPECTED BACTERIAL CAUSE BASED ON PRELIMINARY GRAM STAIN RESULTS AND SUSPECTED SOURCE OF INFECTION

SOURCE/TYPE OF INFECTION	MOST COMMON BACTERIAL CAUSES OF INFECTION BASED ON GRAM STAIN RESULTS
Meningitis	**Gr + bacilli:** Listeria mycytogenes **Gram + cocci:** Streptococcus agalactiae **Gram neg cocci:** Neisseria meningitidis
UTI	**Gram + cocci:** Enterococcus faecalis* & Enterococcus faecium* **Gram neg bacilli:** Escherichia coli, Klebsiella, Proteus, Enterobacter
PNA	**Gr + bacilli:** Nocardia, Bacillus antracis **Gram + cocci:** Pseudomonas aeruginosa (immunocompromised hosts) Enterobacter, Klebsiella, Serratia*
Bacteremia	**Gram + bacilli:** Listeria mycytogenes **Gram + cocci:** Enterococcus faecalis & Enterococcus faecium, Streptococcus agalactiae (in neonates), Staphylococcus aureus **Gram neg bacilli:** Escherichia coli, Klebsiella, Enterobacter
Diarrhea	**Gram neg bacilli:** Campylobacter, Escherichia coli, Salmonella, Shigella **Anaerobic Gram +:** Propionibacterium acnes, Clostridium difficile
Typhoid fever	**Gram neg bacilli:** Salmonella
Tetanus	**Anaerobic Gram +:** Clostridium tetani
Intraabdominal infections	**Anaerobic Gram neg:** Prevotella, Bacteroides fragilis
Soft tissue/Skin	**Gr + bacilli:** Nocardia, Bacillus antracis **Gram + cocci:** Staphyococcus aureus, Streptococcus pyogenes (group A β-hemolytic Streptococcus) **Gram neg bacilli:** Vibrio **Anaerobic Gram +:** Clostridium perfringens **Anaerobic Gram neg:** Prevotella, Fusobacterium
Diptheria	**Gr + bacilli:** Corynebacterium diphtheriae

(continued)

TABLE 83.2: SUSPECTED BACTERIAL CAUSE BASED ON PRELIMINARY GRAM STAIN RESULTS AND SUSPECTED SOURCE OF INFECTION (*continued*)	
SOURCE/TYPE OF INFECTION	**MOST COMMON BACTERIAL CAUSES OF INFECTION BASED ON GRAM STAIN RESULTS**
Brain abscess	**Gr + bacilli:** Nocardia
Bioterrorism	**Gr + bacilli:** Bacillus antracis
Toxic shock syndrome	**Gram + cocci:** Staphylococcus aureus
Pharyngitis	**Gram + cocci:** Streptococcus pyogenes (group A β-hemolytic Streptococcus)
Immuno-compromised hosts	**Gram neg bacilli:** Pseudomonas aeruginosa (PNA), Acinetobacter baumanii
Diabetic foot wound*	**Gram + cocci:** Staphylococcus aureus, streptococcus **Gram neg bacilli:** Pseudomonas
Endocarditis	**Gram + cocci:** Staphylococcus lugdunensis
Foreign body	**Anaerobic Gram +:** Propionibacterium
Other	**Gram neg bacilli:** Brucella, Bordetella, Haemophilis, Legionella, Helcobacter, Neisseria gonorrhoeae, Moraxella catarrhalis **Anaerobic Gram +:** Actinomyces israelii

*Diabetic foot wounds are often polymicrobial.

+, positive; neg, negative; PNA, pneumonia; UTI, urinary tract infection.

Sources: Data from Hall G, Woods G. 58. Medical bacteriology. In: McPherson RA, Pincus MR, eds. *Henry's Clinical Diagnosis and Management by Laboratory Methods.* 23rd ed. Elsevier; 2017:1114–1152; Lipsky BA, Berendt AR, Cornia PB, et al. Executive summary: 2012 Infectious Diseases Society of America clinical practice guideline for the diagnosis and treatment of diabetic foot infectionsa. *Clin Infect Dis.* 2012;54(12):1679–1684. doi:10.1093/cid/cis460

be done for both anaerobic bacteria and aerobic bacteria.[6,7] In the absence of bacterial growth, bacterial cultures may be retained to incubate longer than 120 hours to evaluate if fungi could be present, although when clinician suspicion is high it should be communicated to laboratory personnel as not all laboratories operate under this protocol.[3,8] Additionally, cultures of suspected fungi may require up to 4 weeks of incubation and special growth medium to obtain microbes for identification.

After identification of bacteria, susceptibility testing can be performed and is particularly useful to identify antibiotic-resistant organisms. This is one advantage of performing cultures over newer molecular microbial testing, although molecular testing techniques are being designed to identify resistant microbes.[9] Antibiotics chosen in susceptibility testing are decided by a laboratory leadership team comprised of medical staff, infectious disease specialists, and laboratory clinicians using guidance from the Clinical & Laboratory Standards Institute (CLSI) and knowledge of local antimicrobial resistance patterns.[9] Minimum inhibitory concentrations (MIC) are determined, which are defined as the least antibiotic concentration that limits the visible growth of the organism outside the body (in vitro).[9] MIC thresholds are predetermined

TABLE 83.3: CULTURE MEDIUMS REQUIRED BASED ON DIFFERENTIAL DIAGNOSIS	
DIFFERENTIAL DIAGNOSIS	**CULTURE MEDIUM USED BY LABORATORY PERSONNEL**
Neisseria gonorrhea; Haemophilus	Chocolate blood agar
Legionella/nocardia	Charcoal yeast medium
N. gonorrhoeae; Haemophilus	Thayer-Martin media
Fungal	Glucose agar/potato dextrose agar
Bordetella	Regan-Lowe or Bordet-Gengou agar
Nonfastidious gram negative: Shigella, pseudomonas, proteus, salmonella, Escherichia coli, Enterobacter, and Klebsiella	MacConkey
Most others (standard culture medium)	Blood agar

Sources: Data from Hall G, Woods G. 58. Medical bacteriology. In: McPherson RA, Pincus MR, eds. *Henry's Clinical Diagnosis and Management by Laboratory Methods.* 23rd ed. Elsevier; 2017:1114–1152; Snyder LM, Rao LV, Wallach JB. *Wallach's Interpretation of Diagnostic Tests: Pathways to Arriving at a Clinical Diagnosis.* Wolters Kluwer; 2021; de la Maza LM, Pezzlo MT, Bittencourt CE, Peterson EM. *Color Atlas of Medical Bacteriology.* Wiley; 2020:338–366. doi:10.1128/9781683671077.ch41; Willinger B. Culture-based techniques. In: Lion T, ed. *Human Fungal Pathogen Identification.* Vol 1508. Methods in Molecular Biology. Springer Publishing Company; 2017:195–207. doi:10.1007/978-1-4939-6515-1_10

using disc diffusion methods to categorize the concentration of antibiotic needed to limit growth. Based on these thresholds, the bacterium will be categorized as susceptible, intermediate, or resistant to antimicrobial therapy.[9]

Other tests can be used to complement Gram stain and culture when specific microbes are suspected. One example is the acid-fast test for acid-fast bacteria like *Mycobacterium tuberculosis*, atypical mycobacterium (e.g., *Mycobacterium abscessus*), and nocardia. In this test, a stain is applied and then an acid alcohol is applied which should remove the stain. However, acid-fast bacteria can resist the acid alcohol that normally decolors the original stain.[10] A coagulase test is a second example, and is performed to differentiate between *Staphylococcus (s.) aureus* and other types of staphylococcus (*S. epidermis* and *S. saprophyticus*).[10] The latter do not produce the enzyme, coagulase, which causes plasma to clot.

Clinicians should take care to develop a complete differential diagnoses list when ordering cultures and communicate the diagnoses of concern to the laboratory since specific pathogens of interest may require unique culture mediums or laboratory procedures (Table 83.3).[6] Viral, fungal, aerobic, and/or anaerobic bacterial cultures can be ordered using individual or concurrent orders for each based on the differential diagnosis list. Gram stain and sensitivities are usually included as part of aerobic and anaerobic cultures.

INDICATIONS FOR GRAM STAIN, CULTURE, AND SENSITIVITIES OF BLOOD

Screening

- Universal screening is not indicated.
- Blood cultures may be used in targeted screening for bacteremia in conditions with a known risk (Table 83.4).

TABLE 83.4: RISK OF BACTEREMIA BY CONDITION		
LOWER RISK*	**INTERMEDIATE RISK***	**HIGH RISK**
Complicated UTI in adult	Pyelonephritis	Ventricular shunts
Pediatric UTI	Nonvascular shunts	Discitis
	Prostethic vertebral osteomyelitis	Catheter-associated bloodstream infection

* Blood culture is used in these instances, mostly when there is a risk for endovascular infection or if primary site of infection cannot be cultured.

UTI, urinary tract infection.

Source: Data from Fabre V, Sharara SL, Salinas AB, Carroll KC, Desai S, Cosgrove SE. Does this patient need blood cultures? A scoping review of indications for blood cultures in adult nonneutropenic inpatients. *Clin Infect Dis.* 2020;71(5):1339–1347. doi:10.1093/cid/ciaa039.

Diagnosis and Evaluation

■ A Gram stain with follow-up blood culture is the current gold standard test to evaluate for suspicion of bacteremia as in the case of sepsis, endocarditis, or endovascular infections.[3,11]

Monitoring

■ Use to document resolution of bacteremia in children when bacteremia is caused by *Staphylcoccus aureus* respiratory infection. It is not generally recommended to document resolution of other causes of bacteremia related to pneumonia (i.e., pneumococcus).[12]
■ Used in monitoring, at 48 hours after initial blood culture, to check for clearance of bacteremia in the following circumstances[11]:
  ● Infection with candida, *S. aureus*, and *S. lugdunensis*
  ● Catheter-related bloodstream infections before replacing catheters
  ● Infective endocarditis/endovascular infection

INDICATIONS FOR GRAM STAIN, CULTURE, AND SENSITIVITIES OF SKIN/WOUNDS

Screening

■ Not indicated.

Diagnosis and Evaluation

■ Due to improved patient outcomes when used, Gram stain, culture, and sensitivities are recommended to guide antibiotic treatment after abscess incision and drainage.[13–16] Culture is likely unnecessary for mild abscesses.[14,17]
■ Can be used (but often not required) for ecthyma and impetigo-like lesions to help differentiate between *S. aureus* and beta hemolytic strep.[14]
■ Used in the presence of wounds with purulent exudate, warmth, erythema, and edema. These signs are not always present so Gram stain, culture, and sensitivities should also be considered in the setting of increased pain, wound necrosis, prolonged wound healing, and wound bed deterioration.[18]

Monitoring

- Not used.

INDICATIONS FOR GRAM STAIN, CULTURE, AND SENSITIVITIES OF OROPHARYNX AND SPUTUM

Screening

- Not indicated.

Diagnosis and Evaluation

- In suspected streptococcal sore throat, a throat culture is indicated to follow-up negative rapid antigen tests in children and is optional in adults. Throat culture is not needed if a molecular testing for streptococcal sore throat is chosen instead of rapid antigen tests.[2]
- Sputum samples for acid-fast bacteria smear and culture can be used to evaluate for suspected tuberculosis (TB) in patients with suspicious signs/ symptoms: Cough for longer than 3 weeks, hemoptysis, chest pain, loss of appetite, night sweats, fever, fatigue, and unexplained weight loss.[19] Recognize that false positives and false negatives are both common and three specimens should be collected in addition to molecular tests.[20]
- Sputum samples can be used to evaluate for suspected community acquired pneumonia (CAP) or healthcare-associated pneumonia:
  - In hospitalized adults and children who can produce random sputum specimens[12]
  - Through tracheal aspirates obtained at the time of endotracheal intubation[12]
- Sputum samples can be used to evaluate for hospital-acquired pneumonia/ ventilator-associated pneumonia (VAP) using:
  - Noninvasive methods in non-intubated patients[21,22]
  - Endotracheal aspirates or bronchial aspirates in intubated patients Endotracheal aspirates have more risk of contamination, however.[21]

Monitoring

- Sputum cultures are not used in monitoring of infection, even in patients with tuberculosis.[23]

INTERPRETATION

- Gram stains report bacteria as gram negative or gram positive and as rods or cocci. Cultures are reported as positive or negative, based on the ability to grow microbes and will also include a report of the number and amount of microbes identified (colony count). Sensitivities will report susceptibility of organisms to a variety of antibiotics as susceptible, resistant, or indeterminate.
- When interpreting blood culture reports, interpret in the context of both sets together. For example, one positive culture out of two sets may represent contamination, especially if positive for certain microbes associated with

Box 83.1: Results on Blood Culture Representing Possible Contamination

- Coagulase negative staph
- Corynebacterium species
- Propionibacterium acnes
- Bacillus species
- Viridans streptococci
- Clostridiium perfringens

Sources: Data from Hall KK, Lyman JA. Updated review of blood culture contamination. *Clin Microbiol Rev.* 2006;19(4):788–802. doi:10.1128/CMR.00062-05; Hall G, Woods G. 58. Medical bacteriology. In: McPherson RA, Pincus MR, eds. *Henry's Clinical Diagnosis and Management by Laboratory Methods.* 23rd ed. Elsevier; 2017:1114–1152.

contamination (Box 83.1). Two positive cultures are more likely to represent true bactermeia.[24]
- Interpret blood culture in concordance with gram stain. If a gram stain is positive for an organism, but the culture is negative, consider the possibility of bacteremia caused by a bacteria that may have been missed due to incorrect media use or slow growth (fastidious bacteria or anerobic).[5,25]
- When identified on blood cultures, the following should always be considered a true positive: *Streptococcus pyogenes, Streptococcus agalactiae, Listeria monocytogenes, Neisseria meningitidis, Neisseria gonorrhoeae, Haemophilus influenzae, Bacteroides fragilis, Candida, Cryptococcus neoformans; Staphylococcus aureus, Streptococcus pneumoniae, Escherichia coli, Enterobacteriaceae,* and *Pseudomonas aeruginosa.*[1,24,26,27]

FOLLOW-UP

Blood Cultures
- Perform another set of blood cultures at 48 hours for a patient with one of two blood cultures positive for coagulase negative staphylocci if the patient is immunocompromised, has suspected bacteremia, or has a prosthesis or intravascular catheter.[11]
- Perform another set of blood cultures if there is persistent bacteremia without ability to address the source (retained vascular catheter).[11]
- Microbial tests that look for multiple organisms can be used as an adjuvant to Gram stain and culture when needed.[28] One example includes a test for 19 bacteria and six fungal pathogens, which provides results in 5 hours or less.[29,30]

Wound Cultures
- Patients with wound infection should be monitored for signs or symptoms of systemic inflammatory response syndrome and sepsis.[14]

Sputum/Oropharynx
- Molecular tests are used as adjuvants or as replacements for Gram stain, culture, and sensitivities.

PEARLS & PITFALLS

Blood Cultures

- Blood cultures should be obtained concurrently with culture of intravenous catheters. Five centimeters of the catheter tip should be provided to the laboratory.[6]
- Concurrent blood cultures should be performed at the time of cerebrospinal fluid (CSF) culture.[6]
- It is possible that low concentrations of microbes (fewer than 10,000 org/mL) can cause clinically important infections that may be missed by Gram stain and culture.[5]
- Always remember to only order cultures if results will impact management.[11]
- In patients with sepsis, blood cultures are usually mandated by the U.S. Centers for Medicare and Medicaid Services (CMS) as part of a severe sepsis management bundle even though blood cultures may only be positive in 25% of patients with sepsis.[11]
- Fever and leukocytosis have low association with bacteremia and are not considered indications for blood cultures on their own.[11]
- Blood cultures are rarely needed for fever within 48 hours of surgical procedures, community-acquired pneumonia, healthcare associated pneumonia, cystitis, prostatitis, and cellulitis unless unique situations exist (e.g., immunocompromise).[11]
- Proper collection is paramount since many microbes (especially anaerobic) are part of normal skin flora.[1] For blood cultures, skin cleansing with chlorhexidine gluconate (CHG), iodine tincture, or chlorine peroxide provides less risk of contamination compared to povidine iodine as long as CHG and iodine are allowed to dry for 30 seconds.[6,31] If povidine iodine is the only option (infants younger than 2 months), 90 seconds is required for drying time.[6]
- Blood cultures are subject to both false positives (contamination rates as high as 50% to 85% in one review)[24,32] and false negatives (up to 70% in one study).[3]
- It is important to stay tuned to local facility quality control measures and blood culture contamination rates to help maintain a goal of less than 2% of all blood cultures being contaminated.[33]
- Blood cultures may be least sensitive in patients already receiving antibiotic therapy or when bacteremia is due to slow growing microbes.[3] Always strive to obtain culture prior to initiation of antibiotic therapy.
- It is challenging to grow yeast from blood cultures. In cases of suspected candidemia, cultures can be negative in up to half of patients.[1]
- Always interpret culture results in the context of the patient's clinical situation. The possibility of contamination must always be considered when interpreting blood culture results.[24] Conversely, low colony counts do not always equate to contamination.[1]
- When it is determined that blood cultures are indicated, two sets (each set includes one bottle with aerobic medium and one with anaerobic medium) should be drawn, each from a separate site. There is no optimal time frame

between each set of blood cultures, but they should ideally be collected within 24 hours of each other.[34]

- Greater than two sets of blood cultures may be required in the presence of endocarditis.[11]

Wound

- Do not perform cultures for cellulitis unless there is presence of neutropenia or immunocompromise.[14]
- Cultures are likely not needed for mild abscesses as long as there are no underlying medical conditions.[1,5,6]
- For diabetic foot infections or other wounds without an abscess, superficial wound cultures lack adequate sensitivity/specificity.[35] Deep tissue culture obtained through curettage or biopsy is recommended after appropriate wound debridement, especially for complicated wounds.[13,36-39] Needle aspirate could also be used.[18,40] If osteomyelitis is suspected, bone biopsy should be obtained at the time of debridement.[13]
- When there is no other choice, superficial wound culture is acceptable[41] and should be obtained from the deepest part of the wound using the Levine (rotating the swab over a 1- to 2-cm area of the wound) or zig-zag ("Z") technique. Care should be used to not touch the edge of the wound.[40,42] When swabbing is required, consider using flocked swabs (fibers of multiple lengths) or swabs coated in a way to enhance collection of pathogens.[6,40]
- Order both aerobic and anaerobic cultures for patients with diabetes.[13,38]
- Samples for culture and sensitivity should be collected before starting antibiotics.[6]
- Be specific when labeling wound samples for Gram stain and culture. For example, use "plantar aspect of left great toe, puncture wound" instead of "left great toe."[6]
- Extensive biofilms can cause false-negative wound cultures.[36]
- If candidiasis is a differential and fungal culture is required, samples should be obtained from satellite lesions, scaling borders, or moist areas as they are most likely to yield positive culture.[8]
- Make sure to remove any topical treatments before obtaining cultures.[8]

Sputum/Throat Cultures

- Mycobacterium sputum cultures require 1 to 2 weeks of incubation.[20]
- Collecting three sputum samples still only results in 70% sensitivity for tuberculosis.[20]
- In some studies, using sputum Gram stain and cultures to guide CAP treatment shortened length of stay and reduced costs.[43]
- Sputum samples can be obtained through one of four sampling methods:
  - Spontaneous samples are obtained as a single spot sputum specimen, first morning sputum specimen, or as several specimens over time (pooled)[44] For this method, patients should rinse with water and gargle before providing the specimen.[45] As many samples as possible should be early morning specimens,[19,20] although in one study random sputum samples provided similar accuracy as early morning samples.[44]

- ● Induction samples involve inducing a cough through nebulized aerosols containing water and saline.[45]
- ● Flexible bronchoscopic sampling involves bronchoscopy with bronchial alveolar lavage or bronchoscopic brush sampling.
- ● Invasive sampling involves percutaneous lung aspiration, or open lung biopsy.
- ■ Molecular testing has largely replaced the role of sputum culture, especially for lower respiratory track pathogens.

PATIENT EDUCATION

- ■ https://www.health.state.mn.us/diseases/tb/basics/factsheets/sputeng.pdf
- ■ https://www.who.int/csr/disease/plague/collecting-sputum-samples.PDF

RELATED DIAGNOSES AND ICD-10 CODES

Cough	R05	Sepsis	A41.9
Tuberculosis	A15.0	Osteomyelitis	M86.9

REFERENCES

Full list of references can be accessed through Springer Publishing Company Connect™ at the following link: http://connect.springerpub.com/content/reference-book/978-0-8261 -8843-4/part/part03/toc-part/ch083

---

84. GROUP B STREP

Cara A. Busenhart

PHYSIOLOGY/PATHOPHYSIOLOGY REVIEW

Group B Streptococcus (GBS or group B strep), or *Streptococcus agalactiae*, is a bacteria that colonizes the gastrointestinal and genital tracts of an estimated 20% to 30% of pregnant patients.[1-6] These patients do not feel sick and do not have any symptoms, yet newborns that are exposed to the GBS bacteria during pregnancy, labor, or birth may develop GBS disease, which can cause bacteremia, sepsis, pneumonia, or meningitis.[1,6,7] Ascending spread of the bacteria from the vagina to the amniotic fluid, uterus, or infant is the suspected mode of transmission.[6,8,9]

OVERVIEW OF LABORATORY TESTS

Using nucleic acid amplification to screen for GBS colonization (CPT codes 87081 and 87150) in the vagina and rectum of pregnant patients near the end of pregnancy has been identified as a method to prevent GBS transmission to neonates. If GBS is identified, antibiotics can be given while the patient is in labor.[10] To test for GBS colonization during pregnancy, a sterile swab is used to collect a sample for bacterial culture.[10] The sample is collected between 36 and 37 weeks' gestation from the pregnant patient's vagina and rectum.[11] Correct specimen collection is imperative.[12] The swab should be inserted 2 cm into the vagina, then the same swab is inserted 1 cm into the anus (through the anal sphincter)—a speculum is not necessary and specimens from the cervix, rectum, and perineum are not acceptable.[13]

INDICATIONS

Screening

■ Universal screening of all pregnant patients for GBS colonization should be performed once between 36 and 37 weeks' gestation (36 0/7 to 37 6/7 weeks) using vaginal-rectal culture.[2,8,10,12]
  ● If the pregnant patient has had GBS bacteriuria during pregnancy, a sample does not need to be collected and the patient should be treated with antibiotics during labor.[12]

Diagnosis and Evaluation

■ Vaginal-rectal culture for group B strep is not routinely used for evaluation of signs or symptoms.

Monitoring

■ Not used.

INTERPRETATION

■ Reported as positive or negative.
■ Screening considered positive when:
  ● GBS colonization identified by antenatal vaginal-rectal culture OR GBS bacteriuria identified at any point during the pregnancy.[2]
■ Patients who have had a positive screen are at increased risk of having a baby that will develop GBS disease[10]
  ● For a patient who tested positive for GBS bacteria during pregnancy AND received antibiotics in labor, the infant has a one in 4,000 chance of developing GBS disease.[10]
  ● For a patient who tested positive for GBS bacteria during pregnancy and did NOT receive antibiotics in labor, the infant has a one in 200 chance of developing GBS disease.[10]
■ Screening considered negative when:
  ● No GBS colonization is identified by antenatal vaginal-rectal culture AND no GBS bacteriuria is identified at any point during the pregnancy.[5]

FOLLOW-UP

■ Up to 40% of GBS bacterial colonization may be resistant to traditional antibiotic therapy; thus, sensitivity testing is necessary for all GBS isolated from routine screening.[11] Sensitivity testing is especially important for patients with penicillin allergy.[5,11]

- Infants born to pregnant patients who have GBS colonization may require blood cultures and close monitoring for development of GBS disease.[2,6]
- If an individual, pregnant patient, or neonate has suspected GBS disease, cultures may be collected to determine if the amniotic fluid, placenta, blood, urine, or cerebrospinal fluid samples grow the GBS bacteria.[5,7] Occasionally, a chest x-ray may help to diagnose GBS disease.[7]
- For the newborn exposed to GBS colonization during the birth process, their condition at birth and during the subsequent 12 to 24 hours are strong predictors of early-onset GBS disease; providers should monitor for abnormal vital signs, supplemental oxygen requirement, need for continuous positive airway pressure (CPAP), mechanical ventilation, or blood pressure support.[2]

PEARLS & PITFALLS

- GBS colonization and disease rates are substantially higher among Black patients and their neonates.[6,8]
- Antibiotic treatment/prophylaxis should be administered as soon as the patient with GBS colonization is determined to be in labor.[12]
- In the patient who presents in term labor with no GBS universal screening, the patient should be treated with intrapartum antibiotic prophylaxis if they develop risk factors during labor (rupture of membranes at 18 hours or more or maternal temperature 100.4 °F [38 °C] or higher).[2]
- Pregnant patients with GBS colonization in a prior pregnancy have an approximately 50% risk of colonization in subsequent pregnancies.[2]

PATIENT EDUCATION

- https://www.acog.org/womens-health/faqs/group-b-strep-and -pregnancy?utm_source=redirect&utm_medium=web&utm_campaign=otn
- https://onlinelibrary.wiley.com/doi/full/10.1111/jmwh.13125

RELATED DIAGNOSES AND ICD-10 CODES

Maternal diagnoses:		Neonatal diagnoses:	
Streptococcus B carrier state complicating pregnancy	O99.820	Streptococcus, group B, as the cause of disease classified elsewhere	B95.1
Streptococcus B carrier state complicating childbirth	O99.824	Newborn affected by maternal infectious and parasitic diseases	P00.2
Carrier of group B streptococcus	Z22.330	Sepsis of newborn due to streptococcus, group B	P36.0

REFERENCES

Full list of references can be accessed through Springer Publishing Company Connect™ at the following link: http://connect.springerpub.com/content/reference-book/978-0-8261 -8843-4/part/part03/toc-part/ch084

85. HAPTOGLOBIN

Barbara Rogers and Beth Faiman

PHYSIOLOGY REVIEW

Haptoglobin is a glycoprotein produced primarily in the liver. It is used by the body to clear free hemoglobin that is released from hemolyzed red blood cells (RBCs).[1] Free hemoglobin scavenges nitric oxide, which is an important regulator of smooth muscle relaxation, the expression of adhesion molecules by vascular endothelium, and activation and aggregation of platelets. In addition, free hemoglobin interacts with and disrupts lipid membranes and other lipophilic structures. There are three major genotypes of haptoglobin: Hp1-1, Hp2-1, and HP-2-2.[1] These three genotypes have different molecular weights, and their properties vary in binding strength, anti-oxidative ability, and rate of clearance. The strength of binding is greatest with HP1-1; however, the HP-2 genotypes bind to a larger number of hemoglobin alpha-beta dimers.[1] Multiple clinical trials have shown an increased incidence of cardiovascular events (e.g., myocardial infarction, stroke) and death among patients with diabetes mellitus and the Hp2-2 genotype. A 2018 meta-analysis by Asleh et al. confirmed this relationship.[2]

Haptoglobin has also been detected in the lungs and mRNA has been detected in the kidney, spleen, thymus, and heart.[1] The haptoglobin test measures the amount of haptoglobin in the blood. It serves as a protectant by irreversibly binding free hemoglobin from lysed red cells. Haptoglobin levels become depleted in the presence of large amounts of free hemoglobin. When RBCs are damaged, they release haptoglobin, making haptoglobin a marker for hemolysis. Because haptoglobin binds to free hemoglobin, it prevents the occurrence of free hemoglobin-induced vascular dysfunction or injury. The haptoglobin-hemoglobin complex is then degraded by the reticuloendothelial system. Haptoglobin also has additional roles. It is an acute-phase reactant, and its production is increased by inflammatory cytokines (e.g., IL-1, IL-6).[1] It can increase 3 to 8 times the normal range in response to an acute or chronic bacterial or parasitic infection.[3] It may provide antioxidant and antimicrobial effects and can suppress the proliferation of lymphocytes and B-cell mitogenesis. In addition, it modulates macrophage function by inhibiting viral hemagglutination and prostaglandin synthesis. Haptoglobin can also function as an immune system modulator by altering the distribution of helper T-cells. It also has been found to induce angiogenesis. In addition to hemolysis, haptoglobin can also be decreased in parenchymatous liver disease (e.g., cirrhosis), protein loss via the kidney, GI tract, skin, infancy, pregnancy, and malnutrition.[1]

OVERVIEW OF LABORATORY TESTS

There are two common laboratory tests used to measure haptoglobin: spectrophotometry and immunoreactive methods. Spectrophotometry identifies hemoglobin–haptoglobin complexes in hemolysis. It measures light absorption at two different wavelengths to determine the concentration of hemoglobin–haptoglobin complexes. The calculation of the change of absorption and the ratio of these changes determines the presence of hemoglobin–haptoglobin complexes, free hemoglobin, and free haptoglobin. Limitations of spectrophotometry include the potential interference of bilirubin and chylomicrons.[1]

Immunoreactive methods (CPT code 83010) use antisera against haptoglobins that produce a precipitated product that is measured by radial immunodiffusion, nephelometry, or turbidimetry. Nephelometry and turbidimetry involves applying a light beam to haptoglobin–hemoglobin–antibody complexes that is suspended in solution and a detector measures the different properties of the reflected light. Using a cutoff value of 25 mg/dL or less, the sensitivity and specificity were 83% and 96% and there was an 87% probability of predicting hemolysis when levels were below 25 mg/dL.[1,4]

INDICATIONS

Screening
■ Universal and targeted screenings are not recommended.

Diagnosis and Evaluation
Haptoglobin testing is primarily used to assist in the diagnosis of hemolytic anemia and distinguish hemolytic anemia from other causes of anemia. It is not diagnostic in itself but provides additional information to the overall clinical scenario of the patient.

Testing for haptoglobin should be considered in the following[5-7]:

■ Symptoms/signs of anemia including pale skin, jaundice, dark-colored urine, tachycardia, shortness of breath, weakness, and/or fatigue
■ Suspected acute hemolytic transfusion reaction

Monitoring
Haptoglobin level can be repeated after the cause of hemolysis is treated to determine if the increased destruction of RBCs persists and the response to treatment.[8] Time to repeat testing will vary based on the determined intervention and underlying etiology.

INTERPRETATION

Table 85.1 provides normal reference values for haptoglobin by age but can vary by laboratory.

The best cutoff between hemolytic and non-hemolytic disorders is 25 mg/dL or lower. Sensitivity increases especially when used in conjunction with an increased serum LDH.

There is no gold standard for testing for hemolysis. Therefore, the diagnosis of hemolysis relies on a combination of clinical factors and correlation with other laboratory markers. Extravascular and intravascular hemolysis can both decrease haptoglobin; therefore, the level of haptoglobin cannot be used

TABLE 85.1: HAPTOGLOBIN REFERENCE INTERVALS BY AGE		
AGE	MALE (mg/dL)	FEMALE (mg/dL)
0 to 6 m	Not established	Not established
7 m to 1 y	23–218	23–218
2 to 5 y	10–212	10–212
6 to 12 y	10–182	10–182
13 to 17 y	20–191	22–208
18 to 40 y	17–317	33–278
41 to 50 y	23–355	42–296
51 to 60 y	29–370	33–346
61 to 70 y	32–363	37–355
71 to 80 y	34–355	42–346
>80 y	38–329	41–333

Source: Data from Lab Tests Online. Haptoglobin. https://labtestsonline.org/tests/haptoglobin

to differentiate the origin of the hemolysis. Using other clinical parameters can help to determine whether it is extravascular or intravascular hemolysis.[1] Decreased levels occur more often with intravascular hemolysis than extravascular hemolysis (Table 85.2).[5]

During hemolysis, the haptoglobin is expected to be decreased, and the reticulocyte increased. Haptoglobin levels have low specificity. Normal individuals may have very low levels. In addition, both increased and decreased haptoglobin levels can occur in the absence of hemolysis due to a variety of conditions and medications (Table 85.3).

The haptoglobin level can be decreased in congenital haptoglobin but this is not related to hemolysis or liver disease. Congenital haptoglobin deficiency is seen in the general population in about 0.1% of Caucasians and 4% of Black individuals.[6]

TABLE 85.2: INTERPRETATION OF TESTING TO DETERMINE THE LOCATION OF THE HEMOLYSIS			
POSSIBLE LOCATION OF HEMOLYSIS	HAPTOGLOBIN	RETICULOCYTE COUNT	RBC, HEMOGLOBIN, HEMATOCRIT
Intravascular	Significantly decreased	Increased	Decreased
Extravascular	Normal or slightly decreased	Increased	Decreased

Source: Evidence Based Medicine Consult. Haptoglobin. https://www.ebmconsult.com/articles/lab-test-haptoglobin-level; Reproduced with permission from https://labtestsonline.org/tests/haptoglobin

TABLE 85.3: CAUSES OF ALTERED HAPTOGLOBIN LEVELS

INCREASED HAPTOGLOBIN	DECREASED HAPTOGLOBIN
Inflammatory diseases—ulcerative colitis, acute rheumatic disease, heart attack, severe infection, rheumatoid arthritis	Congenital haptoglobin deficiency
Drugs—androgens, corticosteroids	Normal finding in newborns and infants younger than 6 months
Aging	Pregnancy
Hypersplenism	Intravascular hemolysis (e.g., hereditary spherocytosis, PK deficiency, autoimmune hemolytic anemia, transfusion reactions)
Smoking	Extravascular hemolysis (e.g., large retroperitoneal hemorrhage)
Diabetes mellitus	Intramedullary hemolysis (e.g., thalassemia, megaloblastic anemias, sideroblastic anemias)
Megaloblastic anemia	Parenchymatous liver disease (especially cirrhosis)
Obstructive biliary disease	Kidney disease
Aplastic anemia	Drugs—isoniazid, quinine, streptomycin, birth control pills, chlorpromazine, diphenhydramine, indomethacin, nitrofurantoin,
Red cell membrane or metabolic defects (e.g., G6PD deficiency, hereditary spherocytosis, paroxysmal nocturnal hemoglobinuria)	Disseminated ovarian carcinomatosis
	Pulmonary sarcoidosis
	Elevated estrogen levels
	Hemodilution
	Malnutrition
	Improper phlebotomy technique or specimen handling
	Cardiac surgery: Cardiopulmonary bypass

Sources: Data from Evidence Based Medicine Consult. Haptoglobin. https://www.ebmconsult.com/articles/lab-test-haptoglobin-level; Lab Tests Online. Haptoglobin. https://labtestsonline.org/tests/haptoglobin; Marchand A, Galen RS, Van Lente F. The predictive value of serum haptoglobin in hemolytic disease. *JAMA*. 1980;243(19):1909–1911. doi:10.1001/jama.1980.03300450023014; Nagalla S, Besa E. What lab levels should be monitored inn patients with hemolytic anemia? *Medscape.* 2021. https://www.medscape.com/answers/201066-27091/what-lab-levels-should-be-monitored-in-patients-with-hemolytic-anemia; Shih A, McFarlane A, Verhovsek M. Haptoglobin testing in hemolysis: measurement and interpretation. *Am J Hematol.* 2014;89:443–447. doi:10.1002/ajh.23623.

FOLLOW-UP

Haptoglobin is commonly used in conjunction with other tests such as CBC, reticulocyte count, lactate dehydrogenase (LDH), bilirubin (indirect), direct antiglobulin test, and a peripheral blood smear.

It is a sensitive test for hemolytic anemia but cannot be used to determine the cause of the anemia; therefore, other tests, such as autoantibodies, sickle cell tests, or G6PD, might need to be completed to determine the underlying etiology.

If a transfusion reaction is suspected, a direct antiglobulin test is also ordered (Chapter 50).

PEARLS & PITFALLS

- False positives (decreased level) can occur in the following circumstances[1,5–7,9]:
  - Improper specimen preparations
  - Cirrhosis
  - Elevated estrogen states
  - Hemodilution
  - Drugs: chlorpromazine, diphenhydramine, indomethacin, isoniazid, nitrofurantoin, oral contraceptives, quinidine, streptomycin
- False negatives (increased level) can occur in the following circumstances:
  - Hypersplenism
  - Medications:

androgens

corticosteroids

  - Malignancy
  - Inflammatory disorders
  - Biliary obstruction

PATIENT EDUCATION

- https://medlineplus.gov/lab-tests/haptoglobin-hp-test/
- https://www.merckmanuals.com/home/blood-disorders/anemia/autoimmune-hemolytic-anemia

RELATED DIAGNOSES AND ICD-10 CODES

Acquired hemolytic anemia, unspecified	D59.9
Autoimmune hemolytic anemia	D59.1
Drug-induced hemolytic anemia	D62

REFERENCES

Full list of references can be accessed through Springer Publishing Company Connect™ at the following link: http://connect.springerpub.com/content/reference-book/978-0-8261-8843-4/part/part03/toc-part/ch085

86. *HELICOBACTER PYLORI* TESTS

Christine Colella and Kelly Small Casler

PHYSIOLOGY REVIEW

Helicobacter pylori (*H. pylori*) is a gram-negative bacterium causing an infection that can result in peptic ulcer and gastric cancer.[1] Diagnosis of *H. pylori* is crucial to treating the infection and inflammation that can result in these complications. Some estimates suggest that 50% of the population is infected with *H. pylori* and that the infection can be acquired at an early age and more frequently in developing countries.[2-4] *H. pylori* has unique physiology through the production of urease which allows conversion of urea to ammonia and therefore elevation of the gastric pH to allow its survival.[5]

OVERVIEW OF LABORATORY TESTS

There are three noninvasive tests and one invasive test used to evaluate for *H. pylori*. Table 86.1 compares these tests.

TABLE 86.1: SUMMARY OF NONINVASIVE TESTS

	PROS	CONS	SENSITIVITY*[23,24]
UBT	Can use as TOC High accuracy	Avoidance of PPI/bismuth needed Most expensive Can be used as TOC Complicated to perform	92%–94%
serology	Do not have to avoid PPIs/bismuth	Falling out of favor Cannot tell past from present infection Insurances starting to deny coverage due to accuracy issues Cannot be used as TOC	84%
SAT	Can use as test of cure Inexpensive High accuracy if monoclonal product used	*Samples must be refrigerated/frozen after collection Avoidance of PPI/bismuth needed	83%
EGD RUT	Can rule out do not miss diagnoses (cancer)	Invasive Requires pathologist	93%

*Calculated based on a 90% specificity.

EGD RUT, esophagogastroduodenoscopy rapid urease test; PPI, proton pump inhibitors; SAT, stool antigen test; TOC, test of cure; UBT, urea breath test.

Sources: Data from Chey WD, Leontiadis GI, Howden CW, Moss SF. ACG clinical guideline: treatment of *Helicobacter pylori* infection. *Am J Gastroenterol.* 2017;112(2):212–239. doi:10.1038/ajg.2016.563; Dore MP, Pes GM, Bassotti G, Usai-Satta P. Dyspepsia: when and how to test for *Helicobacter pylori* infection. *Gastroenterol Res Pract.* 2016;2016:8463614. doi:10.1155/2016/8463614; Best LM, Takwoingi Y, Siddique S, et al. Non-invasive diagnostic tests for *Helicobacter pylori* infection. *Cochrane Database Syst Rev.* 2018;3(3):CD012080. doi:10.1002/14651858.CD012080.pub2.

Urea Breath Test (CPT Code 83013)

Available since 1996, urea breath tests (UBTs) detect the presence of urease that is produced by *H. pylori*.[6] For this test, patients ingest a solution containing a mixture of urea and carbon and exhale 15 minutes later into a plastic container which can be evaluated up to 7 days later.[6] If *H. pylori* is present in the gastrointestinal (GI) tract, urease breaks down the urea–carbon mixture and produces carbon dioxide, which is excreted through exhalation and detected by the UBT.[7,8] This type of test can use one of two carbon atoms, either carbon-13(C-13) or carbon-14 (C-14). The differences are important since C-14 is radioactive and, therefore, cannot be used in pregnant individuals or children.[9–11] C-13 is not radioactive, and so C-13–based UBTs have been Food and Drug Administration (FDA) approved for use in children as young as age 3 since 2012.[6] However, UBTs are generally discouraged from use in children under 6 years of age due to difficulty with swallowing the solution appropriately, which could lead to false positives from solution interaction with urease producing normal flora of the oropharynx.[10] UBT can be performed using CLIA-waved POCTs or performed in the laboratory.[12] The UBT has a 0.96 to 0.97 sensitivity and 0.91 to 0.94 specificity in adults and performs with similar accuracy in children.[9] One caveat to UBT is the preclusion from patient use of antibiotics for 4 weeks prior, proton pump inhibitors (PPIs) or bismuth products for 2 weeks prior, and histamine-2 receptor blockers for 2 days prior to the test due to the possibility of false-negative tests.[10,13]

H. Pylori Serum Antibody Test (CPT Code 86677)

In this test, a nonfasting serum sample is tested for presence of antibodies, specifically IgG. This has not been tested in pediatric populations, and a positive test does not differentiate between an active infection and colonization;[6] it only indicates the presence of IgG antibodies to the *H. pylori* infection. Results may be negative (less than 0.80), equivocal (0.80 to 0.89), or positive (greater than 0.89). Serology can be tested using CLIA-waved POCTs or laboratory-performed tests.[12]

H. Pylori Stool Antigen Test (SAT) (CPT Code 87338)

SATs are structured as enzyme immunoassays or lateral assays using either monoclonal antibodies or polyclonal antibodies. Stool antigens (SATs) based on monoclonal antibodies tend to be more accurate (and offer sensitivity/specificity similar to UBT), but are also more expensive.[14–16] This test can be used in children and adults and detects *H. pylori* antigens in a stool sample. As with UBTs, there may also be false-negative results if any antibiotics, PPIs, or bismuth preparations have been taken within the 2 weeks prior to testing or if histamine-2 receptor blockers have been taken within the last 2 days.[10,13] SATs can be performed as CLIA-waved POCTs or laboratory-performed tests.[12] There are more laboratory-based stool tests on the market and they tend to perform better than rapid POCT SATs.[10,12]

Rapid Urea Test

Rapid urea tests (RUTs) are performed after biopsy is obtained during endoscopy. This method is invasive.

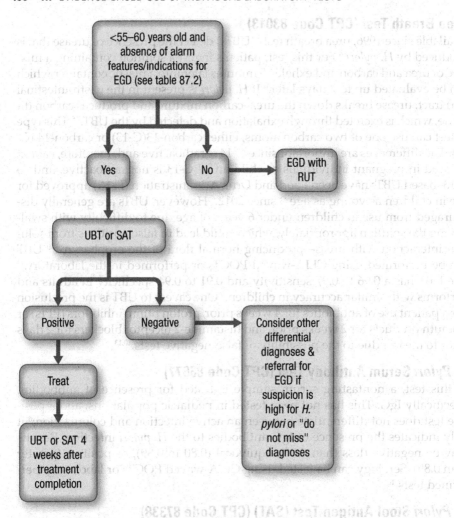

FIGURE 86.1. Algorithm for testing of patient with dyspeptic symptoms. EGD, esophagogastroduodenoscopy; RUT, rapid urease test; SAT, stool antigen test; UBT, urea breath test. *Sources:* Data from Chey WD, Leontiadis GI, Howden CW, Moss SF. ACG clinical guideline: treatment of *Helicobacter pylori* infection. *Am J Gastroenterol.* 2017;112(2):212–239. doi:10.1038/ajg.2016.563; Sjomina O, Pavlova J, Niv Y, Leja M. Epidemiology of *Helicobacter pylori* infection. *Helicobacter.* 2018;23(suppl 1):e12514. doi:10.1111/hel.12514.

INDICATIONS

Screening

- Some areas outside the United States use *H. pylori* tests to screen patients at high risk of gastric cancer (history of gastric cancer in a first-degree relative).[17]
- Screening for patients on long-term acetylsalicylic acid (ASA) or nonsteroidal anti-inflammatory drug (NSAID) use is supported by guidelines.[1,15]

Diagnosis and Evaluation

- Diagnostic testing is indicated in individuals with suggestive symptoms, which usually manifest in three primary ways:
  - Epigastric pain and dyspepsia
  - Dysmotility-like dyspepsia (feeling of fullness, early satiety, bloating, and/or nausea)
  - Unspecified dyspepsia (ill-defined gastric complaints)[18]
- For diagnostic testing in individuals older than 55 to 60 years old or with alarm features (Box 86.1, Figure 86.1), use EGD with RUT and biopsy over noninvasive methods in order to co-evaluate for other more serious differential diagnoses of dyspepsia.[1,2]
- Invasive testing methods are rarely used in children.[19]

Monitoring

- Because up to 20% of patients fail therapy,[20] a test of cure is indicated 4 weeks after treatment completion and after 1 to 2 weeks of proton pump inhibitor therapy completion.[1,10]

INTERPRETATION

- UBT: negative or positive for *H. pylori*
- Serum antibody test: negative, equivocal, or positive for *H. pylori*.[14]
- SAT: negative or positive for *H. pylori*

FOLLOW-UP

- If a noninvasive test is negative, but suspicion for *H. pylori* remains high, refer for EGD with biopsy and RUT.

Box 86.1: Indications for Invasive *H. pylori* Testing Over Noninvasive Tests

- Abdominal mass
- Adult >55–60 years of age
- Dysphagia
- First-degree relative with gastric cancer
- Idiopathic thrombocytopenic purpura*
- Iron deficiency anemia
- Overt GI bleeding
- Past history of gastric cancer or gastric lymphoma
- Vitamin B12 deficiency
- Weight loss

*Can use UBT for these patients.

Sources: Data from Dore MP, Pes GM, Bassotti G, Usai-Satta P. Dyspepsia: when and how to test for *Helicobacter pylori* infection. *Gastroenterol Res Pract.* 2016;2016:8463614. doi:10.1155/2016/8463614; Malfertheiner P, Megraud F, O'Morain CA, et al. Management of *Helicobacter pylori* infection—the Maastricht V/Florence Consensus Report. *Gut.* 2017;66(1):6–30. doi:10.1136/gutjnl-2016-312288.

PEARLS & PITFALLS

■ One analysis found a test and treat strategy (with noninvasive testing) cost $389 less per patient than using EGD to confirm diagnosis.[21]

■ The cost of serology and SAT are roughly equivalent with UBT costing about twice the amount of both.[22]

■ UBTs appear to be the most accurate tests of the noninvasive methods for children and adults, although the comparison studies are of lower quality.[23]

■ In extremely complicated cases, culture and sensitivity may be used to test for *H. pylori* antibiotic resistance.[1]

■ Individuals with *H. pylori* infection have a 2- to 6-fold increased risk of mucosal associated-lymphoid-type (MALT) lymphoma and gastric cancer.[4]

■ Testing is rarely needed in children under the age of 6 since *H. pylori* treatment is not indicated in these children.[10]

PATIENT EDUCATION

■ https://www.meridianbioscience.com/diagnostics/disease-areas/gastrointestinal/h-pylori/breathtek-ubt-for-h-pylori/

RELATED DIAGNOSES AND ICD-10 CODES

Helicobacter pylori [*H. pylori*] as the cause of diseases classified elsewhere	B96.81
Duodenal ulcer, unspecified as acute or chronic, without hemorrhage or perforation	K26.9
Peptic ulcer, site unspecified, unspecified as acute or chronic, without hemorrhage or perforation	K27.9
Acute gastritis without bleeding	K29.00
Chronic atrophic gastritis without bleeding	K29.40
Unspecified chronic gastritis without bleeding	K29.50
Other gastritis without bleeding	K29.60
Gastritis, unspecified, without bleeding	K29.70
Gastroduodenitis, unspecified, without bleeding	K29.90
Functional dyspepsia	K30
Other diseases of stomach and duodenum	K31.89

REFERENCES

Full list of references can be accessed through Springer Publishing Company Connect™ at the following link: http://connect.springerpub.com/content/reference-book/978-0-8261 -8843-4/part/part03/toc-part/ch086

87. HEMOGLOBIN A1C

Bridget O'Brien

PHYSIOLOGY REVIEW

Hemoglobin A1c (HbA1c) is also known as the measurement of glycosylated hemoglobin. It measures a minor fraction of hemoglobin in which glucose is attached. Red cells are highly permeable to glucose. Hemoglobin A1c denotes the concentration of the blood glucose that is irreversibly attached to the red blood cell during its life span. The life span of the red blood cell is approximately 120 days. This value provides a sense of the glycemic history over this time frame. The attachment of glucose to hemoglobin is nonlinear and measures the levels during the preceding 3 to 4 months, but the more recent glucose exposure in the preceding 4 weeks contributes to additional glycosylation. The higher the exposure of hemoglobin to blood glucose, the higher the fraction of glycosylated hemoglobin, and therefore a higher percentage will be expressed in the A1c value. The value expressed as HbA1c is more weighted toward reporting values from the most recent 4 weeks, but commonly represents the value over the last 3 months.[1-3] Overall HbA1c is most useful for the long-term measurement of glycemic control.

While it is a helpful index across the life span, during pregnancy HbA1c measurement every 4 to 6 weeks rarely suggests change for management and should not be used for insulin adjustment in pregnancy.[4] There are factors that may adversely influence the accuracy of HbA1c such as conditions that alter the survival of red blood cells, for example, hemolytic anemia. These alterations in red blood cells may play a factor in the usefulness of measurement in the pregnant female.

OVERVIEW OF LABORATORY TESTS

HbA1c (CPT code 83036)[5] is commonly utilized for screening, diagnosis, and for monitoring of diabetes mellitus. It is considered the standard of care for testing and monitoring diabetes. Hb A1c is widely used to estimate the mean blood glucose over a 3-month period. Since daily fluctuations do not affect the glucose concentration in the hemoglobin, a fasting test is not required. Without the presence of persistent hyperglycemia, elevations in HbA1c would not be found. Normal findings of glucose concentration are approximately 4% to 6% of total hemoglobin, depending on the assay.[6]

The other area of study for this test has been regarding the benefits of improved glycemic control in overall long-term outcomes. A landmark study based on data from the Diabetes Control and Complications Trial (DCCT) revealed that intensive therapy for diabetes delays onset and slows progression of the development of neuropathy, nephropathy, and retinopathy.[7] As a result, HbA1c is widely used for evaluation of intensive therapy and is the primary endpoint in many drug approval trials.

INDICATIONS

Screening

Adults

■ The United States Preventive Services Task Force recommends screening with HbA1c every 3 years for asymptomatic adults ages 35 to 70 years old who are overweight or obese (body mass index [BMI] of 25 or greater).[8]
  ● Screenings should be considered earlier in the following populations: positive family history of diabetes, personal history of gestational diabetes or polycystic ovarian syndrome, Black individuals, American Indians, Alaskan Natives, Asian individuals, Hispanics or Latinos, Native Hawaiians, or Pacific Islanders.

■ The International Expert Committee appointed by members of the American Diabetes Association, the European Association for the Study of Diabetes, and the International Diabetes Federation recommended HbA1c for diagnosis of diabetes, as well as screening for progression to diabetes. Testing should be performed when there is a clinical suspicion for diabetes. In children and adolescents, HbA1c is recommended if diabetes is in the differential without common symptoms, or a fasting plasma glucose greater than 200 is noted.[9]

■ The American Diabetes Association (ADA) recommends screening for diabetes with HbA1c for all people starting at age 45 every 3 years or sooner if symptoms develop.[10]

■ The ADA recommends screening adults, regardless of age, who are overweight or obese (BMI 25 kg/m² or higher) and who have one or more risk factors for diabetes mellitus. Asians should have a screening if their BMI is 23 kg/m² or higher. Risk factors include first-degree relative with diabetes, high risk race/ethnicity (see the previous text for a list), personal history of cardiovascular disease, personal history of hypertension, low HDL (less than 35 mg/dL), triglyceride level greater than 250 mg/dL, females with polycystic ovarian syndrome, history of physical inactivity, and other conditions associated with insulin resistance.[10]

■ A systematic review evaluating validity of using HbA1c as a screening tool for type 2 diabetes demonstrated that at some values, there is lower sensitivity and higher specificity than fasting plasma glucose. Conclusions were that HbA1c is equally effective to fasting plasma glucose for screening.[11]

Pregnancy-Related

■ Individuals with a history of gestational diabetes should be screened for diabetes mellitus at least every 3 years.

■ HbA1c is not considered the standard screening for gestational diabetes due to alterations in interpretation of values.

■ Testing for prediabetes/diabetes should be considered for individuals who are planning pregnancy and are overweight.

Children/Adolescents

■ Diabetes mellitus screening should be considered for children 10 years of age, or at puberty, whichever is earlier. With normal results, testing should be repeated every 3 years or more frequently if BMI or clinical risk

Box 87.1: Criteria for Diagnosis of Diabetes

- Fasting plasma glucose of 126 mg/dL or higher
- 2-hour plasma glucose of 200 mg/dL or higher during oral glucose tolerance test
- HbA1c of 6.5% or higher using a method that is NGSP* certified
- In a patient with symptoms of polyuria, polydipsia, polyphagia, or a random plasma glucose of 200 mg/dlL or higher

Source: Adapted from American Diabetes Association. 6. Glycemic targets: standards of medical care in diabetes-2021. *Diabetes Care*. 2021;44(suppl 1):S73–S84. doi:10.2337/dc21-S006

is increasing. Testing before the age of 10 years should only be considered with multiple risk factors.[10]

- Risk-based screening in asymptomatic children for prediabetes or type 2 diabetes should be considered if BMI is greater than 85% and there are one or more of the following risk factors: maternal history of gestational diabetes, family history of diabetes in first- or second- degree relative, or signs of insulin resistance.[10]

Diagnosis and Evaluation

HbA1c reflects the average glucose measurements over a 3-month period. It is widely accepted as an option for diagnosing diabetes in comparison to fasting or random blood glucose (Box 87.1). Averages of blood glucose results were studied with over 2,700 readings of patients with type 1, type 2, and no diabetes. The correlation of these numbers can help clinicians estimate mean glucose numbers with HbA1c (Table 87.1). There is also a highly statistically significant correlation between HbA1c and mean glucose levels in children with type 1 diabetes.[12]

- Signs and symptoms of diabetes include the following: polyphagia, polydipsia, polyuria, blurry vision, unexplained weight loss, fatigue, numbness/tingling in hands and feet, dry skin, slow healing, and more prone to infections.

TABLE 87.1: ESTIMATION OF AVERAGE GLUCOSE COMPARED TO HBA1C

HbA1c (%)	AVERAGE BLOOD GLUCOSE (mg/dl)
5	97
6	126
7	154
8	183
9	212
10	240
11	269
12	298

Source: Adapted from American Diabetes Association. 6. Glycemic targets: standards of medical care in diabetes-2021. *Diabetes Care*. 2021;44(suppl 1):S73–S84. doi:10.2337/dc21-S006.

- There may be false positivity or false negativity impacting the diagnostic decision-making.[13]
- Consider differential diagnoses including diabetic ketoacidosis, secondary hyperglycemia, diabetes insipidus, and insulin resistance.

Monitoring

Standardization of the assay was established by the National Glycohemoglobin Standardization Program (NGSP) to make sure that 99% of the assays are standardized for accuracy.[14] When there is a disparity between glucose and HgA1c, glucose should be prioritized. Fasting blood glucose can be used as diagnostic, and an oral glucose tolerance test is utilized in gestational diabetes. Glycemic control can also be monitored by glucose serial self-monitoring.

- HbA1c should be monitored at least twice a year in patients with diabetes mellitus who have stable glycemic treatment goals.[12]
- HbA1c should be tested quarterly in patients with changes to their treatment regimen or when they are not meeting intended goals.[12]
- Point-of-care testing can be performed for established patients to ensure timely results for treatment planning. Point-of-care testing is also commercially available and certified by NGSP.[12,14]
- HbA1c goals for many nonpregnant adults is less than 7%, although lower if tolerated.[12]
- Higher goals lower than 8% may be considered if patients have severe hypoglycemia, multiple comorbidities, or limited life expectancy.[12]

INTERPRETATION

See Tables 87.2 and 87.3 for interpretation of test results.

FOLLOW-UP

- All tests to declare a diagnosis of diabetes require a second measurement for confirmation although point-of-care testing should not be utilized for diagnosis.
- Additional laboratory tests to consider with a new diagnosis are the following: fasting lipid profile, liver function tests, urine albumin to creatinine ratio, and serum creatinine. In type 1 diabetes mellitus, thyroid-stimulating hormone (TSH) and celiac antibodies should also be considered.
- Autoantibodies (IA-2, GAD-65) can also be tested to differentiate type 1 from type 2 diabetes.

TABLE 87.2: DIABETES DIAGNOSTIC CRITERIA BY HBA1C	
Normal	Below 5.7%
Prediabetes	5.7 to 6.4%
Diabetes	6.5% or greater*

*Value is based on AACE guidelines.

TABLE 87.3: TARGET HBA1C VALUES FOR CHILDREN, ADULTS, AND PREGNANT INDIVIDUALS	
	HbA1c VALUE
ADA guidelines for nonpregnant adults[12]	<7.0%
ADA guidelines for all pediatric age groups[15]	<7.0% adjusting for risk of hypoglycemia
ADA guideline for pregnancy[16]	Target between 6%–6.5%
	Adjust to below 6% if without hypoglycemia or to below 7% if needed to prevent hypoglycemia.
AACE Consensus Statement[17] for nonpregnant adults	A1c level of 6.5% or below is optimal if it can be achieved in a safe and affordable manner. Higher targets can be individualized.

AACE, American Association of Clinical Endocrinologists.

PEARLS & PITFALLS

- HbA1c values have been reported as relatively higher in some racial groups including Black, Hispanic, and Asian Americans compared to Caucasian persons. These differences are insignificant, and studies have been limited. It is known that race is a social construct, and therefore race should not be added to the interpretation of these values.[18]
- HbA1c is often used as an outcome measure to determine efficacy of treatment. All factors that could influence results should be considered.
- For older adult patients with shorter life expectancy or multiple comorbidities, or patients with frequent hypoglycemia, less strict goals for HbA1c should be considered.
- A limitation of HbA1c is that it does not account for large changes in glucose concentrations during the day which may be frequently measured by glucose readings. If multiple daily readings consistently range from 50 to 250 mg/dL throughout the day, the average would still be 150 mg/dL. If another similar patient stayed within the 100 to 200 mg/dL range, they also would have an average of 150 mg/dL. Their HbA1c levels would likely be similar, yet one patient has much less glucose control.
- Patients who have received a blood transfusion likely will have false HbA1c levels. They may be decreased due to dilution, or the HbA1c level may reflect the donor's glucose levels.[19]
- HbA1c can decline in pregnancy due to alterations in erythrocytes. It can also increase later in pregnancy due to some insulin resistance.
- HbA1c values can be altered with chronic kidney disease or hemodialysis in patients with type 2 diabetes, especially in the setting of erythropoietin treatment.[20]
- Data from the National Health and Nutrition Examination Survey (NHANES) determined that for a HbA1c value of 5.7%, sensitivity was 39% and specificity was 91%.[21]
- Inaccurate results have been identified in the following conditions: sickle cell anemia, kidney failure, liver disease, or with those who have received a blood transfusion.[22]
- In addition, alcoholism, folic acid deficiency, severe hypertriglyceridemia, severe hyperbilirubinemia, and vitamin C supplementation can alter results.[23]

PATIENT EDUCATION

- https://www.diabetes.org/a1c
- https://www.aace.com/disease-and-conditions/diabetes/what-you-need -know-about-diabetes

RELATED DIAGNOSES AND ICD-10 CODES

Abnormal blood glucose level	R73.09	Type 1 diabetes mellitus	E10
Diabetes mellitus	E08	Type 2 diabetes mellitus	E11
Drug or chemical induced diabetes mellitus	E09	Other specified diabetes mellitus	E13

REFERENCES

Full list of references can be accessed through Springer Publishing Company Connect™ at the following link: http://connect.springerpub.com/content/reference-book/978-0-8261 -8843-4/part/part03/toc-part/ch087

88. HEMOGLOBINOPATHIES

Oralea A. Pittman

PHYSIOLOGY REVIEW

Hemoglobin is a tetramer made up of two alpha globin chains and two beta globin chains which are combined with heme to transport oxygen in the blood.[1] Normal adult hemoglobin is expressed as alpha$^A_2$ beta$^A_2$. Genetic abnormalities of hemoglobin can affect either the alpha genes or the beta genes. More than 1,000 hemoglobin variants have been identified worldwide.

Hemoglobinopathies and thalassemias are due to amino acid substitutions, insertions, and deletions.[1] They can vary in severity according to how many deletions occur on a gene. Deletions in thalassemia affect the quantity of hemoglobin produced. One and two deletions do not usually cause health problems for the individual with deletions on a gene, although they can pass the deletions on to subsequent children. Three deletions (HbH), however, can cause varied clinical and hematologic problems. Four deletions, called Hb Barts hydrops fetalis, is not compatible with life.

Common alpha globin variants include Hb Barts, Hb Constant Spring, HbH, and HbJ. Beta globin variants commonly seen include HbS, HbC, HbD, HbE, and HbG.[1] Beta globin variants are structural. A mutation in one beta globin subunit results in a combination of variant and normal hemoglobin and results in a carrier, or trait status. This is also known as the heterozygous state. Mutations that affect both beta globin subunits result in disease, the severity of which depends on whether the mutation is homozygous like the HbSS in sickle cell anemia or heterozygous such as those found in HbSE, HbSC, or HbS/beta thalassemia. Some mutations can also affect both alpha and beta globin genes such as HgM. Hb disorders show autosomal recessive or autosomal dominant patterns in families.

Fetal hemoglobin (HbF) is the primary hemoglobin throughout gestation and the first 10 days of life. By 6 months of age, fetal hemoglobin has fallen below 1%.[2]

OVERVIEW OF LABORATORY TESTS

There are two overall types of laboratory tests currently in use: protein (also called hematologic/biochemical methods) and molecular methods.[1,2] Although hemoglobin electrophoresis was commonly used in the past, there are now faster and more sensitive tests. Protein chemistry methods include isoelectric focusing (IEF) (CPT code 83020), high performance liquid chromatography (HPLC) (CPT code 83021), and capillary zone electrophoresis (CZE) (CPT code 83020). These can be used for both screening and diagnosis. Abnormal results must be confirmed by a second, different test. All tests can be done on a dried blood spot collected on filter paper during newborn testing or on a liquid blood sample.

Molecular (DNA sequencing) methods, the second type of test, are currently used primarily for diagnosis.[1,2] Commonly used tests include restriction fragment length polymorphism (RFLP), allelic discrimination (AD), and DNA sequencing (CPT codes 81259, 81364, 81363, 81479),[2] although there are multiple molecular tests in use. Abnormal results on protein chemistry tests must also be confirmed with DNA tests. Prenatal and pre-implantation genetic testing with chorionic villus sampling, amniocentesis, and fetal blood sampling is also used as a testing method.

Any abnormal findings should be confirmed by another method. Currently for screening of newborns, most laboratories are using IEF and HPLC.[1] Although it can be part of the total workup, a blood smear alone is inadequate for screening or diagnosis.

INDICATIONS

Screening

- Universal screening is completed on all newborns in the United States and in much of the rest of the world.[1-3] It should be noted that in a Cochrane review in 2010, no randomized controlled studies were found to support universal screening of newborns, but the authors recommended screening because of the risk benefit ratio.[3]
- Preconception and prenatal screening of parents who are high risk or who have a child with a hemoglobinopathy is recommended but not required.[2,4]
- In the past, certain ethnic groups were targeted for screening. These ethnic groups included Black individuals, Africans, Southeast Asians, and persons from India, China, the Mediterranean, and the Pacific Islands. Screening by ethnic group is no longer considered a useful strategy due to migration and the frequency of conception between two members of different ethnic groups. It can be helpful in choosing tests to know the ethnicity of the

parents in addition to their carrier status in preconception, prenatal, and pre-implantation genetic testing.[1,2]

Diagnosis and Evaluation

Consider testing in the following populations:

- Testing is advised for adults with persistent microcytosis without iron deficiency or other unexplainable anemias.
- Testing is advised for adults with abnormal results on their CBC or blood smear that suggest an abnormal form of hemoglobin.
- Testing of the fetus should be preceded by testing of the parents.
- Testing should also include a CBC and smear and iron studies including iron, total iron binding capacity, ferritin, transferrin, and B12 and folate.[2]

INTERPRETATION

Hemoglobin AA is the normal state. Results reporting will depend on the laboratory and test used. Typically the laboratory report includes an interpretation by a hematopathologist.[2] The report typically includes the following elements (Table 88.1):

- Percentage of normal hemoglobin
- Any abnormal forms of hemoglobin including HbS, HbC, HbE, HbH, HbF, HbD, HbG, HbJ, Hb Barts, Hb Constant Spring, and HbM
- Percentage of abnormal forms detected

TABLE 88.1: EXEMPLAR OF HEMOGLOBINOPATHY EVALUATION

RESULTS SEEN	CONDITION	GENES
Slightly decreased Hb A Moderate amount Hb S (about 40%)	Sickle cell trait	One gene copy for Hb S (heterozygous)
Majority Hb S Increased Hb F (up to 10%) No Hb A	Sickle cell disease	Two gene copies for Hb S (homozygous)
Majority Hb C No Hb A	Hemoglobin C disease	Two gene copies for Hb C (homozygous)
Majority Hb A Some Hb H	Hemoglobin H disease (alpha thalassemia)	Three out of four alpha genes are mutated (deleted)
Majority Hb F Little or no Hb A	Beta thalassemia major	Both beta genes are mutated
Majority Hb A Slightly increased Hb A2 (4%–8%) Hb F may be slightly increased	Beta thalassemia minor	One beta gene is mutated, causing slight decrease in beta globin chain

Source: Reproduced with permission from https://labtestsonline.org/tests/hemoglobinopathy-evaluation.

RBC count can also help to distinguish between iron deficiency and thalassemia with thalassemia showing erythrocytosis to compensate for a chronically low mean cell hemoglobin (MCH).

FOLLOW-UP

■ If the first protein screening test is abnormal, a second protein test is necessary. If abnormal, DNA (molecular) testing is the next step.[1,2]
■ With the diagnosis of any hemoglobinopathy regardless of age, genetic counseling and possible referral to a hematologist is important.[2]

PEARLS & PITFALLS

■ Hemoglobinopathies and the testing done for them are complicated. After protein testing, consulting with a hematologist is necessary to help choose which type of DNA testing is best.
■ Different tests are best for diagnosing different hemoglobinopathies.[2]
■ Many laboratories have protocols in place for which tests they do. Find out which tests they do before ordering.[1,2]

PATIENT EDUCATION

■ https://www.cdc.gov/ncbddd/sicklecell/index.html
■ https://www.cdc.gov/ncbddd/thalassemia/index.html

RELATED DIAGNOSES AND ICD-10 CODES

Microcytic anemia	D50.9
Sickle cell disease	D57.9
Hemoglobin C	D57.20
Other thalessemias	D56.8

REFERENCES

Full list of references can be accessed through Springer Publishing Company Connect™ at the following link: http://connect.springerpub.com/content/reference-book/978-0-8261 -8843-4/part/part03/toc-part/ch088

---

89. HEPATITIS (INFECTIOUS) TESTING

Pam Kibbe, Kelly Small Casler, and Amanda Chaney

PHYSIOLOGY/PATHOPHYSIOLOGY REVIEW

There are five types of hepatitis viruses: hepatitis A, B, C, D, and E. All are RNA viruses except for hepatitis B, which is a DNA virus. Hepatitis A, B, and C are the most common types of hepatitis (Table 89.1). In the United States, the use of universal precautions and screening along with the availability of vaccinations have cause the incidence of hepatitis A and hepatitis B to decrease significantly over time.[1] On the other hand, the incidence of hepatitis C has increased over time, thought to be due partly to the opioid epidemic.[2,3] Hepatitis A virus (HAV) causes an acute viral hepatitis in which symptoms are typically mild and self-limited in healthy people. In those who are immunocompromised or have underlying chronic diseases, HAV severity may be worse. It does not cause chronic disease.[3,4] Hepatitis B virus (HBV) causes an acute, short-term illness that becomes chronic in some individuals and hepatitis C virus (HCV) causes a short-term illness that may become chronic in about half of individuals.[3] In the United States, most cases of HCV are transmitted by sharing intravenous drug use equipment.[3] Hepatitis D virus (HDV) is called the "satellite virus" since it only infects individuals who have HBV, either as co-infection or secondary infection during HBV chronicity. Like HBV, HDV can cause chronic illness in some patients.[5] Hepatitis E is rare in developed countries, but common in countries with poor sanitation and water supply. It almost always causes acute illness only, though in patients with immunocompromise, it can become chronic in rare situations.[6]

OVERVIEW OF LABORATORY TESTS

Hepatitis tests can be done to detect antigens (Ag), antibodies, and viral RNA/DNA using samples of whole blood, saliva (HCV only), serum, or plasma.[7] Testing for hepatitis A is typically done through total HAV antibodies (CPT code 86708), which combines IgG and IgM antibodies for a total count. IgM Abs appear early at symptom onset and may persist for as long as a year after infection. IgG Abs appear as early as the convalescent phase and persist for decades. If differentiation is needed between acute (IgM) versus chronic (IgG) infection, the antibodies can be tested separately. Tests for HBV and HCV are summarized in Tables 89.2 and 89.3.

TABLE 89.1: KEY FACTS ABOUT HEPATITIS A, HEPATITIS B, AND HEPATITIS C

CHARACTERISTIC	HEPATITIS A	HEPATITIS B	HEPATITIS C
Main route(s) of transmission	Fecal–oral	Blood, sexual	Blood
Incubation period	15–20 days (average: 28 days)	60–150 days (average: 90 days)	14–182 days (average range: 14–84 days)
Symptoms of acute infection	Symptoms are similar and can include one or more of the following: jaundice, fever, fatigue, loss of appetite, nausea, vomiting, abdominal pain, joint pain, dark urine, clay-colored stool, diarrhea (hepatitis A only)		
Perinatal transmission	No	Yes	Yes
Vaccine available	Yes	Yes	No
Treatment	Supportive care	Yes, not curative	Yes, not curative

Source: From CDC. https://www.cdc.gov/hepatitis/statistics/2019surveillance/Introduction.htm.

TABLE 89.2: TESTS FOR HEPATITIS B VIRUS

TEST	DESCRIPTION
HBV surface antigen (HBsAg)	Tests for a surface protein. Detected during acute illness. Indicates that the person is infectious.
Hepatitis B surface antibody (anti-HBs)	Indicates recovery and immunity from HBV infection. Indicates successful response to HBV vaccination.
Hepatitis B core total IgG/IgM antibodies (anti-HBc)	Present with the onset of symptoms in HBV infection, persists for lifetime. If detected, means ongoing or previous HBV infection.
Hepatitis B core IgM antibody (anti-HBcIgM)	Present with onset of symptoms in HBV infection, persists for up to 6 months. Used to detect active infection.
Hepatatis B virus PCR	Provides quantitative level of HBV DNA. Detects active infection.
Hepatitis B-e Antigen (HBeAg)	Used to detect the highly infective stage of HBV. If persists after acute illness, indicated chronic liver disease from HBV.
Hepatitis B-e Antibody (HBeAb)	Used to detect recovery of infection (HBeAg normally converts to HBeAb)

HBV, hepatitis B virus; PCR, polymerase chain reaction.

Sources: Data from Centers for Disease Control and Prevention. Interpretation of hepatitis B serologic test result. https://www.cdc.gov/hepatitis/HBV/PDFs/SerologicChartv8.pdf; Schillie S, Vellozzi C, Reingold A, et al. Prevention of hepatitis B virus infection in the United States: recommendations of the Advisory Committee on Immunization Practices. *MMWR Recomm Rep.* 2018;67(1):1–31. doi:10.15585/mmwr.rr6701a1.

TABLE 89.3: TESTS FOR HEPATITIS C VIRUS

TEST	DESCRIPTION
HCV Antigen (HCV-Ag)	Tests for part of the viral capsid. Used to detect/monitor virologic response during HCV therapy. May lack sensitivity in early infection. More often, HCV RNA is performed instead of this test.
HCV Antibody (HCV-Ab)	If detected, equates to either current infection or past infection that has resolved. Can be performed as POC or laboratory-based test. Positive test should be followed with HCV RNA testing.
HCV RNA, quantitative (also called quantitative viral load)	Signals current, active infection. Can detect as little as 5 IU/mL of HCV RNA
HCV RNA, qualitative	Qualitative (detected/not-detected) molecular test for HCV RNA
HCV Genotyping	Identifies genotype 1–6 to determine appropriate pharmacotherapy.

HBV, hepatitis B virus; POC, point of care.

Sources: Data from Kamili S, Drobeniuc J, Araujo AC, Hayden TM. Laboratory diagnostics for hepatitis C virus infection. *Clin Infect Dis.* 2012;55(suppl 1):S43–S48. doi:10.1093/cid/cis368; Rao LV, Snyder LM, Wallach JB. *Wallach's Interpretation of Diagnostic Tests.* Wolters Kluwer; 2021.

Some hepatitis tests can be performed at the point-of-care (POC). While POC tests for hepatitis B are available in some countries,[8] they are not yet approved for use in the United States.[9] However, a POC test for HCV is available in the United States and offers 100% specificity and 98% sensitivity compared to laboratory-based tests.[10] One advantage of the HCV POC tests is that the faster turnaround results in improved linkages to HCV treatment and care.[11]

INDICATIONS

Screening

- Screening for HAV, HDV, and HEV is typically not needed.
- Screening recommendations for HBV and HCV infection are summarized in Table 89.4 and Box 89.1.
- In some instances, screening for proof of immunity (healthcare workers) to HBV may be warranted. Use HBsAb for this indication.

TABLE 89.4: RECOMMENDATIONS FOR SCREENING FOR HEPATITIS B AND C INFECTION

HEPATITIS B^	HEPATITIS C#
Periodic screening for individuals 12 years old and older who are at risk and not vaccinated. This includes people born in regions with a greater than 2% infection rate, people living with HIV, people using intravenous drugs, household contacts or sexual partners of those infected with HBV, people with a compromised immune system, and those receiving hemodialysis	One-time, opt-out, universal screening for all individuals 18 years old and older as well as younger than 80 years old
At first prenatal visit, with each pregnancy*	At first prenatal visit, with each pregnancy
Before starting immunosuppressive treatment	One time for individuals younger than 18-year-old with risk factors+
	Annually for persons who inject IV drugs, MSM if taking PrEP, HIV-infected MSM when sex is unprotected
	Periodically (frequency unspecified) for individuals with risk factors

*See also: https://www.cdc.gov/hepatitis/hbv/pdfs/perinatalalgorithm-prenatal.pdf

^Guidelines vary on whether to use HBsAg alone for screening or with anti-HBc and anti-HBs. Guidelines for screening in pregnancy agree to use HBsAg as the sole test.

Using hepatitis C virus antibody tests

+For risk factors see Table 88.5.

anti-HBC, antibody to hepatitis B core antigen; anti-HBs, antibody to hepatitis B surface antigen; HBsAg, hepatitis B surface antigen; HBV, hepatitis B virus; HIV, human immunodeficiency virus; IV, intravenous; MSM, men who have sex with men; PrEP, pre-exposure prophylaxis.

Sources: Data from Abara WE, Qaseem A, Schillie S, McMahon BJ, Harris AM, High Value Care Task Force of the American College of Physicians and the Centers for Disease Control and Prevention. Hepatitis B vaccination, screening, and linkage to care: best practice advice from the American College of Physicians and the Centers for Disease Control and Prevention. *Ann Intern Med.* 2017;167(11): 794–804. doi:10.7326/M17-1106; American College of Obstetricians and Gynecologists. Routine hepatitis C virus screening in pregnant individuals. Practice Advisory. Published May 2021. https://www.acog.org/clinical/clinical-guidance/practice-advisory/articles/2021/05/routine-hepatitis-c-virus-screening-in-pregnant-individuals; Schillie S, Wester C, Osborne M, Wesolowski L, Ryerson AB. CDC recommendations for hepatitis C screening among adults—United States, 2020. *MMWR Recomm Rep.* 2020;69(2):1–17. doi:10.15585/mmwr.rr6902a1; Terrault NA, Lok ASF, McMahon BJ, et al. Update on prevention, diagnosis, and treatment of chronic hepatitis B: AASLD 2018 hepatitis B guidance. *Hepatology.* 2018;67(4):1560–1599. doi:10.1002/hep.29800; United States Preventive Services Task Force; Krist AH, Davidson KW, et al. Screening for hepatitis B virus infection in adolescents and adults: US Preventive Services Task Force Recommendation Statement. *JAMA.* 2020;324(23):2415–2422. doi:10.1001/jama.2020.22980; United States Preventive Services Task Force; Owens DK, Davidson KW, et al. Screening for hepatitis C virus infection in adolescents and adults: US Preventive Services Task Force Recommendation Statement. *JAMA.* 2020;323(10):970. doi:10.1001/jama.2020.1123.

Box 89.1: Risk Factors for Hepatitis C Virus Infection

- Current or past injection/intranasal drug use
- Men who have sex with men
- Current or past use of long-term hemodialysis
- Parenteral exposure to blood/mucus of HCV-infected individual
- Infant born to individuals with HCV infection
- Solid organ transplant recipients and donors
- Infection with HBV
- Recipient of transfusion or organ transplant before 1987
- Current or previous incarceration
- HIV infection
- Plans to start PrEP for HIV
- Chronic liver disease
- Persistent elevations in ALT levels
- End-stage renal disease/dialysis

ALT, alanine aminotransferase; HBV, hepatitis B virus; HCV, hepatitis C virus; HIV, human immunodeficiency virus; PrEP, pre-exposure prophylaxis.

Sources: Data from Abara WE, Qaseem A, Schillie S, McMahon BJ, Harris AM, High Value Care Task Force of the American College of Physicians and the Centers for Disease Control and Prevention. Hepatitis B vaccination, screening, and linkage to care: best practice advice from the American College of Physicians and the Centers for Disease Control and Prevention. *Ann Intern Med.* 2017;167(11):794–804. doi:10.7326/M17-1106; American Association for the Study of Liver Diseases, Infectious Diseases Society of America. *HCV Guidance: Recommendations for Testing, Managing, and Treating Hepatitis C.* 2021. https://www.hcvguidelines.org/contents.

Diagnosis and Evaluation

- Use HBV PCR (DNA levels) to confirm infection in HBsAg-positive pregnant individuals and others with positive screening.[12]
- HCV RNA (usually, quantitative) level is used to confirm infection in those testing positive on HCV-Ab tests.[2]
- HCV genotyping is used to diagnose specific virus type if a patient is not a candidate for pan-genome pharmacotherapy.
- HAV, HBV, and HCV tests are used in the diagnosis of individuals with signs/symptoms suspicious for acute hepatitis including jaundice, fatigue, malaise, headache, abdominal pain (especially right upper quadrant), nausea, vomiting, diarrhea, arthralgias, dark-colored urine, and/or clay-colored stool.
- HBsAg, anti-HBc, and anti-HBs and HCV-Ab tests are used to evaluate for infectious hepatitis in patients presenting with elevated liver enzymes.

Monitoring

- HBV PCR is used to monitor HBV pharmacotherapy. Baseline levels are also obtained.[7]
- Quantitative HCV RNA tests are used for monitoring HCV pharmacotherapy.[13,14]
- Anti-HBs and HBsAg are used to confirm immunity for postvaccination testing (1 to 2 months after vaccination completion) in infants whose mothers tested positive for HBsAg.[12]

INTERPRETATION

- Antigen, antibody, and qualitative viral testing are usually reported as detected/not-detected.
- Quantitative viral testing will report a quantifiable amount of viral load.
- HCV test interpretation
  - +HCV-Ab with negative HCV RNA = false-positive HCV-Ab test or recent past (in the last 6 months) infection that is no longer active (has cleared).[2]
  - +HCV-Ab with +HCV RNA = current infection and needs linkage to HCV care center.
- HBV test interpretation
  - Summarized in Table 89.5.
  - Anti-HBs 10 mIU/mL or above is the reference limit for proof of adequate immunity to HBV.
  - Chronic inactive HBV: HBV DNA less than 2,000 IU/mL.[15] Active HBV: HBV DNA greater than 20,000 IU/mL[1,15]

FOLLOW-UP

- Repeat HCV-Ab tests in 6 months if there was possible exposure in the 6 months preceding testing.[2]
- Follow-up +HbsAg in pregnant individuals with HBV DNA testing.[12] Positive results should trigger linkage to care. If HBV DNA is 200,000 mIU/mL or greater, patient requires treatment.

TABLE 89.5: INTERPRETATION OF HEPATITIS B TESTING				
HBsAg	**ANTI-HBc**	**ANTI-HBs**	**INTERPRETATION**	**MANAGEMENT**
+	+	–	HBV infection	Additional testing and management needed. Perform IgM anti-HBc: if positive, it indicates acute infection; if negative, it indicates chronic infection
–	+	+	Post HBV infection, resolved and immune	No further management unless immunocompromised or undergoing chemotherapy or immunosuppressive therapy
–	+	–	Could be either: false-positive result, resolving acute infection, low level chronic infection, or resolved past infection	HBV DNA testing if immunocompromised
–	–	+	Immune due to vaccination	No further testing
–	–	–	Uninfected; not immune; susceptible	No further testing, consider immunization

Anti-HBs, antibody to hepatitis B surface antigen; Anti-HBc, antibody to hepatitis B core antigen; DNA, deoxyribonucleic acid; HBsAg, hepatitis B surface antigen; HBV, hepatitis B virus.

Sources: Data from Centers for Disease Control and Prevention. Interpretation of hepatitis B serologic test result. https://www.cdc.gov/hepatitis/HBV/PDFs/SerologicChartv8.pdf; Terrault NA, Lok ASF, McMahon BJ, et al. Update on prevention, diagnosis, and treatment of chronic hepatitis B: AASLD 2018 hepatitis B guidance. *Hepatology.* 2018;67(4):1560–1599. doi:10.1002/hep.29800.

- Transient elastography is used as follow-up in some instances to evaluate for fibrosis/cirrhosis.
- It is preferable for HCV-Ab tests to be ordered with automatic reflex to quantitative or qualitative HCV molecular tests if positive.[16] Follow-up with these tests in patients with positive HCV-Ab tests if automatic reflex was not performed.

PEARLS & PITFALLS

- Chronic hepatitis B is defined as the presence of the HBsAg for greater than 6 months.
- Acute hepatitis B is confirmed with the presence of the anti-HBc IgM and is present for less than 6 months.
- Guidelines conflict on the extent of testing needed for screening/diagnosis of HBV. The American College of Physicians recommends HbsAg, anti-HBc, and anti-HBs;[17] the United States Preventive Services Task Force recommends HBsAg;[18] and the American Association for the Study of Liver Disease recommends HBsAg and anti-HBs.[15] It is recommended to check local facility guidelines and practices.
- A small percentage of individuals who receive vaccination for HBV may be nonresponders and antibodies for HBsAg may be undetectable.[19,20] These patients may need to be re-vaccinated.

PATIENT EDUCATION

- https://www.cdc.gov/hepatitis/hcv/HepatitisCTesting.htm

RELATED DIAGNOSES AND ICD-10 CODES

Hepatitis A with hepatic coma	B15.0	Unspecified viral hepatitis B with hepatic coma	B19.11
Hepatitis A without hepatic coma	B15.9	Unspecified viral hepatitis C without hepatic coma	B19.20
Other specified acute viral hepatitis	B17.8		
Acute viral hepatitis, unspecified	B17.9	Unspecified viral hepatitis C with hepatic coma	B19.21
Chronic hepatitis C	B18.2		
Chronic viral hepatitis, unspecified	B18.9	Unspecified viral hepatitis without hepatic coma	B19.9
Unspecified viral hepatitis B without hepatic coma	B19.10		

REFERENCES

Full list of references can be accessed through Springer Publishing Company Connect™ at the following link: http://connect.springerpub.com/content/reference-book/978-0-8261-8843-4/part/part03/toc-part/ch089

90. HERPES SIMPLEX VIRUS

Joan E. Zaccardi and Kelly Small Casler

PATHOPHYSIOLOGY REVIEW

Herpes simplex virus (HSV) is a DNA virus with two serotypes: HSV-1 and HSV-2. It is most commonly known for causing sexually transmitted genital infections but can also cause other ocular, cutaneous, and neurologic syndromes from keratitis or gingivostomatitis to life threatening encephalitis.[1] HSV-1 and HSV-2 are similar in genetic makeup and replicate rapidly. Following the primary infection, the virus remains latent in the nerve cells and can reactivate along the neuron. Reactivation may occur without symptoms.[1-4]

Genital HSV is a lifelong recurrent infection of the anogenital tract characterized by vesicles of the genital mucosa and area occurring 2 to 21 days following primary infection. Transmission occurs with skin-to-skin contact with the virus entering through breaks in the skin and/or the mucous membranes of the oropharyngeal and/or anogenital area.[1-4] Genital HSV can be spread from infected mothers to the neonate during delivery.[1,5]

OVERVIEW OF LABORATORY TESTS

Viral Culture
Until recently, viral culture (CPT code 87255) had been the traditional gold standard diagnostic test for samples from vesicular fluid or other body fluids, like cerebrospinal fluid. However, culture use is limited by its poor sensitivity, especially compared to newer molecular tests.[6,7] Culture is most accurate in primary infections and in the early stages of vesicular development (when lesions are fluid filled). Accuracy decreases as vesicles start to heal.[2-4] Results are typically available within 2 to 5 days.[2-4,8]

Cytology and Antigen Tests
The Tzanck smear (CPT code 88161) detects characteristic cell changes (multinucleated giant cells) under the microscope. To perform the test, cells are scraped from active genital lesions and treated with Giemsa stain. This test has low sensitivity (30% to 67%) and specificity and cannot differentiate HSV-1 or HSV-2 infection.[5,7,9] Characteristic Tzanck smear cell changes are also seen in Varicella and herpes zoster, so this test does not definitively diagnose HSV.[7,10]

The direct fluorescent antibody (DFA) (CPT codes 87273 and 87274) test is an antigen detection test used to detect HSV-1 or HSV-2 in cells from lesion samples.[2,4,5] Testing process is labor intensive and therefore only performed in some laboratories.[11] Accuracy is poorer than culture and it has a high false-negative rate, limiting its use.[11,12]

Molecular Testing
Polymerase chain reaction (PCR) assays are the most sensitive and specific methods to confirm HSV infection and have generally replaced viral culture and

cytology/antigen tests.[13,14] Results can be obtained in as quick as 2 hours.[14] There are multiple brands of molecular HSV tests on the market and different brands have different approval for type of use (specimen tested).[14] A summary list of approved sample types across all brands is listed in Box 90.1. PCR is considered by most experts to be the new gold standard for diagnostic testing of active lesions due to its superior sensitivity/specificity and ability to differentiate between type 1 and type 2.[7] Like culture, samples from primary lesions are more likely to produce positive results than samples from reactivation outbreaks.[15]

Serology

Type-specific serology using immunoassay techniques for IgG antibodies against HSV glycoproteins is available to diagnose HSV-1 and HSV-2.[16] Serology can be used for testing an asymptomatic person with a history suspicious for genital herpes with negative or never performed diagnostic testing. Antibodies appear in the serum within 3 weeks after primary infection and have 80% to 98% sensitivity for the detection of HSV-2, depending on the brand used.[9] Point-of-care (POC) serology antibody testing can also be done with capillary or serum specimens.[9] POC testing is beneficial in assisting in rapid diagnosis in order to limit disease transmission.[8] A recent study highlighted that these POC tests may have poor positive and negative predictive values, which is a limitation of their use.[17] In some studies, the positive predictive value of serology is only about 50%.[18]

INDICATIONS

Screening

- The United State Preventive Services Task Force (USPSTF), Centers for Disease Control and Prevention (CDC), American College of Obstetricians and Gynecologists (ACOG), and two Choosing Wisely documents recommend against HSV screening in asymptomatic individuals.[8,9,15,18,19]
- Routine screening of pregnant individuals is not recommended, nor evidence-based.[9,15] However, the CDC states serologic screening could be offered to pregnant individuals with an unknown HSV status even though this practice has not been shown to be cost-effective in preventing neonatal HSV transmission.
- Screening of neonates is indicated 24 hours after delivery if the mother had characteristic genital HSV lesions at the time of birth. Culture or

---

Box 90.1: FDA Approved Uses (Specimen Types) for Molecular Herpes Simplex Virus Tests

- Anogenital
- Cerebrospinal fluid
- Cutaneous
- Dermal
- Ocular mucocutaneous
- Oral
- Vesicular lesions

Note: Not all brands are approved for all types of use.

PCR testing of blood (not FDA approved, but guideline recommended), conjunctiva, mouth, nasopharynx, rectum, and scalp electrode sites is indicated. Testing of CSF is indicated if suspicion of transmission is high.[20]

Diagnosis and Evaluation

■ Molecular testing is indicated in patients with signs or symptoms of genital HSV infection, specifically, those with painful, multiple grouped vesicular lesions with acute onset. Diagnostic testing should include typing differentiation between HSV-1 and HSV-2.[19]
■ Site-specific testing using molecular methods is indicated in patients with signs or symptoms of cutaneous HSV, herpes keratitis, or HSV encephalitis/meningitis.

Monitoring
■ This is not used.

INTERPRETATION

■ Culture/Molecular test: reported as positive or negative.
■ Serology: reported as positive, negative, or equivocal. Additional pearls for interpretation follow:
  ● Site of infection cannot technically be determined with serologic tests;[18] be cautious about the usual assumptions that if HSV-2 antibodies are detected, it is likely that the patient has genital HSV. If antibodies to HSV-1 or HSV-2 are detected, it may indicate either orolabial or genital HSV.[9]
  ● False-negative results can occur in the first 3 weeks of infection.

FOLLOW-UP

■ In patients with symptoms of genital herpes simplex infection but negative diagnostic testing, follow-up testing should be guided by differential diagnoses which include primary syphilis, chancroid, lymphogranuloma, herpes zoster, and Behcet's syndrome.
■ Patients with genital HSV should undergo screening for other sexually transmitted infections.

PEARLS & PITFALLS

■ Because of the psychosocial and lifelong ramifications of a HSV diagnosis (risk of neonatal exposure for pregnant individuals; risk of lifelong suppressive medication; etc.), testing of lesions to confirm clinical suspicion of HSV is always recommended.[3]
■ To collect a sample from a lesion, unroof the vesicle and sample the base of the lesion for best accuracy. Lesions are exquisitely painful for patients, so reassurance and support are imperative.
■ Serologic testing of IgM antibodies is not useful; only order IgG antibodies.

PATIENT EDUCATION

■ https://www.cdc.gov/std/herpes/screening.htm

RELATED DIAGNOSES AND ICD-10 CODES

Herpes viral infection of the lower urogenital system, unspecified	A60.00	Herpes viral infection of perianal skin and rectum	A60.1
Herpes viral infection, unspecified	B00.9	Herpes viral cervicitis	A60.03
Disorders of the male genital organs	N51	Herpes viral vulvovaginitis	A60.04
Herpes simplex infection of the penis	A60.01		

REFERENCES

Full list of references can be accessed through Springer Publishing Company Connect™ at the following link: http://connect.springerpub.com/content/reference-book/978-0-8261 -8843-4/part/part03/toc-part/ch090

91. HOMOCYSTEINE

Audra Hanners

PHYSIOLOGY REVIEW

Homocysteine is an amino acid intermediary product formed during metabolism of methionine. Elevated homocysteine levels are associated with an increased risk of cardiovascular disease (CVD), specifically stroke, coronary heart disease, and peripheral vascular disease.[1-3] Hyperhomocysteinemia (15 µmol/L or greater) causes endothelial damage and promotes atherosclerosis. Homocysteine concentrations in the blood are influenced by many nutritional factors, such as B vitamins, folate, vitamin B12 ,and vitamin B6 into other metabolism products the body needs. These nutritional factors break down homocysteine. Dietary deficiency of vitamin B12, vitamin B6, and folate are common causes of elevated homocysteine. Folic acid, as well as vitamins B6 and B12, have been used in studies to successfully lower homocysteine levels.[4] Evidence suggests a two-fold increase in chances of a myocardial infarction among individuals with a total homocysteine concentration of 15 µmol/L or more. This association did not differ by race or ethnicity.[1,2] Homocysteine levels may increase with age, smoking, and low intake of B vitamins. Low levels of homocysteine may be due to abnormalities in metabolic pathways due to lack of availability or ability of the body to produce certain metabolites.[5]

OVERVIEW OF LABORATORY TESTS

Laboratory evaluation of homocysteine status can be assessed by a fasting plasma homocysteine level (CPT code 83090). Testing for homocysteine is expensive and there are no current guidelines recommending routine testing.

INDICATIONS

Screening

- No universal screening indications. Targeted screening may be used for family members of patients with homocysteinuria.[6]
- Although limited research shows vitamin B12, B6, and folic acid therapy can decrease homocysteine levels, studies do not indicate that these therapies indicate a reduction in heart disease risk.[4,7] Therefore, homocysteine screening is not useful as a prevention measure for heart disease.

Diagnosis and Evaluation

- Testing is warranted in neonates with acidosis, failure to thrive, neutropenia, seizure, and irritability, as these may be symptoms of newborn homocystinuria.[8,9]
- Testing is also warranted in children and adolescents with developmental delay, cardiovascular disease, thromboembolism, osteoporosis, or ocular abnormalities, as these may be symptoms of homocystinuria.[8]
- Homocysteine levels can assist in the diagnosis of vitamin B12 or folate deficiencies when results from vitamin B12 or folate levels are borderline low. Elevated homocysteine levels are seen with folate and vitamin B12 vitamin deficiencies.[6]

Monitoring

- No evidence exists to support routine monitoring.

INTERPRETATION

- Normal reference interval for homocysteine is between 5 and 14 µmol/L.
- Hypohomocysteinemia occurs when homocysteine is below 5 µmol/L.
- Classifications for hyperhomocysteinemia are as follows[6,10]:
  - Moderate: 15 to 30 µmol/L
  - Intermediate: 30 to 100 µmol/L
  - Severe: greater than 100 µmol/L

FOLLOW-UP

- Increased homocysteine may be caused by the following; therefore, follow-up testing is warranted to evaluate for[1,2,4,10]:
  - Cardiovascular disease
  - Cerebrovascular disease
  - Peripheral vascular disease
  - Folate deficiency or b12 deficiency
  - Chronic kidney disease

PEARLS & PITFALLS

- Hypohomocysteinemia due to metabolic pathway changes may result in secondary neuropathy.[5]
- Hyperhomocysteinemia should be further investigated for possible results of certain drug effects, genetic factors, lifestyle determinants, and clinical comorbid conditions[6,9]

■ Drugs used in hypercholesterolemia may raise homocysteine levels in addition to metformin or methotrexate.[11,12]

■ Cigarette smoking can cause elevated homocysteine levels.[13]

PATIENT EDUCATION

■ https://www.webmd.com/heart-disease/guide/homocysteine-risk

RELATED DIAGNOSES AND ICD-10 CODES

Homocystinuria	E72.11
Homocystinemia	E72.11

Note: No ICD-10 code distinguishes between homocystinuria and homocystinemia.

REFERENCES

Full list of references can be accessed through Springer Publishing Company Connect™ at the following link: http://connect.springerpub.com/content/reference-book/978-0-8261 -8843-4/part/part03/toc-part/ch091

92. HUMAN CHORIONIC GONADOTROPIN

Randee L. Masciola

PHYSIOLOGY/PATHOPHYSIOLOGY REVIEW

Human chorionic gonadotropin (hCG) is commonly called the pregnancy hormone and is secreted by the trophoblastic cells of the early embryo, specifically the placenta.[1] In the absence of pregnancy, smaller amounts of hCG are secreted from the pituitary gland monthly and trigger the corpus luteum (CL) to sustain progesterone levels which, in turn, maintain the stability of the endometrium. When fertilization does not occur, the CL regresses and progesterone production decreases, leading to menstruation. When pregnancy is achieved, the embryo produces large amounts of hCG, signaling the CL to produce more progesterone to maintain the endometrium and uterine environment to promote implantation and pregnancy establishment.[1] In the first 6 weeks of pregnancy, the CL produces most of the progesterone in response to the hCG produced by the embryo.[1] High levels of hCG are required for the CL to produce enough progesterone to maintain the endometrium environment for implementation and placenta development. After 6 weeks, the placenta takes over the responsibility of producing progesterone and the hCG level will begin to decrease.[1] In addition to facilitating progesterone production by the CL, hCG is also responsible for an increase in maternal thyroid activity during pregnancy,[2] fetal testes and adrenal development,[3] and endometrial function.[4]

In a normal pregnancy, serum hCG levels are detectable by 1 day after implementation and 8 days after ovulation, after which they double every 2 to 3 days until they peak at 60 to 90 days gestation.[1] The levels will then plateau for the remainder of the pregnancy. In urine, hCG levels can be detected 12 to 15 days after ovulation.

While hCG is almost exclusively found during normal pregnancy, it can be detected in other conditions. Very high levels occur with an ectopic or molar pregnancy. In these conditions where the placenta and CL are absent, high hCG levels are produced by the aberrant fertilized eggs and will continue to be produced; they will elevate rapidly.[5] Very low levels of hCG can be detected in men and women, with no known function. Low levels of hCG can also be seen in perimenopause, cancers (liver, lung, pancreatic, or stomach), and chemotherapy.[6]

OVERVIEW OF LABORATORY TESTS

There are two ways to detect hCG. The most common method uses a urine sample to qualitatively detect hCG in the urine through immunoassay. Urine hCG tests are less expensive, less invasive, more convenient, and faster, with a turnaround time of 5 to 10 minutes.[7] They also can be obtained and completed by the patient without a clinician order. Urine hCG or "urine pregnancy" tests (CPT code 81025) can detect hCG in urine up to 7 days prior to a missed period, and the over-the-counter FDA-approved home pregnancy tests work as well as the healthcare-based products. Urine pregnancy tests can be up to 99% accurate, if used correctly (i.e., timing, follow instructions, read results properly) and are the gold standard test to confirm pregnancy.[8] Home pregnancy tests, however, do have a large variation in detectable lower limit of hCG, which can create a variation in specificity.[9]

hCG can also be detected using a serum blood sample. Serum hCG tests are more sensitive and specific than urine testing. Serum levels can be detected at as low as 1 to 2 milli-international units/mL, whereas urine detection occurs at a level of 20 to 50 milli-international units/mL.[10] This is significant since if a pregnancy test is completed too early it could provide a false-negative result. The serum test is often ordered with a quantitative reflex (CPT code 84703) which, if positive qualitatively, will reflex to give a quantitative value. The quantitative value is useful to evaluate length of gestation in a normal pregnancy or to monitor levels to guide determination of normal/viable pregnancy or alternative diagnoses.[11] Serum hCG testing is the only testing method that can provide quantitative values.

INDICATIONS

Screening

■ Universal pregnancy screening in not indicated for routine primary care visits.
■ Even though universal preoperative pregnancy testing is often the standard, a retrospective review of universal preoperative pregnancy screening demonstrated very low utility to this requirement.[12] In 2016, the

American Society of Anesthesiologists (ASA) reiterated that there is no need for this practice.[9]

Diagnosis, Evaluation, and Monitoring

▪ Qualitative hCG testing is used in the differential diagnosis of amenorrhea or abdominal pain to evaluate for the possibility of pregnancy.

▪ Serial serum hCG levels are monitored to rule out a differential diagnosis that would not align with a viable pregnancy. Viable pregnancies show doubling of hCG every 48 hours, and so serial serum hCG levels should be monitored according to this interval when evaluating for a differential diagnosis that could be life threatening or may need intervention. Signs/ Symptoms that warrant testing include:
  ● Spotting during previously diagnosed pregnancy to rule out ectopic or molar
  ● Severe pain during previously diagnosed pregnancy to rule out ectopic or molar
  ● Diagnosed spontaneous abortion to rule out ectopic or molar pregnancy

▪ In ectopic pregnancy, decreasing serum hCG values should be followed until nonpregnant levels (less than 5 mIU/mL) are achieved due to the possibility of spontaneous rupture while levels are decreasing.[5]

INTERPRETATION

▪ Table 92.1 lists expected serum quantitative hCG results based on gestation age for a singleton pregnancy.

▪ Serum hCG tests are qualitative and can measure hCG as low as 1 to 2 mIU/mL.[7] A qualitative serum hCG test is considered negative for pregnancy if the hCG level is less than 5 mIU/mL and positive if the level is above 25 mIU/mL.[7]

TABLE 92.1: REFERENCE RANGES FOR HUMAN CHORIONIC GONADOTROPIN	
GESTATIONAL AGE	**EXPECTED hCG VALUES (mIU/mL)**
<1 Week	5–50
1–2 Weeks	50–500
2–3 Weeks	100–5,000
3–4 Weeks	500–10,000
4–5 Weeks	1,000–50,000
5–6 Weeks	10,000–100,000
6–8 Weeks	15,000–200,000
8–12 Weeks	10,000–100,000

Source: Data from Williamson MA, Snyder LM. *Wallach's Interpretation of Diagnostic Tests.* Lippincott Williams and Wilkins; 2021.

- Quantitative serum hCG levels are reported as milli-international units of hCG hormone per milliliter of blood, or mIU/mL, but can also be reported as international unit per liter (IU/L) and can detect hCG as low as 1 to 2 mIU/mL. If there is concern for viable pregnancy and the hCG level is between 6 and 24 mIU/mL, the patient is retested in 48 hours to confirm a normal intrauterine pregnancy.[7]
- Whether at home or in a clinic, urine hCG testing is a qualitative result, reporting only a positive or negative result. The urine test detects hCG levels as low as 20 to 50 mIU/mL, which correlates to approximately 4 weeks post-conception.[7]
- hCG levels should double every 29 to 53 hours during the first 30 days after implantation for a viable, intrauterine pregnancy and to rule out any differential diagnosis.[8] Failing to double every 48 hours is an early sign of potential spontaneous abortion and warrants further testing.
- Decreasing serum hCG values indicate a failing pregnancy and can be used to evaluate spontaneous abortion resolution.[5] This decrease should not be considered diagnostic and should be coupled with transvaginal ultrasound evaluation.[5]
- Significantly high hCG levels (more than doubling every 48 hours) could indicate multiples, ectopic, or molar pregnancy and requires further testing, usually with ultrasound.
- A negative urine hCG does not rule out ectopic pregnancy, and if the potential of pregnancy is suspected a serum hCG should be evaluated.[13]
- Table 92.2 reviews false positives and false negatives that should be considered when interpreting hCG results.

FOLLOW-UP

- Serum hCG alone should never be used to diagnose (or when suspicion is high, exclude) a molar or ectopic pregnancy and should be used in conjunction with ultrasound, as a ruptured ectopic can lead very quickly to a medical emergency.[5]

TABLE 92.2: CAUSES OF FALSE POSITIVES AND FALSE NEGATIVES IN HUMAN CHORIONIC GONADOTROPIN INTERPRETATION

URINE hCG	SERUM hCG
False positives	**False positives**
• Blood in urine	• Recent blood transfusions
• Human error	• Chronic renal failure
• Drugs	• IgA deficiency
	• Rheumatoid factors
False negatives	**False negative**
• Sample taken too early	• Sample taken too early
• Diluted sample	

Source: Data from Betz D, Fane K. Human Chorionic Gonadotropin. [Updated 2020 Aug 30]. In: *StatPearls* [Internet]. StatPearls Publishing; 2021. https://www.ncbi.nlm.nih.gov/books/NBK532950/

- Urine hCG testing may be repeated if it was determined the test may have been done incorrectly or too early.
- If amenorrhea and/or pregnancy symptoms continue, a urine pregnancy test should be repeated in 1 week. If symptoms continue, a serum hCG test should be considered.
- hCG levels are often followed down to less than 5 mIU/mL to assure a complete abortion has occurred or the treatment for a molar or ectopic pregnancy has been successful.

PEARLS & PITFALLS

- All patients of childbearing age with delayed menses onset, unexplained pelvic pain, or undiagnosed uterine bleeding/spotting should receive a hCG test.
- Consider ultrasound if hCG testing results do not align with history and physical assessment or a viable intrauterine pregnancy.
- A patient with vaginal spotting/bleeding and/or pelvic pain and a positive pregnancy test (urine or serum) without ultrasound confirmation of intrauterine location should be promptly evaluated for the possibility of an ectopic pregnancy.
- Serum hCG levels do not rise normally in ectopic pregnancies and ectopic pregnancies can rupture at very low hCG levels (under 100 mIU/mL).[13]

PATIENT EDUCATION

- https://www.plannedparenthood.org/learn/pregnancy/pregnancy-tests
- https://www.hormone.org/your-health-and-hormones/glands-and-hormones-a-to-z/hormones/human-chorionic-gonadotropin-hormone-hcg

RELATED DIAGNOSES AND ICD-10 CODES

Normal pregnancy	Z34	Multiple gestations	O30
Secondary amenorrhea	N911	Familial hCG syndrome (inappropriate change in quantitative hCG)	O0281
Abnormal uterine bleeding (vaginal spotting/bleeding)	N93		
		Cancer	Dependent on location
Abdominal/pelvic/adnexal pain	R10		
Ectopic pregnancy	O00	Perimenopause/menopause	
Molar pregnancy	O08	Premature menopause	E2831
		Asymptomatic menopausal state	Z780
Spontaneous abortion	O03		

REFERENCES

Full list of references can be accessed through Springer Publishing Company Connect™ at the following link: http://connect.springerpub.com/content/reference-book/978-0-8261-8843-4/part/part03/toc-part/ch092

93. HUMAN IMMUNODEFICIENCY VIRUS AND CD4

Courtney DuBois Shihabuddin and Stephanie L. Marrs

PHYSIOLOGY REVIEW

HIV is an opportunistic infection resulting from CD4 cell depletion.[1] HIV most commonly enters the body through the anogenital tract. HIV has several targets including dendritic cells, macrophages, and CD4+ T cells. HIV-1 most often enters the host through the anogenital mucosa, where the viral envelope protein, glycoprotein (GP)-120, binds to the CD4 molecule on dendritic cells and the virus enters the cell.[2]

HIV-infected cells fuse with CD4+ T cells, leading to spread of the virus. HIV is detectable in regional lymph nodes within 2 days of mucosal exposure and in plasma within another 3 days.[3] Once the virus enters the blood, there is widespread dissemination to organs such as the brain, spleen, and lymph nodes. HIV RNA levels rapidly increase to a peak level that usually coincides with seroconversion of HIV status.[4,5] When a patient is initially infected with the HIV virus, they have a large number of susceptible CD4+ T cells and no HIV-specific immune response. Viral replication is therefore rapid.[6]

As previously mentioned, there are two types of the HIV virus. HIV type 1 (HIV-1) causes faster disease progression than HIV type 2 (HIV-2).[7] HIV-1 contributes to the most HIV infections worldwide. HIV-2 is often seen in the following geographic areas: West Africa or areas with historic ties to West Africa, such as Portugal, Spain, and Goa, India. The natural history of HIV-2 infection is similar to that of HIV-1 infection (i.e., acute infection followed by prolonged, asymptomatic chronic infection and ultimate immunosuppression with greater risk for additional infection and other comorbidities) but is characterized by lower levels of viremia, slower declines in the CD4 cell count, and a longer asymptomatic period of chronic infection.[7]

OVERVIEW OF LABORATORY TESTS

Testing for HIV should be completed using the fourth-generation antigen/antibody combination of HIV-1/2 immunoassay (CPT codes 87389, 86701, 86702). In addition, a confirmatory HIV-1/HIV-2 antibody differentiation immunoassay should be performed.[8]

Plasma HIV RNA (CPT code 87536), also referred to as HIV viral load (HIV VL), should be measured in all patients upon entry into care and at regular intervals during treatment, as it is the most accurate indicator of response to antiretroviral therapy (ART) and is useful in predicting disease progression.[9,10]

A CD4 cell is a type of lymphocyte that helps to coordinate the body's immune response by stimulating other immune cells, such as macrophages, B lymphocytes (B cells), and CD8 T lymphocytes (CD8 cells), to fight infection.

HIV weakens the immune system by destroying CD4 cells. Therefore, CD4 cell counts (CPT code 86361) correlate with a patient's immune response. In patients who achieve and maintain viral suppression, immunologic improvement is progressive over many years.[11] The CD4:CD8 ratio (CPT code 86360) test can also be ordered and it includes the percentage of CD4 cells, the absolute CD4 count, the percentage of CD8 cells, the absolute CD8 count, the CD4:CD8 ratio, and a CBC with differential.

INDICATIONS

Screening

There are universal and targeted HIV screenings recommended.

- Patients without risk factors for HIV should receive at least one-time HIV screening between the ages of 13 to 75 years.[12]
- All pregnant individuals should be tested for HIV early in pregnancy using an "opt-out" approach, even if they have been screened during a previous pregnancy.[12]
- Men who have sex with men (MSM) may benefit from HIV testing every 3 to 6 months, depending on sexual activity.[13,14]

The following patient categories would also benefit from frequent (every 3 to 6 months) screening[12,13]:

- Injection drug users
- Persons who exchange sex for drugs or money
- Sex partners of people who are HIV-infected, bisexual, or inject drugs
- People who have sex with partners whose HIV status is unknown

Diagnosis and Evaluation

Symptoms of acute retroviral syndrome should alert the clinician to test for HIV. These symptoms include[15-17]:

- Fever
- Lymphadenopathy (may be minimal)[18]
- Sore throat
- Myalgias
- Diarrhea
- Weight Loss
- Headache
- Rash of the upper chest to face

Patients may not present with multiple symptoms, but many will have at least one.[18]

Differential diagnoses for HIV should include:

- Mononucleosis due to Epstein-Barr virus (EBV) or cytomegalovirus (CMV)
- Toxoplasmosis
- Rubella
- Syphilis
- Disseminated gonococcal infection

- Viral hepatitis
- Other viral infections

Monitoring

Long-term monitoring for immune status function is completed with CD4 cell counts and HIV RNA testing. CD4 T-cell count and plasma HIV RNA are two of the key tests needed to assess and monitor the status of an HIV patient's disease progression and treatment success.

Plasma HIV RNA

Plasma HIV RNA, also referred to as HIV VL, should be measured in all patients upon entry into care and every 3 to 4 months during the first 2 years of HIV treatment. After this monitoring phase and following a persistently suppressed viral load, it can be monitored every 6 months.[9,19] HIV VL is the most accurate indicator of response to ART and is useful in predicting disease progression.[9,10]

CD4 T-Cell Count

After initial HIV diagnosis, CD4 count should be monitored every 3 to 6 months. Patients with higher levels of CD4 counts and consistently suppressed HIV viral loads require less frequent monitoring. An annual CD4 count is sufficient once the patient's CD4 count is greater than 500. However, the CD4 count would require more frequent monitoring if the HIV viral load is no longer suppressed. HIV viral loads of less than or equal to 200 are considered fully suppressed and usually do not require action.[20,21]

The following patient categories should continue to receive CD4 count monitoring every 3 to 6 months[20,21]:

- Patients with an opportunistic infection
- Those undergoing immunosuppressive therapy
- Patients with a viral load of more than 200 copies/mL and receiving ART

INTERPRETATION

HIV-1/HIV-2 Antibody Differentiation Immunoassay

Results of the HIV-1/HIV-2 antibody differentiation immunoassay can be interpreted as follows[4,5] (Figure 93.1)[22]:

- If the fourth-generation combination assay is negative, the person is not infected with HIV and no additional testing is warranted.
- If the fourth-generation combination assay is positive, an HIV-1/HIV-2 antibody differentiation immunoassay should be performed. This test confirms the result of the combination assay and determines if the patient is infected with HIV-1, HIV-2, or both HIV-1 and HIV-2.
- A plasma HIV RNA level should be ordered to evaluate for acute infection if the fourth-generation combination assay is positive and the confirmatory antibody differentiation immunoassay is indeterminate or negative.

Plasma HIV RNA

- Upon initiation of ART therapy, HIV RNA should achieve substantial ($2 \log_{10}$ or more) decline by 2 to 4 weeks of treatment. Anything less than a $2\text{-}\log_{10}$ or greater decrease is suggestive of poor medication adherence (Table 93.1)[23].

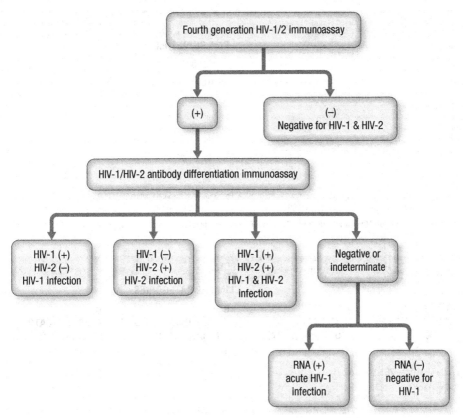

FIGURE 93.1. Interpretation of results of the HIV-1/HIV-2 antibody differentiation immunoassay.
Source: Modified from CDC and Prevention and Association of Public Health Laboratories. Laboratory
esting for the diagnosis of HIV infection: updated recommendations. Published June 27, 2014. http://
stacks.cdc.gov/view/cdc/23447.

- The viral load should be near undetectable or undetectable by 8 to 24 weeks
  of antiretroviral drug therapy, regardless of prior treatment experience. The
  higher the initial load, the longer it will take to become undetectable.[24–26]
- Viral blips of up to 400 copies per milliliter are not of clinical significance
  in individuals with otherwise well controlled HIV. Less than 200 copies per
  milliliter is consistent with appropriate HIV control.[9,19]

CD4 T-Cell Count

- Normal values for a CD4 absolute count range from 500 to 1,600.
- Normal percentages of CD4 lymphocytes are about 30% to 60%.
- Patients with a CD4 count of 200 cells/mm³ or lower blood meet
  the diagnostic criteria for AIDS and are considered at most risk for
  opportunistic infections (OI's).[19]
- See Table 93.2 for HIV staging information based on CD4 counts.

FOLLOW-UP

Depending on the viral load and CD4 cell count, the patient may need additional testing, especially if there are any "AIDS defining illnesses" (Box 93.1).

TABLE 93.1: HIV RNA VIRAL LOAD LOG VALUE-NUMBER CONVERSION

LOG*10	RNA COPIES/mL
7	10,000,000
6	1,000,000
5	100,000
4	10,000
3	1,000
2	100
1	10

* A log is a mathematical term used to describe changes in HIV RNA. For example, if the viral load is 2,000,000 copies/mL, then a 1-log decrease equals a 10-fold (10 times) decrease, or 200,000 copies/mL. A 2-log decrease equals a 100-fold decrease, of 20,000 copies/mL.

Source: Data from HIV/AIDS Glossary: Log10. NIH's Office of AIDS Research. https://clinicalinfo.hiv.gov/en/glossary/log10.

TABLE 93.2: CDC CLASSIFICATION SYSTEM FOR HIV INFECTION

CD4+ T-CELL COUNT (CELLS/μl.) (CD4%)	CLINICAL CATEGORIES		
	A ASYMPTOMATIC, ACUTE (PRIMARY) HIV	B SYMPTOMATIC, (NOT A OR C CONDITIONS)	C AIDS-INDICATOR CONDITIONS
>500 (28%)	A1	B1	C1
200–499 (15%–28%)	A2	B2	C2
<200 (14%)	A3	B3	C3

Notes: Category A: Asymptomatic HIV infection, persistent generalized lymphadenopathy.

Category B: Oropharyngeal and vulvovaginal candidiasis, constitutional symptoms such as fever (38.5 °C) or diarrhea lasting longer than 1 month, herpes zoster (shingles).

Category C: Mycobacterium tuberculosis (pulmonary or disseminated), Pneumocystis carinii pneumonia, candidiasis of bronchi; trachea or lungs, extrapulmonary cryptococcosis, CMV, HIV-related encephalopathy, Kaposi's sarcoma, wasting syndrome due to HIV.

Consider screening for other sexually transmitted infections, including gonorrhea, chlamydia, syphilis, and trichomonas if the patient is at high risk, even with a negative HIV test.

PEARLS & PITFALLS

■ Opt-out screening should be used for HIV testing.[12]
  ● Patients should be informed via signage, hand out, or discussion that an HIV test will be done. The patient can decline, or "opt-out."
  ● No special counseling or consent form is needed.
  ● Patients may not be aware of risk factors, and asymptomatic infection can be identified early, adding years to an individual's life.
  ● Opt-out screening lowers barriers to testing and normalizes the screening.
  ● HIV-related stigma is a barrier to testing for many individuals and communities. Healthcare clinicians can help by including this test with other routine laboratory tests.
  ● Reduction in transmission occurs when status is known and people are in care for HIV.

Box 93.1: AIDS Defining Illnesses

- Bacterial infections, multiple or recurrent
- Candidiasis of esophagus, bronchi, trachea, or lungs (not oral)
- Cervical cancer, invasive
- Coccidioidomycosis, disseminated or extrapulmonary
- Cryptococcosis, extrapulmonary
- Cryptosporidiosis, chronic intestinal
- Cytomegalovirus (other than liver, spleen, or nodes)
- Cytomegalovirus retinitis (with vision loss)
- Encephalopathy (HIV)
- Herpes simplex virus, chronic or bronchitis, pneumonitis, or esophagitis
- Histoplasmosis, disseminated or extrapulmonary
- Isosporiasis, chronic
- Kaposi sarcoma
- Lymphoma
- *Mycobacterium avium* complex or *Mycobacterium kansaii*, disseminated or extrapulmonary
- Mycobacterium tuberculosis, any site
- Mycobacterium, other species or unidentified, disseminated or extrapulmonary
- Pneumocystis pneumonia (PCP)
- Pneumonia (recurrent)
- Progressive multifocal leukoencephalopathy
- Salmonella septicemia
- Toxoplasmosis (brain)
- Wasting syndrome

PATIENT EDUCATION

- https://www.cdc.gov/hiv/basics/index.html
- https://hivinfo.nih.gov/understanding-hiv/fact-sheets

RELATED DIAGNOSES AND ICD-10 CODES

Human immunodeficiency syndrome	Z21
Acquired immunodeficiency syndrome	B20
Encounter for screening for human immunodeficiency virus	Z11.4
Human immunodeficiency virus (HIV) disease complicating pregnancy	O98.7
Contact with and suspected exposure to HIV	Z20.6
High risk sexual activity	Z72.5

REFERENCES

Full list of references can be accessed through Springer Publishing Company Connect™
at the following link: http://connect.springerpub.com/content/reference-book/
978-0-8261-8843-4/part/part03/toc-part/ch093

94. HUMAN LEUKOCYTE ANTIGEN

Elyssa Power

PHYSIOLOGY REVIEW

The major histocompatibility complex (MHC) is a group of genes that encode a variety of cell surface markers, antigen-presenting molecules, and other proteins involved in immune function. In humans, the MHC is synonymous with the human leukocyte antigen (HLA) complex. These cell membrane glycoproteins, which are found on the short arm of chromosome 6, reside on the surface of almost every cell in the human body and play a key role in the initiation of the immune response. Each person has a unique set of human leukocyte antigens, half of which are inherited from each parent. In the context of transplantation, biologic parents are a "half-match" with their children, whereas siblings of the same biologicparents have a one in four chance of being a full HLA match.[1] With the knowledge of HLA typing, it was now possible to tissue match organ donors to recipients, increasing the probability of a successful transplant without rejection. Since the first HLA gene was discovered, thousands of HLA alleles have been identified and the names and sequences of all known alleles have been curated in the IMGT/HLA database.[2]

The HLA genes are known to be the most polymorphic genes of the human genome (e.g., over 6,500 alleles are known for HLA-B and over 2,500 alleles for HLA-DRB1). The HLA region (Figure 94.1) has been subdivided into three regions: class I, class II, and class III; the HLA genes are located within the class I and class II regions. This polymorphism is predominantly found within the six classical HLA genes: the class I genes HLA-A, -B, and -C and the class II genes HLA-DRB1, -DQB1, and -DPB1. Each gene contains numerous gene loci, including expressed genes and pseudogenes.[3] While the class III region does not contain any of the HLA genes, it does contain many genes of importance in the immune response (e.g., complement, tumor necrosis factor, heat shock protein).[1]

HLA typing is predominantly used in transplant medicine as pre-transplant testing to assess compatibility of recipients and donors of hematopoietic stem cell or bone marrow transplants and kidney transplants. Due to advancements in the field, HLA testing can now identify HLA alleles and allele groups associated with specific diseases as well as diagnose certain HLA-related drug hypersensitivity reactions when the testing is supported by the literature.[3]

OVERVIEW OF LABORATORY TESTS

■ HLA testing is obtained via a tissue sample, either via a blood test or a cheek swab.
■ Current methods for HLA typing (CPT codes 81370 to 81383) define HLA alleles and allele groups using DNA-based methods.

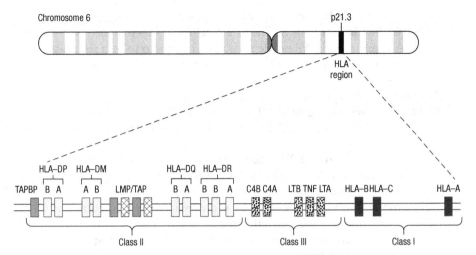

FIGURE 94.1. Gene structure of the human leukocyte antigen (HLA).

■ All typing methods rely on DNA extraction from the nucleated cells following cell lysis and protein digestion.[4]
■ Different clinical scenarios present different HLA typing requirements.
■ Next generation sequencing (NGS) (CPT codes 81445, 81450, 81455), the latest molecular technology introduced in clinical tissue typing laboratories, has demonstrated advantages over other established methods.[5]

INDICATIONS

The text that follows includes the clinical indications in which a clinician may order HLA typing. The most common application of histocompatibility testing remains the selection of compatible donors for recipients who require hematopoietic stem cell/bone marrow transplantation or solid organ transplantation.

1. Allogeneic hematopoietic stem cell transplantation (HSCT)
   ● Allogeneic transplants are when cells are collected from a person other than the patient (either a related or unrelated donor) and are infused after the patient receives chemotherapy. This is as opposed to autologous transplants which are when the patient's own cells are collected and then re-infused after chemotherapy. Allogeneic hematopoietic cell transplantation is a potentially curative therapy for a wide variety of malignant and non-malignant hematologic disorders.
   ● All recipients and potential donors should have high-resolution HLA typing, screening, and identification of HLA antibodies in the recipient, and detection of antibodies in the recipient that are reactive with lymphocytes of a prospective donor (i.e., crossmatching).
   ● Matching donor and recipient for HLA class I (-A, -B, and -C) and class II (-DR and -DQ) haplotypes is key to a successful allogeneic HSCT.

■ HLA class I (A, B, and/or C) allele mismatch causes a significantly higher incidence of engraftment failure than HLA match.[6]

■ HLA-A and/or HLA-B allele mismatch is known to be a significant factor for the occurrence of acute and chronic graft-versus-host-disease (GVHD).

● Potential donor options

■ Identical twin (syngeneic, HLA identical = 6 of 6)

■ Sibling, relative, or unrelated donor (HLA identical, haploidentical, or mismatched).

● Siblings: There is a 25% chance that a sibling will be fully HLA matched at the A, B, and DR loci, which are principal loci evaluated in this setting.

● An HLA-haploidentical donor is one who shares, by common inheritance, exactly one HLA haplotype with the recipient and is mismatched for a variable number of HLA genes, ranging from zero to six, on the unshared haplotype.

■ HLA-haploidentical donors are typically biologic parents or biologic children of the recipient.

■ Haploidentical grafts allow for additional grafts if needed but have a higher rate of graft-versus-host-disease and/or relapse depending on the approaches utilized.[7]

■ There are advantages and disadvantages with this donor source that should be taken into consideration.

■ Umbilical cord blood (UCB)

● Recipients of UCB transplants are able to tolerate greater HLA disparity than those of other graft sources.

● Minimum matching criteria for an unrelated donor transplant requires at least a seven of eight HLA match, while UCB transplant allows for a four of six match. However, there are disadvantages to UCB including a greater risk of graft failure; UCB transplants do not allow for additional grafts from the same donor if needed.

● In addition to the clinical benefits of a fully matched sibling, these donors are preferred over other sources due to the speed of identification and initiation of cell collection.

■ Approximately one-third of patients in the United States have a sibling who can serve as their donor.

● When an HLA-matched or partially mismatched acceptable related donor is not available, the transplant center will proceed with an unrelated donor search through the registry. The National Marrow Donor Program (NMDP) was founded in the United States in 1986 to establish a volunteer marrow donor registry and to serve as a source of HLA-matched unrelated marrow and stem cell donors. The NMDP now contains more than 19 million donors.[7]

● Choosing among several equally matched donors (related and/or unrelated) is further narrowed based on the type of graft planned (bone marrow versus peripheral blood), the mismatched HLA gene, further typing of other HLA genes, and an evaluation of the recipient for specific HLA antibodies. In addition, donor selection among several equally matched donors must take into account other donor characteristics such as age, cytomegalovirus (CMV) status (matching for CMV status is preferred), sex (males and nulliparous females preferred), and blood type.[7]

- Donor selection is a complicated process that requires the clinical expertise of a transplant center.

2. Solid organ transplantation
   - Kidney transplantation
     - The benefits of HLA matching are well established in kidney transplantation.
     - There is a clear relationship between the degree of HLA matching and kidney graft survival from living related donors.
     - Kidney transplantation from a living unrelated donor shows graft survival superior to deceased donor transplantation (except for a six of six match) despite a greater degree of HLA mismatch.[8]
     - Better results are obtained from an HLA-matched sibling donor than with HLA-haploidentical parents, siblings, or children.[9]
   - Heart transplantation
     - Allocation of donors with regard to HLA is controversial in this patient population.
     - The potential benefits of HLA matching on cardiac transplant survival have generally been obscured by the short cardiac cold ischemia time, donor-recipient cardiac size constraints, absence of a long-term life support alternative to transplantation, and the severe prognosis of refractory cardiac failure.
     - HLA typing is not routinely performed in heart transplantation.[10]
   - Liver and thoracic organ transplantation: The influence of HLA matching on the survival of these organs is uncertain and further research is needed.
     - Pretransplant crossmatching is not routinely performed prior to liver transplant because of the urgent need of organs and the unclear benefits of a crossmatch-negative transplant.[9]
   - Deceased donor organ transplant candidates
     - All deceased organ donor candidates are registered with UNOS and each organ donor is HLA typed and screened for preformed HLA antibodies.[11]
     - Pretransplant crossmatching is performed by the patient's transplantation center.
   - The specific methodology used for HLA typing in solid organ transplantation differs between HLA laboratories.

3. Pharmacogenetics
   - Pharmacogenetic testing is not widely used in routine clinical practice to optimize drug choice or clinical management.

- This is most likely due to the fact that the successful incorporation of a pharmacogenetic test into routine clinical practice requires a combination of high-level evidence that can be generalized to diverse clinical settings, widespread availability of cost-effective and reliable laboratory tests, and effective strategies to incorporate testing into routine clinical practice.
- HLA testing may be used for selected pharmacogenomics testing, specifically for risk assessment of drug hypersensitivity reactions.
- It is known that the HLA genes of a specific individual influence select drug responses; more recently, severe and even fatal drug hypersensitivity reactions linked to particular HLA alleles have been discovered.
- Numerous studies have shown a relationship between HLA class I and class II molecules and DIH; the most well-established of such relationships is the association of HLA-B with carbamazepine-induced Stevens-Johnson syndrome/toxic epidermal necrolysis (SJS/TEN) in Southeast Asian populations and HLA-B*57 with abacavir hypersensitivity.[4]
  - Carbamazepine (see Chapter 38)
    - Severe hypersensitivity reactions including SJS/TEN may occur in 5% to 10% of patients taking the anti-epileptic drug carbamazepine if they carry the *HLA-B*1502* allele.
    - The U.S. FDA recommends screening for the *HLA-B*1502* allele prior to administration of carbamazepine for all patients of Asian ancestry.[12]
  - Abacavir
    - Serious and sometimes fatal hypersensitivity reactions with multi-organ involvement may occur in *HLA-B*57:01* positive patients taking the antiretroviral drug, abacavir.
    - The U.S. FDA recommends prescreening patients for *B*57:01* prior to starting treatment with abacavir.[4]

4. Disease association

Certain diseases, especially of autoimmune nature, have been found to be associated with particular HLA types in the general population; however, the association level varies among diseases, and there is a lack of strong concordance between the HLA type and the disease. Despite these associations, the mechanism of the association with certain HLA types remains under investigation and future research is needed to understand the clinical utility of HLA typing in this context. Ethnic differences must also be taken into account as the frequency of a particular allele in one population can be very different from that in another population.[13]

- The presence of a disease-associated HLA type alone is not sufficient to trigger disease.
- A small number of diseases have shown strong associations with specific HLA genes; however, HLA typing for disease association is not currently recommended.

■ Ankylosing spondylitis (AS) with HLA-B27
- HLA-B27 is commonly present in patients with ankylosing spondylitis, but many individuals who have HLA-B27 are without disease because HLA-B27 is a relatively common antigen and ankylosing spondylitis is an uncommon disease.[13]

■ Rheumatoid arthritis (RA) with HLA-DRB1: Despite association, HLA typing has not been found useful for diagnosis or screening of RA.[14]

■ Celiac disease with HLA-DQ2 or DQ8: HLA testing is only useful to rule out celiac disease.[15]

5. Platelet refractoriness
- When a patient consistently has an insufficient response to platelet transfusions, they are deemed to be platelet refractory.
- Refractoriness to platelet transfusion is often multifactorial and can be classified into non-immune and immune causes.
- Approximately two-thirds of refractory episodes are due to non-immune causes, such as fever, infection/sepsis, bleeding, splenomegaly, disseminated intravascular coagulation (DIC), hepatic veno-occlusive disease, graft-versus-host disease (GVHD), and medications (e.g., vancomycin, amphotericin B and heparin).
- The remaining one-third of cases are due to immune causes which include alloimmunization to HLA and/or human platelet-specific antigens (HPA), which are due to prior exposure via transfusion, transplantation, or pregnancy. Immune refractoriness is most commonly the result of HLA antibodies (either single or multiple specificities), not HPAs.
- For patients who appear to be alloimmunized, a tissue sample from the patient should be tested for the presence of antibodies to the HLA system (i.e., anti-HLA antibodies).
- Once antibodies to HLA or HPA are identified, the transfusion service will work with the clinical team and community blood center to find compatible platelet products.[16]
- Options include:
  ■ HLA-matched platelets
  1. The traditional management of patients with HLA antibodies is to provide platelets from donors who are HLA-matched for the HLA-A and HLA-B loci.
  2. HLA-matched donors are frequently unavailable for many patients.
  ■ HLA-antigen negative compatible platelets
  1. Platelet units that lack the HLA antigens react specifically with the patient's antibodies.
  2. This approach has further increased the available donor pool significantly.
  3. At many institutions nationwide this is now the standard approach given the greater likelihood of finding a compatible unit.[16]

Screening

■ Universal screening is not indicated.

HLA typing should be considered in the following individuals:

■ All potential recipients and potential donors of hematopoietic bone marrow or stem cell transplantation.[6]
■ All potential recipients and potential donors of kidney transplantation.[11]
■ Screening for the *HLA-B*1502* allele prior to administration of carbamazepine for all patients of Asian ancestry.[12]
■ Screening patients for *HLA-B*57:01* prior to starting treatment with abacavir.[4]
■ Patients with platelet refractoriness once non-immune causes are ruled out.[16]

Diagnosis and Evaluation

■ Not applicable

Monitoring

■ This is not applicable.

INTERPRETATION

■ This is not applicable. All results are considered normal.

FOLLOW-UP

■ No follow-up testing is required.

PATIENT EDUCATION

■ https://bethematch.org/transplant-basics/matching-patients-with -donors/how-donors-and-patients-are-matched/hla-basics/
■ https://www.mskcc.org/cancer-care/patient-education/human-leukocyte -antigen-typing

RELATED DIAGNOSES AND ICD-10 CODES

Stem cell transplant status	Z94.84
Graft-versus-host disease, unspecified	D89.813
Unspecified transplanted organ and tissue rejection	T86.91
Unspecified donor, stem cells	Z52.001

REFERENCES

Full list of references can be accessed through Springer Publishing Company Connect™ at the following link: http://connect.springerpub.com/content/reference-book/ 978-0-8261-8843-4/part/part03/toc-part/ch094

95. HUMAN PAPILLOMAVIRUS TESTS AND CERVICAL CYTOLOGY

Kymberlee Montgomery

PHYSIOLOGY/PATHOPHYSIOLOGY REVIEW

Human papillomavirus (HPV) is a group of more than 200 small, double-stranded DNA viruses that infect the squamous epithelium and are transmitted through skin-to-skin contact.[1] The majority of HPV types invade the cutaneous layer of the epithelium causing skin warts, while approximately 40 HPV types infect the mucosal epithelium and possess oncogenic properties.[1,2] Spread through intimate contact such as vaginal, anal, and oral sexual activity, HPV is the most common sexually transmitted infection (STI) in the United States.[1] Penetrative intercourse in not necessary for transmission.

Categorized by their epidemiologic association with cancer, genital-specific HPV types are grouped into low-risk and high-risk categories. Low-risk HPV types, such as the prevalent strains 6 and 11, cause 90% of benign anogenital warts, low grade cervical cell abnormalities, and respiratory tract papillomas.[1] High-risk HPV (hrHPV) types are responsible for both low-grade and high-grade cervical cell abnormalities. High-risk types can be precursors to oncogenic disease and cause anogenital (skin of the penis, vulva, cervix, and anus) and oropharyngeal cancers (lining of the mouth, back of the tongue, throat, and tonsils).[3]

While the majority of HPV infections are asymptomatic and/or become undetectable within 2 years, persistent infection with the hrHPV types is the most important factor for serious and potentially fatal disease.[1]

Anogenital Warts

Anogenital warts, also known as condylomata, are usually flat, papular, or pedunculated growths found in the anogenital epithelium or skin or within the anogenital mucosa caused mainly by HPV types 6 and 11.[4] They can be flesh-toned, pink, or brown. Larger external warts may have a cauliflower-like shape. The lesions are usually asymptomatic but can be painful, pruritic, or bleed depending on the location.[4] Developing approximately 2 to 3 months after initial infection, anogenital warts should be assessed by a clinician and can be treated. Approximately 25% of warts can spontaneously regress and approximately 30% may reoccur.[5]

Recurrent Respiratory Papillomatosis

Recurrent respiratory papillomatosis (RRP) is a disease in which benign wart-like growths or tumors (HPV type 6 and 11) are found in the respiratory tract of individuals across the life span.[6] Children acquire the virus mainly through vertical transmission during childbirth while adults contract the RRP after oral exposure to HPV types 6 and 11. These growths are commonly found in the vocal folds (laryngeal papillomatosis) and can cause hoarseness, sore throat, and difficulty breathing.

Human Papillomavirus-Related Cancers

Cervical cancer is the fourth most common cause of cancer and the fourth most common cause of death from cancer in females (and transgender males who have not yet surgically transitioned) worldwide.[7] High-risk HPV infection is detected in 99% of all cervical cancer cases.[7] HPV types 16 and 18 together are responsible for 70% of invasive cervical cancer, with HPV-16 causing over 70% of cervical cancer cases and HPV-18 accounting for 10% to 15%.[8,9] The additional 12 high-risk types (31, 33, 35, 39, 45, 51, 52, 56, 58, 59, 66, and 68) are responsible for another 15% of cervical cancers and 11% of all HPV-associated cancers.[1]

Infection with hrHPV is necessary for cervical cancer development; however, other high-risk factors are contributory (smoking, sexual history, birth control use, immune system deficiencies/immunosuppression, exposure to diethylstilbestrol (DES), history of STIs, long-term oral contraceptive usage, and history of more than three pregnancies).[10] The usual time between initial HPV infection and development of cervical cancer can be years to decades. The median age at diagnosis for cervical cancer in the United States is age 49 years.[11] However, the majority of women with any type of HPV infection do not develop cancer. HPV is also responsible for 91% of anal cancers, 69% of vulvar cancers, 75% of vaginal cancers, 63% of penile cancers, and 70% of oropharyngeal cancers.[12]

OVERVIEW OF LABORATORY TESTS

Pap Smear

A Pap smear is a liquid-based cytology test done to screen for cervical cancer. This test is not a diagnostic test and any abnormal physical examination findings regarding the cervix warrant referral for colposcopy. Studies that compare the Pap test with repeat Pap testing have found that the sensitivity of any abnormality on a single test for detecting high-grade lesions is 55% to 80%.[13] This range is wide due to patient demographics and health history, to collection and sampling, laboratory, and interpretation errors as well as provider failure for not following up properly on previous abnormalities.

Human Papillomavirus Molecular Testing

HPV is not cultured by conventional methods and its presence is identified by detection of HPV DNA or messenger RNA (mRNA) from clinical specimens. Tests for HPV detection differ considerably in their sensitivity and specificity, and detection is also affected by the anatomic region sampled, as well as the method of specimen collection.[1] HPV testing is approved for use in two contexts: as a stand alone test for hrHPV (primary HPV screening) and for cotesting in conjunction with cervical cytology. Testing for low-risk HPV types does not identify females at risk of precancer (CIN 2 or CIN 3) or cancer.[13] Utilizing hrHPV testing alone may detect more precancer and cancer than cytology testing.[13]

The Food and Drug Administration (FDA) has approved numerous tests to detect up to 14 hrHPV strains (HPV 16, 18, 31, 33, 35, 39, 45, 51, 52, 56, 58, 59, 66, 68). The tests are considered positive when the presence of any combination of these strains is detected.[1] Additionally, some tests will only specify HPV-16 and HPV-18 strains. HPV testing used with Pap testing can increase the sensitivity of the Pap test to almost 100%.[13]

HPV DNA test: Real-time polymerase chain reaction (PCR) assay amplifies all mucosal HPV types and it is the most common HPV test utilized. This can be used in conjunction with the Pap smear (co-test), alone (primary testing), or management of an abnormal Pap smear in cervical cancer screening to detect the hrHPV strains and their genotype.[14]

The HPV mRNA E6/E7 test: uses mRNA E6/E7 oncoproteins in the HPV genome to detect hrHPV stains; more specific than the HPV DNA test; leads to fewer false positives; more specific in determining the presence of HSIL and cervical cancer.[15] This test can be used in co-testing or primary testing.

INDICATIONS

Screening

■ The United States Preventive Services Task Force,[16] the American Cancer Society,[17] the American College of Obstetricians and Gynecologists,[18] and the American Society for Colposcopy and Cervical Pathology[19] have recommendations regarding cervical cancer screening rooted in evidence. Although similar, the recommendations differ in age of initiation of Pap smear screenings and type of testing (Pap alone, co-testing, or primary HPV testing) and are summarized in Table 95.1. Clinicians may use the recommendations for either organization based on clinical judgment and expertise. For females age 30 or older, both HPV/Pap co-testing and HPV testing alone are more sensitive than Pap testing alone. Consider more frequent Pap test screening with HPV DNA for those with high risk factors[16-19]:

- History of cervical or endometrial cancer
- HIV diagnosis
- Immunocompromised/immunosuppressed
- Exposure to DES
- Women with limited access to healthcare

■ There are no current recommendations for routine anal cancer screening for the general population. However, anal Pap screening should be considered for high-risk groups[20]:

- Men who have sex with men (MSM)
- Women who have receptive anal sex
- Females with a history of abnormal cervical Pap results
- All people infected with HIV who have genital warts (condylomas)
- Females who have had vaginal, vulvar, or cervical cancer
- Anyone who has had an organ transplant
- Anyone with a history of genital warts

Diagnosis and Evaluation

Signs and symptoms of HPV include the following:

■ High-risk HPV is typically asymptomatic.
■ Genital warts are soft, fleshy bumps found around the genitals and anus that can resemble cauliflowers.
■ Common symptoms/signs of RRP are chronic hoarseness, stridor, and respiratory distress.

TABLE 95.1: SUMMARY OF CERVICAL CANCER SCREENING RECOMMENDATIONS

POPULATION	UNITED STATES PREVENTIVE SERVICES TASK FORCE (USPSTF) 2018	AMERICAN CANCER SOCIETY (ACS) 2020	AMERICAN COLLEGE OF OBSTETRICIANS AND GYNECOLOGISTS (ACOG) & AMERICAN SOCIETY FOR COLPOSCOPY AND CERVICAL PATHOLOGY 2016
Initial screening	Age 21	Age 25	Age 21
Females with average cervical cancer risk	**Age 21 to 29 years:** • Every 3 years with cervical cytology alone **Age 30 to 65 years:** • Every 3 years with cervical cytology alone OR • Every 5 years with high-risk human papillomavirus (hrHPV) testing alone OR • Every 5 years with hrHPV testing in combination with cervical cytology (co-testing)	**Age 25 to 65 years:** • Every 5 years with FDA-approved HPV test (preferred) • Every 3 years with cervical cytology alone OR • Every 5 years with hrHPV testing in combination with cervical cytology (co-testing)	**Age 21 to 29 years:** • Every 3 years with cervical cytology alone **Age 30 to 65 years:** • Every 5 years with hrHPV testing in combination with cervical cytology (co-testing) (preferred) OR • Every 3 years with cervical cytology alone OR • Every 5 years with hrHPV testing alone
Females aged 65 and older	Discontinue screening females who have had adequate prior screening[a] and are not otherwise at high risk for cervical cancer.	Discontinue screening females who have had adequate prior screening[b] and are not otherwise at high risk for cervical cancer. Individuals aged >65 years without documentation of prior screening should continue screening until criteria for cessation are met.	Discontinue screening females who have had adequate prior screening[a] and are not otherwise at high risk for cervical cancer.

TABLE 95.1: SUMMARY OF CERVICAL CANCER SCREENING RECOMMENDATIONS (*continued*)

POPULATION	UNITED STATES PREVENTATIVE SERVICES TASK FORCE (USPSTF) 2018	AMERICAN CANCER SOCIETY (ACS) 2020	AMERICAN COLLEGE OF OBSTETRICIANS AND GYNECOLOGISTS (ACOG) & AMERICAN SOCIETY FOR COLPOSCOPY AND CERVICAL PATHOLOGY 2016
Females who have had a hysterectomy	Discontinue screening females who have had a hysterectomy with removal of the cervix and without a history of a high-grade precancerous lesion (CIN 2 or 3 or cervical cancer, diethylstilbestrol [DES], or a compromised immune system)	Discontinue screening for individuals without a cervix and without a history of CIN2 or a more severe diagnosis in the past 25 years or cervical cancer.	
Females with a history of high-risk conditions	No specific recommendation	**Diethylstilbestrol exposed (DES) females:** annual cytology and consideration of colposcopy **HIV infections:** follow recommendations from the Centers for Disease Control and Prevention, the National Institutes of Health, the HIV Medicine Association of the Infectious Diseases Society of America, and the U.S. Department of Health and Human Services. **Immunocompromised states/Immunosuppressant therapy:** follow HIV guidelines.	

Notes: [a] Females with limited access to care, females from racial/ethnic minority groups, and females from countries where screening is not available may be less likely to meet criteria for adequate prior screening.

[b] Adequate negative prior screening is currently defined as two consecutive, negative high-risk HPV tests, or two negative co-tests, or three negative cytology tests within the past 10 years, with the most recent test occurring within the past 3 to 5 years.

CIN, cervical intraepithelial neoplasia; HIV, human immunodeficiency virus; hrHPV, high-risk human papillomavirus.

Differential diagnoses for genital HPV include:

- Herpes simplex
- Seborrhea
- Chancroid
- *Molluscum contagiosum*
- Psoriasis
- *Condyloma latum*
- Corns/calluses

Differential diagnoses for RRP include:

- Asthma
- Acute laryngitis
- Upper respiratory infection
- Bronchitis

Monitoring

- Pap smear and HPV molecular testing are used to monitor individuals with a cervix as summarized in Table 95.1 and the ASCCP guidelines (https://www.asccp.org/management-guidelines).

INTERPRETATION

- Tables 95.2, 95.3, and 95.4 review interpretation of Pap smear cytology.

TABLE 95.2: NORMAL RESULTS	
RESULT	**INTERPRETATION**
Negative for intraepithelial lesion or malignancy	Negative result

TABLE 95.3: ABNORMAL RESULT: SQUAMOUS EPITHELIAL ABNORMALITIES	
RESULT	**INTERPRETATION***
Atypical squamous cells of undetermined significance (ASC-US)	Indeterminate; can be related to infection, douching, menses, HPV infection, cancer precursor, or cancer.
Atypical squamous cells in which a high-grade squamous intraepithelial lesion cannot be excluded (ASC-H)	Mixture of true high-grade squamous intraepithelial lesion cells and other cells that might mimic this type of lesion; finding concerning for high-grade lesion.
High-grade squamous intraepithelial lesion (HSIL)	Concerning for precancerous or cancerous lesions
Squamous cell carcinoma	Highly suspicious for squamous cell carcinoma

*Refer to https://www.asccp.org/management-guidelines for management

HPV, human papillomavirus.

TABLE 95.4: ABNORMAL RESULTS: GLANDULAR CELL ABNORMALITIES*^	
RESULT	**INTERPRETATION**
Atypical glandular cells not otherwise specified (AGC-NOS)	Indeterminate; can be related to IUD, severe inflammation, vigorous sampling, radiation, cancer precursor, or cancer.
Atypical glandular cells, endocervical (AGC-EC)	Lack unequivocal features of endocervical adenocarcinoma in situ or invasive adenocarcinoma.
Atypical glandular cells, endometrial (AGC-EM)	Lack unequivocal features of endometrial adenocarcinoma in situ or invasive adenocarcinoma.
Atypical glandular cells, favor neoplastic endocervical or endometrial (AGC-FN)	Unable to interpret as endocervical adenocarcinoma in situ or invasive adenocarcinoma; highly suspicious.
Adenocarcinoma in situ (AIS)	Highly suspicious for cancer
Adenocarcinoma	

*Any glandular abnormality will be reported with the specific origin of the abnormality noted.
^Refer to https://www.asccp.org/management-guidelines for management.
IUD, intrauterine device.

HPV testing interpretation:

- **Positive HPV test:** A positive test result indicates the presence of hrHPV, which has the potential to cause cervical cancer. Depending on the test selected, the result will show which hrHPV genotype is present.
- **Negative HPV test:** A negative test result indicates the absence of hrHPV.

FOLLOW-UP

Management and follow-up testing is dependent on the Pap and/or HPV test results. Algorithms for follow-up cervical cancer screening can be found at https://www.asccp.org/management-guidelines. Clinicians can also also download the ASCCP Management Guidelines App for use on their mobile devices for a fee.

Biopsy is indicated if the lesions are pigmented, indurated, affixed to underlying tissue, bleeding, or ulcerated to exclude a carcinoma diagnosis.[21] Additionally, biopsy may be indicated in the following circumstances:

- The diagnosis is uncertain.
- The lesions do not respond to standard therapy.
- The disease worsens during therapy.
- The individual is immunocompromised, immunosuppressed, or pregnant.

Internal genital warts can only be visualized by colposcopy (internal vagina and cervix) and anoscopy (anal).

If RRP is suspected by clinical history, visualization of the vocal cords through flexible laryngoscopy is needed. A biopsy may be performed to both confirm the diagnosis of RRP and also to make sure that the lesions do not show precancerous changes.[22]

PEARLS & PITFALLS

- Virtually all cervical cancer is caused by HPV.
- Individuals vaccinated should still have a Pap screening and HPV testing per current guidelines.
- When performing a Pap test, be sure to follow the specific laboratory instructions on the proper way to send the specimen; be certain that the correct and complete information is filled out on the requisition form.
- Avoid ordering screening tests for low-risk HPV.

PATIENT EDUCATION

- https://www.cdc.gov/std/hpv/facts-brochures.htm
- https://www.cdc.gov/std/hpv/HPV-FS-July-2017.pdf

RELATED DIAGNOSES AND ICD-10 CODES

Anogenital warts	A63.0
Recurrent respiratory papillomatosis	D14.4
Pap smear only: screening for malignant neoplasm of the cervix	Z12
Pap smear screening as part of the annual gynecologic examination	Z01.4
Pap smear of the vagina only (hysterectomy)	Z12.72
Encounter for screening for human papillomavirus	Z11.51
Encounter for screening for malignant neoplasm of the rectum	Z12.12

REFERENCES

Full list of references can be accessed through Springer Publishing Company Connect™
at the following link: http://connect.springerpub.com/content/reference-book/
978-0-8261-8843-4/part/part03/toc-part/ch095

---

96. IMMUNOGLOBULIN E AND SKIN ALLERGY TESTING

Heidi Bobek

PHYSIOLOGY REVIEW

Immunoglobulin E or IgE-mediated reactions are associated with type 1 hypersensitivity reactions which have a reproducible acute onset of symptoms that can affect multiple body systems causing symptoms such as urticaria, wheezing, nausea, and hypotension.[1,2]

There are four main allergy groups: inhalants (such as pollens, dust mites), foods, venoms, and drugs. When certain allergens are presented to the body, B cells and T lymphocyte cells are activated and transform into antibody-secreting cells or plasma cells. These plasma cells produce IgE antibodies and are capable of binding a specific allergen. The IgE then bind to receptors on mast cells and basophils. When re-exposure occurs, the binding of the specific allergen to IgE initiates the immune system, resulting in a more aggressive and rapid response.[3]

OVERVIEW OF LABORATORY TESTS

Laboratory evaluation of immediate hypersensitivity testing can be assessed by allergen-specific serum IgE (CPT code 86003) via blood serum (in-vitro) testing or by performing and evaluating percutaneous and intracutaneous (in-vivo) testing, also referred to as skin prick testing. It is important to note that patient history must be assessed in relationship to the IgE testing for accurate results and consideration of possible allergic diagnoses.

Sensitization refers to the detection of IgE via skin prick or blood serum testing. However, the term "allergy" refers to a clinical history suggestive of an immediate onset of reproducible symptoms AND the detection of specific IgE via skin prick or in-vitro testing.[1,4-6]

Skin prick testing is a procedure commonly performed by a trained allergist; therefore, in-vitro testing is more accessible to general healthcare clinicians. Skin prick testing technique involves pricking the skin with a specific allergen along with a positive and negative control. A trained medical clinician should interpret the skin test results 15 to 20 minutes post application (Figure 96.1).[1,7]

Common examples of in-vitro testing include ELISA (enzyme-linked immunosorbant assay), FAST (fluorescent allergosorbant test), RAST (radioallergosorbent test), and ImmunoCAP (allergens linked to polyurethane caps).

The gold standard of food allergy testing is an oral food challenge (OFC).[1,4,6,8] During an oral food challenge, the suspected food is gradually introduced with close supervision. Graded challenges can be time consuming and anaphylaxis can occur. Therefore, food challenges should be performed by a clinician specially trained in allergy to identify candidates appropriate for food challenges and treatment of allergic reactions should they occur.[4]

Approximately 30% of the general population reports a food allergy. However, with appropriate testing only 4% to 8% of the pediatric population and 1% to 6% of the adult population demonstrate signs and symptoms of a true food allergy.[1,4]

INDICATIONS

Screening

- **Universal screening is not indicated and is discouraged by several groups due to lack of evidence to support**[1,9-12]
  - The American Academy of Allergy, Asthma, and Immunology (AAAAI) recommends against IgE food testing without a history consistent with potential IgE-mediated food allergy.[11]

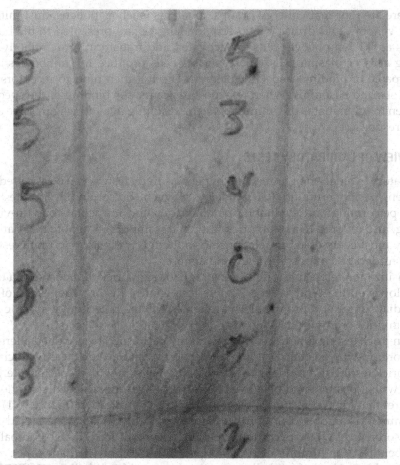

FIGURE 96.1. Skin Prick Test. This picture demonstrates a positive skin test and a control. The skin labeled "0" measures a 0-mm wheal and can serve as the control. Any 3-mm or greater wheal compared to the control is considered a positive skin test suggesting sensitization. The wheals labeled 3,4,5 on this image all indicate wheals equal to or greater than 3 mm. It is important to note that wheal size does not indicate severity; however, wheal size can be used to indicate clinical relevance. *Source*: Sampson HA, Aceves S, Bock SA, et al. Food allergy: a practice parameter update-2014. *J Allergy Clin Immunol.* 2014;134(5):1016–1025.e43. doi:10.1016/j.jaci.2014.05.013; Courtesy of Stephany Roseberry.

Their Choosing Wisely statements emphasize "IgE testing for specific foods must be driven by a history of signs or symptoms consistent with an IgE-mediated reaction after eating a particular food" and "Ordering IgE testing in individuals who do not have a history consistent with or suggestive of a food allergy based on history frequently reveals positive tests that are unlikely to be relevant."[11]

● The National Institute of Allergy and Infectious Disease (NIAID) food allergy guidelines warn against indiscriminate use of IgE tests.[4]

● The AAAAI, the American College of Allergy, Asthma, and Immunology (ACAAI), and the Joint Council of Allergy, Asthma, and Immunology

(JCAAI) collaborated to develop the Joint Task Force on Food Allergy Practice Parameters. Recommendations include:

■ Summary Statement 23: The clinician should use IgE tests (skin prick tests, serum tests, or both) to foods as diagnostic tools; however, testing should be focused on foods suspected of provoking the reaction, and test results alone should not be considered diagnostic of food allergy (Strength of recommendation: Strong; B evidence).[1]

■ The Joint Task Force on Food Allergy Practice Parameters caution, "The clinician should be aware that a relatively small number of foods are responsible for the majority of IgE-mediated food reactions, and therefore panel testing to a large number of allergens should not be conducted."[1]

■ Summary Statement 25: The clinician should consider OFCs to aid in the diagnosis of IgE-mediated food allergy (Strength of recommendation: Strong; A Evidence).[1]

● The American Academy of Pediatrics recommends against IgE screening panels. Their Choosing Wisely statements emphasize "Don't perform screening panels for food allergies without previous consideration of medical history."[10]

Targeted screenings should include individuals with risk factors including a family history of atopy and atopic dermatitis as these are associated with the development of food allergy; however, it is not recommended to perform allergic testing on the general population *prior* to ingestion of highly allergic foods.[1,4]

■ Consider testing for cow's milk, egg, peanut, wheat, and soy in children less than 5 years old with moderate to severe atopic dermatitis if they experience one of the following:
  ● Persistent atopic dermatitis despite optimal management including topical therapy
  ● History of allergic reaction after ingestion of a specific food[4]

Diagnosis and Evaluation

■ Common food allergens include cow's milk, egg, soy, wheat, peanut, tree nuts, finned fish, and shellfish, which are responsible for over 90% of food allergies; allergies to meat, fruits, vegetables, and spices are uncommon.[4,13]

■ Perform IgE testing (in-vitro, skin prick testing) with a history suggestive of reproducible allergy reaction symptoms presenting immediately or up to 120 minutes after exposure involving two or more body systems that can progress to life threatening anaphylaxis. Symptoms may include pruritis, urticaria, angioedema, wheezing, cough, nasal congestion, nausea, vomiting, cramping, hypotension, sense of impending doom, and syncope.[4,14]

■ Skin testing for respiratory inhalants and foods in patients with chronic idiopathic urticaria is of limited use and is not recommended.[15,16]

■ There are several non–IgE-mediated food intolerances worth mentioning. A detailed history will help to differentiate these conditions from IgE-mediated reactions:

● Non–IgE-mediated food intolerance/allergy refers to acute or chronic symptoms mostly affecting the gastrointestinal tract with varying severity of symptoms. Anaphylaxis does not occur with non-IgE reactions and therefore epinephrine is not needed.[4,14] Examples of non–IgE-mediated food allergies include food protein-induced enterocolitis syndrome (FPIES), food protein-induced enteropathy (FPE), and food protein-induced allergic proctocolitis (FPIAP). Symptoms may include abdominal pain, cramping, bloating, diarrhea, and constipation. Non-IgE food allergy diagnosis is based on patient history, clinical decision-making, and elimination of the specific food into the diet. Treatment involves avoidance of triggering food with occasional oral food challenges. Resolution of hypersensitivity typically occurs within the first few years of life.[17,18]

● Celiac disease is an autoimmune, non–IgE-mediated delayed hypersensitivity, caused by ingestion of gluten in genetically susceptible individuals; this causes damage to the intestine. Serologic testing such as tTG-IGA and intestinal biopsy are used to confirm diagnosis, and strict lifelong avoidance of gluten is required.[17]

Monitoring

■ Once an IgE-mediated food allergy is detected, perform repeat testing in 1 to 2 years via SPT or in-vitro testing, which helps to determine a trend over time for possible tolerance (Strength of recommendation: Strong; C Evidence).[1]

■ Food allergy in adults is unlikely to change; however, a periodic re-evaluation, every 2 to 5 years, is recommended depending on the food allergy (Strength of recommendation: C Evidence).[1]

INTERPRETATION

■ Both in-vitro testing and skin prick testing have high rates of false positives.[1]

■ Both in-vitro and skin prick testing have low specificity and low positive predictive value. For this reason, allergy should not be assumed solely with positive test results.[1]

■ Differences in accuracy may depend upon the system being used and the quality of the allergen. In-vitro test results should be validated using the Clinical Laboratory Standards Institute guidelines.[19] Historically, in-vitro results of greater than 0.35 kU/L were considered positive; however, many laboratories presently use greater than 0.1 kU/L as the positive threshold (Table 96.1).[20]

FOLLOW-UP

■ Trained allergy specialists may utilize a combination of testing (e.g., in-vitro, skin prick testing, oral food challenge, component testing) to determine diagnosis and management of allergic diseases.

TABLE 96.1: COMPARISON OF ALLERGY TESTING

MEASURE OF COMPARISON	IN-VITRO[1,4,13,21]	SKIN PRICK[1,4,13,21]	ORAL FOOD CHALLENGE[1,4,20]
Interpretation of Results	>0.1 kU/L–0.35 kU/L[3,13,22] can indicate sensitization	3 mm or greater wheal than the negative control can indicate sensitization	Tolerate food without reaction OR present with signs of reaction after eating specific food
Sensitivity and Specificity	General sensitivity is high from 60%–95% depending upon history but low specificity Positive predictive value of 95% with history of reaction Negative predictive value in absence of IgE-mediated reaction is 90%–95%	General sensitivity is high 60%–95% depending upon history but low specificity Positive predictive value of 95% with history of reaction Negative predictive value in absence of IgE-mediated reaction is 90%–95%	100% specificity
Risk	No risk of reaction, more expensive, results after a few days depending upon laboratory	Relatively safe, cheap, results within 20 minutes, more accurate	High-risk, typically performed by allergy specialist in a monitored medical setting with appropriate equipment/medication for treatment of anaphylaxis; results within a few hours
Preparation	Results unaffected by medications use; may use with skin conditions such as urticaria and severe atopic dermatitis; requires needle stick	Must stop certain medications such as antihistamines for 3–7 days prior to testing; contraindicated to perform skin testing over rashes and hives; mild discomfort	Some medications must be stopped prior to challenge that can interfere with challenge results or anaphylaxis treatment

PEARLS & PITFALLS

- Children may outgrow their allergies to cow's milk, egg, wheat, and soy. Peanut, tree nut, fish, and shellfish allergies can resolve; however, they are more likely to persist lifelong.[23]
- Once a diagnosis of food allergy is made, strict avoidance and possession of epinephrine for emergent treatment of anaphylaxis is advised.[23]
- Panels of food-specific IgE tests should not be used as a screening tool due to risk of false positives. Testing should focus on specific foods associated on positive clinical history and symptoms associated with an IgE-mediated response.[5,12,24]
- Do not eliminate foods with positive IgE testing if the individual currently consumes these foods in their diet without symptoms or signs of reaction.[14]
- Dietary restrictions based on the presumption of food allergy can lead to malnutrition, increased medical costs, and decreased quality of life for the individual and their family.[12,24,25]
- IgG testing represents a normal immune response to food and does not predict allergy or hypersensitivity. IgG testing is not recommended when evaluating potential food allergy.[13,16]

- Panel tests may be performed for respiratory aeroallergens such as pollens and molds. However, consideration of cross reactivity and elimination of allergens that are not relevant to the individual's specific geographical region should be taken into account. Testing may be indicated when there is poor control despite medication use for atopic conditions such as asthma and allergic rhinitis.[3,26]
- Total IgE has limited use; elevated levels indicate general atopic conditions, not specific food allergy.[4,20]
- It is a myth that individuals with a diagnosed shellfish or fish allergy should avoid iodine-based contrast. There is no increased risk of allergic reaction unless specifically allergic to iodine. Additionally, there are no studies documenting a relationship between shellfish/fish allergy and iodine.[1]

PATIENT EDUCATION

- https://www.choosingwisely.org/wp-content/uploads/2015/02/AAAAI-Choosing-Wisely-List.pdf
- https://www.foodallergy.org/

RELATED DIAGNOSES AND ICD-10 CODES

Allergic rhinitis, unspecified	J30.8
Anaphylactic reaction due to a food	T78.0
Allergy to peanuts	Z91.010
Allergy to eggs	Z91.012
Allergy to milk	Z91.011
Atopic dermatitis	L20.9

REFERENCES

Full list of references can be accessed through Springer Publishing Company Connect™ at the following link: http://connect.springerpub.com/content/reference-book/978-0-8261-8843-4/part/part03/toc-part/ch096

97. INFLUENZA

Kimberly R. Joo

PHYSIOLOGY REVIEW

Influenza is a viral upper respiratory illness that typically affects the nose and throat. In some cases, the virus can migrate to the lower respiratory tract where it can affect the lungs as well.[1] The pathogens that cause influenza, also known as flu, are influenza viruses that are single-stranded, negative sense, enveloped viruses that belong to the *Orthomyxoviridae* family.[2,3] Due to the number of differing influenza viruses, the World Health Organization (WHO) created a standard nomenclature for identification of these viruses in 1980. This nomenclature includes the antigenic type (A, B, or C); host of origin; geographical region of origin; number of lineages; year of isolation; and subtypes (HA and NA) for influenza A only.[2] Most influenza testing is focused on types A and B since these types are responsible for global outbreaks and represented in seasonal influenza vaccine.[3]

Influenza is known to cause numerous complications in patients of all ages including pneumonia, exacerbation of other chronic conditions, respiratory failure, and death.[4] The populations with the highest morbidity and mortality include children younger than or equal to 2 years of age and adults greater than or equal to 65 years of age.[3]

Influenza virus is transmitted from person to person primarily through large respiratory droplets. The incubation period is 1 to 2 days and can range from 1 to 4 days.[2]

OVERVIEW OF LABORATORY TESTS

There are several types of diagnostic tests available for influenza A and B. They can be categorized into two broad categories: respiratory specimen tests and serologic tests.[5]

Respiratory Specimen Testing

Respiratory specimen tests play a large role in the diagnosis of influenza at the point of care. Respiratory specimen tests include molecular assays, antigen detection tests, and viral cultures (VCs).[5]

Molecular Assays
Rapid Molecular Assays

Rapid molecular assays (CPT code 87502) detect influenza A or B viral RNA. These tests are simple to perform and can yield results in as fast as 15 minutes; however, their cost can be a limitation.[6,7]

Nucleic Acid Amplification Test

Nucleic acid amplification tests (NAATs; CPT code 87631) detect influenza A or B viral RNA. These tests are the "new gold standard" test for influenza due to their high sensitivity and quick results (less than 3 hours).[8] Their disadvantages are their higher cost, specialized equipment, and need for specialized training.[8]

Reverse Transcription Polymerase Chain Reaction

Reverse transcription polymerase chain reaction tests (rt-PCRs; CPT codes 87502 and 87503) detect influenza A or B viral RNA. Disadvantages of traditional rt-PCR testing include long result times and often they are not available on nights or weekends.[9]

Antigen Detection Tests
Rapid Influenza Detection Tests

Rapid influenza detection tests (RIDT; CPT code 87804) detect influenza A or B antigens. They are widely used in the outpatient clinical setting due to their advantages of low cost, quick results (15 to 30 minutes), and ease of use. The disadvantage of these tests is their low and varied sensitivity (10% to 80%).

One systematic review and meta-analysis gave an overall pooled sensitivity of 61.1% and specificity of 98.9% for these tests.[10]

Immunofluorescence Antibody Tests

Immunofluorescence antibody tests (CPT codes 87275 and 87276) detect influenza A or B antigens. The advantage of these tests includes a higher sensitivity. The disadvantages of these tests are the complicated processing that requires a skilled technician, and they can take up to 3 hours to result.[11]

Viral Culture

VCs (CPT code 87254) detect influenza A or B through virus isolation on a culture agar. The VC has been the "gold standard" in the past for influenza testing due to its high sensitivity. The big disadvantage of this test is the long resulting time that can range from 2 to 14 days.[12] Refer to Table 97.1 for sensitivities and specificities for each test.

Serologic Testing

Serologic tests can have an important role in influenza surveillance, vaccine development and evaluation, and, to a less extent, diagnosis.[3] They are not recommended for diagnosis since they require two samples that are taken several weeks

TABLE 97.1: SENSITIVITIES AND SPECIFICITIES OF INFLUENZA TESTS

INFLUENZA TEST CATEGORY BY SPECIMEN TYPE	INFLUENZA TEST CATEGORY	SPECIFIC INFLUENZA TEST NAME	SENSITIVITY	SPECIFICITY
Respiratory Specimen Tests	Molecular Assay	Rapid Molecular Assay	90.5%–97%	97.6%–99.4%
Respiratory Specimen Test	Molecular Assay	Nucleic Acid Amplification Test (NAAT)	98.4%	99.7%
Respiratory Specimen Test	Molecular Assay	Reverse Transcription Polymerase Chain Reaction (rt-PCR)	98%	99%
Respiratory Specimen Test	Antigen Detection Test	Rapid Influenza Detection Test (RIDT)	61.1%	98.9%
Respiratory Specimen Test	Antigen Detection Test	Immunofluorescence Antibody Test	85.3%–93.8%	100%
Respiratory Specimen Test	Viral Culture	Viral Culture	82.3%	100%

Sources: Data from Antoniol S, Fidouh N, Ghazali A, et al. Diagnostic performances of the Xpert® Flu PCR test and the OSOM® immunochromatographic rapid test for influenza A and B virus among adult patients in the emergency department. *J Clin Virol*. 2018;99–100:5–9. doi:10.1016/j.jcv.2017.12.005; El Feghaly RE, Nolen JD, Lee BR, et al. Impact of rapid influenza molecular testing on management in pediatric acute care settings. *J Pediatr*. 2021;228:271–277.e1. doi:10.1016/j.jpeds.2020.08.007; López Roa P, Catalán P, Giannella M, et al. Comparison of real-time RT-PCR, shell viral culture, and conventional cell culture for the detection of the pandemic influenza A (H1N1) in hospitalized patients. *Diagn Microbiol Infect Dis*. 2011;69(4):428–431. doi:10.1016/j.diagmicrobio.2010.11.007; Nguyen AVT, Dao TD, Trinh TTT, et al. Sensitive detection of influenza a virus based on a CdSe/CdS/ZnS quantum dot-linked rapid fluorescent immunochromatographic test. *Biosens Bioelectron*. 2020;155:112090. doi:10.1016/j.bios.2020.112090; Otto CC, Kaplan SE, Stiles J, et al. Rapid molecular detection and differentiation of influenza viruses A and B. *J Vis Exp*. 2017;(119):54312. doi:10.3791/54312; Rebelo-de-Andre H, Zambon MC. Different diagnostic methods for detection of influenza epidemics. *Epidemiol Infect*. 2000;124(3):515–522. doi:10.1017/S0950268899003751; Yu ST, Thi Bui C, Kim DTH, Nguyen AVT, Thi Trinh TT, Yeo SJ. Clinical evaluation of rapid fluorescent diagnostic immunochromatographic test for influenza A virus (H1N1). *Sci Rep*. 2018;8(1):13468. doi:10.1038/s41598-018-31786-8.

apart and cannot be reliably interpreted.[5] Serologic tests include hemagluttination inhibition assays, virus neuralization assays, and enzyme immunoassays.[3]

INDICATIONS

Signs and symptoms of influenza can vary based on immune status, age, and chronic health conditions. The most common symptoms of influenza include fever, cough, sore throat, runny/stuffy nose, muscle/body aches, headache, and fatigue. Gastrointestinal symptoms such as vomiting and diarrhea are more commonly seen in children but can also be found in adults.[1] It is difficult to distinguish between influenza and other upper respiratory illnesses due to shared symptoms. The Infectious Disease Society of America (IDSA) sets clinical practice guidelines for the diagnosis, testing, and treatment of influenza.[13] However, it is important to note that testing for influenza is not a requirement for antiviral treatment in patients with symptoms that are consistent with influenza when it is currently prevalent in the community.[5]

Screening

There are no universal or targeted screenings for influenza.

Diagnosis and Evaluation

These tests (molecular assays, NAAT, rt-PCR, VC, RIDT, direct fluorescent antibody tests, and serologic testing) are used to rule in or rule out the following diagnoses[14]:

- Influenza A
- Influenza B

These tests can also be used to rule out influenza when the following diagnoses are suspected: COVID-19, respiratory syncytial virus (RSV), parainfluenza virus, adenovirus, rhinovirus, enterovirus, pneumonia, strep throat, and rhinosinusitis.

Infectious Diseases Society of America Criteria for Influenza Testing During Influenza Activity

- High-risk patients, including immunocompromised persons who present with flu-like symptoms if the test result will influence clinical management
- Patients who present with acute onset of respiratory symptoms with or without fever, and either exacerbation of chronic medical condition or known complications of influenza if the testing result will influence clinical management
- Consider testing for patients not at high risk for influenza complications who present with flu-like symptoms and who are likely to be discharged home if the results might influence antiviral treatment or chemoprophylaxis decisions for high-risk household members.[13]

Infectious Diseases Society of America Criteria for Influenza Testing During Low Influenza Activity

- Consider testing for patients with acute onset of respiratory symptoms with or without fever, especially for immunocompromised and high-risk patients.[13]

Infectious Diseases Society of America Criteria for Influenza Testing for Hospitalized Patients During Influenza Activity

- Test all patients on admission with acute respiratory illness, including pneumonia with or without fever.

- Test all patients on admission with acute worsening of chronic cardiopulmonary disease since influenza can be associated with acute exacerbation of underlying conditions.
- Test all patients on admission who are immunocompromised or at high risk of complications and present with acute respiratory symptoms with or without fever, as the manifestations of influenza in such patients are frequently less characteristic than in immunocompetent individuals.
- Test all patients who, while hospitalized, develop acute onset of respiratory symptoms, with or without fever, or respiratory distress, without a clear alternative diagnosis.[13]

Infectious Diseases Society of America Criteria for Influenza Testing for Hospitalized Patients During Low Influenza Activity

- Test all patients for influenza on admission who present with acute respiratory illness with or without fever, who have an epidemiologic link to a person diagnosed with influenza, an influenza outbreak, or an outbreak of acute febrile respiratory illness of uncertain cause, or who recently traveled from an area with known influenza activity.
- Consider testing for patients with acute, febrile respiratory tract illness, especially children and adults who are immunocompromised or at high risk of complications, or if the results might influence antiviral treatment or chemoprophylaxis decisions for high-risk household contacts.[13]

Algorithms have been created to assist with clinical decision-making when ordering influenza tests. The Centers for Disease Control and Prevention (CDC) has a "guide for considering influenza testing when influenza viruses are circulating in the community" which is regardless of influenza vaccination status (Figure 97.1).[5]

Monitoring

- Monitor patients with a diagnosis of influenza for symptom improvement within 7 to 10 days of onset due to the numerous complications associated with influenza.
- Monitor for side-effects of antiviral agents when prescribed.

INTERPRETATION

- Positive RIDT, PCR for influenza A: Diagnosis is influenza A.
- Positive RIDT, PCR for influenza B: Diagnosis is influenza B.

FOLLOW-UP

- Positive RIDT, PCR for influenza A: No follow-up testing recommended.
- Positive RIDT, PCR for influenza B: No follow-up testing recommended.
- Negative RIDT, PCR for influenza A: No follow-up testing recommended.
- Negative RIDT, PCR for influenza B: No follow-up testing recommended.

PEARLS & PITFALLS

- Clinical suspicion by clinicians for patients presenting with signs and symptoms of influenza has been found to be inaccurate. One research study showed that 69% of providers changed their treatment plans for patients who presented with signs and symptoms of influenza once they were given the results of the influenza rt-PCR results.[15]

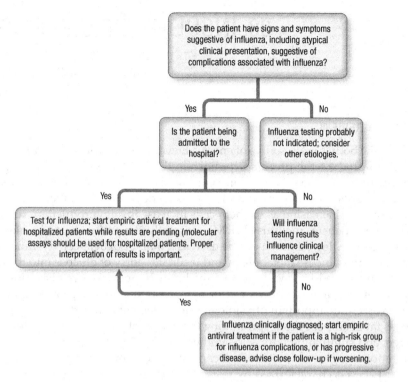

FIGURE 97.1. Guide for considering influenza testing when influenza viruses are circulating in the community. *Source*: Adapted from Overview of influenza testing methods. Updated August 31, 2020. https://www.cdc.gov/flu/professionals/diagnosis/overview-testing-methods.htm.

- One research study showed a decrease in antibiotic use and decreased return visits in a 2-week period after rapid point-of-care influenza tests.[16]
- Due to the low sensitivities of many RIDTs, caution should be used with negative tests, especially in high-risk populations. If there is a high suspicion for influenza in a high-risk patient with a negative RIDT, it is recommended to treat the patient with an antiviral agent.[4,17]

PATIENT EDUCATION

- http://www.cdc.gov/flu/about/index.html
- https://www.cdc.gov/flu/resource-center/freeresources/print/index.htm

RELATED DIAGNOSES AND ICD-10 CODES

Influenza due to certain identified influenza viruses	J09
Influenza due to other identified influenza viruses	J10
Influenza due to unidentified influenza virus	J11

REFERENCES

Full list of references can be accessed through Springer Publishing Company Connect™ at the following link: http://connect.springerpub.com/content/reference-book/978-0-8261-8843-4/part/part03/toc-part/ch097

98. INSULIN AND C-PEPTIDE

Cara Harris and Kathleen Wyne

PHYSIOLOGY REVIEW

Glucose is the body's main source of energy. Elevated glucose levels stimulate the beta cells to produce the precursor proinsulin that undergoes intracellular processing, resulting in C-peptide and insulin (the mature hormone) being secreted in equal amounts.[1] A small amount of proinsulin does end up in the circulation with the amount increasing as the beta-cells increase insulin production, such as in early type 2 diabetes mellitus (T2DM). Normally, the proinsulin-to-insulin ratio should be very low; if not, it can be used as a marker of beta-cell dysfunction. Insulin regulates glucose metabolism and facilitates entry of glucose into the cell where it can be used for energy to fuel the body. In normal physiology, insulin and its counterregulatory hormone, glucagon, work together to provide glucose homeostasis. Other important physiologic effects of insulin include the storage of energy as fat in adipose tissue, promoting the liver to store glucose in the form of glycogen, and stimulating fatty acid synthesis for lipid metabolism.[1-3]

Alterations in glucose metabolism can lead to one of two types of diabetes mellitus. T2DM is characterized by resistance to insulin, which causes elevated glucose and insulin levels early in diagnosis, eventually leading to a relative deficiency of insulin from progressive beta-cell failure. Type 1 diabetes (T1D) is an absolute deficiency of insulin, most commonly due to autoimmune destruction of the pancreatic beta-cell.[1,2,4]

OVERVIEW OF LABORATORY TESTS

Insulin (CPT code 83525) is measured in the blood serum but is not clinically useful except in the evaluation of hypoglycemia. Pitfalls of measuring insulin levels include:

- Insulin has a rapid removal and short half-life of about 5 minutes.[3]
- Insulin levels can come from endogenous insulin (pancreas) or exogenous insulin (pharmaceutical).[3] Therefore, insulin levels may be falsely elevated due to cross reactivity of the insulin assays with both endogenous and exogenous insulin.[5]
- Administration of exogenous insulin may suppress endogenous production, making measurement of serum insulin levels less useful.[4,6]

Instead of insulin, C-peptide (CPT code 84681) should be used to reflect insulin production. C-peptide is also used in the assessment of hypoglycemia. Characteristics of C-peptide include:

- C-peptide circulates in the body longer than insulin and has a more stable half-life of about 30 minutes.[3,5]
- C-peptide and insulin are co-secreted, so C-peptide can be used to assess insulin secretion.[5]

- C-peptide is not contained in commercial insulin preparations. However, exogenous insulin administration may suppress C-peptide production.[3]

Some available methods for assessing C-peptide level as a surrogate for beta-cell function include serum C-peptide measurement, glucagon stimulation test (GST), mixed meal tolerance test (MMTT), oral glucose tolerance test (OGTT), and either 24-hour urine or random urine for urine to c-peptide/creatinine ratio (UCPCR).[5]

- Serum C-peptide assays are easy to perform and have good sensitivity and specificity. However, measurements must always have a simultaneous glucose measurement to determine if the C-peptide level is appropriate to the glucose level. To minimize variability, it is recommended to use the same method/laboratory to compare trends.[5,6]
- GST and MMTT provide assessments of a stimulated C-peptide level that are very sensitive and specific for assessing beta-cell function. However, the test can cause nausea and is time consuming.
- OGTT can be practical if C-peptide is also measured, but evidence is limited regarding the predictive value of the test for long-term beta cell function.[5]
- Although primarily still a research tool, UCPCR has been shown to be comparable to serum testing and is both sensitive and specific in differentiating T1D from T2DM or maturity onset diabetes of the young (MODY). As an emerging tool, UCPCR is limited by the small size of the populations studied and possible variations with gender as well as inaccuracy in the presence of kidney disease.[5,7-9] Limitations of 24-hour UCPCR include the challenge of obtaining accurate collections and variations in the fraction of C-peptide secretion in urine.[5,6] Random samples for UCPCR provide more practical convenience.

INDICATIONS

Screening
- There are no screening indications for C-peptide or insulin.

Diagnosis and Evaluation
- C-peptide and insulin are used in the diagnosis of T1D. Prior to exogenous insulin initiation, C-peptide and insulin are low and glucose levels are high.[1]
- Insulin, proinsulin, and C-peptide are used in evaluate the etiology of persistent hypoglycemia.[3]
- Insulin levels assist in identifying factitious hypoglycemia. Synthetic insulin preparations do not contain C-peptide so typically a patient taking excess exogenous insulin will have low glucose, a high insulin level (if the exogenous insulin is detectable in that assay), and a low C-peptide level.[4,10]

Monitoring
- Insulin levels are not monitored on a regular basis.
- C-peptide could be monitored over time to evaluate beta cell function and insulin secretion. This can be especially useful during initial diagnosis of T1D when glucose levels may revert to near normal (honeymoon period). However, evidence is limited on using C-peptide to predict insulin requirements in these instances.[5,6]

- C-peptide could be assessed to determine if there is adequate endogenous insulin production for a planned non-insulin therapeutic regimen. The evidence for the accuracy of this use is mixed, however. Ongoing studies are trying to determine a threshold level that predicts success with non-insulin therapies.[5,6]
- C-peptide is typically monitored post-pancreas transplantation to assess organ function.[6]

INTERPRETATION

- C-peptide reference intervals: 1.1 to 4.4 ng/mL[11]
- Insulin reference intervals: 2.6 to 24.9 mcIU/mL[12]
- In classifying the type of diabetes, C-peptide and insulin levels can be considered but are not diagnostic.[6,13] Both C-peptide and insulin must be interpreted in context of the glucose level as summarized in Table 98.1.
- The following caveats should be considered when interpreting C-peptide and insulin levels.[1,3–5]
  - The presence or absence of C-peptide does not confirm or refute T1D.
  - If C-peptide levels are low, T1D is usually more likely than T2DM.
  - If C-peptide levels are high, T2DM is more likely than T1D.
  - Having a detectable C-peptide does not exclude the diagnosis of T1D.
  - C-peptide and insulin can be falsely high with acute severe hyperglycemia.
  - C-peptide and insulin can be low or undetectable with hypoglycemia.
  - C-peptide can be present in T1D, even after many years of diagnosis.

FOLLOW-UP

- Autoantibodies for T1D can be used to help evaluate for T1D.

TABLE 98.1: RELATION OF GLUCOSE, INSULIN, AND C-PEPTIDE TO ENDOCRINE CONDITIONS

CONDITION	GLUCOSE	INSULIN	C-PEPTIDE
T1D	High	Low	Low
T2DM	High	High^	High
Insulinoma	Low	High	High
Factitious Hypoglycemia	Low	High	Low or normal
Malnutrition	Low	Low	Low
Hypoglycemia from Sulfonylurea or Glinide	Low	High	High

^May be 10 to 20× above reference limit.

*Also will have high proinsulin and high proinsulin/insulin ratio.

Sources: Data from Lavin N. *Manual of Endocrinology and Metabolism.* 2002; McDermott MT. *Endocrine Secrets.* 4th ed. Elsevier Health Sciences; 2005; Neal JM. *How the Endocrine System Works.* Blackwell, Science Inc.; 2002; Wilcox G. Insulin and insulin resistance. *Clin Biochem Rev.* 2005;26(2):19–39. https://www.ncbi.nlm.nih.gov/pmc/articles/PMC1204764

- If abnormal or conflicting results occur with insulin and C-peptide levels, patients should be referred to an endocrinologist or diabetes specialist for interpretation and recommendations.[3,4,6]
- Persistent, symptomatic unexplained blood sugars under 50 mg/dL warrant detailed hypoglycemia evaluation. This includes testing for possible adrenal insufficiency, thyroid disease, autoimmune hypoglycemia, or insulinoma. Indicated tests include C-peptide, insulin, proinsulin, serum acetone, anti-insulin antibodies, am cortisol with simultaneous adrenocorticotropic hormone (ACTH) followed by ACTH stimulation test, and thyroid function studies.[3,10,14]

PEARLS & PITFALLS

- Acute or chronic renal failure leads to artificially elevated C-peptide levels because renal filtration is the mechanism of clearance of C-peptide.[5,6]
- Acute illness, hepatic dysfunction, and malnutrition are all conditions that may have unexpected insulin resistance leading to wide fluctuations in glucose and difficult to interpret C-peptide and insulin levels.[6,10]
- Insulin resistance is found in people with prediabetes or T2DM where high levels of insulin are needed to maintain glucose homeostasis. Insulin resistance occurs when the cells become resistant to the action of insulin and are unable to use insulin well. The body tries to compensate for the insulin resistance by secreting more insulin to maintain normoglycemia. Over time, the pancreas is unable to meet the demands, resulting in a relative deficiency of insulin, hyperglycemia, and a diagnosis of T2DM.[15]
- In prediabetes, insulin levels are not usually drawn due to its variability, short half-life, and because results do not change treatment or therapy (lifestyle modifications). Additionally, in prediabetes, hyperinsulinemia is expected since the pancreas overproduces insulin to prevent hyperglycemia.[15,16]

PATIENT EDUCATION

- https://medlineplus.gov/lab-tests/c-peptide-test/
- https://medlineplus.gov/lab-tests/insulin-in-blood/

RELATED DIAGNOSES AND ICD-10 CODES

Type 1 diabetes mellitus	E10.
Type 2 diabetes mellitus	E11.
Hypoglycemia, unspecified	E16.2
Long-term current use of insulin	Z79.4
Insulinoma	E16.1

REFERENCES

Full list of references can be accessed through Springer Publishing Company Connect™ at the following link: http://connect.springerpub.com/content/reference-book/978-0-8261-8843-4/part/part03/toc-part/ch098

99. INSULIN-LIKE GROWTH FACTOR AND GROWTH HORMONE

Lisa Ward

PHYSIOLOGY REVIEW

Insulin growth factor 1 (IGF1) is a polypeptide hormone produced mainly by the liver in response to growth hormone (GH) levels.[1,2] The main effects of IGF1 are to stimulate linear growth in children, promote glucose metabolism, and increase lean muscle mass while decreasing fat mass. IGF1 is bound to IGF-binding proteins (IGFBP), making the levels more constant than that of GH with longer half-lives of up to 15 hours.[3] GH secretion from the pituitary occurs approximately 10 times a day, with a half-life of only 20 minutes.[1,4] Therefore, the IGF1 is a more accurate measurement of growth hormone production and is the preferred test when evaluating GH deficiencies or excess.[1,5,6] GH levels by themselves are not clinically useful.[3,7] Figure 99.1 describes the normal process of GH and IGF1 production.

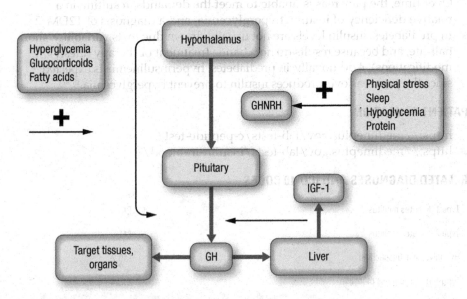

FIGURE 99.1. IGF1 negative feedback loop. Release of GH is regulated by a negative feedback loop. GH, secreted in the pituitary gland, stimulates the liver to produce IGF1, which then promotes bone and organ growth and glucose metabolism. GH secretion inhibition is then regulated by IGF1, glucose, and glucocorticoid levels. This balance release and inhibition of GH occurs in a pulsatile fashion throughout the day. *Source:* Data from Siebert DM, Rao AL. The use and abuse of human growth hormone in sports. *Sports Health.* 2018;10(5):419–426. doi:10.1177/1941738118782688.

OVERVIEW OF LABORATORY TESTS

Laboratory evaluation of GH status can be done with GH (CPT code 83003) but is most often done with IGF1 (CPT code 84305). IGF1 mirrors GH excesses and deficiencies, but unlike GH, it is stable throughout the day.[6] Therefore, IGF1 has superior diagnostic sensitivity and specificity and should be used as the primary test.[8] Although IGF1 also has minimal diurnal fluctuation and can be collected at any time of the day, for the most accurate results, patients should fast after midnight, with the specimen collected at 8 a.m. Large variability can exist between the different IGF1 assays and comparing results across assays is difficult; therefore, ordering clinicians should use the same assay/laboratory when monitoring IGF1 levels over time.[8-11] IGF1 is used to diagnose acromegaly, growth hormone deficiency, and to monitor response to treatment for growth hormone deficiency.[1,4] Low levels can be seen in children younger than 6 years old and in advanced age and is considered a normal variant.[6] Adolescent growth spurts will also cause elevated IGF1 levels and is a normal variant.[1,4]

INDICATIONS

Screening

- Screening for growth hormone deficiency is warranted in the following cases[1,2,12]:
    1. Adults with changes in muscle mass, surgery, or radiation to the hypopituitary region, or those with traumatic brain injury
    2. Patients with other pituitary hormone deficiencies
    3. History of pituitary gland trauma, surgery, or radiation
    4. History of pediatric radiation to the central nervous system

Diagnosis and Evaluation

- IGF1 testing is indicated to diagnose GH deficiency or excess when a patient demonstrates symptoms as summarized in Table 99.1

TABLE 99.1: SIGNS AND SYMPTOMS THAT WARRANT IGF1 TESTING

GROWTH HORMONE DEFICIENCY	GROWTH HORMONE EXCESS
Child whose height is below the third percentile or decreased growth velocity	Child with gigantism
Delayed puberty	Delayed puberty
Adults with poor memory, emotional lability, and poor physical/mental energy	Adults: acromegaly, coarse facial features, enlarged hands/feet, enlarged internal organs

Sources: Data from Bolanowski M, Ruchała M, Zgliczyński W, Kos-Kudła B, Hubalewska-Dydejczyk A, Lewiński A. Diagnostics and treatment of acromegaly—updated recommendations of the Polish Society of Endocrinology. *Endokrynol Pol.* 2019;70(1):2–18. doi:10.5603/EP.a2018.0093; Ergun-Longmire B, Wajnrajch MP. Growth and growth disorders. In: Feingold KR, Anawalt B, Boyce A, et al., eds. *Endotext*. MDText.com; October 31, 2020; Katznelson L, Laws ER Jr, Melmed S, et al. Acromegaly: an Endocrine Society clinical practice guideline. *J Clin Endocrinol Metab.* 2014;99(11):3933–3951. doi:10.1210/jc.2014-2700; Lexicomp Online. *Lab Tests and Diagnostic Procedures*. UpToDate, Inc; 2019; Yuen KC. Adult growth hormone deficiency guidelines: more difficult than it seems to incorporate into clinical practice universally [published online ahead of print, 2021 Feb 1]. *Eur J Endocrinol.* 2021;184(4):C5–C7. doi:10.1530/EJE-20-1455; Yuen KCJ, Biller BMK, Radovick S, et al. American Association of Clinical Endocrinologists and American College of Endocrinology guidelines for management of growth hormone deficiency in adults and patients transitioning from pediatric to adult care. *Endocr Pract.* 2019;25(11):1191–1232. doi:10.4158/GL-2019-0405.

Monitoring

■ Serum IGF1 is the best single test to monitor adequacy of GH replacement therapy.[13] Repeat IGF1 testing every 3 months in children[14] and every 6 to 12 months in adults.[13]
■ In patients surgically treated for acromegaly, IGF1 levels should not be checked until 12 weeks after surgery.[7,11,15]
■ Malnutrition can cause decreased levels of IGF1 and can be used for monitoring for food deprivation.[1,8]

INTERPRETATION

■ Reference intervals are listed in Tables 99.2 and 99.3.
■ An IGF1 level lower than the gender- and age-specific lower limit of normal in a patient with pituitary disease confirms the diagnosis of GH deficiency.[12]
■ Low levels can be seen in hypopituitarism, malnutrition, delayed puberty, DM, old age, and cirrhosis.[1,16]

TABLE 99.2: NORMAL IGF1 RANGES BASED ON AGE

AGE	MALE (ng/mL)	FEMALE (ng/mL)
2 mo–5 y/o	17–248	17–248
6–8 y/o	88–474	88–474
9–11 y/o	110–565	117–771
12–15 y/o	202–957	261–1,096
16–24 y/o		182–780
25–39 y/o		114–492
40–54 y/o		90–360
≥55 y/o		71–290

Source: Data from Lexicomp Online. *Lab Tests and Diagnostic Procedures.* UpToDate, Inc; 2019.

TABLE 99.3: NORMAL IGF1 RANGES BASED ON TANNER STAGE

TANNER STAGE	MALE (ng/mL)	FEMALE (ng/mL)
I	109–485	128–470
II	174–512	186–695
III	230–818	292–883
IV	396–776	394–920
V	402–839	308–1,136

Source: Data from Lexicomp Online. *Lab Tests and Diagnostic Procedures.* UpToDate, Inc; 2019.

- Elevated levels can be seen during adolescent growth spurts (which is a normal variant), precocious puberty, pregnancy, obesity, diabetes mellitus, and acromegaly.[1,4]
- An equivocal IGF1 level in a patient with suspected GH deficiency requires dynamic/provocative testing (see follow-up testing) to confirm the diagnosis.[1,9,17]
- All tests for GH secretion are more likely to give false-positive results in obese patients[12] The GH cutoff to diagnose GH deficiency should be lower for obese patients than for normal weight patients.[13]
- Differential diagnosis of decreased IGF1 levels: normal aging, hypopituitarism, short stature.
- Differential diagnosis of increased IGF1 levels: acromegaly, gigantism.

FOLLOW-UP

- Abnormally low IGF1 levels should be followed up with appropriate dynamic testing to confirm diagnosis. The gold standard dynamic test for growth hormone deficiency is the insulin tolerance test (ITT).[1] However, there is risk for seizures and angina secondary to hypoglycemia with the ITT. This test is described in the text that follows.
  - Patient fasts for 8 hours, then a baseline GH and glucose level are drawn and 0.1 U/kg of insulin is given. Blood sugar and GH levels are drawn at 30, 45, 60, 90, and 120 minutes. Performance of the test is considered adequate when the blood glucose level decreases below 50% of its baseline value. If GH levels do not increase with hypoglycemia, GH deficiency is diagnosed.
- All cases of elevated IGF1 levels require confirmation with an oral glucose tolerance test (OGTT) to diagnose with acromegaly/gigantism.[9,16]
  - For this test, a baseline GH and glucose level are drawn, the patient drinks a 75-g glucose drink, and GH and glucose levels are drawn 2 hours later. A GH level of 1 mcg/liter or less rules out acromegaly.[3,9,12] A GH level of greater than 2 mcg/L confirms the diagnosis of acromegaly. GH levels between 1 mcg/L and 2 mcg/L are equivocal and must be interpreted in the context of clinical suspicion.[12] Patients with equivocal results should be referred to an endocrinologist for further testing if clinically indicated.

PEARLS & PITFALLS

- Normal aging is not a reason to evaluate for GH deficiency.[13] GH and IGF1 levels decrease normally with age; however, these declines have not been associated with clinical consequences.
- No one test can definitively diagnose GH deficiency.[2]
- Hypothyroidism should be ruled out prior to IGF1 testing as hypothyroid symptoms can mimic GH deficiencies and are more common.[1]
- GH promotes muscle growth in adults; therefore, GH supplements may be used by athletes as performance-enhancing drugs.[4] GH supplements have been banned by many sports organizations including NCAA, International Olympic Committee, and Major League Baseball and the World Anti-Doping Agency (WADA).[2,18]

- GH therapy in otherwise healthy older individuals is not recommend[2] and off-label use of recombinant human GH as anti-aging intervention is illegal in the United States.[12]
- During normal pregnancy, serum IGF1 increases almost two-fold.[8]

PATIENT EDUCATION

- https://kidshealth.org/en/parents/somatomedin-test.html

RELATED DIAGNOSES AND ICD-10 CODES

Growth hormone deficiency/hypopituitarism	E23.0
Acromegaly/gigantism	E22.0
Pituitary adenoma	D35.2
Short stature	R62.52

REFERENCES

Full list of references can be accessed through Springer Publishing Company Connect™ at the following link: http://connect.springerpub.com/content/reference-book/978-0-8261-8843-4/part/part03/toc-part/ch099

100. INTERFERON-GAMMA RELEASE ASSAYS

Oralea A. Pittman

PHYSIOLOGY REVIEW

Interferon gamma release assays (IGRAs) are an alternative test to the tuberculin skin test (TST) used in the diagnosis of latent tuberculosis infection (LTBI). Both TST and IGRA are indirect tests of immune response to tuberculosis antigens.[1] Tuberculosis is a disease on a continuum that includes those who breathe in the bacteria and eliminate the disease with their own immune system, those for whom the body's immune system isolates the disease (LTBI), and those who develop tuberculosis.[2] The reasons that some people may eliminate the bacteria on their own and others develop LTBI or tuberculosis are poorly understood but are likely immunologic.[2] Only a small percentage of those with LTBI go on to develop tuberculosis disease.[2]

IGRAs were developed to address some of the false-positive issues with the TST including exposure to non-tuberculosis bacteria, bacillus Calmette-Guerin (BCG) vaccination, and infections cleared through immunologic mechanisms.[2]

It was also hoped that IGRAs would better diagnose LTBI, including in those who are immunocompromised or at risk for immunocompromise, although IGRAs have not proved superior to TST except in the case of persons who received BCG vaccine after 1 year of age or repeated BCG vaccines.[2] IGRAs measure the T-cell release of interferon-gamma (IFN-gamma) after stimulation by antigens more specific to *M. tuberculosis*, making them slightly more specific in persons who have received BCG. These antigens are not produced by the BCG strains or most other mycobacterium species, although there are a few mycobacterium that have the same antigens.[2] Overall, in multiple systematic reviews, IGRAs have not proven to be a better test than TST for the diagnosis of LTBI.[3-5]

IGRAs are more likely to be falsely negative in persons over 40 years of age.[6] This is due to a decrease in peripheral lymphocytes. Because the T-SPOT.TB does not involve peripheral lymphocytes, it could be more accurate in older persons, but this has not been well studied.[6]

In infants under 5 years old, the TST is currently recommended rather than the IGRA though the IGRA is used by some experts in younger children.[1]

OVERVIEW OF LABORATORY TESTS

Two IGRAs are currently marketed in the United States, QuantiFERON Gold In-Tube (QFT-GIT) and T-SPOT.TB.[2] For the QFT-GIT (CPT code 86480), whole blood is placed in three different tubes. The first tube, a negative control tube, measures IFN-gamma response. The second tube is the antigen tube that measures antigen-specific response. The antigens used are early secreted antigenic target 6 (ESAT-6) and culture filtrate protein-10 (CFP-10).[2] The third tube is a positive control tube which measures non-specific T-cell response.

T-SPOT.TB (CPT code 86481) is an enzyme-linked immunospot assay which is performed on blood mononuclear cells incubated with the ESAT-6 and CFP-10 antigens. The result is the number of IFN—gamma-producing T cells. The QFT-GIT is more commonly used. Both procedures have several steps at which errors can occur.[7]

In general, specificity and sensitivity of IGRAs has been lower than hoped and they do not help distinguish latent TB from active TB. In patients without HIV, pooled sensitivity of the IGRAs is 69% to 83% and specificity is 50% to 52%. In persons with HIV infection, the pooled sensitivity is 60% to 76% and the specificity is 50% to 52%.[1]

INDICATIONS

Screening

- There is no indication for universal screening among low-risk groups where false positives are more common.[1,8]
- Targeted screenings should be completed in groups at high risk for infection with *M. tuberculosis* including[1,4,8]:
  - Contacts with known or presumed TB
  - Persons born in or who travel frequently to countries where TB disease is common (See the Centers for Disease Control and Prevention [CDC]

website for the most up-to-date list. Includes immigrants and refugees from these countries.)
- Persons who live or have lived in congregate living situations like homeless shelters, prisons, jails, and nursing homes, as well as employees of these settings
- Healthcare workers who care for patients with TB disease
- Healthcare workers upon hire[2]
- Locally defined high-risk populations such as the medically underserved and those who abuse substances such as drugs or alcohol
- Infants, children, and adolescents exposed to high-risk adults
- Persons at high risk for developing TB disease if infected with *M. tuberculosis*[2]
  - People living with HIV
  - Children younger than 5 years of age
  - People recently infected with *M. tuberculosis*
  - People with inadequate previous treatment
  - People receiving immunosuppressive therapy including (TNF)-alpha antagonists, systemic corticosteroids, and immunosuppressive drug therapy after organ transplantation
  - People with silicosis, chronic renal failure, leukemia, or cancer of the head, neck, or lung
  - People with diabetes
  - People who have had a gastrectomy or jejunoileal bypass
  - People who have low body weight

Diagnosis and Evaluation

These tests will assist in making the diagnoses of LTBI and/or tuberculosis disease but definitive diagnosis requires additional testing (e.g., chest x-ray).

Monitoring

The IGRAs are not used in the monitoring of LTBI or tuberculosis disease treatment because the interferon gamma responses do not reflect treatment.[9]

INTERPRETATION

- For the QFT-GIT, a test is considered positive if the IFN-gamma response to the TB antigens minus the background IFN-gamma is above the test cutoff value.[7]
- Tests can also be resulted as negative or indeterminate.
- Indeterminate tests are due to unusually high or low IFN-gamma response in the positive or negative controls.[10]
- For the T-SPOT.TB, the test is positive if the number of T-cells exceeds a threshold relative to the negative control.[2]

FOLLOW-UP

- Complete a thorough health history to determine if the patient has had a previous positive test(s), or previous treatment(s) for LTBI or TB before testing with IGRA. If the test is positive, this history should be reviewed and include a risk assessment for liver disease.[2]

- Physical examination focusing on signs of respiratory TB or nonrespiratory TB should also be done.
- In the case of an indeterminate test, repeating the IGRA or a TST may be warranted.[2]
- A chest x-ray is the next step in testing when the IGRA is positive. The chest x-ray may indicate active TB or nodular or fibrotic lesions consistent with old TB infection (LTBI), which may convert to TB disease.
- If the patient has respiratory symptoms or an abnormal chest x-ray and a positive IGRA, sputum testing for acid-fast bacilli smear and culture must be done. In the patient with HIV, sputum testing should be considered even if the chest x-ray is normal.
- Some new tests are available that simultaneously test for active TB and rifampin resistance on a sputum specimen. There are two versions of this test available, the Xpert MTB/RIF and the Xpert Ultra. Both are nucleic acid amplification tests (NAAT). Compared to current culture and drug resistance testing, which take several weeks, results of the new tests are available in 2 hours.[2,3]
- A Cochrane review determined that there are not yet enough studies across diverse populations to have confidence in the results of the test except in those with HIV infection.[3,4]

PEARLS & PITFALLS

- IGRAs avoid the "booster phenomenon" that is sometimes seen with the use of the TST. In this phenomenon, a TST is given to someone who may have had TB. If their immune system destroyed it long ago, they may have an initially negative TST followed by a positive TST (two-step testing).[1,4]
- Serial testing in healthcare workers with IGRAs in high resource countries is not recommended because there is a high rate of conversions and reversions when repeated tests are performed.[2]
- The website www.bcgatlas.org provides information about whether BCG is commonly administered in a particular country. IGRAs are the better test if the patient previously vaccinated for BCG.
- In patients with advanced HIV or AIDS not on antiretroviral therapy (ART), who have a negative IGRA or TST, testing should be repeated after the initiation of ART.[2] If either a TST or IGRA is positive in the case where both are done, further assessment for LTBI and TB must be done.[2]

PATIENT EDUCATION

- https://www.cdc.gov/tb/publications/factsheets/testing/tb_testing.htm

RELATED DIAGNOSES AND ICD-10 CODES

Contact and exposure to tuberculosis	Z20.1
Encounter for testing for latent TB	Z86.15
Personal history of latent TB	Z22.7

Encounter for screening for respiratory TB	Z11.1
Latent tuberculosis (LTBI)	Z22.7
Respiratory TB	A15.9

REFERENCES

Full list of references can be accessed through Springer Publishing Company Connect™ at the following link: http://connect.springerpub.com/content/reference-book/978-0-8261-8843-4/part/part03/toc-part/ch100

---

101. LACTATE

Carolyn McClerking

PHYSIOLOGY REVIEW

The production of lactate occurs in numerous tissues in the body; however, the majority of lactate production takes place in the muscle.[1] Lactate is primarily cleared by the liver, with the remainder of the clearance occurring through the kidneys.[1] Lactate is a product of anaerobic metabolism and considered an indicator for tissue hypoxia.[2] In aerobic conditions, lactate production is bypassed when pyruvate is produced by glycolysis and enters the Kreb cycle.[1,2] If tissue energy needs are unmet by aerobic respiration, lactate concentration will increase from the anaerobic metabolism. In anaerobic conditions, lactate is an end product of glucose breakdown and acts to influence the Cori cycle (lactic acid cycle) as a substrate for gluconeogenesis.[1]

Lactate levels are elevated due to either overproduction, decreased ability for clearance, or a combination of the two.[1] The upper limit of normal for lactate is approximately 2.5 mmol/L and levels that increase above 4.0 mmol/L are considered hyperlactatemia.[3] Lactic acidosis, which is oftentimes used interchangeably with lactate, occurs in the setting of hyperlactatemia and a low systemic blood pH.[3,4] Normally lactic acidosis is produced due to tissue hypoperfusion and hypoxia, which is seen with such conditions as respiratory distress, moderate anemia hypermetabolic states, and varying types of shock.[4] In a comparison of arterial, peripheral venous, and capillary blood lactate, studies found venous blood to be just as accurate in assessing sepsis severity.[5] As blood lactate is primarily elevated in tissue hypoxia, other conditions not associated with hypoxia can cause elevation in lactate as well.[3] These additional conditions linked to lactate elevation include but are not limited to trauma, malignancy, and cardiac abnormalities.[3] Although some evidence shows point-of-care (POC) testing leads to faster identification of patients with sepsis, there are no current, randomized controlled trials for the utilization of lactate POC in the community setting.[6]

OVERVIEW OF LABORATORY TESTS

Lactate can be measured in the plasma (CPT code 83605) via spectrophotometry, cerebral spinal fluid, or via electrode-based biosensors that evaluate tissue oxygenation.[7] The incorporation of biosensors in blood gas analyzers and similar POC testing instruments allows lactate to be measured and easily obtained outside the laboratory in a small amount of time and are often used in critical care settings.[7] If evaluation will take place in later than half an hour, the sample should be preserved on ice.[7] In order to avoid falsely elevated lactate levels, samples should be processed within 15 to 30 minutes. Studies suggest that a tourniquet should not affect the levels as long as the samples are processed quickly.[8]

INDICATIONS

Screening

- Universal screening of lactate is not recommended.
- Targeted screening is recommended in patients with conditions predisposing them to hyperlactatemia (Box 101.1)[1,9–12].

Diagnosis and Evaluation

Consider diagnostic testing for the following patients:

Box 101.1: Conditions Commonly Associated With Hyperlactatemia

- Acid–base disturbances
- Congestive heart failure
- Diabetes uncontrolled (DKA)
- Malignancy
- Medications
- Meningitis (CSF)
- Myocardial infarction
- Overdose
- Kidney failure
- Seizure
- Sepsis
- Septic shock
- Severe anemia
- Severe asthma
- Toxins
- Trauma

Sources: Data from Andersen LW, Mackenhauer J, Roberts JC, Berg KM, Cocchi MN, Donnino MW. Etiology and therapeutic approach to elevated lactate levels. *Mayo Clin Proc.* 2013;88(10):1127–1140; Khodashahi R, Sarjamee S. Early lactate area scores and serial blood lactate levels as prognostic markers for patients with septic shock: a systematic review. *Infect Dis (Lond).* 2020;52(7):451–463; Lou Isenberg A, Jensen ME, Lindelof M. Plasma-lactate levels in simulated seizures—an observational study. *Seizure.* 2020;76:47–49; Marik PE. Lactate guided resuscitation-nothing is more dangerous than conscientious foolishness. *J Thorac Dis.* 2019;11(suppl 15):S1969–S1972; Ren D, Wang X, Tu Y. The prognostic role of lactate in patients who achieved return of spontaneous circulation after cardiac arrest: a systematic review and meta-analysis. *Cancer Translat Med.* 2019;5(1):1–9.

Box 101.2: Signs/Symptoms of Hyperlactatemia

- Abdominal pain
- Coma
- Diaphoresis
- Dyspnea
- Hypoxia
- Muscle weakness
- Nausea
- Pallor
- Tachypnea

Source: Data from Ferreruela M, Raurich JM, Ayestarán I, Llompart-Pou JA. Hyperlactatemia in ICU patients: incidence, causes and associated mortality. *J Crit Care*. 2017;42:200–205.

- Chronic liver disease[13]
- Hyperlacticaemia during cardiac surgery[14]
- Sepsis and septic shock[15,16]
- Amniotic fluid lactate in prolonged labor[17]
- Signs/symptoms that could be due to hyperlactatemia (Box 101.2)[18]
- Signs/symptoms that indicate hypoxia including shortness of breath, tachypnea, paleness, diaphoresis, muscle weakness, abdominal pain, nausea, and/or coma.

Monitoring
- Used for lactate clearance for effective resuscitation target[10,19,20]
- Used for resuscitation and recovery for surviving sepsis guidelines[21,22]

INTERPRETATION
- Reference range for lactate: 0.2 to 2.2 mmol/L.[23]
- Lactate level greater than 2.0 requires immediate medical attention in children.
- Late level greater than 4.0 in adults requires immediate medical attention.
- Common causes of elevated lactate are reviewed in Box 101.1.

FOLLOW-UP
- Follow-up testing will depend on the medical condition identified.
- Complete blood count, urinalysis, procalcitonin, and blood cultures can further assist with diagnosis of sepsis and/or other infectious etiology.[24]

PEARLS & PITFALLS
- A study evaluating the validity of a POC handheld device, Lactate Pro 2, saw no difference between healthy and acute critically ill patients using arterial blood; however, less agreement was seen using venous blood in the two groups.[25]
- One study assessed whether tourniquets as compared to no tourniquet use during lactate blood draw altered the results; findings suggested there was no major impact on the results and recommended institutional guidelines should likely be changed.[8]

- Authors studied whether initiating and trending lactate levels had an impact on the outcomes of septic patients. Results suggested repeating the lactate within 3 hours was appropriate if the initial level was drawn within 1 hour of admission to the intensive care unit.[26]
- Randomized controlled trials were conducted to determine if lactate testing as opposed to pH testing of fetal blood from the scalp were effective after detection of abnormal heart rate patterns and posed less risk. Results suggested lactate fetal blood scalp sampling was likely to have more success than pH testing.[27]
- Elevated blood lactate increases the risk of mortality in critically ill patients; patients presenting to the emergency department in septic shock with an elevated lactate level above 2.5 mmoL/L were at greater risk of death.[18,28,29]
- A randomized controlled study evaluated the correlation between hyperlactatemia and patients given albuterol for acute asthma exacerbation and found a significant association between plasma albuterol concentration and elevated lactate concentration.[30,31]
- Higher lactate levels are associated with presentation of patients receiving CPR and 1 month mortality.[32]
- One study concluded that sepsis screening algorithms designed to determine adverse patient outcomes should use a beginning serum lactate level of 2 mmol/L or greater as a threshold to initiate treatment interventions and continued monitoring.[33]
- A study evaluated the association between lactate clearance and mortality in septic shock patients with hyperbilirubinemia. The study found increased lactate clearance was associated with decreased 28-day mortality.[34]
- A meta-analysis sought to determine if lactate level or lactate clearance were associated with predicting neurologic outcomes after cardiac arrest. Lactate levels were significantly associated with neurologic outcomes; however, lactate clearance was not as stable.[35]
- Serum lactate level predicts long-term and short-term mortality in all patients; however, patients with sepsis have a higher mortality with any lactate level.[36]
- A study found that ongoing elevated lactate post veno-arterial extracorporeal membrane oxygenation (VA-ECMO) initiation for patients with cardiogenic shock predicted in-hospital mortality and acute cerebrovascular strokes.[37]

PATIENT EDUCATION

- https://labtestsonline.org/tests/lactate

RELATED DIAGNOSES AND ICD-10 CODES

Other specified abnormal findings of blood chemistry	E87.2
Synonyms: Lacticaemia, excessive; lactic acidosis	

REFERENCES

Full list of references can be accessed through Springer Publishing Company Connect™ at the following link: http://connect.springerpub.com/content/reference-book/ 978-0-8261-8843-4/part/part03/toc-part/ch101

102. LACTATE DEHYDROGENASE

Barbara Rogers and Beth Faiman

PHYSIOLOGY REVIEW

Lactate dehydrogenase (LDH) is an enzyme that catalyzes the formation of lactate from pyruvate in the anaerobic metabolic pathway (of glucose).[1] It is important in maintaining homeostasis when there is a lack of oxygen. LDH is in the cytoplasm of all cells and is an important checkpoint of gluconeogenesis and DNA metabolism. When cells are in an anaerobic or hypoxic state, there is disruption of the production of adenosine triphosphate (ATP) by oxidative phosphorylation. This then leads to cells needing to produce energy by alternate metabolism processes. As a consequence of the need to produce energy, LDH is upregulated. LDH becomes more active during extreme muscular activity.[1]

While LDH is predominantly in the cytoplasm of various tissues, it also has significant mitochondrial activity. The highest concentration of LDH is found in the heart, liver, lungs, kidneys, skeletal muscle, red blood cells and lymphocytes. LDH can be fractionated to five major isoenzymes (LDH_{1-5}) to help distinguish the site of origin of the LDH. LDH_1 is primarily found in the heart. While LDH_2 is also noted in the heart, it is, to a lesser degree than LDH_1, primarily in the reticuloendothelial system and red blood cells (RBCs). LDH_3 is the major isoenzyme of the lungs. LDH_4 is primarily in the lungs and LDH_5 has significant expression in the liver and skeletal muscle. LDH_5 is the isoenzyme that is expressed in cancer cells, whereas LDH_1 is usually down-regulated in cancer cells.[1,2] Routine isoenzyme measurement is usually not available in clinical laboratories. Therefore, other tests are needed to determine the site of disease that may be causing the elevated LDH (e.g., creatine kinase [CK] for muscle, alanine aminotransferase (ALT) for liver, troponin for heart diseases). Very high levels of LDH seem to correlate with severe disease or multiple organ failure. In cancer cells, the function of LDH is different than that of LDH in normal cells. Cancer cells employ LDH to increase their aerobic metabolism. The cancer cells benefit from switching to anaerobic metabolic process (Warburg effect) by avoiding the generation of oxidative stress. The Warburg effect seems to be important for the tumorigenic potential of malignant cells.[1,2] High LDH levels are noted to be associated with advanced stages of cancer. LDH is an important prognostic factor for different tumors and can be used as a marker for staging of a disease.[2-17]

OVERVIEW OF LABORATORY TESTS

LDH assays (CPT code 83615) measure the amount of LDH present in the serum. LDH can be used as a marker for diverse tissue injuries. Upon tissue damage, the cells release LDH in the serum due to organ destruction and cause elevation of serum LDH. The elevation of LDH in blood can remain high for up to 7 days depending on the type of tissue damage. LDH levels can also be used in the evaluation of body fluids from sources other than the blood and can be analyzed from peritoneal fluid, cerebral spinal fluid, or pleural fluid.[1]

INDICATIONS

Screening
No universal or targeted screenings of LDH are recommended.

Diagnosis and Evaluation
LDH may be ordered as part of a diagnostic workup along with a comprehensive metabolic panel (CMP) and other testing when an individual has a condition that is believed to be causing some degree of cellular or tissue damage such as malignancies.

Table 102.1 reviews the common causes for increased and decreased levels of LDH.

Some diagnostic considerations for malignancies are as follows:

- LDH is a nonspecific marker for certain tumors; however, it is not useful in the identification of the type of cancer.[1,2]
- Serum LDH has been noted to be a clinical biomarker in lymphoid malignancies. The elevation of LDH has been associated with high tumor burden and more aggressive clinical behavior. LDH is a strong adverse prognostic factor (shorter survival time) in aggressive B-cell lymphomas (e.g., diffuse large cell lymphoma), mantle cell lymphomas, and follicular lymphomas. Increased level of LDH is associated with high tumor mass in patients with multiple myeloma.[2]
- The level of elevation of serum LDH correlates with bulky tumor mass; therefore, it represents an independent prognostic factor for hematologic diseases and solid tumors. It has been used for years as part of the clinical evaluation of malignancies.[2]
- LDH is one of the most useful serum biomarkers for assessing metastatic melanoma since it has been found to be an independent prognostic factor.[2]
- LDH has been noted to correlate with disease state, response to treatment, and survival in lung cancer and has indicated an increased risk of tumor recurrence and poor survival. It is also an important prognostic marker and is related to poorer survival rates.[2]
- Central nervous system (CNS) lymphoma, leukemia, and metastatic carcinoma can be noted to have LDH of more than 40 U/L over the upper limit of normal.[1]
- LDH is an important diagnostic marker for cutaneous lymphoma.[4]
- LDH is used as a staging marker in non-seminomatous testicular cancer.[1]
- The concentration of LDH_5 has been demonstrated to be a predictor of radiotherapy and chemotherapy response in malignancy.[1]
- LDH plays an important role in resistance of breast cancer cells to paclitaxel. Higher levels of LDH in breast cancer cells are associated with high cell proliferation.[2]
- Refer to Table 102.2 for more information about the role of LDH in malignancies.

TABLE 102.1: CAUSES OF ALTERED LACTATE DEHYDROGENASE LEVELS

INCREASED LDH	DECREASED LDH
Cardiac diseases (e.g., MI)	Irradiation
Liver diseases	Genetic deficiency of subunits of LDH
Hematologic diseases (e.g., hemolytic anemia, pernicious anemia)	Medications-vitamin C
Diseases of lung	
Malignancy (testicular cancer, lymphoma, and other cancers)	
Muscle diseases including injuries from trauma	
Renal diseases	
Bone fractures	
Infections: encephalitis, meningitis, encephalitis, HIV	
Other conditions: parasitic diseases, hypothyroidism, collagen vascular diseases, acute pancreatitis, intestinal obstruction, intestinal obstruction, sarcoidosis, CNS conditions, hypoxia, shock	
Drugs/Medications: anesthetics, aspirin, alcohols, certain narcotics, procainamide	
Pediatric age-infants and young children have higher normal levels of LDH as compared to older children and adults	

CNS, central nervous system; LDH, lactate dehydrogenase; MI, myocardial infarction.

Sources: Jurisic V, Radenkovic S, Konjevic G. The actual role of LDH as tumor marker, biochemical and clinical aspects. *Adv Exp Med Biol.* 2015;867:115–124. doi:10.1007/978-94-017-7215-0_8; National Comprehensive Cancer Network. *NCCN Clinical Practice Guidelines in Oncology- B-Cell Malignancies. Version 3.2021.* 2021. https://www.nccn.org/professionals/physician_gls/pdf/b-cell.pdf; National Comprehensive Cancer Network. *NCCN Clinical Practice Guidelines in Oncology-Chronic Lymphocytic Leukemia. Version 3.2021.* 2021. https://www.nccn.org/professionals/physician_gls/pdf/cll.pdf; National Comprehensive Cancer Network. *NCCN Clinical Practice Guidelines in Oncology-Hairy Cell Leukemia. Version 2.2021.* 2021. https://www.nccn.org/professionals/physician_gls/pdf/hairy_cell.pdf; National Comprehensive Cancer Network. *NCCN Clinical Practice Guidelines in Oncology-Histiocytic Neoplasms. Version 1.2021.* 2021. https://www.nccn.org/professionals/physician_gls/pdf/histiocytic_neoplasms.pdf; National Comprehensive Cancer Network. *NCCN Clinical Practice Guidelines in Oncology-Hodgkin Lymphoma. Version 3.2021.* 2021. https://www.nccn.org/professionals/physician_gls/pdf/hodgkins.pdf; National Comprehensive Cancer Network. *NCCN Clinical Practice Guidelines in Oncology-Melanoma. Version 2021.* 2021. https://www.nccn.org/professionals/physician_gls/pdf/cutaneous_melanoma.pdf; National Comprehensive Cancer Network. *NCCN Clinical Practice Guidelines in Oncology-Multiple Myeloma. Version 5.2021.* 2021. https://www.nccn.org/professionals/physician_gls/pdf/myeloma.pdf; National Comprehensive Cancer Network. *NCCN Clinical Practice Guidelines in Oncology-Myelodysplastic Syndrome. Version 3.2021.* 2021. https://www.nccn.org/professionals/physician_gls/pdf/mds.pdf; National Comprehensive Cancer Network. *NCCN Clinical Practice Guidelines in Oncology-Myeloproliferative Disorders. Version 1.2020.* 2021. https://www.nccn.org/professionals/physician_gls/pdf/mpn.pdf; National Comprehensive Cancer Network. *NCCN Clinical Practice Guidelines in Oncology -Ovarian Cancer. Version 1.2021.* 2021. https://www.nccn.org/professionals/physician_gls/pdf/ovarian.pdf; National Comprehensive Cancer Network. *NCCN Clinical Practice Guidelines in Oncology-Primary Cutaneous Lymphomas. Version 2.2021.* 2021. https://www.nccn.org/professionals/physician_gls/pdf/primary_cutaneous.pdf; National Comprehensive Cancer Network. *NCCN Clinical Practice Guidelines in Oncology-Small Cell Lung Cancer. Version 2.2011.* 2021. https://www.nccn.org/professionals/physician_gls/pdf/sclc.pdf; National Comprehensive Cancer Network. *NCCN Clinical Practice Guidelines in Oncology-Systemic Light Chain Amyloidosis. Version 2.2021.* 2021. https://www.nccn.org/professionals/physician_gls/pdf/amyloidosis.pdf; National Comprehensive Cancer Network. *NCCN Clinical Practice Guidelines in Oncology-Testicular Cancer. Version 1.2021.* 2021. https://www.nccn.org/professionals/physician_gls/pdf/sclc.pdf.

TABLE 102.2: THE ROLE OF LACTATE DEHYDROGENASE LEVELS IN MALIGNANCIES

DISEASE	WORKUP	PROGNOSTIC USE	ONGOING MONITORING
HEMATOLOGIC MALIGNANCIES			
CLL	X • Elevated LDH = suspicion of transformation	X	While at risk of TLS
Non-Hodgkin Lymphoma	X • Included in work-up of most types of NHL • Elevated LDH = suspicion of transformation of low grade lymphomas	• Component of FLIPI score • Component of IPI • Prognostic indicator for assessment of risk of CNS disease in DLBCL • Prognostic indicator for Burkitt's lymphoma	
Hairy Cell Leukemia	X		
Hodgkin Lymphoma	X		
Multiple Myeloma	X (Reflects tumor cell characteristics)	X (Component of revised ISS)	X
Systemic Light Chair Amyloidosis	X		
Waldenström's Macroglobulinemia	X	X (Component of revised IPSS)	
MDS	X	X (Component of IPSS and IPSS-R)	
MYELOPROLIFERATIVE NEOPLASMS			
• Myelofibrosis	X (Minor criteria for diagnosis)		Obtain LDH before starting therapy with JAK Inhibitor and every 2–4 weeks until dose stabilized
• Post ET Myelofibrosis	X (Minor criteria for diagnosis)		Obtain LDH before starting therapy with JAK inhibitor and every 2–4 weeks until dose stabilized
Rosai-Dorfman Disease	X		
Melanoma	X (surrogate of overall tumor burden)-Component of AJCC staging system	X (Predicts poor outcome in patients with stage IV disease)	

(*continued*)

TABLE 102.2: THE ROLE OF LACTATE DEHYDROGENASE LEVELS IN MALIGNANCIES (*continued*)

DISEASE	WORKUP	PROGNOSTIC USE	ONGOING MONITORING
Ovarian	X (added as tumor marker for germ cell tumors)	X (Predicts poor outcome in germ cell tumors)	
Small Cell Lung Cancer		X (Elevated LDH poor prognostic indicator)	
Systemic Mastocytosis	X		
Testicular Cancer	X (Part of AJCC staging system)	X	X (Markers followed until normalization or plateau)

AJCC, American Joint Committee on Cancer; CLL, chronic lymphocytic leukemia; CNS, central nervous system; DLBCL, diffuse large B cell lymphoma; ET, essential thrombocytosis; FLIPI, follicular lymphoma international prognostic index; IPI, international prognostic index; IPSS, International Prognostic Scoring System; IPSS-R, International Prognostic Scoring System-Revised; LDH, lactate dehydrogenase.

Sources: National Comprehensive Cancer Network. *NCCN Clinical Practice Guidelines in Oncology- B-Cell Malignancies. Version 3.2021.* 2021. https://www.nccn.org/professionals/physician_gls/pdf/b-cell.pdf; National Comprehensive Cancer Network. *NCCN Clinical Practice Guidelines in Oncology-Chronic Lymphocytic Leukemia. Version 3.2021.* 2021. https://www.nccn.org/professionals/physician_gls/pdf/cll.pdf; National Comprehensive Cancer Network. *NCCN Clinical Practice Guidelines in Oncology-Hairy Cell Leukemia. Version 2.2021.* 2021. https://www.nccn.org/professionals/physician_gls/pdf/hairy_cell.pdf; National Comprehensive Cancer Network. *NCCN Clinical Practice Guidelines in Oncology-Histiocytic Neoplasms. Version 1.2021.* 2021. https://www.nccn .org/professionals/physician_gls/pdf/histiocytic_neoplasms.pdf; National Comprehensive Cancer Network. *NCCN Clinical Practice Guidelines in Oncology-Hodgkin Lymphoma. Version 3.2021.* 2021. https://www.nccn.org/professionals/physician_gls/pdf/hodgkins.pdf; National Comprehensive Cancer Network. *NCCN Clinical Practice Guidelines in Oncology-Melanoma. Version 2021.* 2021. https://www.nccn.org/professionals/physician_gls/pdf/cutaneous_melanoma.pdf; National Comprehensive Cancer Network. *NCCN Clinical Practice Guidelines in Oncology-Multiple Myeloma. Version 5.2021.* 2021. https://www.nccn.org/professionals/physician_gls/pdf/myeloma.pdf; National Comprehensive Cancer Network. *NCCN Clinical Practice Guidelines in Oncology-Myelodysplastic Syndrome. Version 3.2021.* 2021. https://www.nccn.org/professionals/physician_gls/pdf/mds.pdf; National Comprehensive Cancer Network. *NCCN Clinical Practice Guidelines in Oncology-Myeloproliferative Disorders. Version 1.2020.* 2021. https://www.nccn.org/professionals/physician_gls/pdf/mpn.pdf; National Comprehensive Cancer Network. *NCCN Clinical Practice Guidelines in Oncology -Ovarian Cancer. Version 1.2021.* 2021. https://www.nccn.org/professionals/physician_gls/pdf/ovarian.pdf; National Comprehensive Cancer Network. *NCCN Clinical Practice Guidelines in Oncology-Primary Cutaneous Lymphomas. Version 2.2021.* 2021. https://www.nccn.org/professionals/physician_gls/pdf/primary_cutaneous.pdf; National Comprehensive Cancer Network. *NCCN Clinical Practice Guidelines in Oncology-Small Cell Lung Cancer. Version 2.2011.* 2021. https://www.nccn.org/professionals/physician_gls/pdf/sclc.pdf; National Comprehensive Cancer Network. *NCCN Clinical Practice Guidelines in Oncology-Systemic Light Chain Amyloidosis. Version 2.2021.* 2021. https://www.nccn.org/professionals/physician_gls/pdf/amyloidosis.pdf; National Comprehensive Cancer Network. *NCCN Clinical Practice Guidelines in Oncology-Testicular Cancer. Version 1.2021.* 2021. https://www.nccn.org/professionals/physician_gls/pdf/sclc.pdf; National Comprehensive Cancer Network. *NCCN Clinical Practice Guidelines in Oncology-Waldenströms Macroglobulinemia. Version 1.2021.* 2021. https://www.nccn.org/professionals/physician_gls/pdf/waldenstroms.pdf.

Some diagnostic considerations for other conditions:

- In CSF, LDH increases in bacterial meningitis, but is normal in viral meningitis.[1]
  The ratio of LDH from body fluid compared to the upper limit of normal of LDH in serum indicates an inflammatory process.[1]
  A high LDH indicates that pericardial fluid, peritoneal fluid, or pleural fluid is an exudate which can be from multiple causes and usually requires additional workup. A low level of LDH indicates transudate that is usually from congestive heart failure or cirrhosis.[1]

- LDH can indicate muscle response to training by demonstrating an increase in skeletal and cardiac muscles after 3 to 5 hours of training.[1]
- LDH can be markedly elevated during intracranial hemorrhage.[1]
- In hepatitis with jaundice, a raised LDH to ten-times the upper limit of normal may be noted.[1]
- LDH can be increased during effusions such as pericardial and peritoneal fluids or in cerebral spinal fluids (CSF).[1]

Monitoring

- LDH is used for monitoring prognosis or response to treatment for various conditions (e.g., malignancy, hemolytic anemia).[1]
- LDH can be used to monitor progressive conditions such as muscular dystrophy or HIV infections.[1]
- A decrease in LDH during treatment indicates better prognosis and/or a good response to treatments in certain conditions (e.g., acute myocardial infarction or liver injury).[1]

INTERPRETATION

An elevated LDH indicates some type of tissue damage. The LDH level increases at the start of cellular destruction, peaks after some time, and then begins to decline. With some chronic and progressive conditions, moderately elevated LDH levels may persist. Low levels of LDH, or LDH deficiency, are rare and are not felt to be harmful.[1]

See Table 102.3 for standard reference values for LDH.

FOLLOW-UP

- Follow-up testing will depend on the medical condition identified.

TABLE 102.3: REFERENCE VALUES FOR LACTATE DEHYDROGENASE	
AGE	**NORMAL LDH VALUE**
1–30 days	135–750 U/L
31 days–11 months	180–435 U/L
1–3 years	160–370 U/L
4–6 years	145–345 U/L
7–9 years	143–290 U/L
10–12 years	120–293 U/L
13–15 years	110–283 U/L
16–17 years	105–233 U/L
≥ 18 years	140–280 U/L

Note: Normal value ranges may vary slightly among different laboratories.

PEARLS & PITFALLS

- The major limitation of LDH is its lack of specificity since it is found in numerous organs and tissues.[1]
- RBC contain much more LD than serum; therefore, hemolysis can cause false-positive results.[1]
- A hemolyzed specimen is not acceptable for testing LDH since the level of LDH is affected by hemolysis of the blood sample.[1]
- Hemolysis elevates LDH results.[1]
- LDH test can be affected by medications and ascorbic acid.[1]
- While previously, the measurement of LDH_1 and the ratio of LDH_1 and LDH_2 were used as part of determination of a myocardial infarction (MI), there are now better cardiac-specific markers for this purpose.[1]

PATIENT EDUCATION

- https://labtestsonline.org/tests/lactate-dehydrogenase-ld

RELATED DIAGNOSES AND ICD-10 CODES

Elevation of LDH	R74.02

REFERENCES

Full list of references can be accessed through Springer Publishing Company Connect™ at the following link: http://connect.springerpub.com/content/reference-book/978-0-8261-8843-4/part/part03/toc-part/ch102

---

103. LEAD

Rosie Zeno

PHYSIOLOGY REVIEW

Lead (Pb) is a toxic, heavy metal organically occurring in the environment (air, soil, water). The majority of toxic environmental exposures are attributed to inorganic lead compounds found in industrial products like paint, gasoline, and plumbing. Lead is mainly absorbed through the respiratory or gastrointestinal (GI) tract. Cutaneous exposure to organic lead also occurs but transdermal absorption is relatively inefficient. Adults are more likely to absorb toxic levels of lead from inhaled occupational exposures whereas children are more likely to ingest sources of lead from environmental exposures.

Lead is more readily absorbed when dietary iron (Fe) or calcium (Ca) is insufficient and also during times of fasting as the presence of food in the GI tract decreases absorption. Approximately 40% to 50% of ingested lead is absorbed by infants and children versus 3% to 10% in adults.[1] The mechanism by which lead crosses cell membranes is not well explicated, but distribution is essentially the same regardless of the route of absorption. Lead is similarly distributed to blood, bone, and lead-responsive soft tissues such as the kidneys, liver, brain, and placenta.

In blood, 99% of lead is bound to heme while 1% remains in the plasma and is readily exchanged with body tissues. The largest proportion of the body's total lead burden resides in bone, although to a greater degree in adults (94%) compared to children (73%).[1] The half-life of lead ranges from 28 to 40 days in blood and soft tissue to greater than 25-years in mineralized bone.[1] During periods of accelerated bone resorption (such as hyperthyroidism, bone fracture, menopause, pregnancy, lactation, or immobility), the bones become an endogenous source of lead exposure as retained lead is more rapidly released from demineralizing bone. Ultimately, lead is primarily excreted in urine and feces, and, to a minor extent, sweat, saliva, hair, nails, breast milk, and semen. The rate of lead clearance is relatively dependent on its biologichalf-life and ultimately influenced by chronicity of exposure and kidney function.

Lead interferes with a wide variety of biochemical reactions causing widespread physiologic effects that lead to irreversible damage at the cellular level and cell death, particularly in the central nervous system.[2,3] The effects of lead toxicity on the brain include delays or regression in development, permanent cognitive disabilities, seizures, coma, and death. The permeability of the blood-brain barrier of fetuses and young children (compared to adults) increased their risk of permanent neurobehavioral disorders from lead exposure. The most significant and long-term effects of lead exposure occur during the first 3 years of life when the brain is undergoing a period of critical development.

OVERVIEW OF LABORATORY TESTS

- Human exposure to lead is evaluated by blood lead level (BLL) analysis. Venous BLL testing is the most useful screening and diagnostic test for recent and ongoing exposure.[1,10] Capillary blood specimens are appropriate for screening, but venous blood specimens are required for BLL confirmation and clinical decision-making due to the high potential of contamination with capillary samples.[3]
- Lead testing (CPT code 83655) is indicated in the screening, evaluation, and monitoring of lead exposure and toxicity. BLLs may also be evaluated by obtaining a heavy metal profile when clinical suspicion for heavy metal poisoning warrants evaluation. In addition to lead, a heavy metal profile may include testing for arsenic (CPT code 82175), mercury (CPT code 83825), and cadmium (CPT code 82300).
- Erythrocyte protoporphyrin (EP), or zinc protoporphyrin (ZPP), was formerly the recommended test for screening asymptomatic children for lead exposure, but it is not adequately sensitive at lower BLLs and therefore no longer useful.[1]
- Do not perform hair or nail testing for "metal poisoning" screening in patients with nonspecific symptoms as hair and nail testing are rarely required, frequently unreliable, and provide limited utility after metal exposures.[4]

INDICATIONS

Screening

- The United States Preventive Services Task Force (USPSTF) finds current evidence insufficient to assess the balance of benefits and harms of screening for elevated BLL in asymptomatic children aged 5 years and younger or asymptomatic pregnant individuals (I statement).[5]
- The American Academy of Family Physicians (AAFP) recommends against routine screening for elevated BLLs in (a) asymptomatic children younger than 5 years old who are at average risk, and (b) asymptomatic pregnant individuals; and cites insufficient evidence for making recommendations on the routine screening of children at higher risk.[6]
- The American Academy of Pediatrics' Bright Futures recommends (a) screening in accordance with state law, and (b) universal screening for all children aged 12 and 24 months in states without screening programs.[7]
- The Early and Periodic Screening, Diagnostic and Treatment (EPSDT) program administered by the Centers for Medicare and Medicaid Services (CMS) requires universal BLL screening of all children at ages 12 and 24 months, as well as children aged 24 to 72 months who have not been previously screened.[8]
- The Centers for Disease Control and Prevention (CDC) and the American College of Obstetricians and Gynecologists (ACOG) recommend targeted screening during pregnancy and lead testing in pregnant and lactating individuals with one or more risk factors for lead exposures.[9-11]
- The CDC recommends BLL screening in children at increased risk for lead exposure.[9,10]
- The American Academy of Pediatrics recommends BLL screening in accordance with federal and state requirements; in children living in high-prevalence areas; and in children with identified risks for lead exposure (Table 103.1).[12]

Diagnosis and Evaluation

- Consider lead screening in those with risk factors for lead exposure (see Table 103.1) and in any individual exhibiting signs or symptoms of lead toxicity (Table 103.2).
- Symptoms of lead toxicity appear on a continuum relative to the level, frequency, and duration of lead exposure and may vary from person to person. Many patients initially present asymptomatically or with nonspecific neurologic concerns; hence, the importance of screening when indicated.
- Consider testing young children for lead exposure when a sibling or close contact is being monitored or treated for lead exposure.[9,12]
- With the exception of lead testing when indicated, do not routinely test blood or urine for heavy metal levels to guide clinical decision-making.[13] People encounter environmental chemicals in food, air, water, soil, dust, and commercial products each day. Presence does not mean toxicity.

TABLE 103.1: RISK FACTORS FOR LEAD EXPOSURE

Populations at higher risk:	Children <6 years old
	Internationally adopted children
	Pregnant individuals
	Refugees
	Industrial workers
Primary sources of child lead exposure:	Lead-based paint, lead-contaminated dust, and soil
	Social determinants:
	• Housing inequity in communities of color
	• Households living at or below the federal poverty level and living in housing built before 1978
Sources of industrial lead exposures:	Plumbers or pipe fitters
	Lead manufacturers, miners, refiners, smelters
	Steel workers and welders
	Radiator and auto repairers
	Recyclers and solid waste incinerators
	Construction workers, painters, and ship builders
	Gunsmiths, firing range workers
	Manufacturers of glass, batteries, plastics, rubber, bullets, ceramics
Sources of international lead exposures:	Leaded gasoline
	Ceramic or metal cookware
	Environmental contamination from mining or smelting
	Drinking water from metal pipes or containers
	Industrial emissions
	Traditional medicines
	Cosmetics

Sources: Data from Advisory Committee on Childhood Lead Poisoning Prevention. *Low Level Lead Exposure Harms Children: A Renewed Call for Primary Prevention.* Centers for Disease Control and Prevention; 2012; Centers for Disease Control and Prevention. *CDC Response to Advisory Committee on Childhood Lead Poisoning Prevention Recommendations in Low Level Lead Exposure Harms Children: A Renewed Call of Primary Prevention.* Centers for Disease Control and Prevention; 2012

■ Do not order heavy metal screening tests to assess nonspecific symptoms in the absence of a history of excessive metal exposure. Only order specific metal testing when there is concern for a specific poisoning based on history and physical examination findings.[14]

■ Do not order "chelation challenge" urinary analysis for children with suspected lead poisoning.[15] This test has no clinical utility in treatment of childhood lead toxicity. Instead, children should undergo tailored testing for a specific metal exposure based on the clinical evaluation.

■ Do not routinely test urine for metals and minerals in children with autistic behaviors. Toxicologic exposures have not been conclusively associated with the development of autistic behaviors in children. Testing for metals and minerals may be harmful if treatment is guided on the basis of these results.[16–18]

TABLE 103.2: RANGE OF SYMPTOMS OF ONGOING LEAD EXPOSURE	
Lowest exposure	May appear asymptomatic
	Impaired cognitive abilities:
	• Decreased learning and memory
	• Decreased verbal ability
	• Impaired speech and hearing functions
	• Lowered IQ
Low exposure	Irritability, lethargy, mild fatigue
	Myalgia or paresthesia
	Abdominal discomfort
Moderate exposure	Arthralgias
	Headache, tremor, difficulty concentrating
	Vomiting, constipation, weight loss, diffuse abdominal pain
	Fatigue
High exposure	Colicky abdominal pain
	Paresis or paralysis
	Encephalopathy, seizures, coma, death

BLL, blood lead level.

Sources: Data from Advisory Committee on Childhood Lead Poisoning Prevention. *Low Level Lead Exposure Harms Children: A Renewed Call for Primary Prevention*. Centers for Disease Control and Prevention; 2012; Agency for Toxic Substances and Disease Registry. *Toxicological Profile for Lead*. U.S. Department of Health and Human Services, Public Health Service; 2020. doi:10.15620/cdc:95222; Cantor AG, Hendrickson R, Blazina I, Griffin J, Grusing S, McDonagh MS. *Screening for Elevated Blood Lead Levels in Children: A Systematic Review for the U.S. Preventive Services Task Force: Evidence Synthesis No. 174*. Agency for Healthcare Research and Quality; 2019; Cantor AG, Hendrickson R, Blazina I, Griffin J, Grusing S, McDonagh MS. Screening for elevated blood lead levels in childhood and pregnancy: updated evidence report and systematic review for the US Preventive Services Task Force. *JAMA*. 2019;321(15):1510–1526. doi:10.1001/jama.2019.1004; Centers for Disease Control and Prevention. *CDC response to Advisory Committee on Childhood Lead Poisoning Prevention Recommendations in Low Level Lead Exposure Harms Children: A Renewed Call of Primary Prevention*. Centers for Disease Control and Prevention; 2012.

■ Do not order hair analyses for "environmental toxins" in children with behavioral or developmental disorders including autism.[19]

Monitoring

■ For those identified with BLLs of 5 µg/dL or more, ongoing monitoring of BLL is indicated during and after appropriate medical, educational, and environmental interventions (Tables 103.3, 103.4).[1,9,12,20]

INTERPRETATION

■ An elevated BLL is defined as 5 µg/dL or more of whole blood (venous sample).[9,20-22]
■ No BLL threshold for adverse health effects has been established. Adverse effects, such as neurocognitive effects, lower IQ, language delay, learning problems, and impaired motor skills, have been observed in young children with BLLs less than 10 µg/dL from chronic low-level exposure.[2,3,12] Hence, any BLL above the reference standard should be investigated.
■ The geometric mean BLL for children aged 1 to 5 years and adults older than 20 years is less than 3 µg/dL (2.765 µg/dL and 2.895 µg/dL respectively).[20,23]

TABLE 103.3: TIME FRAME FOR CONFIRMATION OF CAPILLARY SCREENING RESULTS

CAPILLARY BLL (µg/dL) SCREENING	MAX TIME TO CONFIRMATION TESTING
5–9 µg/dL	1–3 months
10–19 µg/dL	1 week–1 month
20–44 µg/dL	48 hours
45–60 µg/dL	24 hours
≥ 70 µg/dL	Urgently, STAT

BLL, blood lead level.

Sources: Data from Advisory Committee on Childhood Lead Poisoning Prevention. *Low Level Lead Exposure Harms Children: A Renewed Call for Primary Prevention.* Centers for Disease Control and Prevention; 2012; American Academy of Pediatrics, Council on Environmental Health. Prevention of childhood lead toxicity. *Pediatrics.* 2016;138(1):e20161493. doi:10.1542/peds.2016-1493; Centers for Disease Control and Prevention. *CDC response to Advisory Committee on Childhood Lead Poisoning Prevention Recommendations in Low Level Lead Exposure Harms Children: A Renewed Call of Primary Prevention.* Centers for Disease Control and Prevention; 2012.

TABLE 103.4: TIME FRAME FOR ONGOING FOLLOW-UP TESTING

VENOUS BLL (µg/dL)	EARLY FOLLOW-UP TESTING	LATE FOLLOW-UP TESTING (AFTER BLL STARTS TO DECLINE)
5–9 µg/dL	3 months*	6–9 months
10–19 µg/dL	1–3 months*	3–6 months
20–24 µg/dL	1–3 months*	1–3 months
55–44 µg/dL	2 weeks–1 month	1 month
≥ 45 µg/dL	As soon as possible	As soon as possible

* For new patients, consider follow-up testing within 1 month to ensure BLL is not rising more quickly than anticipated.

BLL, blood lead level.

Sources: Data from Advisory Committee on Childhood Lead Poisoning Prevention. *Low Level Lead Exposure Harms Children: A Renewed Call for Primary Prevention.* Centers for Disease Control and Prevention; 2012; American Academy of Pediatrics, Council on Environmental Health. Prevention of childhood lead toxicity. *Pediatrics.* 2016;138(1):e20161493. doi:10.1542/peds.2016-1493; Centers for Disease Control and Prevention. *CDC response to Advisory Committee on Childhood Lead Poisoning Prevention Recommendations in Low Level Lead Exposure Harms Children: A Renewed Call of Primary Prevention.* Centers for Disease Control and Prevention; 2012.

- Elevated BLL with a capillary screening result must be confirmed by venous sample due to the higher likelihood of contamination during capillary sample collection.[1,3,21] See Table 103.3 for the recommended time frames for confirmation testing following a capillary result.
- BLLs respond rapidly to abrupt changes in lead absorption; however, for those with high or chronic past exposures, BLLs often underrepresent the total body burden of lead since the majority of lead is stored in mineralized bone.[1] Conversely, those with a high body burden of lead may experience more rapid increases in BLL during times of physiologic stress and accelerated bone resorption.

FOLLOW-UP

■ Following confirmation of an elevated BLL, the source of exposure should be promptly identified as well as the initiation of medical, educational, and environmental interventions.

■ The goal of ongoing follow-up testing is to observe a decline in BLL. If the BLL does not decline as expected, consider the potential for a remaining, unidentified source of exposure, an ineffective environmental lead abatement, or a redistribution of lead stores within the body from bone to blood and soft tissue.

■ See Table 103.4 for recommended time frames for follow-up testing.

PEARLS & PITFALLS

■ The CDC and the National Institute of Occupational Safety and Health (NIOSH) lowered the BLL reference value from 10 μg/dL or more to 5 μg/dL or more (in 2012 and 2015, respectively) based on population surveillance data for children and adults.[20,22,24]

■ BLL of 5 μg/dL or more is the reference value adopted by laboratories and clinical guidelines for the evaluation and management of lead-exposed children and adults.[5,9–12,25–27]

■ In contrast, the Occupational Safety and Health Administration (OSHA) lead standards allow those who have been removed from work-based lead exposure to return to work when their BLL drops below 40 μg/dL; however, NIOSH recommends that exposed adults be managed according to the current CDC/NIOSH reference value of 5 μg/dL.[23]

■ Chelation therapy is considered the mainstay of medical management for those BLLs greater than 45 μg/dL; however, this is a guideline for consideration, not a threshold value. Chelation should be used with caution.[1]

PATIENT EDUCATION

■ https://kidshealth.org/en/parents/lead-poisoning.html
■ https://www.cdc.gov/nceh/lead/prevention/populations.htm

RELATED DIAGNOSES AND ICD-10 CODES

Abnormal lead level in blood	R78.71
Contact with and (suspected) exposure to lead	Z77.011
Toxic effect of lead and its compounds, accidental (unintentional)	T56.1
Lead-induced gout, unspecified site	M10.10

REFERENCES

Full list of references can be accessed through Springer Publishing Company Connect™ at the following link: http://connect.springerpub.com/content/reference-book/978-0-8261-8843-4/part/part03/toc-part/ch103

104. LEIDEN FACTOR V ANALYSIS (R506Q)

John Prickett

PHYSIOLOGY REVIEW

Factor V Leiden (FVL) is the most common inheritable thrombophilia mutation, with heterozygous mutations estimated to be present in around 5% in American Caucasians.[1] It is estimated that about 5% of individuals with a heterozygous mutation will have pathologic venous thromboembolism (VTE) at some point in their life, and it may be a risk factor for late pregnancy loss.[2-4] Despite its role in thrombophilia risk, heterozygous FVL has not been shown to significantly affect overall mortality. While studies show an increased risk of first thrombosis to be around 3- to 7-fold higher in a heterozygous state and 25- to 50-fold higher in a homozygous state, it has not been shown to be helpful in predicting recurrent VTE.[5-7]

Leiden Factor represents a point mutation that causes a conformational change in Factor V, affecting protein C binding. This diminishes the activity of protein C inactivation of FVa (by 20-fold) which allows for the dysregulated generation of thrombin. Before identification of the altered gene, it was known as protein C resistance, due to abnormal clotting studies. Other non-Leiden Factor V mutations exist that may also cause protein C resistance and thrombophilia.[8-10]

OVERVIEW OF LABORATORY TESTS

Functional Assay

An activated protein C (APC) resistance ratio assay (CPT code 85307), which is available in some laboratories, utilizes activated partial thromboplastin (aPTT) techniques. Two assays are completed. The first assay is completed as normal. The second is completed with the addition of a standardized amount of APC. The difference between the two tests is reported as a ratio. However, functional assays may be inaccurate due to their insensitivity to detect FVL when other interfering factors are present (anticoagulants, acute thrombosis, protein S deficiency, elevated FVIII, estrogens, antiphospholipid antibodies, cancer, nephrotic syndrome, elevated body mass index [BMI], and smoking). Additionally, though 95% of APC is due to FVL, there are other mutations that cause APC resistance.[11-13]

Molecular Gene Analysis

Detection of the *FVL* or *R506Q* gene by molecular testing methods including polymerase chain reaction (PCR) (CPT code 81241) have become standard practice. It is done in the event of a positive functional assay as confirmation or can be done in place of the less specific functional APC resistance testing.[12]

INDICATIONS

Screening

Targeted screenings should be considered in individuals with the following[14]:

■ Testing for FVL mutation in unselected patients presenting with their first episode of VTE is not indicated as it does not reduce recurrence of VTE.

■ Asymptomatic relatives should not be screened.

Diagnosis and Evaluation

As with other hypercoagulable laboratory tests, consider testing for FVL mutation in the following patients[14]:

■ First VTE younger than 40 years old

■ VTE in an unusual location (portal, mesenteric, or cerebral vein)

■ Recurrent VTE

■ Pregnant females with a previous VTE due to a minor provoking factor (e.g., travel)

■ Asymptomatic pregnant females with a family history of venous thrombosis in a first-degree relative that was unprovoked, or provoked by pregnancy, oral contraceptive use, or a minor provoking factor.

Monitoring

No routine monitoring of FVL is recommended.

INTERPRETATION

Functional APC resistance is reported as a ratio with a value of 2.3 or greater representing a positive result.

The molecular gene study is typically reported as positive or negative for the presence of the R506Q mutation. If the mutation is present, hetero- or homozygosity is also reported.

FOLLOW-UP

FVL is often co-ordered with prothrombin gene mutation.[15,16]

Depending on the patient's presentation and risk factors, FVL is typically ordered with other tests for hypercoagulation including but not limited to prothrombin time (PT), aPTT (partial thromboplastin time), homocysteine, protein C, antithrombin, and, as previously noted, prothrombin gene mutation testing.

PEARLS & PITFALLS

■ Though testing for the previous indications is generally acceptable practice, there is growing evidence that testing for FVL may not be beneficial.[17]

■ Other mutations of the *F5* gene can cause a "pseudo-homozygous" state, leading to one copy of the *FVL* gene (*R506Q*) and another mutation that causes a reduction in Factor V, leading to a greater thrombotic risk.[18]

■ When present along with prothrombin gene mutation, the risk of thrombosis increases significantly.[15]

- The thrombophilic risk associated with FVL appears to be predominantly for VTE. Data have been mixed regarding FVL as a risk for arterial thromboses (myocardial infarction [MI] and stroke) with the greatest risk seeming to be in people who smoke or females with FVL.[19-24]

PATIENT EDUCATION

- https://www.stoptheclot.org/wp-content/uploads/2014/02/FactorVLeiden-lw.pdf
- https://rarediseases.info.nih.gov/diseases/6403/factor-v-leiden-thrombophilia

RELATED DIAGNOSES AND ICD-10 CODES

Activated protein C resistance, FVL   D68.51

REFERENCES

Full list of references can be accessed through Springer Publishing Company Connect™ at the following link: http://connect.springerpub.com/content/reference-book/978-0-8261-8843-4/part/part03/toc-part/ch104

---

105. LEVETIRACETAM (KEPPRA)

Candice Short and Ryan Short

PHYSIOLOGY REVIEW

Levetiracetam (Keppra) is an antiepileptic drug and is used as an adjuvant or monotherapy for partial onset seizures in children and adults.[1] Levetiracetam is not related to any other antiepileptic drugs; therefore, it belongs to its own drug class.[1] The antiepileptic effect for levetiracetam is unknown; however, it is known that levetiracetam inhibits burst firing without affecting normal neuronal excitability.[2] After oral administration, levetiracetam is almost entirely absorbed; however, the absorption rate is reduced by co-ingestion with food.[1,3] Peak concentration is reached in about an hour for immediate release and 3 hours for extended release.[1] Metabolism of levetiracetam occurs by enzymatic hydrolysis of the acetamide group[1,4] and does not use the cytochrome P450 enzyme.[4] Levetiracetam has a half-life of 7 hours in adults and approximately 67% is excreted renally.[1,4]

Levetiracetam should be considered as an antiepileptic treatment choice for both older adults and pediatric populations. In older adult patients, levetiracetam is a good anticonvulsant choice for numerous reasons, including safety, low side effect profile, reduced interactions with other drugs, and efficacy.[5] Levetiracetam has been proven as an effective antiepileptic drug in pediatric patients.[6] It should be noted that levetiracetam clears more quickly in this population; therefore, pediatric patients require a higher dosage and frequent monitoring.[6]

OVERVIEW OF LABORATORY TESTS

High performance liquid chromatography (HPLC) is used to measure levetiracetam in serum plasma (CPT code 80177). Due to the complexity of this methodology, immediate results are not possible, making this laboratory test very difficult to use in clinical practice.[3] The Ark levetiracetam assay is a rapid and automated test which is more suitable for clinical practice.[6] The Quantitative Enzyme Immunoassay is reported within 24 hours (CPT code 80177).

INDICATIONS

Screening

■ There is no universal or targeted screening recommended.

Diagnosis and Evaluation

■ Evaluate levetiracetam levels if failure to respond to treatment.[3]
■ Evaluate levetiracetam levels for signs of toxicity including agitation, aggression, drowsiness, somnolence, decreased level of consciousness, or respiratory depression.[7]

Monitoring

■ Levetiracetam is easily dosed and well tolerated among most individuals. In some instances, therapeutic drug monitoring may be indicated; these include pregnancy, pediatric dosing, renal failure, noncompliance, and limited response with high doses (Table 105.1).[3,4]
■ Routine therapeutic monitoring of levetiracetam is not supported in the literature,[8] except in the populations and circumstances that were previously listed.

TABLE 105.1: DOSE ADJUSTMENT REGIMEN FOR ADULT PATIENTS WITH RENAL IMPAIRMENT			
GROUP	**CREATININE CLEARANCE (mL/min/1.73 m²)**	**DOSAGE (mg)**	**FREQUENCY**
Normal	>80	500–1,500	Every 12 hours
Mild	50–80	500–1,000	Every 12 hours
Moderate	30–50	250–750	Every 12 hours
Severe	<30	250–500	Every 12 hours
end-stage renal disease (ESRD) patients using dialysis	____	500–1,000*	Every 24 hours*

*Following dialysis, a 250- to 500-mg supplemental dose is recommended.

Source: Data from Food and Drug Administration. Highlights of prescribing information. Accessed May 17, 2021. https://www. accessdata.fda.gov/drugsatfda_docs/label/2017/021872s023lbl.pdf.

INTERPRETATION

- A trough level of 12 to 46 mcg/mL is considered a therapeutic range of levetiracetam.[3,4]
- Optimal response is noted with serum levels between 10.0 to 40 mcg/mL.[9]
- Clinical evaluation is necessary to interpret response, as some patients may show signs of toxicity while in therapeutic range, while others will show response outside of therapeutic levels.[4,9]

FOLLOW-UP

- Supratherapeutic level: lower the dose (based on clinical response).[10]
- Therapeutic level: maintain current dosing (based on clinical response).[10]
- Subtherapeutic level: raise the dose (based on clinical response).[10]

PEARLS & PITFALLS

- Clinical judgment is paramount when determining the effectiveness of antiepileptic drugs such as levetiracetam.[10]
- Levetiracetam may increase the incidence of suicidal ideation.[7]
- The level of levetiracetam may decrease during pregnancy, resulting in the possibility of requiring an increased dose adjustment.[7]
- Levetiracetam is pregnancy category C.[7]
- Levetiracetam is excreted in breast milk.[7]
- Levetiracetam clearance is reduced in patients with renal impairment and relates to creatinine clearance (see Table 105.1).[7]
- In clinical trials, drowsiness was the only adverse effect noted in overdose cases of levetiracetam. In post-marketing use, somnolence, agitation, aggression, depressed level of consciousness, respiratory depression, and coma were observed in overdose cases.[7]
- There is no known antidote for overdoses of levetiracetam.[7]

PATIENT EDUCATION

- https://medlineplus.gov/druginfo/meds/a699059.html
- https://www.merckmanuals.com/professional/neurologic-disorders/seizure-disorders/drug-treatment-of-seizures?query=%E2%80%A2Levetiracetam

RELATED DIAGNOSES AND ICD-10 CODES

Partial onset seizure	G40.009
Myoclonic seizures	G40.309
Primary generalized tonic-clonic seizures	G40.4

REFERENCES

Full list of references can be accessed through Springer Publishing Company Connect™ at the following link: http://connect.springerpub.com/content/reference-book/978-0-8261-8843-4/part/part03/toc-part/ch105

106. LIPASE AND AMYLASE

Kelly Small Casler

PHYSIOLOGY REVIEW

Amylase and lipase are both digestive enzymes. The key role of amylase is to break down carbohydrates while the key role of lipase is to break down triglycerides into glycerol and free fatty acids. Amylase can be found in the salivary glands, ovaries, intestines, muscles, and pancreas.[1] Lipase is found in the liver, pancreas, endovascular tissues, and various other locations. Pancreatic lipase is made and stored in the acinar cells of the pancreas.

OVERVIEW OF LABORATORY TESTS

Amylase (CPT code 82150) and lipase (CPT code 83690) are measured using blood serum to evaluate for acute pancreatitis as a cause of abdominal pain. Amylase elevations are noted within 12 to 72 hours after acute pancreatitis onset and lipase elevations are noted after 24 hours of onset. Amylase levels return to baseline in 3 to 5 days whereas lipase levels return over 8 to 14 days.[2] The longer duration of lipase elevations makes this test particularly helpful for evaluation of abdominal pain with long duration.[2] Amylase testing is rarely used in evaluation of abdominal pain since it can be elevated even in cases of normal pancreatic function, such as can be seen in parotitis.[2] Because laboratory tests for lipase use additives to inactivate all but pancreatic lipases, they have replaced amylase as a test of choice due to their specificity for pancreatic dysfunction.

INDICATIONS

Screening
- Neither test is indicated.

Diagnosis and Evaluation
- Amylase is not used due to poor specificity.[3,4]
- Lipase is used for the diagnostic evaluation of abdominal pain, especially epigastric pain, to look for pancreatitis as a cause.[1]
- Lipase levels are used as part of the Atlanta classification for acute pancreatitis diagnosis. The classification requires two of the three findings for a diagnosis: characteristic epigastric pain, lipase 3 times the upper limit of normal (ULN) or higher, and findings characteristic of pancreatitis on computerized tomography scan or magnetic resonance imaging.[5] In some delayed presentations of acute pancreatitis, 3× ULN may not be reached.[5]

Monitoring

- Neither test is indicated.[2]
- Amylase/Lipase may have a limited role when monitoring for pancreatic injury in pediatric blunt trauma,[6] being used most often for this role in resource-limited locations (where access to imaging is unavailable).[7]

INTERPRETATION

- Lipase: 0 to 50 U/L[8]
- Amylase: 5 to 125 U/L[8]
- A lipase result greater than 3 times the ULN diagnoses acute pancreatitis with 79% to 88% sensitivity and 89% to 93 % specificity.[9]
- Besides pancreatitis, differential diagnosis for lipase elevations include pancreatic cancers, trauma to the pancreas, bowel obstructions, renal disease, appendicitis, cholecystitis, diabetes, and mumps.[7,10–12]
- Low lipase and amylase levels may be seen in chronic pancreatitis, but have poor sensitivity when used to identify it.[13,14]
- May need higher cutoff in chronic kidney disease (CKD) and renal disease, appendicitis, cholecystitis, and diabetes since lipase is high in these conditions[12]

FOLLOW-UP

- Complete blood count, complete metabolic counts, and lactate dehydrogenase may also be used in the evaluation for pancreatitis.[1]
- Acute pancreatitis is most often related to gallstone disease or extensive alcohol use. If neither is present in the patient with pancreatitis diagnosis per lipase, a triglyceride level to evaluate for hypertriglyceridemia as the cause of pancreatitis is warranted. Triglyceride (TG) levels greater than 1,000 mg/dL are diagnostic of hypertriglyceridemia-induced pancreatitis.[12]

PEARLS & PITFALLS

- Severity of disease does not correlate with degree of lipase elevation.[2,12]
- Lipase is less accurate the longer symptoms have been present.[9]
- Do not forget to consider other differentials of lipase elevations, such as bowel perforations.[9]
- Use of amylase in the diagnostic work of abdominal pain is discouraged since lipase has higher sensitivity and specificity.[15–18]
- Amylase as an additional test to lipase offers no added benefit.[2,3,17] This practice wasted 19.4 million Medicare dollars during 2011 to 2014 and can adversely affect patients, subjecting them to unnecessary diagnostic tests or longer NPO status.[3]
- Amylase testing is not recommended by Choosing Wisely[4] and should be removed from the panel of laboratory test options, according to many experts.[3,19,20]

PATIENT EDUCATION

■ https://medlineplus.gov/lab-tests/lipase-tests/

RELATED DIAGNOSES AND ICD-10 CODES

Epigastric pain	R10.13
Epigastric abdominal tenderness	R10.816
Epigastric rebound abdominal tenderness	R10.826
Acute pancreatitis	K85.90
Alcohol dependence	F10.2

REFERENCES

*Full list of references can be accessed through Springer Publishing Company Connect™
at the following link:* http://connect.springerpub.com/content/reference-book/
978-0-8261-8843-4/part/part03/toc-part/ch106

---

107. LIPID PROFILES AND LIPOPROTEIN TESTS

Kelly Small Casler and Matthew Granger

PATHOPHYSIOLOGY REVIEW

Lipid profiles measure the amounts of lipids in the blood and usually focus on two primary lipids: cholesterol and triglycerides (TG). Lipids are packaged together with apoproteins to form a water-soluble lipoprotein, allowing transport of lipids in the bloodstream. Each lipoprotein has a unique makeup of apoproteins on its cell wall to allow binding to various hepatic or cell receptors to allow for energy delivery and lipid transport. Some advanced lipid profiles may also measure these apoprotein amounts in addition to cholesterol and triglycerides. Table 107.1 summarizes the relationships between lipids, apoproteins, and lipoproteins.[1]

TG and cholesterol are absorbed from the diet by the small bowel and are packaged with apoproteins to form the lipoprotein chylomicron. Chylomicrons circulate through the body to deliver TG for energy use in fat and muscles. Lipoprotein lipase (LPL) removes TG from chylomicrons for energy use and the chylomicron remnants go back to the liver for either excretion or synthesis into very low-density lipoproteins (VLDLs). VLDLs contain mostly TG, but also some cholesterol. Like chylomicrons, VLDLs circulate through the body and deliver TG to the body for energy use. Again,

TABLE 107.1: LIPOPROTEIN, APOPROTEIN, AND LIPID RELATIONSHIPS		
LIPOPROTEIN	**PRIMARY APOPROTEINS**	**PRIMARY LIPID**
Chylomicrons	Apoprotein B48 Apolipoprotein C2 Apoprotein E	Triglycerides*
Very Low-Density Lipoproteins (VLDL)*	Apoprotein B-100 Apolipoprotein C2	Triglycerides*
Intermediate-Density Lipoproteins (IDL)	Apoprotein B100	Cholesterol*
Low-Density Lipoprotein (LDL)*	Apoprotein B100	Cholesterol*
High-Density Lipoprotein (HDL)*	Apoprotein A-1	Cholesterol*
Lipoprotein (a)	Apoprotein (a) Apoprotein B100	

*Denotes lipids and lipoproteins reported on a minimal lipid profile.

LPL helps in cleaving off the TG when TG is needed for energy use. After it loses TG, VLDL particles diminish in size to become intermediate-density lipoprotein (IDL), which now contain mostly cholesterol. IDL delivers some of its cholesterol to the body for cellular functions and becomes smaller, turning into low-density lipoprotein (LDL). LDL can either be absorbed by the liver for excretion through hepatic LDL receptors or it can become an initiator of atherosclerotic disease. LDL and remnant cholesterol including IDL and VLDL are known to cause atherosclerotic cardiovascular disease.[2] High-density lipoprotein (HDL) is synthesized by the liver and is responsible for reverse cholesterol transport, picking up excess cholesterol from the body and delivering it back to the liver for excretion. Lipoprotein a [Lp(a)] is a lipoprotein that is very similar in structure to LDL. However, Lp(a) has an extra apoprotein, called apoprotein (a), added to it which changes its physiologic activity to promote thrombosis and inhibit thrombolysis. Lp (a) is 80% to 90% genetically determined and elevated levels have been identified as having a major role in cardiovascular disease.[3]

Normally, the lipoproteins LDL, IDL, and VLDL are able to freely cross the endothelial layer of arteries and are not necessarily pathologic. However, injury and inflammation in the arterial walls can result in oxidative modification of the lipoproteins, causing them to become entangled in the vascular wall, rather than freely returning to the bloodstream. The oxidative modification cascade ultimately results in the development of an atherosclerotic plaque.[4]

OVERVIEW OF LABORATORY TESTS

A minimal lipid profile reports total cholesterol (CPT code 82465) and TG (CPT code 84478), only. A standard lipid profile (CPT code 80061) reports total

---

Box 107.1: Friedwald Equation

Total cholesterol − HDL − (TG/5)

---

cholesterol and TG as well, but also subdivides by and reports the cholesterol present in three of the lipoproteins: VLDL, LDL, and HDL. It is important to note, that the standard lipid profile measures the amount of cholesterol within the lipoproteins and not the actual number of VLDL, HDL, and LDL lipoproteins. When reporting TG and cholesterol, laboratories directly measure TG, total cholesterol, and the amount of cholesterol in HDL. Cholesterol levels associated with LDL may also be directly measured but are also often estimated through a calculation like the Friedewald Equation (Box 107.1) or the Martin/Hopkins method. LDL cholesterol should always be directly measured when TGs are greater than 400 mg/dL; laboratory protocol usually dictates direct measurements of LDL in these instances. Both the standard lipid profile and minimal lipid profile can be performed as CLIA waved point-of-care tests in addition to the traditional laboratory method. Both methods have similar accuracy.[5]

An advanced lipid profile includes the previously noted parameters with the addition of other measurements depending on the laboratory providing the test. These measurements in an advanced lipid profile can also be ordered as individual laboratory tests. Particle number (CPT code 83704), apoprotein B (CPT code 82712), and Lp(a) (CPT code 83695) are the most common measurements used with an advanced lipid profile. Particle number is ordered to determine if there is an excess number of smaller LDLs that are packed tightly with cholesterol, since, in a standard lipid profile, LDL cholesterol is measured, but not every LDL particle carries the same amount of cholesterol. The smaller, denser LDL are concerning, since they are more atherogenic (Figure 107.1) Apoprotein B testing provides similar information to particle number since there is only one apoprotein B per each LDL particle. However, apoprotein B is also present on the other atherogenic lipoproteins like IDL and VLDL. Thus, measuring apoprotein B can provide an overview of the number of all atherogenic lipoprotein particles in circulation, not just LDL. Finally, Lp (a) can be evaluated in patients with normal VLDL, cholesterol, TG, and HDL since some patients may still have a high cardiovascular risk related to an excessive amount of Lp(a). There are limited indications for use of each of the advanced lipid profile tests, which are discussed under indications.[6,7]

INDICATIONS

Screening

- For children, universal screening for hyperlipidemia/dyslipidemia with a standard lipid profile is recommended once between the ages of 9 and 11 years and again between the ages of 17 and 21, by the American Academy of Pediatrics.[8] The United States Preventive Services Task Force has found insufficient evidence to either support or refute this recommendation.[9]

Patient 1	Patient 2
Total LDL cholesterol (Total LDL-c) = 135 mg/dL Packed densely in many, small LDL particles	Total LDL cholesterol (Total LDL-c) = 135 mg/dL Packed loosely in fewer, larger LDL particles

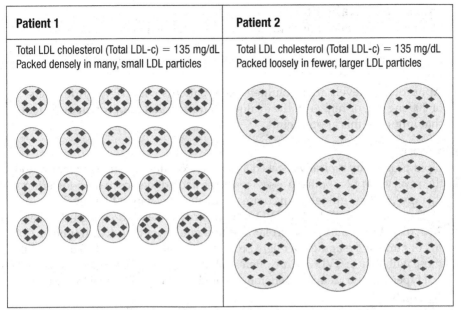

FIGURE 107.1. Depiction of two patients with total LDL cholesterol of 135 mg/dL on standard lipid profile. One with densely packed versus one with lightly packed LDL. Due to their size, the smaller LDL are able to enter the lining of the blood vessels and cause atherosclerosis. The gray circles represent LDL and the diamonds represent cholesterol. LDL, low-density lipoprotein; LDL-c, low-denisty lipoprotein cholesterol.

- For adults, universal screening for hyperlipidemia/dyslipidemia with a standard lipid profile is recommended to be conducted every 5 years, starting at age 20.[10]
- For adults, a one-time universal screening for elevated Lp(a) levels is recommended, especially if there is premature atherosclerotic cardiovascular disease (ASCVD) (occurrence at 55 years of age or younger in males and 65 years of age or younger in females) in a family member. One-time targeted screening is also recommended for patients with personal history of early ASCVD or disease progression despite moderate intensity statin therapy.[6,11,12]
- Particle size or apoprotein B levels may be used for targeted screening in individuals with ASCVD or other high-risk factors.[13]
- For adults, targeted screening for hyperlipidemia/dyslipidemia with a standard lipid profile is recommended for patients with hypertension, diabetes, cigarette smoking, or family history of premature ASCVD. Generally, rescreening is completed yearly if values are normal.[11]
- For children, targeted screening for hyperlipidemia/dyslipidemia is conducted as early as ages 1 to 4 years old, if there is family history of premature ASCVD. Other indications for screening children include a history of hypertension, chronic kidney disease, smoking, Kawasaki disease history, obesity, and chronic inflammatory disease.[14]

Diagnosis and Evaluation

■ Standard or advanced lipid profiles are used for diagnostic purposes when patients have signs or symptoms of lipid disorders (arcus senilus, xanthelasma, or xanthomas) and have not previously had assessment of lipid levels.

■ Apoprotein B levels are recommended in patients with triglyceride levels of 200 mg/dL or higher in the evaluation for familial lipoprotein disorders that influence this apoprotein.

Monitoring

■ Lipid profiles are typically checked 4 to 12 weeks after initiation of therapy and then every 3 to 12 months to assess response and adherence to lipid-lowering therapy.[11,15] Some guidelines recommend treating to a target LDL level.[15]
  ● Those with established ASCVD, a 10-year risk of heart disease greater than 20%, diabetes mellitus, glomerular filtration rate lower than 45 mL/min/1.73 m^2, or familial dyslipidemia might be treated to a goal LDL-C of 55 to 70, while those with less ASCVD risk are often treated to a goal of 100 mg/dL or less.[15]
  ● Hypertriglyceridemia is generally treated to a target TG level lower than 150 mg/dL.

■ Some guidelines do not recommend treating to a target lipid level, and instead patients are observed for the expected amount of improvement in lipid levels.[11] Expected improvement responses by pharmacotherapy are listed in the text that follows[11,15,16]:
  ● Moderate-intensity statins should be expected to lower LDL by 29% to 52% and high-intensity statins should lower levels by 50% or more.
  ● Cholesterol absorption inhibitors used as add-on therapy to statins lower LDL levels by another 12% to 17%.
  ● Proprotein convertase subtilisin/kexin type 9 (PCSK9) inhibitors lower LDL levels by 48% to 71%.
  ● Bile acid sequestrants lower LDL levels by 8% to 16%.

INTERPRETATION

■ Normal and abnormal lipid profile results are summarized in Tables 107.2 and 107.3. Lipid profile results are almost always interpreted in context with patient risk factors using the evidence-based equations described in the text that follows.
  ● The pooled cohort equations used with lipid panel results to calculate ASCVD risk scores were validated in non-Hispanic White and Black patients and have limited evidence to support estimating risk in other ethnic/race groups.[13,17] The pooled cohort equation calculator for 10-year ASCVD risk is available at https://tools.acc.org/ascvd-risk-estimator-plus/#!/calculate/estimate/
  ● The MESA (Multi-Ethnic Study of Atherosclerosis) equation utilizes patient history and lipid panel results along with coronary artery calcium scoring to calculate ASCVD risk and may provide more accurate risk stratification in Hispanic and Chinese-Americans.[18] The MESA calculator is available at https://www.mesa-nhlbi.org/MESACHDRisk/MesaRiskScore/RiskScore.aspx

TABLE 107.2: INTERPRETATION OF LIPID PROFILES

COMPONENT	NORMAL/DESIRABLE	ABNORMAL
Lipoprotein a	<50 mg/dL	≥50 mg/dL
Apoprotein B	<130 mg/dL	≥130 mg/dL (the risk of this level is similar to a LDL of ≥160 mg/dL)
HDL	≥40 mg/dL for females ≥50 mg/dL males	
Non-HDL cholesterol (total cholesterol minus HDL)	<130 mg/dL	≥220 mg/dL*
LDL	<130 mg/dL	≥130 mg/dL
Fasting triglyceride	<150 mg/dL	>200 mg/dL*

Note: Interpretation varies based on past medical history and whether pharmacotherapy is already initiated for dyslipidemia.

*If value is checked non-fasting, recheck a fasting level in 2 to 4 weeks.

HDL, high-density lipoprotein; LDL, low-density lipoprotein.

TABLE 107.3: INTERPRETATION OF LIPID PROFILES IN CHILDREN*

CATEGORY	ACCEPTABLE	BORDERLINE	HIGH+
TC	<170 mg/dL	170–199 mg/dL	≥200 mg/dL
LDL-C	<110 mg/dL	110–129 mg/dL	≥130 mg/dL
Non-HDL-C	<120 mg/dL	120–144 mg/dL	≥145 mg/dL
ApoB	<90 mg/dL	90–109 mg/dL	≥110 mg/dL
TG 0–9 years 10–19 years	<75 mg/dL <90 mg/dL	75–99 mg/dL 90–129 mg/dL	≥100 mg/dL ≥130 mg/dL
HDL-C	>45 mg/dL	40–45 mg/dL	<40 mg/dL
ApoA-1	>120 mg/dL	115–120 mg/dL	<115 mg/dL

Note: Values given are in mg/dL. Top convert to SI units, divide the results for total cholesterol (TC), low-density lipoprotein cholesterol (LDL-C), high-density lipoprotein cholesterol (HDL-C), and non-HDL-C by 38.6; for triglycerides (TG), divide by 88.6.

*Values for plasma lipid and lipoprotein levels are from the National Cholesterol Education Program (NCEP) Expert Panel on Cholesterol Levels in Children. Non-HDL-C values from the Bogalusa Heart Study are equivalent to the NCEP Pediatric Panel cutpoints for LDL-C. Values for plasma ApoB and ApoA-1 are from the National Health and Nutrition Examination Survey III.

+The cutpoints for high and borderline high represent approximately the 95th and 75th percentiles, respectively. Low cutpoints for HDL-C and ApoA-1 represent approximately the 10th percentile.

Source: National Heart Lung and Blood Institute. *Expert Panel on Integrated Guidelines for Cardiovascular Health and Risk Reduction in Children and Adolescents Summary Report.* National Heart Lung and Blood Institute; 2012. https://www.nhlbi.nih.gov/files/docs/peds_guidelines_sum.pdf

FOLLOW-UP

- Evaluate for hyperlipidemic pancreatitis in those with TG greater than 500 mg/dL.
- Evaluate for metabolic syndrome in those with TG levels greater than 150 mg/dL and HDL lower than 40 mg/dL for men or lower than 50 mg/dL in women.
- Evaluate for familial (genetic) lipoprotein disorders in those with:[19,20]
  - LDL of 160 to 190 mg/dL or higher
  - A 1-to-1 TG-to-total cholesterol ratio
  - A fasting TG and cholesterol of both 300 mg/dL or higher (suggests dysbetalipoproteinemia)
  - A fasting, non-HDL level of 220 mg/dL or higher
  - A fasting TG greater than 500 to 1,000 mg/dL
  - LDL-to-apoB ratio of less than 1.2 (normal value greater than 1.4).
  - ApoB concentration is greater than 120 mg/dL

PEARLS & PITFALLS

- Since 2016, global guidelines have endorsed non-fasting lipid profile testing due to cost and time savings and increased safety due to decreased hypoglycemia risks.[21-24] When non-fasting and fasting levels of lipid profile results were compared, they did not vary in a statistically significant way. Compared to fasting testing, TG in the non-fasting state increased by 26 mg/dL, LDL decreased by 8 mg/dL, total cholesterol decreased by 8 mg/dL, and non-HDL decreased by 8 mg/dL. Some studies have also shown better correlation to CV events with non-fasting lipid profiles.[22,25]
- Lp (a) and apoprotein levels are not significantly different in fasting versus non-fasting states.[21]
- Indications for performing fasting lipid profiles are:[22-24,26]
  - Family history of genetic hyperlipidemia or premature ASCVD.
  - Non-fasting TG greater than 200 mg or non-HDL cholesterol greater than 220 mg/dL should be repeated fasting.
- Most lipid profile abnormalities are due to secondary causes: poor nutrition, obesity, lack of exercise, hypothyroidism, diabetes mellitus, or medication side effects (steroids).[1]
- Hypothyroidism can cause abnormal lipid profiles. Generally, hypothyroidism should be controlled prior to interpretation of lipid profile results, unless hyperlipidemia or dyslipidemia has been previously diagnosed.
- Persistently elevated ApoB levels greater than 130 mg/dL are considered a risk-enhancing factor for ASCVD.
- An elevated TG should be repeated before interpreting it as a persistent elevation.
- Advanced lipid testing with lipoprotein subfractions, apoprotein levels, or phenotyping are not cost effective and not considered clinically useful.
- Lp(a) levels vary little over the lifetime of an individual, so it is recommended to only perform this test once in a lifetime.[6]

■ Elevated levels of lipids are termed "hyperlipidemia." When a term is needed to encompass abnormally low HDL levels, "dyslipidemia" can be used.

PATIENT EDUCATION

■ https://www.lipid.org/sites/default/files/advanced-lipid-testing-tear
-sheet_0.pdf

RELATED DIAGNOSES AND ICD-10 CODES

Hyperlipidemia, unspecified (Dyslipidemia)	E78.5
Elevated lipoprotein(a)	E78.41
Other hyperlipidemia	E78.49
Mixed hyperlipidemia	E78.2
Pure hyperglyceridemia (Hypertriglyceridemia)	E78.1
Familial hypercholesterolemia	E78.01
Metabolic syndrome	E88.81
Encounter for screening of lipid disorder	Z13. 220
Family history of other endocrine, nutritional, and metabolic diseases	Z83.49
Family history of ischemic heart disease and other diseases of the circulatory system	Z82.49

REFERENCES

Full list of references can be accessed through Springer Publishing Company Connect™ *at the following link:* http://connect.springerpub.com/content/reference-book/ 978-0-8261-8843-4/part/part03/toc-part/ch107

108. LITHIUM

Shannon L. Linder

PHYSIOLOGY REVIEW

Lithium (Li) is a type of salt known as an alkali metal on the periodic table in the group IA. It is a monovalent ion where the mechanism of action in psycho-pharmacology is unknown. The IA group of periodic elements also includes sodium, potassium, rubidium, cesium, and francium.[1] Li has been used to treat bipolar disorder for more than 50 years.[2] Originally, it was not used for a period of time due to its high toxicity. It was officially approved by the Food and Drug Administration (FDA) in 1970 for the treatment of mania, and then in 1974 for the treatment of maintenance therapy for a history of mania.[1] Li was the first and only treatment approved by the FDA for both acute and maintenance treatment for several years. Unfortunately, concerns about the toxicity of Li limit its use in the United States. Better understanding of monitoring Li levels, side effects, and signs of toxicity will improve utilization.

In addition to FDA treatment of manic episodes associated with bipolar disorder and maintenance treatment for patients with manic depression with a history of mania, Li has off-label indications for use in bipolar depression, adjunctive treatment for major depressive disorder, vascular headache, and neutropenia.[3] Several studies have also shown that Li treatment may decrease self-harm behaviors, suicidal ideations, and suicide in bipolar disorder I and II, and also unipolar major depressive disorder.[3,4] Li may also be used in psychiatry for patients with specific symptoms of episodic and recurrent rage, anger, violence, and self-destructive behaviors.[3] Remission of symptoms is the goal of treatment; thus, treatment can be indefinite. Regular monitoring of Li levels is therefore essential when patients are on Li pharmacotherapy, in addition to monitoring of kidney function tests, thyroid function tests, electrocardiogram (specifically for patients over 50), and metabolic monitoring during treatment.[3]

Li pharmacologic actions include rapid and full absorption after ingestion of the medication. However, for antimanic effects, Li onset of action is typically 1 to 3 weeks. Li is not protein bound, is not metabolized, and is excreted through the kidneys.[1] Renal insufficiency will decrease clearance of Li. It is also important to note that the blood-brain barrier of Li only permits a slow passage at a time; therefore, overdose toxicity is less likely to happen from a single dose and indicates why long-term Li toxicity is slow to resolve. Li concentrations are higher in thyroid and renal tests than serum levels.

OVERVIEW OF LABORATORY TESTS

Laboratory evaluation of Li status can be assessed by Li serum level (CPT code 80178). Li levels should be ordered as a trough, meaning 12 hours post-dose of medication. For example, if a patient takes their last dose of Li in the evening around 8 p.m., they should skip their a.m. Li dosage if they take one and have the laboratory level drawn at 8 a.m.

INDICATIONS

Screening
Universal and targeted screenings are not indicated.

Diagnosis and Evaluation
- Evaluate Li levels for routine monitoring of Li therapy.
- Evaluate Li levels if failure to respond to treatment occurs.
- Evaluate Li levels if side effects are present.

▪ Evaluate Li levels for signs of toxicity. Mild toxicity includes nausea, vomiting, diarrhea, worsening of tremor, and dry mouth.[1,5,6] As toxicity worsens into the moderate intoxication level, persistent gastrointestinal side effects are noted, along with onset and worsening of neurologic effects such as blurred vision, muscle fasciculations, hyperactive deep tendon reflexes, delirium, ataxia, dizziness, dysarthria, nystagmus, lethargy, or excitement and muscle weakness.[1]

▪ See Table 108.1 for a complete list of Li side effects and signs of toxicity.

Monitoring

▪ Li serum concentration levels are monitored for patients receiving Li medication pharmacotherapy to ensure Li levels are in the therapeutic dosage range.[6]

▪ Prior to starting Li, patients should have the following laboratory tests: serum creatinine concentration, 24-hour urine creatinine if any suspicion for impaired renal function, blood urea nitrogen (BUN), electrolyte panel, thyroid function starting with thyroid-stimulating hormone (TSH), urinalysis, complete blood count (CBC), electrocardiogram (ECG), fasting lipid profile, and a human chorionic gonadotropin (HCG) in childbearing individuals.[1,5]

TABLE 108.1: SIDE EFFECTS AND SIGNS OF TOXICITY WITH LITHIUM USE	
DOSE-RELATED SIDE EFFECTS	**SERIOUS SIDE EFFECTS/SIGNS OF TOXICITY**
Polyuria	Renal impairment (interstitial nephritis or nephrogenic diabetes insipidus) due to decreased concentrating capacity because of reduced renal response to antidiuretic hormone (ADH) arrhythmia
Polydipsia	
Nausea	
Diarrhea	Cardiovascular changes
Weight gain (may or may not be associated with increased appetite)	Sick sinus syndrome
	Bradycardia
Cognitive side effects	Hypotension
Ataxia	T wave flattening and inversion on EKG
Sedation	Lithium toxicity
Dysarthria	Pseudotumor cerebri
Tremor	Seizures
Hair loss	
Acne	
Edema	
Elevated thyroid-stimulating hormone (TSH) and reduced thyroxine level	
Benign leukocytosis	

Sources: Data from Hirschfeld RMA, Bowden CL, Gitlin MJ, et al. *Work Group on Bipolar Disorder.* 2010:82; Stahl SM, Grady MM. *Stahl's Essential Psychopharmacology: Prescriber's Guide.* 6th ed. Cambridge University Press; 2017.

- Due to potential weight gain from Li, metabolic screening should also be completed prior to initiating Li treatment and at regular intervals throughout treatment: weight, height, body mass index (BMI), waist circumference, blood pressure, fasting glucose, and fasting lipid profile.[5]
- Renal function should be monitored in patients treated with Li. Elevations in BUN are seen with impaired clearance of Li. Creatinine is a less sensitive measure of renal function but can indicate extensive renal impairment. Cr clearance is also monitored in patients taking Li; during this, urine is collected for 24 hours with a serum Cr level obtained at the midpoint of the 24-hour collection period.[1] Renal function including BUN, creatinine, and estimated glomerular filtration rate (eGFR) should be tested every 2 to 3 months during the first 6 months, then every 6 to 12 months subsequently or when clinically indicated.[3,5,7,8] Long-term morphologic kidney changes occur in 10% to 20% of patients on Li.[7]
- TSH should be tested every 2 to 3 months for the first 6 months, and then every 6 to 12 months subsequently or when clinically indicated.[5,7,8] Hypothyroidism is caused by Li treatment in 5% to 35% of cases.
- The National Institute for Health and Care Excellence (NICE) also recommends calcium levels being routinely monitored prior to initiation of Li and then tested every 6 months routinely for long term Li treatment.[8]
- Evaluate Li levels 5 to 7 days after starting Li. This is referred to as steady-state Li dosing which is typically after 5 days of constant dosing.[1] The level is monitored 5 to 7 days after a dosage change. In older adult patients or those patients with impaired renal function, it may take longer to achieve steady state; therefore, assessing at 10 to 12 days is more appropriate.[9]
- When continuing Li after the first therapeutic level is achieved, recheck in 1 month, then every 2 to 3 months for maintenance for the first 6 months, and then every 3 to 6 months indefinitely.[9] If a patient is experiencing a physical illness or changes in other medications, more frequent monitoring is required.[4]

INTERPRETATION

- There can be slight variations of normal levels; however, due to the narrow therapeutic level of lithium, these variations are negligible. Table 108.2 summarizes current interpretation guidelines. The overall consensus of the Li therapeutic range is 0.6 to 0.8 mEq/L.[9]
- It is imperative with Li levels to monitor trends. For example, if a patient is trending toward a toxic level, lowering the dosage must be considered.
- There are several guidelines with varying follow-up recommendations for monitoring of Li serum blood level. The consensus is as follows: it is recommended that Li levels are monitored within 5 days to 1 week of initiation, with a change in dosage and until levels are stable.[3,7,8] Routine monitoring should then occur every 2 to 3 months during the first 6 to 12 months of treatment, and then every 6 months for subsequent years.[3,5,8]
- NICE recommends indefinite 3-month testing for special populations including older adults; patients on medications with drug interactions with Li or change in medications; patients with risk of renal, thyroid, or elevated

TABLE 108.2: INTERPRETATION OF LITHIUM DRUG LEVEL				
REFERENCE	**NORMAL**	**SUB-THERAPEUTIC**	**HIGH**	**TOXIC**
Nolen[9]	0.6–0.8 mEq/L for maintenance once stabilized	0.4–0.6 mEq/L if good response or poor tolerance to higher dosages		
Sadock, Sadock, & Ruiz[1]	0.6–1.2 mEq/L	<0.6 mEq/L	1.3 mEq/L	Mild to moderate 1.5–2.0 mEq/L Moderate to severe 2.0–2.5 mEq/L Severe >2.5 mEq/L
Jacobson[5]	Adult 0.6–1.2 mEq/L		>1.5 mEq/L	
Stahl[3]	Acute mania: 1.0–1.5 mEq/L Depression: 0.6–1.0 mEq/L Maintenance once stabilized: 0.7–1.0 mEq/L			

calcium levels; patients with poor symptom control; patients with risk of poor compliance; and patients whose Li level was 0.8 mE/L or greater at the previous testing.[8]

- Clinical toxicity can occur with certain populations even in the documented therapeutic range; for example, with older adults.[1] Older adult patients may have signs or symptoms of toxicity at levels less than 1.2 mEq/L. Therefore, lower dosages of Li are typically used in older adult population. The therapeutic range for the older adult population is usually 0.4 to 1.0 mEq/L.[6] More recent guidelines on the older adult populations recommend maintenance levels of 0.4 to 0.6 mEq/L with a maximum of 0.7 to 0.8 mEq/L in ages 65 to 79, and if over 80 years of age a maximum level of 0.7 mEq/L.[9]
- Serum concentrations shown to be effective for mania associated with bipolar disorder are 1.0 to 1.5 mEq/L. The maintenance range is usually 0.4 to 0.8 mEq/L.[1,9] Despite these recommendations, it is imperative to treat the patient, not the laboratory value.
- The range of 0.8 to 1.0 mEq/L increases risk of harm to the patient despite increased effectiveness in some patients; therefore, a target range of 0.6 to 0.8 mEq/L is advised.[4] If a patient has good tolerance, but not an optimal response, consideration to increase to 0.8 to 1.0 mEq/L is warranted.[9]
- Critical Li levels are at 1.5 mEq/L or higher. Severe Li intoxication occurs when the level is 2.5 to 3.0 mEq/L or higher.
- Increased levels of Li on interpretation are consistent with overdose, acute renal insufficiency or failure, sodium restriction, co-administration of angiotension-converting enzyme (ACE) inhibitors, thiazide diuretics, nonsteroidal anti-inflammatory medications, or fluoxetine.[5]

■ Decreased levels of Li on interpretation could include co-administration of sodium chloride, sodium bicarbonate, psyllium, fleawort or fleabane (herbal supplements), acetazolamide, aminophylline, or theophylline.[5]

FOLLOW-UP

■ Li serum blood level should be tested in patients who become physically ill.[4]
■ As previously noted, the following laboratory tests should be routinely monitored throughout Li treatment: serum creatinine concentration, 24-hour urine creatinine if any suspicion for impaired renal function, BUN, electrolyte panel, thyroid function starting with TSH, urinalysis, CBC, ECG, fasting lipid profile, and an HCG in childbearing individuals.[1,5]

PEARLS & PITFALLS

■ Li has a very narrow therapeutic index; therefore, clinicians must be familiar with the recommended serum laboratory monitoring schedule and adhere to guidelines. Clinicians should be forthcoming with patients prior to initiating Li pharmacotherapy regarding the absolute necessity of frequent serum blood monitoring.
■ Many medications and other factors may change serum concentrations from well tolerated and therapeutic to developing side effects and toxicity.
■ There were not any studies found suggesting cultural or ethnic variances should change treatment or monitoring of Li.[9]
■ Li toxicity occurs in three forms: acute, chronic, or acute-on-chronic.[5] However, the correlation of Li level and signs and symptoms of acute toxicity is not always accurate. Gastrointestinal side effects predominate with acute toxicity. With chronic toxicity, the correlation of Li level is more accurate and predominates with central nervous symptoms, as well as renal, cardiac, and thyroid effects.[5]
■ Patient education is critical with Li and includes signs and symptoms of toxicity, common side effects, factors that affect Li levels, medication interactions, and how and when to obtain Li laboratory tests.
■ Li inhibits antidiuretic hormone secretion, thereby increasing water loss.[6]
■ Drug–drug interactions, in particular nonsteroidal anti-inflammatory drugs (NSAIDs), ACE inhibitors, diuretics (thiazide diuretics most common), and metronidazole may lead to lithium toxicity due to decreased renal clearance and increased lithium concentration.[1] Other medications that can lead to lithium toxicity include methyldopa, carbamazepine, phenytoin, and calcium channel blockers.[3]
■ Li in combination pharmacotherapy with selective serotonin re-uptake inhibitors (SSRIs) can increase risk of side effects and serotonin syndrome: dizziness, confusion, diarrhea, agitation, and tremor.[3]
■ Fluid changes, particularly with dehydration, require the dosage to be lowered if patients develop signs of infection, sodium restriction, or excessive sweating or diarrhea.[3]

■ Death from overdose has occurred. Signs and symptoms of overdose may include tremor dysarthria, delirium, coma, seizures, and autonomic instability.[3]

■ Li is contraindicated for the following reasons: severe kidney disease, severe cardiovascular disease, severe dehydration, sodium depletion, allergy to Li, and in patients with Burgada syndrome.[3] Burgada syndrome is an inherited condition associated with sudden cardiac death typically by ventricular fibrillation in a normally structured heart.[10] Although very rare, Li can unmask this syndrome.[3,10] If a patient has unexplained syncope or palpitations following initiation of Li treatment, consultation with a cardiologist is recommended.[3]

■ Li side effects are common, affecting up to 75% of patients on Li pharmacotherapy.[7] Recommendations to try to avoid side effects are decreasing dosage, changing timing of dosing schedule, or changing to sustained release formulations.

■ Other factors that may cause alterations in Li levels include sodium intake, mood fluctuations, activity level, body position, and if an alternate tube was used during laboratory collection.[1] If an improper tube was used during collection, for example with a lithium–heparin anticoagulant, results can be falsely elevated by as much as 1 mEq/L.[1] It is important to monitor clinical status in these cases and order a repeat level.

PATIENT EDUCATION

■ https://nami.org/About-Mental-Illness/Treatments/Mental-Health
-Medications/Types-of-Medication/Lithium#:~:text=Lithium%20is%20a%20
mood%20stabilizer%20medication%20that%20works,Bipolar%20disorder%20
involves%20episodes%20of%20depression%20and%2For%20mania.

RELATED DIAGNOSES AND ICD-10 CODES

Bipolar and other bipolar spectrum	F31	Electroconvulsive therapy (ECT)	GZB1ZZZ
Depression and other depressive disorders	F32, F33	Suicidal ideation	R45.851
Cyclothymia	F34.0	Monitoring for therapeutic medication levels	Z51.81

REFERENCES

Full list of references can be accessed through Springer Publishing Company Connect™ at the following link: http://connect.springerpub.com/content/reference-book/978-0-8261
-8843-4/part/part03/toc-part/ch108

109. LIVER ENZYMES/TRANSAMINASES

Pam Kibbe and Kelly Small Casler

PHYSIOLOGY REVIEW

Transaminases are enzymes that catalyze reactions between acids in the body. Alanine transaminase (ALT) and aspartate transaminase (AST) are hepatocyte transaminases that are important in protein metabolism and gluconeogenesis in the liver. Although ALT/AST are referred to as liver enzymes, they are also found in other parts of the body including the heart, skeletal muscle, and kidneys. ALT is found in highest concentrations in the liver and is, therefore, more specific to liver injury than AST. Alkaline phosphatase (ALP) is another liver transaminase. It is found on the surface of the bile duct epithelia but also in the bone, kidneys, and intestines.[1]

ALT and AST are released in excess amounts in the setting of hepatocellular injury or inflammation. Many events can cause injury and inflammation, such as chronic alcohol use, metabolic syndrome, medications, and autoimmune disease. Persistent inflammation may eventually progress to fibrosis, which can progress in severity (from moderate to severe) if inflammation persists. Cirrhosis is fibrosis at its severest stage.

Hepatic ALP is synthesized and released in excess with conditions that block the flow of bile and/or cause accumulation of bile salts. Elevations of ALP can also be seen in skeletal conditions or episodes of rapid growth.

OVERVIEW OF LABORATORY TESTS

ALT (CPT code 84460), AST (CPT code 84450), and ALP (CPT code 84080) are typically ordered and reported as part of a liver profile test (CPT code 80076; will also include protein, albumin, and bilirubin) and serve to provide an overview of the health of the liver. Although sometimes referred to as "liver function tests," this term is misleading and should not be used since these transaminases do not reflect true liver function. These tests are better termed liver enzymes or liver transaminases. These tests do reflect hepatocellular injury/inflammation or cholestasis as they are released during these events. ALP is released predominantly in cholestasis while AST/ALT are released during hepatocellular injury. If reflection of true liver function is desired, tests such as albumin, International Normalized Ratio (INR), and platelets can be assessed. In difficult to interpret cases, ALP can be further evaluated through isoenzyme electrophoresis, which reports the amount of ALP from bone, intestinal, and hepatic sources, in addition to the total level.[2]

INDICATIONS

Screening

- ALT, ALP, and AST are not used to screen for adult nonalcoholic fatty liver disease(NAFLD) in the United States or the United Kingdom, but are used to screen for NAFLD in parts of Europe.[3,4]
- In the United States pediatric population, ALT is used as a screening tool for NAFLD.[5] Screening should be considered in children age 9 to 11 years of age with a body mass index (BMI) greater than the 95th percentile, and in children with a BMI greater than the 85th to 94th percentile who have additional risk factors including central adiposity, insulin resistance, prediabetes or diabetes, hyperlipidemia, sleep apnea, or family history of NAFLD or nonalcoholic steatohepatitis (NASH).[5]

Diagnosis and Evaluation

- ALT, AST, and ALP are used to evaluate for suspected liver dysfunction or cholestasis based on signs and symptoms of abdominal pain (right upper quadrant), jaundice, nausea and vomiting, fatigue, splenomegaly, hemolytic anemia, easy bleeding or bruising, low platelet count, or elevated INR. Liver transaminases are not specific or sensitive for any disease, including cirrhosis.[6] In fact, patients can have normal liver enzymes despite significant disease.[7] This occurred in up to 20% of cirrhosis patients in one study.[8]

Monitoring

- Older guidelines had recommended baseline AST, ALT, and ALP prior to initiating pharmacotherapy with statins;[9] however, newer guidelines and the evidence do not support this practice.[10–12] Additionally, routine monitoring with ongoing statin pharmacotherapy is not needed.[11]
- Low levels of evidence support monitoring ALT, AST, and ALP every 6 weeks for 6 months when potentially hepatotoxic medications are initiated.[13]

INTERPRETATION

Reference Intervals/Limits

- ALT: lower than 33 U/L in adult males and lower than 26 U/L for pediatric males; lower than 25 U/L in adult females and lower than 22 U/L for pediatric females[5,6]
- AST: 10 to 40 IU/L in patients older than 1 year of age and 30 to 80 U/L in those 1 year or younger.[14,15]
- ALP: 30 to 115 IU/L in adults and 30 to 300 IU/L in pediatrics[14,15]

Interpretation of Increased/Decreased Results

- Decreased ALT levels may indicate pyridoxine deficiency and poor nutritional intake.[16]
- Interpretation must always consider the history and physical and other laboratory parameters. A good first step is to assess medications and herbal or alternative supplements to see if drug-induced liver injury (DILI) is possible (Box 109.1).[6]

Box 109.1: Drugs That Can Cause Drug-Induced Liver Injury

- Allopurinol
- Amiodorone
- Amoxicillin-clavulanate
- Azathioprine
- Green tea extract
- Interferon
- Isonizaide
- Lamotrigine, carbamezapine, phenytoin
- Macrolides
- Methotrexate
- Nitrofurantoin
- Non-steroidal anti-inflammatory drugs
- Sulfasalazine
- Trimethoprim/sulfamethoxazole
- Valproate

Source: Data from Chalasani NP, Hayashi PH, Bonkovsky HL, Navarro VJ, Lee WM, Fontana RJ. ACG Clinical guideline: the diagnosis and management of idiosyncratic drug-induced liver injury. *Am J Gastroenterol.* 2014;109(7):950–966. doi:10.1038/ajg.2014.131.

- There are several approaches to interpreting elevations in ALT/AST. The first option is categorizing elevations based on how high above the upper limit of normal (ULN) they are: borderline (lower than 2× ULN), mild (2 to 5× ULN), moderate (5 to 15× ULN), and severe (greater than 15× ULN).[6] Differential diagnoses based on the extent of elevation are reviewed in Table 109.1.
- A second interpretation approach to elevated liver transaminases is to categorize the possible causes as either acute or chronic elevations and as suspected intrahepatic or extrahepatic causes (an accurate history and physical examination will help determine this). Table 109.2[15-17] summarizes interpretation based on these categorizations.
- Ideally, interpretation of liver transaminase elevations should be completed using all laboratory and clinical history/physical examination data.[18,19] Table 109.3[20-27] summarizes tools available to the clinician to assist with liver transaminase interpretation in this fashion.
- When ALT levels are greater than AST levels, this usually signals a problem within the liver whereas AST levels greater than ALT levels may signal alcohol overuse (Table 109.4).[6,28]
- Elevations of ALP often indicate cholestatic liver disease.[29] Differential diagnoses for ALP elevations are found in Table 109.5. Nonhepatic causes for ALP elevation should also be considered and include rapid bone turnover due to pediatric growth, placental synthesis in pregnancy, and consumption of a high fat meal.[2,29-31] Nonhepatic-related causes of elevated ALP can also be seen with rheumatoid arthritis, cardiac surgery, diabetes, pregnancy, multiple sclerosis, or osteomalacia.
- The meaning of a low level of ALP is unclear and in most instances is irrelevant related to a lack of specificity. Low levels may be seen with zinc deficiency, Wilson's disease, cardiac surgery, hypothyroidism, or pernicious anemia.

TABLE 109.1: DIFFERENTIAL DIAGNOSES FOR ALANINE TRANSAMINASE/ASPARTATE TRANSAMINASE BASED ON THE EXTENT OF ELEVATION

<5× ULN*	5–15× ULN	>15× ULN
Viral hepatitis B & C (HCV-Ab, HBsAg)	All conditions from < 5 ULN column	Ischemic hepatitis
Alcoholic liver disease (AUDIT-C)	Acute presentation of infectious hepatitis, including hepatitis A	Acute acetaminophen toxicity
NAFLD (NFS, assess for metabolic syndrome, RUQ US)		
Hemochromatosis (ferritin, iron panel)		
Wilson's disease (ceruloplasmin)		
Alpha-1-antitrypsin deficiency (Alpha-1-antitrypsin level)		
Autoimmune hepatitis (ANA, AMA, SMA)		
DILI (history, LiverTox)		
Celiac disease (celiac panel)		
Tick borne illness		

* Parenthesis denotes follow-up test, calculation, or consideration for the differential diagnosis, https://www.hepatitisc.uw.edu/page/substance-use/audit-c

AMA, antimitochondrial antibodies; ANA, antinuclear antibodies; AUDIT-C, alcohol use disorders identification test; DILI, drug-induced liver injury; HBsAg, hepatitis B virus surface antigen; HCV-Ab, hepatitis C virus antibodies; NFS, nonalcoholic fatty liver disease score; RUQ US, right upper quadrant ultrasound; SMA, smooth muscle antibody.

TABLE 109.2: DIFFERENTIAL DIAGNOSIS FOR ALANINE TRANSAMINASE/ASPARTATE TRANSAMINASE ELEVATIONS BASED ON ACUTE VERSUS CHRONIC PRESENTATION AND INTRAHEPATIC VERSUS EXTRAHEPATIC CAUSES

CHRONIC INTRAHEPATIC	CHRONIC EXTRAHEPATIC
NAFLD/NASH	Hyperthyroidism or hypothyroidism
Autoimmune hepatitis	Rhabdomyolysis
Alcohol	Hemolysis
Hepatitis	Celiac disease
Prescription medications	
Recreational drugs/toxins, herbal medications, or supplements	
Wilson's disease	
Alpha 1 anti-trypsin deficiency	
Hemochromatosis	

(continued)

TABLE 109.2: DIFFERENTIAL DIAGNOSIS FOR ALANINE TRANSAMINASE/ASPARTATE TRANSAMINASE ELEVATIONS BASED ON ACUTE VERSUS CHRONIC PRESENTATION AND INTRAHEPATIC VERSUS EXTRAHEPATIC CAUSES (*continued*)

ACUTE INTRAHEPATIC	ACUTE EXTRAHEPATIC
Acute viral hepatitis (A, B, or C)	Rhabdomyolysis
Ischemic hepatitis	
Prescription medications	
Recreational drugs/toxins, herbal medications, or supplements	
Autoimmune hepatitis	
Fulminant Wilson's disease	
Acute Budd-Chiari syndrome	
Acute biliary obstruction	

NAFLD, nonalcoholic fatty liver disease; NASH, nonalcoholic steatohepatitis.

Sources: Data from Agrawal S, Dhiman RK, Limdi JK. Evaluation of abnormal liver function tests. *Postgrad Med J.* 2016;92(1086):223–234. doi:10.1136/postgradmedj-2015-133715; Pollock G, Minuk GY. Diagnostic considerations for cholestatic liver disease: causes of cholestasis. *J Gastroenterol Hepatol.* 2017;32(7):1303–1309. doi:10.1111/jgh.13738; Schreiner AD, Rockey DC. Evaluation of abnormal liver tests in the adult asymptomatic patient. *Curr Opin Gastroenterol.* 2018;34(4):272–279. doi:10.1097/MOG.0000000000000447.

TABLE 109.3: RESOURCES TO INTERPRET LIVER TRANSAMINASES

NAME OF RESOURCE	ROLE	PARAMETERS USED TO CALCULATE
Alcoholic liver disease/nonalcoholic fatty liver disease index (ANI)[20]	**Diagnosis**: Differentiate NAFLD and ALD	Gender, BMI, MCV, AST, ALT
Accuracy: An ANI < −0.66 predicts NAFLD with specificity of 96.7% and sensitivity of 84.1%[21] **Link:** https://www.mdapp.co/ald-nafld-index-ani-calculator-355/		
Liver Tox	**Diagnosis:** Provides information on causes for and frequency of DILI. Helps determine if medications are a cause of liver transaminase elevations	Does not involve calculations
Link: https://www.ncbi.nlm.nih.gov/books/NBK547852/		
AST to platelet ratio index (APRI)	**Diagnosis:** Helps predict cirrhosis	AST level and AST ULN, platelet count
Accuracy: APRI >1.0 is 76% sensitive and 72% specific for cirrhosis **Link:** https://www.hepatitisc.uw.edu/page/clinical-calculators/apri		
Fibrosis-4 (FIB-4)	**Diagnosis:** Severe liver disease (i.e. fibrosis/cirrhosis) in HBV	AST, ALT, platelet, age
Accuracy: AUROC is 96% for detection of cirrhosis.[22] **Link:** https://www.hepatitisc.uw.edu/page/clinical-calculators/fib-4		

(*continued*)

TABLE 109.3: RESOURCES TO INTERPRET LIVER TRANSAMINASES (*continued*)

NAME OF RESOURCE	ROLE	PARAMETERS USED TO CALCULATE
Nonalcoholic fatty liver disease fibrosis score (NFS)[23]	**Diagnosis:** Helps predict patients at risk of severe forms of NASH in need of referral	Age, BMI, presence of diabetes/prediabetes, AST, ALT, platelet count, albumin

Accuracy: < –1.455 rules out severe NASH and scores >0.676 predict concern for severe NASH with an AUROC of 85%. Scores in between are indeterminate and require further evaluation.[24,25]

Link: https://www.mdcalc.com/nafld-non-alcoholic-fatty-liver-disease-fibrosis-score

AST/ALT ratio[26]	**Diagnosis:** Differentiate ALD from NAFLD (≥ 2 = ALD <1 = NAFLD)	ALT and AST

Accuracy: if ratio >1, additionally assess MCV; if above 90.0 fL the sensitivity for ALD was 97.3% and specificity 88.9%[27]

Link: https://www.optimaldx.com/calculators/ast-alt-ratio-calculator

R value[6,13]	**Diagnosis:** Helps in interpreting the pattern of liver enzyme elevation. >5 = hepatocellular, <2 = cholestatic, 2–5 = mixed (see Table 109.5)	ALT, ALP

Link: https://www.mdcalc.com/r-factor-liver-injury

ALD, alcoholic liver disease; ALP, alkaline phosphatase; ALT, alanine transaminase; AST, aspartate transaminase; AUROC, area under the receiver operating curve; BMI, body mass index; DILI, drug-induced liver injury; HBV, hepatitis B virus; MCV, mean corpuscular volume; NAFLD, nonalcoholic fatty liver disease; NASH, nonalcoholic steatohepatitis; ULN, upper limit of normal.

TABLE 109.4: DIFFERENTIAL DIAGNOSIS OF ELEVATED LIVER TRANSAMINASES BASED ON HEPATOCELLULAR, MIXED, OR CHOLESTATIC PRESENTATION

HEPATOCELLULAR	MIXED	CHOLESTATIC
HCV	Acute viral hepatitis serologies	US
Autoimmune	Autoimmune	
Acute viral hepatitis	HCV	
US	US	

Note: Determining the "R value" helps to categorize elevations as either hepatocellular, mixed, or cholestatic.

HCV, hepatitis C virus; US, ultrasound.

Sources: Data from Kwo PY, Cohen SM, Lim JK. ACG Clinical guideline: evaluation of abnormal liver chemistries. *Am J Gastroenterol.* 2017;112(1):18–35. doi:10.1038/ajg.2016.517; Panteghini M, Adeli K, Ceriotti F, Sandberg S, Horvath AR. American liver guidelines and cutoffs for "normal" ALT: a potential for overdiagnosis. *Clin Chem.* 2017;63(7):1196–1198. doi:10.1373/clinchem.2017.274977

TABLE 109.5: DIFFERENTIAL DIAGNOSIS OF ELEVATED ALKALINE PHOSPHATASE LEVEL CAUSES BASED ON INTRAHEPATIC VERSUS EXTRAHEPATIC CAUSES

INTRAHEPATIC CAUSES OF BILIARY DUCT DISEASE OR CHOLESTASIS	EXTRAHEPATIC CAUSES OF BILIARY DUCT OBSTRUCTION OR CHOLESTASIS
Primary biliary cholangitis	Choledocholithiasis
Primary sclerosing cholangitis	Malignancy: biliary, pancreatic, or metastatic
Autoimmune cholangitis	Pancreatitis/pancreatic pseudocysts
IgG4 cholangiopathy	Secondary sclerosing cholangitis
Medications-induced cholestasis (android steroids and phenytoin)	Lymphoma
HIV/AIDs cholangiopathy	Smoking
Infection- iduced cholestasis	Exercise
Pregnancy-induced cholestasis	Benign familial hyperphosphatemia
Hepatic carcinoma	
Graft-versus-host disease	
Sickle cell disease	
Sarcoidosis	
Tuberculosis	
Amyloidosis	

Sources: Data from Agrawal S, Dhiman RK, Limdi JK. Evaluation of abnormal liver function tests. *Postgrad Med J.* 2016;92(1086):223–234. doi:10.1136/postgradmedj-2015-133715; Pollock G, Minuk GY. Diagnostic considerations for cholestatic liver disease: causes of cholestasis. *J Gastroenterol Hepatol.* 2017;32(7):1303–1309. doi:10.1111/jgh.13738; Schreiner AD, Rockey DC. Evaluation of abnormal liver tests in the adult asymptomatic patient. *Curr Opin Gastroenterol.* 2018;34(4):272–279. doi:10.1097/MOG.0000000000000447; Siraganian PA. Benign familial hyperphosphatasemia. *JAMA.* 1989;261(9):1310. doi:10.1001/jama.1989.03420090074034

FOLLOW-UP

■ Follow-up testing for elevated liver transaminases should be completed in a focused manner based on the most likely differential diagnoses and a thorough history/clinical examination.[32,33] Table 109.1 and 109.6 summarize some of the most common differential diagnoses and the follow-up.

  ● With borderline or mild elevation of ALT/AST (less than 5× ULN) it is a good idea to start with evaluation for hepatitis B and C virus, ALD, and NAFLD when the elevations appear hepatocellular in nature. Use abdominal ultrasound (to assess liver, bile ducts, and hepatic vasculature) when the pattern of elevation is cholestatic in nature.[16]

  ● If evaluation is normal, consider observation and a recheck of liver enzymes in 3 months. Persistent elevation in ALT greater than 2 times the ULN should warrant re-consideration for NAFLD and other causes of chronic hepatitis.[5]

TABLE 109.6: PATIENT CHARACTERISTICS FOR MOST COMMON RELATED DIFFERENTIAL DIAGNOSES FOR ELEVATED LIVER ENZYMES

PATIENT CHARACTERISTICS	DIFFERENTIAL TO CONSIDER	ACTION/FOLLOW-UP
Patient with autoimmune conditions: Hypothyroidism, Inflammatory bowel disease, systemic lupus erythematosus	**Autoimmune liver/biliary tract disease**	ANA, AMA, SMA, ultrasound to assess biliary system, referral[6]
Patient with signs/symptoms of chronic liver disease: Chronic fatigue, gastrointestinal bleeding, spider angiomas, palmar erythema splenomegaly, jaundice, enlarged left lobe of liver, firm liver edge, history of prolonged elevation in ALT (greater than 2 years)[5,6]	**Chronic liver disease**	Look for other laboratory evidence of chronic liver disease (prolonged INR, thrombocytopenia, leukopenia, elevated bilirubin, decreased albumin) Referral to liver specialist
Patient with excessive alcohol intake: Females who consume more than 140 g per week of alcohol or males who consume more than 210 g per week of alcohol[6] Patients who have a positive AUDIT-C screen*	**Alcoholic liver disease**	AST >ALT; AST/ALT ratio >2 Referral to counseling
Patients with diabetes or metabolic syndrome: Presence of three or more of the following[34]: BP >130/85; HDL-C <40 mg/dL (males) or <50 mg/dL (females), TG >150 mg/DL, waist circumference ≥40 inches (males) or ≥35 inches (females); treatment of hyperglycemia or FPG >100 mg/dL	**Nonalcoholic fatty liver disease**	Calculate NFS, referral if elevated; diet, exercise, weight loss, control of hyperglycemia, RUQ US
Patients with risk factors for infectious hepatitis: International travel, intravenous drug use, or high-risk sexual activity	**Hepatitis A (international travel), B (IV drug use, high-risk sexual activity), or C (IV drug use)**	HAV-Ab, HBsAg, HBAb HCV-Ab

*https://www.hepatitisc.uw.edu/page/substance-use/audit-c

ALT, alanine transaminase; AST, aspartate transaminase; AMA, antimitochondrial antibodies; ANA, antinuclear antibodies; AUDIT, alcohol use disorders identification test; BP, blood pressure; FPG, fasting plasma glucose; HAV-Ab, hepatitis A virus antibodies; HBAb, hepatitis B virus antibodies; HBsAg, hepatitis B virus surface antigen; HCV-Ab, hepatitis C virus antibody; HDL-C, high-density lipoprotein-cholesterol; INR, International Normalized Ratio; IV, intravenous; NFS, nonalcoholic fatty liver fibrosis score; SMA, smooth muscle antibody.

- ALP elevations of four times higher than the ULN likely represent cholestasis and the patient should be referred. If the ALP is less than twice the ULN, other liver function tests are normal, and the patient is asymptomatic, observation/monitoring is recommended.[29]
- Follow-up tests for ALP elevations should first consider if bilirubin and other liver transaminases are elevated (Figures 109.1 and 109.2). Elevation in combination with the elevation in other liver chemistries indicates a hepatobiliary origin (as opposed to bone) as the cause of the ALP elevation. If isolated, consider a gamma glutamyl transferase (GGT) test or a fractionated alkaline phosphatase to confirm hepatic causes of ALP elevations.[16] Hepatic causes of ALP elevation should have a concurrent elevation in GGT.[2]

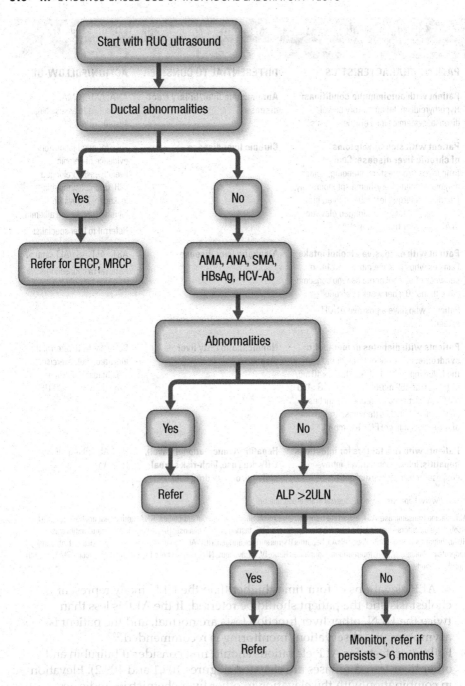

FIGURE 109.1. Approach to elevated serum transaminases when bilirubin is also elevated. ALP, alkaline phosphatase; AMA, antimitochondrial antibodies; ANA, antinuclear antibodies; ERCP, endoscopic retrograde cholangiopancreatography; GGT, gamma-glutamyl transferase; HBsAg, hepatitis B surface antigen; HCV-Ab, hepatitis C virus antibody; MRCP, magnetic resonance cholangiopancreatography; RUQ, right upper quadrant; SMA, smooth muscle antibody.

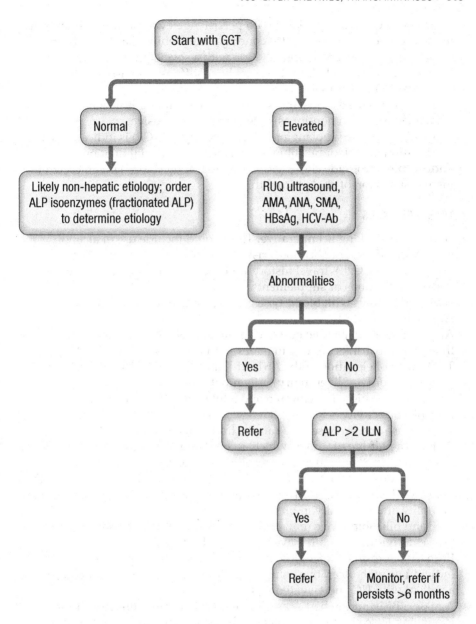

FIGURE 109.2. Approach to elevated serum transaminases when bilirubin is not concurrently elevated. ALP, alkaline phosphatase; AMA, antimitochondrial antibodies; ANA, antinuclear antibodies; GGT, gamma-glutamyl transferase; HBsAg, hepatitis B surface antigen; HCV-Ab, hepatitis C virus antibody; RUQ, right upper quadrant; SMA, smooth muscle antibody.

- Consider referral to a specialist with persistent elevations for 3 to 6 months.
- In the presence of prolonged INR and hyperbilirubinemia, ALP elevations should trigger immediate consultation with a specialist.
- Liver elastography is helpful to assess liver stiffness and assesses for the presence of fibrosis or cirrhosis.
- Liver biopsy is used in instances when tissue sampling is needed to confirm a diagnosis or when non-invasive testing is inconclusive.
- Magnetic resonance cholangiopancreatography (MRCP) is indicated with an elevation in ALP or bilirubin and suspicion for ductal dilation.
- Endoscopic retrograde cholangiopancreatography (ERCP) is completed if there is suspicion of choledocholithiasis.

PEARLS & PITFALLS

- Good history taking is imperative. This should include use of alcohol, recreational drugs, medications, risk factors for infectious hepatitis exposure (A, B, C, E), travel history, and use of supplemental or alternative herbal medications or supplements.
- Some individuals with blood-type group B or O have elevated intestinal ALP without underlying disease.[2]
- Alcohol use of an average of two or more drinks per day in females and three or more drinks per day in males should raise suspicion for ALD.[35]
- The degree of elevation of the AST, ALT, and ALP does not necessarily indicate severity of liver injury/inflammation.
- ALP levels are higher in children and adolescents because of the osteoblastic activity.
- Tobacco use and exercise may cause a transient elevation in ALP.
- ALP has a half-life of 7 days, which accounts for the delay in this enzyme to return to the normal range after resolution of diagnosis.
- In one metanalysis, elevations in AST, ALT, and ALP were associated with higher CVD mortality.[36] ALP elevations are also associated with increased mortality and morbidity in prostate cancer.[37]
- ALP and bilirubin levels may be decreased in oral contraceptive users.[38]
- Obese individuals usually have higher levels of ALT.[6]
- Primary sclerosing cholangitis (PSC) can be present in up to 70% of individuals with ulcerative colitis (UC). Strongly consider this diagnosis in a patient with UC and elevated ALP.
- Age, sex, BMI, and puberty can all influence liver transaminases. Research is ongoing to see if reference intervals based on sex and age or based on percentiles similar to growth charts are needed for children.[39,40] There is also much variation between laboratories, so, for interpretation, clinicians are encouraged to use reference intervals provided by the laboratory.
- INR of 1.5 or greater with hyperbilirubinemia and encephalopathy is suspicious for acute liver failure.[41]
- In one study, the sensitivity and specificity for an ALT greater than 2× the upper limit of normal as a screening test for pediatric NAFLD was 57% and 71%, respectively.[42]

PATIENT EDUCATION

▪ https://www.mayoclinic.org/symptoms/elevated-liver-enzymes/basics/definition/sym-20050830

RELATED DIAGNOSES AND ICD-10 CODES

Abnormal results of liver enzymes	R94.5
Elevated liver enzymes	R79.89
Abnormal alkaline phosphatase test, abnormal AST and ALT	R74.8
Alkaline phosphatase elevation	R74.8
Elevated alkaline phosphatase in a newborn	P09

REFERENCES

Full list of references can be accessed through Springer Publishing Company Connect™ at the following link: http://connect.springerpub.com/content/reference-book/978-0-8261-8843-4/part/part03/toc-part/ch109

---

110. LUPUS ANTICOAGULANT AND ANTIPHOSPHOLIPID ANTIBODIES

John Prickett

PHYSIOLOGY REVIEW

Autoimmune diseases are known to impose varying degrees of thrombophilic risk, particularly lupus anticoagulant (LA) and/or antiphospholipid antibodies (APLA), which may be part of antiphospholipid antibody syndrome (APS). Both LA and APLA refer to a heterogeneous group of antibodies directed at phospholipids and phospholipid-binding proteins including cardiolipin and beta2-glycoprotein I. The terminology regarding these entities has evolved and can be confusing due to lack of terminology standardization.[1,2]

LA was first described in individuals with lupus who had a prolonged activated partial thromboplastin time (aPTT). The term LA is a misnomer as the presence of lupus or other autoimmune disease is not a requisite, though the prevalence of LA is higher in this patient population. Its prevalence may be as high as 30% in patients with autoimmune disease and 2% to 4% of the general population. The term of "anticoagulant" is also misleading as it is not a risk for bleeding, but instead a thrombophilia risk.[3]

Positive testing for LA implies the presence of an antiphospholipid antibody. Testing for the presence of anti-cardiolipin (aCL) antibodies and anti-beta2-glycoprotein I antibodies are attempts to isolate IgG and/or IgM titers of these specific antibodies. When certain clinical and laboratory criteria (detailed in the text that follows) are met, the term "APS" is used.[4] It is a thrombophilic condition that often occurs in individuals with other autoimmune diseases and connotes a risk for both venous and arterial thromboses. The presence of these antibodies in otherwise healthy individuals without a personal history of thrombosis is uncertain.[5] Like other autoimmune diseases, APS may be more likely to exist as part of a familial trend.

OVERVIEW OF LABORATORY TESTS

A diagnosis of LA requires a series of tests that are functional coagulation studies designed to help determine the presence or absence of an LA, other factor inhibitor, or factor deficiency. Partial thromboplastin time (PTT or aPTT) (CPT code 85732), LA-sensitive PTT (contains low levels of phospholipid) (CPT code 85730), and dilute Russell viper venom time test (DRVVT) (CPT code 85613) are the most commonly utilized studies. If initial aPTT or LA-sensitive PTT (PTT-LA) is prolonged, a correction or mixing study is done (hexagonal phase for LA-sensitive PTT). The aPTT mixing study may correct in factor deficiency but may not correct in the presence of LA or a factor-specific inhibitor. The LA-sensitive PTT and DRVVT are better tests to determine presence of LA. Acute clotting events and/or anticoagulation may interfere with testing results.[5,6] An LA comprehensive panel (CPT codes 85613, 85670, 85705, 85732) can also be ordered.

Testing for aCL antibodies (CPT code 86147 x 2) and/or anti-beta2-glycoprotein I antibodies (CPT code 86146 x 2) is done by utilizing enzyme-linked immunosorbent assays (ELISA) to determine the presence of IgG or IgM antibodies. It is reported as a titer of antibody that may additionally be classified as low, intermediate, or high titer. The presence of IgA antibodies or other phospholipid antibodies is of unclear clinical significance.[4,5,7] An antiphospholipid syndrome diagnostic panel (CPT codes 86147, 86146, 85730, 85613) can also be ordered.

INDICATIONS

Screening

Universal screening is not recommended. Target screening should be considered in the following individuals:

■ Prolonged aPTT not due to factor-specific inhibitor (e.g., FVII)

Diagnosis and Evaluation

APS can be described as thrombotic (venous or arterial thrombosis), obstetrical (poor pregnancy outcomes as noted in the text that follows), both, or catastrophic (rare, multi-organ failure).[8,9]

In the diagnosis of APS, the Sapporo or Sydney Criteria[8] is used. Criteria is met when one clinical and one laboratory criteria are both met:

■ Clinical criteria:
  ● Vascular thrombosis (one or more venous, small vessel, or arterial by unequivocal imaging or histology [SVT does not count])
  ● Pregnancy morbidity—one or more unexplained death of morphologically normal fetus at greater than or equal to 10 weeks or one or

more premature births of morphologically normal neonate before 34 weeks' gestation due to preeclampsia or placental insufficiency, or
- Three or more consecutive spontaneous pregnancy losses at less than 10 weeks unexplained by chromosomal abnormalities, maternal anatomic causes, or hormonal causes.
- Laboratory criteria:
  - The presence of one or more antiphospholipid antibodies on two or more occasions at least 12 weeks apart.

Monitoring

As with other autoimmune diseases, testing may be repeated periodically to determine the degree of disease activity, though this may not affect clinical management.

INTERPRETATION

LA activity is defined by the International Society of Thrombosis and Hemostasis (ISTH).[10] All criteria must be met:

1. A positive result in one of the two common phospholipid-dependent coagulation studies (PTT-LA, DRVVT)
2. Prolonged mixing study
3. Correction of coagulation study after adding excess phospholipids
4. Absence of specific coexisting factor inhibitor (e.g., Factor VIII)

For aCL and anti-beta2-glycoprotein antibodies:

IgG or IgM aCL antibodies in moderate or higher titers

- Greater than 40 GPL or MPL units or
- Titer greater than the 99th percentile for laboratory by standardized ELISA

IgG or IgM anti-beta2-glycoprotein I in moderate or high titers

- Greater than 40 GPL or MPL units or
- Titer greater than the 99th percentile for laboratory

The clinical significance of lower-level titers is unclear.[8,9]

FOLLOW-UP

As previously described, positive tests must be validated at an interval of at least 12 weeks apart. Some clinicians will recheck periodically, thereafter.

Depending on the patient presentation and risk factors, an APS workup can be ordered with other tests for hypercoagulation including but not limited to prothrombin time (PT), aPTT (partial thromboplastin time), homocysteine, protein C, protein S, and antithrombin III.

PEARLS & PITFALLS

- The presence of APLA may cause false-positive syphilis testing as VDRL/RPR tests contain cardiolipin.[11]

TABLE 110.1: CAUSES OF TRANSIENT ANTI-CARDIOLIPIN ANTIBODIES			
	BACTERIAL	**VIRAL**	**PARASITIC**
Infectious[15–17] (typically IgM aCL)	(Bacteria) septicemia, leptospirosis, syphilis, Lyme disease (borreliosis), tuberculosis, leprosy, infective endocarditis, post-streptococcal rheumatic fever, and Klebsiella infections	Hepatitis A, B, and C; mumps; HIV; human T-lymphotropic virus type 1 (HTLV-I); MCV; varicella-zoster, Epstein–Barr virus, adenovirus, parvovirus, and rubella	Malaria, *pneumocystis jirovecii*, visceral leishmaniasis
Malignancy[17,19]	Lung, colon, cervix, prostate, kidney, ovary, breast, and bone; Hodgkin ds, NHL, MPN, myeloid and lymphocytic leukemias		
Medications[17,18]	Phenothiazines, phenytoin, hydralazine, procainamide, quinidine, quinine, ethosuximide, alpha interferon, amoxicillin, chlorothiazide, oral contraceptives, and propranolol		

MCV, mean corpuscular volume; MPN, myeloproliferative neoplasm; NHL, non-Hodgkin lymphoma.

- Livedo reticularis, nonbacterial thrombotic endocarditis (NBTE), cognitive deficits with white matter lesions, lupus-like symptoms, and/or mild thrombocytopenia are other findings with APS.[12–15]
- The presence of antibodies directed against phosphatidylserine, phosphatidylcholine, phosphatidylethanolamine, and anti-annexin V is of unknown clinical significance.
- Causes of transient aCL antibodies include some infections, medications, and malignancies (Table 110.1)[16–20]

PATIENT EDUCATION

- https://www.healthline.com/health/lupus-anticoagulant
- https://www.nhlbi.nih.gov/health-topics/antiphospholipid-antibody -syndrome

RELATED DIAGNOSES AND ICD-10 CODES

Antiphospholipid syndrome	D68.61
Raised antibody titer	R76.0
Personal history of diseases of the blood and blood-forming organs and certain disorders involving the immune mechanism APAS	Z86.2
Lupus anticoagulant syndrome	D68.62

REFERENCES

Full list of references can be accessed through Springer Publishing Company Connect™ at the following link: http://connect.springerpub.com/content/reference-book/978-0-8261 -8843-4/part/part03/toc-part/ch110

111. LUTEINIZING HORMONE AND FOLLICLE-STIMULATING HORMONE

Emily Neiman

PHYSIOLOGY REVIEW

The hypothalamic-pituitary-gonadal (HPG) axis is responsible for reproductive development and function in both males and females. The hypothalamus secretes gonadotropin-releasing hormone (GnRH) in a pulsatile fashion approximately every 2 hours. Once released, GnRH stimulates the pituitary gland to produce and release follicle-stimulating hormone (FSH) and luteinizing hormone (LH), both gonadotropic hormones.[1,2]

In females, FSH works to recruit oocytes and helps to develop them into follicles during each menstrual cycle. The most mature follicle continues to develop and becomes the dominant follicle of that cycle, while the other follicles undergo atresia. LH (in combination with FSH) works to trigger ovulation, or the release of the ovum from the dominant follicle, which produces the corpus luteum.[1,3] In males, FSH targets the Sertoli cells of the testes in order to stimulate spermatogenesis while LH attaches to the Leydig cells to regulate the production of testosterone.[1,2,4]

There are cyclical changes in the levels of FSH and LH throughout the month in ovulatory females, corresponding to the menstrual cycle. FSH is at its lowest at the beginning of the cycle and increases throughout the first half of the cycle, otherwise known as the follicular phase. Levels of LH also increase throughout the follicular phase and are highest just prior to ovulation (i.e., the LH "surge"). There continues to be some secretion of FSH at this point in the cycle, and FSH and LH together continue to promote the maturation of the dominant follicle. The ovulatory phase of the menstrual cycle begins midcycle. Ovulation itself occurs approximately 1 to 2 days following the LH surge. Following ovulation, the ruptured follicle becomes the corpus luteum, which is supported by LH and secretes progesterone. Increased progesterone levels inhibit both FSH and LH at the end of each menstrual cycle. If fertilization does not occur, the corpus luteum degenerates, leading to a decrease of both estrogen and progesterone. This removes the negative feedback for FSH and LH, which begin to increase in preparation for the next menstrual cycle. FSH levels for females rise with age and become highest (and constant) in menopause.[1,3,5]

OVERVIEW OF LABORATORY TESTS

FSH is measured by a serum blood draw and can be assessed by ordering FSH (CPT code 83001). LH (CPT code 83002) may be ordered to evaluate serum LH levels. LH is also measured by over-the-counter ovulation predictor kits and is performed at home by the patient through urine testing for the purposes of conception or contraception. Serum FSH may be ordered in combination with other laboratory tests, such as estradiol. If testing any female who is having ovulatory menstrual cycles, it is key to note where the patient is in their menstrual cycle, as the levels normally vary throughout the cycle. If anovulatory, menopausal, or male, FSH and LH may be tested at a random time.[6]

INDICATIONS

Screening
■ There is no current evidence that supports screening with either FSH or LH.

Diagnosis and Evaluation
■ Consider testing FSH and LH to evaluate signs and symptoms listed in Table 111.1[5-13] with the following caveats.
  ● The American Society of Reproductive Medicine (ASRM) recommends against drawing FSH for female patients in their 40s to identify menopause as a cause of abnormal uterine bleeding.[14]
  ● Pediatric endocrine guidelines recommend against testing FSH or LH for children with pubic hair and/or body odor but no other signs of precocious puberty.[15]

TABLE 111.1: INDICATIONS FOR FOLLICE-STIMULATING HORMONE/LUTEINIZING HORMONE TESTING BASED ON SIGNS/SYMPTOMS

FEMALE PATIENTS	MALE PATIENTS
Menstrual irregularities	Infertility
Amenorrhea (primary or secondary)	Galactorrhea
Infertility	Early/delayed puberty
Galactorrhea	
Early/delayed puberty	
Virilization	
Hirsutism	

Sources: Data from Casper RD. Clinical manifestations and diagnosis of menopause. In: Barbieri RL, Crowley WF Jr, eds. *UpToDate.* UpToDate; 2022. https://www.uptodate.com/contents/clinical-manifestations-and-diagnosis-of-menopause; Welt CK, Barbieri RL. Evaluation and management of secondary amenorrhea. In: Crowley WF Jr, Geffner ME, eds. *UpToDate.* UpToDate; 2022. https://www.uptodate.com/contents/evaluation-and-management-of-secondary-amenorrhea; Schuiling KD, Likis FE. *Gynecologic Health Care: With an Introduction to Prenatal and Postpartum Care.* 4th ed. Jones & Bartlett; 2020; Patel S. Polycystic ovary syndrome (PCOS), an inflammatory, systemic, lifestyle endocrinopathy. *J Steroid Biochem Mol Biol.* 2018;182:27–36. doi:10.1016/j.jsbmb.2018.04.008; Practice Committee of the American Society for Reproductive Medicine. Electronic address: asrm@asrm.org. Management of nonobstructive azoospermia: a committee opinion. *Fertil Steril.* 2018;110(7):1239–1245. doi:10.1016/j.fertnstert.2018.09.012; Richard-Eaglin A. Male and female hypogonadism. *Nurs Clin North Am.* 2018;53(3):395–405. doi:10.1016/j.cnur.2018.04.006; Santi D, Crépieux P, Reiter E, et al. Follicle-stimulating hormone (FSH) action on spermatogenesis: a focus on physiological and therapeutic roles. *J Clin Med.* 2020;9(4):1014. doi:10.3390/jcm9041014; Shiraishi K, Matsuyama H. Gonadotoropin actions on spermatogenesis and hormonal therapies for spermatogenic disorders [Review]. *Endocr J.* 2017;64(2):123–131. doi:10.1507/endocrj.EJ17-0001; Ulrich ND, Marsh EE. Ovarian reserve testing: a review of the options, their applications, and their limitations. *Clin Obstet Gynecol.* 2019;62(2):228–237. doi:10.1097/GRF.000000000000044; Welt CK. Clinical manifestations and diagnosis of spontaneous primary ovarian insufficiency (premature ovarian failure). In: Crowley WF Jr, Barvieri RL, eds. *UpToDate.* UpToDate; 2022. https://www.uptodate.com/contents/clinical-manifestations-and-diagnosis-of-spontaneous-primary-ovarian-insufficiency-premature-ovarian-failure

Monitoring

- Ongoing monitoring of FSH and LH may be used during infertility treatment. As the levels may vary from cycle to cycle, one set of values may be insufficient to make a diagnosis. It is useful to assess these levels across several menstrual cycles.[7]
- For transgender people undergoing gender-affirming therapy (feminizing), FSH and LH may be monitored if therapy is used to suppress male puberty. These levels are drawn every 6 to 12 months and demonstrate the desired suppression of gonadtropins.[16,17]

INTERPRETATION

- Reference intervals for FSH and LH vary based on age, sex, stage of puberty, and the menstrual cycle in females. Table 111.2 provides commonly used reference ranges for FSH and LH, but it should be noted that best practice is to follow the reference ranges provided by the laboratory.[18,19]
- Reference intervals for males are based on very scant evidence, with most studies on reference ranges demonstrating that the involved clinical laboratory did not develop their own reference range.[20]
- FSH needs to be interpreted with caution in females younger than 40; positive predictive value for decreased ovarian reserve is higher with age.[5,7]
- Early follicular FSH should be drawn with estradiol for a full picture.[1,6–8]
- Common causes of elevated or decreased FSH/LH are reviewed in Table 111.3,[21] but they are most helpful when interpreted in context with other laboratory tests.
  - An elevated FSH with a low/normal estradiol indicates premature ovarian failure.[6,8]

TABLE 111.2: REFERENCE INTERVALS

	FSH	LH
Female (prepubertal):	0.6–4.1 mIU/mL	<0.02–0.3 mIU/mL
Female (premenopausal): Follicular phase	2.9–14.6 mIU/mL	1.9–14.6 mIU/mL
Female (premenopausal): Midcycle peak	4.7–23.2 mIU/mL	12.2–118.0 mIU/mL
Female (premenopausal): Luteal phase	1.4–8.9 mIU/mL	0.7–12.9 mIU/mL
Female (postmenopausal):	16.0–157.0 mIU/mL (typically > 40 mIU/mL)	5.3–65.4 mIU/mL (typically > 40 mIU/mL)
Male (prepubertal)	<1.5 mIU/mL	<0.02–0.5 mIU/mL
Male (>18 years)	1.2–15.8 mIU/mL	1.3–9.8 mIU/mL

FSH, follicle-stimulating hormone; LH, luteinizing hormone.

Sources: Data from Grimstad F, Le M, Zganjar A, et al. An evaluation of reported follicle-stimulating hormone, luteinizing hormone, estradiol, and prolactin reference ranges in the United States. *Urology.* 2018;120:114–119. doi:10.1016/j.urology.2018.07.024; Mayocliniclabs.com. *LH - Clinical: Luteinizing Hormone (LH), Serum.* https://www.mayocliniclabs.com/test-catalog/Clinical+and+Interpretive/602752.

TABLE 111.3: DIFFERENTIAL DIAGNOSIS OF ABNORMAL FOLLICLE-STIMULATING HORMONE AND LUTEINIZING HORMONE LEVELS

FEMALE

DECREASED FSH	INCREASED FSH
Secondary hypogonadism	Primary hypogonadism
Infertility	Premature ovarian failure
PCOS	Menopause
Dysfunction of pituitary or hypothalamus	Precocious puberty

DECREASED LH	INCREASED LH
Secondary hypogonadism	Primary hypogonadism
Functional hypothalamic amenorrhea	Premature ovarian failure
Primary ovarian hyperfunction	Menopause
Dysfunction of pituitary or hypothalamus	PCOS
	Precocious puberty

MALE

DECREASED FSH	INCREASED FSH
Secondary hypogonadism	Primary hypogonadism
Azoospermia	Precocious puberty
Infertility	Complete testicular feminization syndrome
Dysfunction of pituitary or hypothalamus	

DECREASED LH	INCREASED LH
Secondary hypogonadism	Primary hypogonadism
Primary hypergonadism	Precocious puberty
Dysfunction of pituitary or hypothalamus	Complete testicular feminization syndrome

FSH, follicle-stimulating hormone; LH, luteinizing hormone; PCOS, polycystic ovary syndrome.

Sources: Data from Coss D. Commentary on the recent FSH collection: known knowns and known unknowns. *Endocrinology.* 2020;161(1):bqz035. doi:10.1210/endocr/bqz035; Mayocliniclabs.com. *FSH - Clinical: Follicle-Stimulating Hormone (FSH), Serum.* https://www.mayocliniclabs.com/test-catalog/Clinical+and+Interpretive/602753; Mayocliniclabs.com. *LH - Clinical: Luteinizing Hormone (LH), Serum.* https://www.mayocliniclabs.com/test-catalog/Clinical+and+Interpretive/602752; Practice Committee of the American Society for Reproductive Medicine. Electronic address: asrm@asrm.org. Management of nonobstructive azoospermia: a committee opinion. *Fertil Steril.* 2018;110(7):1239–1245. doi:10.1016/j.fertnstert.2018.09.012; Schuiling KD, Likis FE. *Gynecologic Health Care: With an Introduction to Prenatal and Postpartum Care.* 4th ed. Jones a&Bartlett; 2020; Welt CK, Barbieri RL. Evaluation and management of secondary amenorrhea. In: Crowley WF Jr, Geffner ME, eds. *UpToDate.* UpToData; 2022. https://www.uptodate.com/contents/evaluation-and-management-of-secondary-amenorrhea

- A low/normal FSH with a low/normal estradiol indicates secondary hypogonadism.[6]
- A low/normal FSH with normal prolactin and normal TSH indicates polycystic ovary syndrome (PCOS). If estradiol is also low, functional hypothalamic amenorrhea is more likely than PCOS.[6,12]
- If early follicular FSH is elevated and estradiol is also elevated, this likely indicates diminished ovarian reserve or decreased fertility.[7,8]

■ PCOS, while thought to be associated with obesity, may also be diagnosed in normal-weight females. If PCOS is suspected in a normal-weight female, the ratio of FSH to LH may help distinguish between PCOS and functional hypothalamic amenorrhea. The normal ratio between LH and FSH is 1 to 2. In PCOS, this ratio becomes reversed (increase in LH; decrease in FSH) and can be as high as 2 to 3, leading to anovulatory cycles.[6,22]

FOLLOW-UP

- Follow-up testing will depend on the initial indication for testing.
- For female patients, testing may include an assessment of estrogen status with progestin withdrawal test or endometrial thickness on transvaginal ultrasound, as well as serum estradiol.[1,5,6]
- Other serum tests that may be ordered depending on clinical presentation are total and free testosterone, prolactin, thyroid-stimulating hormone (TSH), fasting blood glucose, or hemoglobin a1c.[1,5,6,8,12]
- To further assess infertility concerns, estradiol and anti-Müllerian hormone (AMH) may be ordered, and an antral follicle count may be performed via transvaginal ultrasound.[7]
- If there is concern for structural anomalies, a pelvic ultrasound to visualize the ovaries may be completed, as well as possible MRI of the pituitary or of the pelvis/ovaries[1,6,11]
- Follow-up testing for male patients may include serum testosterone, estradiol, and prolactin, as well as a semen analysis if infertility is a concern. An MRI may be performed if structural anomalies are suspected.[1,11,13]

PEARLS & PITFALLS

- It is important to recognize that if some ovulatory function is still present, FSH and LH levels may vary widely from cycle to cycle and it can be difficult to make a firm diagnosis based on the results from one menstrual cycle.[5,6,8,12]
- FSH is ideally drawn for female patients on day 2 to 4 of the menstrual cycle when it should be at its lowest basal level (early follicular phase). If prolonged amenorrhea is present, a random draw of FSH is acceptable. Serum estradiol may also be drawn at the same time in order to more fully interpret the FSH result. Estradiol level also provides an assessment of ovarian reserve.[1,6,7]
- LH is commonly self-tested by female patients through urine screening at home.
- For an evaluation of secondary amenorrhea, initial testing should include FSH, serum prolactin, and thyroid-stimulating hormone.[6]
- Pregnancy should always be ruled out first for a complaint of amenorrhea.[1]
- FSH cannot diagnose menopause or predict when it will occur.[5,14]
- Interpreting the results in the context of other laboratory tests is helpful in confirming or refuting a differential diagnosis.

PATIENT EDUCATION

- https://labtestsonline.org/tests/follicle-stimulating-hormone-fsh
- https://labtestsonline.org/tests/luteinizing-hormone-lh

RELATED DIAGNOSES AND ICD-10 CODES

Hypogonadism, male	E29.1
Hypogonadism, female	E28.39
Delayed puberty	E30.0
Precocious puberty	E30.1
Polycystic ovarian syndrome (PCOS)	E28.2
Primary ovarian failure	E28.3
Menopausal and female climacteric states	N95.1
Primary amenorrhea	N91.0
Secondary amenorrhea	N91.1
Female infertility associated with anovulation	N97.0
Encounter for procreative investigation and testing	Z31.4
Azoospermia	N46.0
Testicular hyperfunction	E29.0
Testicular hypofunction	E29.1

REFERENCES

Full list of references can be accessed through Springer Publishing Company Connect™ at the following link: http://connect.springerpub.com/content/reference-book/978-0-8261 -8843-4/part/part03/toc-part/ch111

---

112. LYME ANTIBODIES

Stephanie C. Evans and Kate Sustersic Gawlik

PHYSIOLOGY REVIEW

Lyme disease is a tickborne zoonosis, caused by the bite of an infected tick that carries the bacteria *Borrelia burgdorferi*. *B. burgdorferi* enters the skin at the site of the tick bite and 3 to 30 days later, the organisms migrate locally in the skin around the bite, and cause an inflammatory reaction (*erythema migrans*). *Erythema migrans* or the "bulls-eye" rash is usually greater than the size of a quarter and appears in only 70% of people who are infected with Lyme disease. This happens before a significant antibody response to infection (serologic conversion) occurs.[1] If the rash does not appear or is not identified and treated, there is acute dissemination of the bacteria. The bacteria is spread via the lymphatics to cause regional adenopathy or disseminate in blood to organs or other skin sites. This is characterized by protean manifestations, including potential development of dermatologic, rheumatologic, neurologic, and cardiac abnormalities. If left untreated, this can become chronic or late disseminated Lyme disease where the bacteria have spread throughout the body. The onset of symptoms and complications of late disseminated Lyme disease is usually around 6 to 36 months after the original infection.[2]

OVERVIEW OF LABORATORY TESTS

Testing for Lyme disease uses a two-step process. The two-test methodology uses a sensitive enzyme immunoassay (EIA) or a total or separate immunoglobulin M/immunoglobulin G (IgM/IgG) immunofluorescence assay as the first test for screening. If the first screening test is negative, no further testing is suggested. If the first test is equivocal or positive, the second test completed is the western immunoblot assay or a second EIA, which is the test used for definitive diagnosis for Lyme disease (CPT codes 86617, 86618). The second EIA test was deemed "substantially equivalent to or better than" a legally marketed predicate test.[3,4] IgM immunoblot tests should be disregarded if the patient's symptoms have lasted more than 30 days. If the patient has been sick for longer, only IgG immunoblot tests should be ordered. If the patient is not sure if 30 days have passed, repeat testing may be indicated.[3,4]

According to the American Society of Microbiology and the Choosing Wisely initiative, do not order a Lyme immunoblot without a positive Lyme EIA screening test.[5]

INDICATIONS

Screening

There is no indication for universal or targeted screening of Lyme disease.

Diagnosis and Evaluation

Individuals who have been in areas with a high prevalence of positive infected ticks and present with the following signs/symptoms should be tested[1,2]:

- Fever
- Chills
- Headache
- Fatigue
- Redness, warmth, and swelling in one or a few joints at a time—usually the knees, shoulders, or wrists
- Lymphadenopathy
- Facial palsy
- Arthritis with severe joint pain
- Intermittent pain in muscles, tendons, joints, and bones
- Heart palpitations
- Irregular heartbeat
- Nerve pain
- Inflammation of the spinal cord and brain
- Episodes of dizziness or shortness of breath

The American Society of Microbiology, the American Academy of Pediatrics, and the Choosing Wisely initiative recommend[5,6]:

- Avoiding testing for Lyme disease as a cause of musculoskeletal symptoms without an exposure history or appropriate examination findings and
- Avoiding ordering Lyme serology on patients with a primary *erythema migrans* lesion. At the time of presentation, most patients with primary Lyme disease are seronegative and should be treated regardless of serologicresults. In patients with equivocal or atypical lesions, paired testing with sera collected acutely and 2 to 3 weeks later may be helpful. There is currently no diagnostic method that is highly sensitive in Lyme disease patients with less than 2 weeks of rash or illness.

Monitoring

- Following completion of one or more antibiotic course(s) for Lyme disease:
  - Testing should not be used to monitor response to therapy or determine test of cure.[4,7]
- Monitor for improvement in signs and symptoms during and after completion of treatment. Individuals may have symptoms of pain, fatigue, and difficulty with concentration which last for up to 6 months.

INTERPRETATION

- EIA and immunofluorescence assay screening tests report either a positive or negative result.
- If negative, no second test is recommended.[4,8]
- If positive, a second test (Western Blot or EIA) is needed. Positive or negative is definitive diagnosis.
- Some tests give results for two types of antibodies, IgM and IgG. Positive IgM results should be disregarded if the patient has been ill for more than 30 days.[4,7]
- With over 30 days post symptom onset, only the IgG immunoblot should be performed or interpreted.[4,7]
- The Association of Public Health Laboratories (APHL) has an extensive report titled "Suggested Reporting Language, Interpretation and Guidance Regarding Lyme Disease Serologic Test Results" that reviews and provides interpretation for individual laboratory tests (https://www.aphl.org/aboutAPHL/publications/Documents/ID-2021-Lyme-Disease-Serologic-Testing-Reporting.pdf).[4]

FOLLOW-UP

- After diagnosis and treatment, no further routine monitoring is recommended. Repeat testing is not useful for monitoring treatment response.
- Repeat testing may be useful if initial testing was performed too early in the window period (time period between infection and the development of antibodies that can be detected by serologic assays). If this occurred, the presence or absence of seroconversion may provide additional information for diagnostic decision-making. If seroconversion does not occur, it is

possible that early treatment may have blunted the immune response or signified that another condition may be causing the current symptoms.[4,7]

■ Repeat testing may also be useful if initial test results are unclear (e.g., IgM and IgG results are not consistent between the first- and second-tier tests).[4]

PEARLS & PITFALLS

■ Presence of positive testing in the absence of symptoms may be a false positive; consider the possibility of rheumatic disorders.

■ Lyme disease can be confused with other disorders or diseases; a complete history and potential area of exposure need to be considered for each patient.

■ Late diagnosis should involve an infectious disease specialist.

■ Infection with other diseases, including some tickborne diseases, or some viral, bacterial, or autoimmune diseases, can result in false-positive test results.

■ Antibodies produced by the human immune system to fight off the Lyme disease bacteria (*B. burgdorferi*) can persist long after the infection is gone. Once the patient tests positive and is diagnosed, they will likely continue to test positive for months or years even after the bacteria is gone and antibiotic course has been completed.[9]

PATIENT EDUCATION

■ https://www.cdc.gov/lyme/index.html

RELATED DIAGNOSES AND ICD-10 CODES

Arthritis	A69.23	Granuloma annulare	L92.0
Erythema migrans	L53.9	Ringworm	B35.4
Fever	R50.9	Cellulitis	L03.90
Fatigue	R53.8	Viral illness	B34.9
Myalgia	M79.10	Coxsackie	B97.11
Nummular eczema	L30.0	Arthritis	M13.8

REFERENCES

Full list of references can be accessed through Springer Publishing Company Connect™ at the following link: http://connect.springerpub.com/content/reference-book/978-0-8261-8843-4/part/part03/toc-part/ch112

113. MAGNESIUM

Carolyn McClerking

PHYSIOLOGY REVIEW

As the second most abundant intracellular cation, magnesium is an essential electrolyte which has an important role in maintenance of both physiologic and biochemical processes in the human body. Most of the body's magnesium exists intracellularly. To maintain magnesium homeostasis, the human body must have a functioning gastrointestinal and renal system. Bone metabolism is also important in maintaining normal magnesium levels.[1,2] According to data from the National Health and Nutrition Examination Survey (NHANES), over 60% of females between the ages of 51 and 70 do not meet the Estimated Average Requirement (EAR) for magnesium intake. The number is even less for Black and Mexican American women similar in age. Therefore, older adults are at greater risk for complications associated with magnesium deficiency.[3]

OVERVIEW OF LABORATORY TESTS

Serum magnesium (CPT code 83735) reflects extracellular magnesium and is the most common test used to assess magnesium levels. Ionized magnesium reflects extracellular magnesium that is physiologically active and is less commonly measured. Excretion of magnesium can be measured in a spot or 24-hour urine sample. Some research suggests that the best way to evaluate/manage magnesium status is through simultaneous assessment of serum magnesium level, 24-hour urinary magnesium excretion, and dietary magnesium intake estimation.[4]

INDICATIONS

Screening
- Universal screening for magnesium is not recommended.
- Targeted screening with serum magnesium is recommended for conditions predisposing to hypo- or hypermagnesemia (Table 113.1).[1,5–7]
- Targeted screening with serum magnesium is recommended for patients with hypoparathyroidism, since identification and replacement of low serum magnesium levels can correct hypoparathyroidism and decrease the need for calcium replacement.[8]

Diagnosis and Evaluation
- Used to evaluate for hypomagnesemia as a cause of neuropsychiatric symptoms such as delirium and apathy.[9]
- Used to evaluate for hypomagnesemia as a cause of life-threatening arrhythmias (torsades de Pointes, atrial fibrillation, ventricular tachycardia).[9]

- Used to evaluate other signs/symptoms that could be due to altered magnesium levels (Table 113.2)[1,5,7]

Monitoring

- Monitor magnesium levels in patients with hypoparathyroidism every 3 to 6 months.[10]

TABLE 113.1: CONDITIONS PREDISPOSING TO HYPO- OR HYPERMAGNESEMIA

HYPOMAGNESEMIA	HYPERMAGNESEMIA
Proton pump inhibitor (PPI) use, specifically high dose	Addison disease (adrenal insufficiency)
Use of specific cardiac medications (procainamide, Norpace, or quinidine)	Chronic use of magnesium-containing laxatives or antacids
Malabsorption syndromes	GFR <30 mL/minute/1.73 m²
Diuretics (especially thiazide or loop)	Infusion of intravenous magnesium
Hypocalcemia	Lithium therapy
Extended nasogastric suctioning	
Inflammatory bowel disease	
Alcoholism	
Chronic diarrhea	
Diabetes mellitus	
Vitamin D insufficiency	
Diabetic ketoacidosis	

Sources: Data from Gragossian A, Bashir K, Friede R. Hypomagnesemia. In: *StatPearls.* StatPearls Publishing; 2020. https://www .ncbi.nlm.nih.gov/books/NBK500003/; Hansen B, Bruserud Ø. Hypomagnesemia in critically ill patients. *J Intensive Care.* 2018;6:21. doi:10.1186/s40560-018-0291-y; Srinutta T, Chewcharat A, Takkavatakarn K, et al. Proton pump inhibitors and hypomagnesemia, *Medicine.* 2019;98(44):e17788. doi:10.1097/MD.0000000000017788; Van Laecke S. Hypomagnesemia and hypermagnesemia. *Acta Clin Belg.* 2019;74(1):41–47. doi:10.1080/17843286.2018.1516173

TABLE 113.2: SIGNS AND SYMPTOMS OF HYPO- OR HYPERMAGNESEMIA

HYPOMAGNESEMIA	HYPERMAGNESEMIA
Hypokalemia	Diminished DTRs *
Hypocalcemia	Drowsiness
Tetany	Fatigue
Nystagmus	Bradycardia
Seizures	Nausea/vomiting
Tremor	Muscle weakness
Arrhythmias	ECG changes
Psychosis	Arrythmia
ECG changes	Psychosis

*Complete loss of DTR with severe hypermagnesemia.

DTR, deep tendon reflexes.

Sources: Data from Berg O, Lee RH, Chagolla B. *Magnesium Sulfate.* California Maternal Quality Care Collaborative; 2013; Gragossian A, Bashir K, Friede R. Hypomagnesemia. In: *StatPearls.* StatPearls Publishing; 2020. https://www.ncbi.nlm.nih.gov/books/ NBK500003/; Hansen B, Bruserud Ø. Hypomagnesemia in critically ill patients. *J Intensive Care.* 2018;6:21. doi:10.1186/s40560-018- 0291-y; Van Laecke S. Hypomagnesemia and hypermagnesemia. *Acta Clin Belg.* 2019;74(1):41–47. doi:10.1080/17843286.2018.1516173

- Consider routine monitoring of magnesium levels for patients on long-term PPIs, specifically individuals who are also on other drugs that may cause low magnesium levels, such as diuretics.[7] The best interval for monitoring is unclear.
- Consider routine monitoring of magnesium levels in patients on immunosuppressants such as calcineurin inhibitors (tacrolimus, cyclosporine) as these drugs result in magnesium wasting.[11]
- Consider routine monitoring of magnesium in patients with advanced cancer or chronic diseases.[12]
- Monitor patients on parenteral magnesium sulfate therapy. The interval will vary depending on patient diagnosis and if signs/symptoms of hypermagnesemia are present.

INTERPRETATION

- Reference interval for serum magnesium is 1.5 to 2.5 mg/dL but varies with age.[4,13]
- The differential diagnosis for levels above or below the reference intervals is found in Table 113.1.

FOLLOW-UP

- After identifying hypo- or hypermagnesemia:
  - Evaluate for kidney function, glucose, and other electrolyte abnormalities (especially potassium and calcium).[5,13]
  - Evaluate electrocardiogram to assess for electrophysiologic changes.[13]
- In challenging hypomagnesemia cases, a 24-hour urinary magnesium, a random urine fraction excretion of magnesium, and/or a magnesium tolerance test may be used to determine if etiology is gastrointestinal versus renal losses.[13]

PEARLS & PITFALLS

- Older adults, specifically Black individuals, are at greater risk of low magnesium intake as compared to their Caucasian counterparts.[14]
- Studies have found a link between hypomagnesemia and the development of post-renal transplant diabetes mellitus.[15,16]
- A prospective study conducted in the surgical intensive care unit suggested that ionized magnesium may more accurately reflect magnesium needs in critically ill patients.[17]
- Older adult males with chronic heart failure and left ventricular systolic function have an increased risk of cardiovascular mortality when presenting with hypermagnesemia.[18]
- Hypomagnesemia increases pregnancy and neonatal complications, so magnesium supplementation is often advised in pregnant patients.[19,20]
- International guidelines recommend the use of magnesium sulfate for fetal neuroprotection.[20]
- Magnesium plays a significant role in vitamin D metabolism.[21]
- Studies suggest a link between seizures and hypomagnesemia; therefore, it is critical to measure magnesium levels when patients present with seizure.[22]

- Magnesium must be repleted in order to correct hypokalemia.[6]
- Research is examining the usefulness of a revised evidence-based reference interval for serum magnesium that reflects population diversity and nutrition status.[23]

PATIENT EDUCATION

- https://ods.od.nih.gov/factsheets/Magnesium-Consumer/

RELATED DIAGNOSES AND ICD-10 CODES

Magnesium deficiency	E61.2
Disorders of magnesium metabolism, unspecified	E83.40
Hypermagnesemia	E83.41
Hypomagnesemia	E83.42
Other disorders of magnesium metabolism	E83.49

REFERENCES

Full list of references can be accessed through Springer Publishing Company Connect™ at the following link: http://connect.springerpub.com/content/reference-book/978-0-8261-8843-4/part/part03/toc-part/ch113

114. METHYLENETETRAHYDROFOLATE REDUCTASE

Rachel M. Donner and Tyler Parisien

PHYSIOLOGY REVIEW

Methylenetetrahydrofolate reductase (MTHFR) is an enzyme that plays a key role in regulation of folate and homocysteine metabolism. The body utilizes MTHFR to catalyze the conversion of 5,10-methylenetetrahydrofolate to 5-methyltetrahydrofolate, which is the primary circulatory form of folate and is utilized in the homocysteine remethylation to methionine. Essentially, methylenetetrahydrofolate reductase is important for chemical reactions involving vitamin folate; 5-methyltetrahydrofolate is the primary form found in blood and is necessary for the process that converts homocysteine to methionine, which is utilized to make proteins and other important compounds (Figure 114.1). Deficiencies in MTHFR can cause hyperhomocysteinemia with homocystinuria, or mild hyperhomocysteinemia. Primarily, MTHFR deficiency is identified as

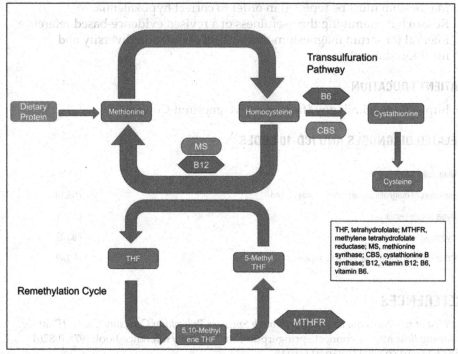

FIGURE 114.1. Methylenetetrahydrofolate reductase is important for chemical reactions involving vitamin folate; 5-methyltetrahydrofolate is the primary form found in blood and is necessary for the process that converts homocysteine to methionine, which is utilized to make proteins and other important compounds.

the most common cause of inborn error of folate metabolism and is still relatively rare. However, genetic testing uncovered a thermolabile variant of MTHFR. This varient has become recognized as the most common genetic cause of hyperhomocysteinemia and has been extensively investigated as a risk factor for several multifactorial disorders associated with disturbances in homocysteine metabolism. cDNA isolation allowed for molecular genetic approaches to study MTHFR deficiencies, which led to the identification of common sequence variants at bp 677 (C → T) and bp 1298 (A → C), which encode the thermolabile form of the enzyme. Since then, many researchers have studied various polymorphisms associated with MTHFR deficiency and their impacts on health and disease.

OVERVIEW OF LABORATORY TESTS

Laboratory testing for MTHFR evaluates the presence or absence of the C677T and/or A1298C mutations (CPT code 81291) by means of DNA analysis. Other possible mutations may be possible but are rarely encountered. MTHFR evaluation is usually ordered in response to elevated homocysteine levels, especially in combination with cardiovascular disease, inappropriate thrombosis, or recurrent pregnancy loss.[1] However, MTHFR testing is not recommended for patients with blood clots due to its limited utility.[2]

INDICATIONS

Screening

- Universal screening is not recommended.
- Consider targeted screening in the following:
  - Infants with neural tube and other related congenital or developmental defects
  - MTHFR should not be ordered as part of a routine clinical evaluation for thrombophilia, recurrent pregnancy loss, or for at risk family members.[3]
  - The utility of screening in other areas is controversial.
- The American Heart Association recommends against screening for common MTHFR gene variants in regard to cardiovascular risk.[4]
- The American College of Obstetricians and Gynecologists recommends against screening for MTHFR due to the lack of association between the MTHFR C677T polymorphism and any negative pregnancy outcomes, or increased risk for blood clots.[5]
- The American College of Medical Genetics/Choosing Wisely recommends against MTHFR genetic testing as part of a recurrent pregnancy loss evaluation.[3,6]

Diagnosis and Evaluation

- Individuals with elevated homocysteine levels of undetermined origin.
- Genetic testing for the *MTHFR* gene is used to find out if a patient has one of two MTHFR mutations (C677T and A1298C).
- MTHFR testing will only confirm whether raised levels are caused by a genetic mutation.

Monitoring

- *MTHFR* gene testing does not need to be repeated or monitored.

INTERPRETATION

Results for the MTHFR C677T and A1298C genetic mutations are typically reported as negative or positive. If the MTHFR genetic test is negative, then neither mutation has been detected and other indications for elevated homocysteine levels should be investigated.[1]

FOLLOW-UP

- If the patient is positive for the homozygous variant C677T, a fasting total plasma homocysteine level should be ordered.

PEARLS & PITFALLS

- Referral to a clinical geneticist is important if the patient is found to have a MTHFR polymorphism.

- Multiple studies suggest that MTHFR polymorphisms may have a correlation to treatment-resistant depression (TRD) due to its role in folate metabolism. Genetic screening for MTHFR for patients with major depression has been proposed. However, due to the high cost of genetic testing, treatment with L-methylfolate has also been suggested to supplement a patient's possible deficiency. Additional studies are needed to determine a future course of action.[7]
- MTHFR polymorphisms, such as C677T, may also have a correlation with male infertility due to the decrease in folate. More analytical studies are needed to validate findings.[8]

PATIENT EDUCATION

- https://rarediseases.info.nih.gov/diseases/10953/mthfr-gene-variant

RELATED DIAGNOSES AND ICD-10 CODES

MTMFR deficiency	E72.12
Hyperhomocysteinemia	E27.11

REFERENCES

Full list of references can be accessed through Springer Publishing Company Connect™ at the following link: http://connect.springerpub.com/content/reference-book/978-0-8261 -8843-4/part/part03/toc-part/ch114

115. METHYLMALONIC ACID

Anthony M. Angelow

PHYSIOLOGY REVIEW

Methylmalonic acid (MMA) is a dicarboxylic acid, which is a breakdown product of protein, fat, and cholesterol metabolism. The amino acids valine, methionine, threonine, and isoleucrine in addition to certain fatty acids and cholesterol are converted to propionyl-CoA through a variety of metabolic processes. Propionyl-CoA is converted into methylmalonyl-CoA. Vitamin B12 is a cofactor, which influences the conversion of methylmalonyl-CoA to succinyl-CoA. Succinyl-CoA is an intermediate in the Krebs cycle (also known as the citric acid cycle). Since vitamin B12 is necessary for the conversion of methylmalonyl-CoA to succinyl-CoA, a lack of vitamin B12 will inhibit this conversion. Methylmalonyl-CoA is then converted to MMA. MMA is commonly used for the detection and evaluation of macrocytic anemia secondary to cobalamin (vitamin B12) deficiency and congenital methylmalonic acidemia, which is seen specifically in infants.[1-3]

OVERVIEW OF LABORATORY TESTS

Laboratory evaluation of MMA can be achieved via serum, plasma, and urine measurements. Elevated MMA levels are recognized in the serum/plasma and, when elevated, MMA is also excreted from the kidneys, causing increased MMA levels in the urine. The most common evaluation of MMA levels is the serum plasma evaluation of MMA. Methylmalonic acid quantitative serum or plasma (CPT code 83921) is readily available and can be obtained through a venipuncture blood drawn with other laboratory specimens. There is also the option of measuring MMA levels using the methylmalonic acid quantitative urine specimen (CPT code 83921). Laboratory analysis of MMA is commonly evaluated with serum homocysteine levels (CPT code 83090) to further evaluate the presence of a macrocytic anemia.[3] When combined with serum homocysteine levels, MMA has a 99.8% sensitivity and specificity for vitamin B12 deficiency.[4,5]

INDICATIONS

Screening
- The U.S. Department of Health and Human Services recommends universal screening of MMA at birth to assess for the presence of methylmalonic acidemia.[3]
- MMA is considered a second-line test for detection of vitamin B12 deficiency so targeted screenings are typically done using serum vitamin B12. See Box 115.1 for risk factors for vitamin B12 deficiency.[4,5]

Box 115.1: Risk Factors of Vitamin B12 Deficiency

- Family history of vitamin B12 deficiency
- Autoimmune disease
- Type 1 diabetes mellitus
- Crohn's disease
- Human immunodeficiency virus
- Gastric surgery requiring removal of the stomach or areas of the small intestine
- Strict vegan diets (rare)
- Exclusively breastfed infants of vegan mothers
- Taking any of the following medications/substances:
  - Colchicine
  - Chloramphenicol
  - Ethanol
  - Histamine 2 receptor antagonists
  - Metformin
  - Proton pump inhibitors

Diagnosis and Evaluation

- Symptoms/signs of B12 deficiency are:[4-6]
  - Megaloblastic anemia and mild pancytopenia
  - Hypersegmented neutrophils
  - Increased levels of indirect bilirubin and lactate dehydrogenase (LDH)
  - Decreased level of haptoglobin
  - Pallor
  - Weakness
  - Fatigue
  - Sensations of pins and needles
  - Paresthesia
  - Glossitis
  - Palpitations
  - Mouth ulcers
  - Breathlessness
  - Dizziness
  - Mood changes (depression, psychosis, irritability)
  - Anorexia
  - Weight loss
  - Walking and vision problems
- Evaluate MMA in infants with unexplained signs of sepsis, acidosis, ketosis, hypoglycemia, hyperglycemia, and neutropenia.[1,6]
- The differential diagnoses for folate deficiency are broad and based on the initial presenting signs/symptoms.

Monitoring

- Serum MMA may be measured every 3 to 6 months to monitor for effectiveness of vitamin B12 replacement therapy.[2]

INTERPRETATION

- Normal value[2] of 40 nmol/mL or lower.
- Vitamin B12 deficiency
  - Serum MMA greater than 40 nmol/mL
  - Serum vitamin B12 lower than 200 to 300 pg/mL
  - Homocysteine greater than 13 mmol/L (females) and greater than 15 mmol/L (males)
- Methylmalonic acidemia
  - Serum MMA greater than 40 nmol/mL (typically will be severely increased)
- Laboratory values will vary based on laboratory.
- Serum B12 is the first-line test for assessing biochemical/functional deficiencies. MMA is second line to help clarify uncertainties like borderline levels. When vitamin B12 is low, MMA is elevated.[5]
- MMA is a more sensitive test than serum B12 for evaluating vitamin B12 status.[4]
- In the clinical scenario where the patient has borderline B12 deficiency results, the clinician should order homocysteine and MMA testing. Homocysteine and MMA are both elevated in B12 deficiency while only homocysteine, and not MMA, is elevated in folate deficiency[7]

- A mean corpuscle volume (MCV) value greater than 115 fL is more specific to vitamin B12 or folate deficiency than other conditions in the differential diagnosis such as hypothyroidism or myelodysplastic syndrome.

FOLLOW-UP

If methylmalonic acidosis is suspected, an evaluation of bicarbonate levels, urine ketones, blood ammonia levels, and glucose levels should also be evaluated.[6]

- For the evaluation of vitamin B12 deficiency, a serum vitamin B12 level, serum folate level, and a complete blood count (CBC) should also be performed.[8]
- May consider evaluating intrinsic factor antibodies or testing for *Helicobacter. pylori* infection with the presence of macrocytic anemias.[8]
- Rule out the presence of folic acid deficiency.[8]
- When vitamin B12 deficiency is suspected or confirmed, evaluate for the presence of diabetes, depression, liver disease, and/or renal disease.[8]

PEARLS & PITFALLS

- MMA evaluation is useful in detecting early and subclinical vitamin B12 deficiency before vitamin B12 levels begin to decrease.[1,2,4,6,9]
- Homocysteine levels increase with both vitamin B12 deficiency and folate deficiency; however, MMA levels only increase with vitamin B12 deficiency and are not affected by folate deficiency.
- MMA levels are not reliable in older adults, who may commonly suffer from vitamin B12 deficiency. In addition, 5% to 15% have a baseline increased MMA level. Over the age of 70 years MMA has a lower specificity for vitamin B12 deficiency.
- Newborns are screened for methylmalonic academia at birth since signs and symptoms of this inherited disorder will not present until the newborn begins to ingest proteins.
- The presence of renal insufficiency may also increase serum MMA levels, which are not indicative of vitamin B12 deficiency.

PATIENT EDUCATION

- https://www.urmc.rochester.edu/encyclopedia/content.aspx?contenttypeid=167&contentid=methylmalonic_acid_blood
- https://www.healthline.com/health/methylmalonic-acid-test

RELATED DIAGNOSES AND ICD-10 CODES[2,10]

Vitamin B12 deficiency	E53.8
Vitamin B12 deficiency anemia	D51
Vitamin B12 deficiency anemia due to selective vitamin B12 malabsorption with proteinuria	D51.1
Transcobalamin II deficiency	D51.2
Other dietary vitamin B12 deficiency anemia	D51.3

Other vitamin B12 deficiency anemias	D51.8
Vitamin B12 deficiency anemia, unspecified	D51.9
Methylmalonic acidemia	E71.120

REFERENCES

Full list of references can be accessed through Springer Publishing Company Connect™ at the following link: http://connect.springerpub.com/content/reference-book/978-0-8261 -8843-4/part/part03/toc-part/ch115

---

116. NEWBORN SCREENING PANELS

Rosie Zeno

PHYSIOLOGY REVIEW

Newborn screening (NBS) aims to identify infants at high risk for congenital disorders that are associated with irreversible morbidity and mortality but for which early diagnosis and intervention can improve outcomes.[1] The conditions identified through laboratory testing include 33 heritable disorders causing dysfunction in an array of metabolic, hematologic, endocrine, immune, and/or exocrine functions that are not typically apparent at birth. Some disorders will become clinically evident over the course of days while others may not fully manifest for months or years.

OVERVIEW OF LABORATORY TESTS

The Health and Human Services (HHS) Advisory Committee on Heritable Disorders in Newborns and Children (ACHDNC) urges state public health NBS programs to screen all neonates for 35 congenital disorders on the national Recommended Uniform Screening Panel (RUSP).[2] Approved RUSP conditions are selected based on evidence supporting the potential net benefit of screening and the availability of effective therapies.[2,3] Core conditions are divided into four categories: metabolic disorders (organic acid, fatty acid oxidation, and amino acid disorders), endocrine disorders, hemoglobin disorders, and other disorders (Table 116.1).[2-4]

Laboratory analysis of a dried blood spot specimen (DBS) (HCPCS Level II code S3620) detects analytes for 33 of the 35 core disorders. Capillary blood samples are obtained via heelstick (CPT code 36416), collected on NBS-specific filter paper cards, and transported to a central state NBS laboratory for analysis.[5-7] Measurement of biomarkers for heritable metabolic disorders is performed on DBS specimens by tandem mass spectrometry (MS/MS). Flow

TABLE 116.1: RECOMMENDED UNIFORM SCREENING PANEL METABOLIC, ENDOCRINE, HEMOGLOBIN, AND OTHER DISORDERS

METABOLIC: ORGANIC ACID CONDITIONS

Propionic acidemia*

Methylmalonic acidemia (methylmalonyl-CoA mutase)*

Methylmalonic acidemia (cobalamin disorders)

Isovaleric acidemia*

3-Methylcrotonyl-CoA carboxylase deficiency

3-Hydroxy-3-methyglutaric aciduria*

Holocarboxylase synthase deficiency*

β-Keothiolase deficiency*

Glutaric acidemia type I*

METABOLIC: FATTY ACID DISORDERS

Carnitine uptake defect/carnitine transport defect

Medium-chain acyl-CoA dehydrogenase deficiency*

Very long-chain acyl-CoA dehydrogenase deficiency*

Long-chain L-3-hydroxyacyl-CoA dehydrogenase deficiency*

Trifunctional protein deficiency*

METABOLIC: AMINO ACID DISORDERS

Argininosuccinic aciduria*

Citrullinemia, type I*

Maple syrup urine disease*

Homocystinuria

Classic phenylketonuria

Tyrosinemia, type I

ENDOCRINE DISORDERS

Primary congenital hypothyroidism

Congenital adrenal hyperplasia*

HEMOGLOBIN DISORDERS

S,S disease (sickle cell anemia)

S, βeta-thalassemia

S,C disease

OTHER DISORDERS

Biotinidase deficiency

Cystic fibrosis

Classic galactosemia*

Glycogen storage disease type II (Pompe)

Critical congenital heart disease (CCHD)**

Severe combined immunodeficiencies

Mucopolysaccharidosis type 1

X-linked adrenoleukodystrophy

Spinal muscular atrophy

Hearing loss**

* Time-critical disorders.

** RUSP disorders screened by a point-of-care procedure rather than DBS analysis.

injection analysis (FIA) and ultra-performance liquid chromatography (UPLC) MS/MS methods produce rapid results with high sensitivity, but the specificity of UPLC-MS/MS is superior.[8]

INDICATIONS

Screening

In the United States, universal NBS is mandated and administered at the state level. Each state determines which conditions will be coded on the state NBS panel and whether newborns will receive one or two screens. As of 2019,

13 states required that a second DBS be routinely collected regardless of the results of the first screen to improve the specificity and minimize false negatives for conditions not detectable on the initial screen.[9] All state NBS programs screened for at least 30 disorders on the RUSP, and six programs screened for all 35 disorders.[6]

■ The ACHDNC routinely evaluates and recommends disorders to be included on the RUSP as well as goals for timeliness of specimen collection and result reporting. Timeliness goals include the following:[10-12]
  ● Initial NBS specimens should be collected in an appropriate time frame for the infant's condition but no later than 48 hours of life.
  ● DBS for NBS should be received as soon as possible but ideally within 24 hours of collection.
  ● All NBS tests should be conducted within the first 7 days of life. Results should be reported to the clinician as soon as possible.
    ■ Presumptive positive results for time-critical disorders should be reported immediately, but no later than 5 days of life (see Table 116.1 for time-critical disorders).
    ■ Presumptive positive results for non-time-critical disorders should be reported immediately, but no later than 7 days of life.
■ DBS should be obtained as close to hospital discharge as possible to permit maximum accumulation of abnormal analytes in the infant's blood and higher likelihood of obtaining a positive result if disease is present.
■ NBS programs individualize screening protocols for premature and critically ill neonates. Delayed screening puts the infant at risk for irreversible morbidity or mortality from an identifiable condition amenable to treatment. However, the risk must be balanced with the increased risk of false-positive results for amino acid and acylcarnitine profiles, especially for neonates receiving parenteral nutrition.[13]
■ If NBS cannot be confirmed for infants born out of the hospital, NBS should be offered at the first routine wellness visit. Clinicians should contact their state public health NBS program for state-specific screening protocols.

Clinicians should be familiar with ongoing policy changes and state-specific requirements for disorders screened, systems processes, and follow-up for out-of-range results. The Newborn Screening Technical assistance and Evaluation Program (NewSTEPs) is funded through a cooperative between the Association of Public Health Laboratories (APHL) and the Genetics Services Branch of the U.S. Health Resources and Services Administration (HRSA). NewSTEPs provides data, both technical and educational resources, for strengthening and improving NBS programs nationally: https://www.babysfirsttest.org/newborn-screening/states

Diagnosis and Evaluation
■ In addition to 35 core disorders, the RUSP lists 26 secondary disorders that can be detected in the differential diagnosis of a core disorder (Table 116.2)[2-4]

TABLE 116.2: RUSP SECONDARY CONDITIONS DETECTED IN THE DIFFERENTIAL DIAGNOSIS OF A CORE DISORDER

METABOLIC: ORGANIC ACID CONDITIONS

Methylmalonic acidemia with homocystinuria	2-Methylbutyrylglycinuria
Malonic acidemia	3-Methylglutaconic aciduria
Isobutyrylglycinuria	2-Methyl-3-hydroxybutyric aciduria

METABOLIC: FATTY ACID DISORDERS

Short-chain acyl-CoA dehydrogenase deficiency	2,4 Dienoyl-CoA reductase deficiency
Medium/short-chain L-3-hydroxyacyl- CoA dehydrogenase deficiency	Carnitine palmitoyltransferase type I deficiency
Glutaric acidemia type II	Carnitine palmitoyltransferase type II deficiency
Medium-chain ketoacyl-CoA thiolase deficiency	Carnitine acylcarnitine translocase deficiency

METABOLIC: AMINO ACID DISORDERS

Argininemia	Biopterin defect in cofactor biosynthesis
Citrullinemia, type II	Biopterin defect in cofactor regeneration
Hypermethioninemia	Tyrosinemia, type II
Benign hyperphenylalaninemia	Tyrosinemia, type III

HEMOGLOBIN DISORDERS

OTHER DISORDERS

Various other hemoglobinopathies	Galactoepimerase deficiency
	Galactokinase deficiency
	T–cell-related lymphocyte deficiencies

Monitoring

- The NBS panel is not recommended for routine monitoring. Disorder-specific analytes should be monitored according to the applicable evidence-based guidelines once confirmatory testing establishes a diagnosis and/or treatment is initiated.

INTERPRETATION

- NBS detects biomarkers for numerous disorders. The results identify which newborns require further testing, not definitive confirmation of diagnosis. Results are reported as:
  - In-range, negative, normal, or low risk
  - Out-of-range, positive, abnormal, or high risk
  - Borderline, inconclusive, or medium risk
- Positive or equivocal NBS results warrant prompt follow-up. Confirmatory testing is imperative and should be performed as soon as possible.[14] Primary care clinicians are responsible for ensuring that NBS has been completed and all positive or equivocal results have been followed up until a diagnosis is confirmed or ruled out.[15]

- Negative results do not rule out the possibility of a disorder. Remain vigilant for signs and symptoms of heritable disease in the newborn and repeat testing as soon as possible if the clinical evaluation and family history raise clinical suspicion.
- The rate of false-positive results is highest in preterm infants born prior to 32-weeks' gestation who are screened for congenital hypothyroidism (CH) and adrenal hyperplasia before 48 hours of life.[16]
- Ethnic variables can affect false-positive rates for Black (glutaric acidemia type 1), Hispanic (methylamalonic acidemia), and White infants (very long-chain acyl-CoA dehydrogenase deficiency and ornithine transcarbamylase deficiency).[17]
- A higher rate of false-positive results has been reported in neonates receiving total parenteral nutrition (TPN).[18]
- False-negative results are more likely in premature infants, infants who were tested at fewer than 24 hours of age, and in infants who received blood transfusions or dialysis therapy.[14]
- NBS testing should be repeated when indicated by clinical symptoms and false-negative results are suspected.
- The state NBS laboratory may require repeat DBS collection and analysis for unsatisfactory specimens due to collection or transport errors.[6]

FOLLOW-UP

Common disorders detected by NBS include the following conditions and consideration for follow-up testing:[14,19,20]

- Metabolic disorders
  - Biochemical markers may indicate a possible enzyme defect in one of the metabolic pathways. Abnormal results may require multiple types of testing including analyte concentrations, enzyme function, and DNA sequencing.
- Hemoglobin disorders
  - Diagnostic testing includes a complete blood count (CBC) (microcytosis) and hemoglobin electrophoresis to differentiate normal and abnormal types of hemoglobin. Some hemoglobinopathies may be difficult to establish before 1 year of life once the conversion from fetal to adult hemoglobin is complete. Presumptive treatment should not be delayed.
  - DNA testing is often necessary to diagnose and characterize a thalassemia.
- Endocrine disorders
  - CH and congenital adrenal hyperplasia (CAH) can have multiple etiologies and varying degrees of severity. Prompt hormone replacement by 1 month of age can improve outcomes, but the diagnosis requires multiple stages of diagnostic testing including thyroid-stimulating hormone (TSH), FT, T4, and 17-hydroxy-progesterone as indicated. Clinical identification of consistent syndromic features is also necessary.

- Cystic fibrosis (CF)
  - Sweat chloride testing by iontophoresis is the diagnostic gold standard for CF.
  - Genotyping for CTFR mutations aids in diagnosis when sweat chloride testing is equivocal to differentiate between carrier and affected status.
  - Some states routinely perform a two-tier test which includes genotyping for two CTFR mutations.
- Severe combined immunodeficiency (SCID)
  - SCID includes genetic conditions characterized by low or absent functional T-cells. Overlapping conditions may be differentiated by genotyping and/or clinical monitoring.

PEARLS & PITFALLS

- The RUSP includes screening for congenital hearing loss (CHL) and critical congenital heart disease (CCHD). These conditions are screened by point-of-care procedures rather than laboratory testing.
  - CHL is screened via an otoacoustic emissions (OAE) and/or auditory brainstem response (ABR) testing depending on state protocol. Neonates should be screened by 1 month of age, with confirmation testing and/or medical intervention by 3 months of age.[21]
  - CCHD is screened by pulse oximetry measurements in the upper and lower extremities. Oxygen saturation of 95% or more in both extremities is required to pass. Failing or equivocal results should be repeated for confirmation.[22]

PATIENT EDUCATION

- https://www.babysfirsttest.org/

RELATED DIAGNOSES AND ICD-10 CODES

Abnormal findings on neonatal screening	P09
Most common disorders detected by NBS are CHL and CCHD[20]	
Unspecified hearing loss	H90.0
Unspecified sensorineural hearing loss	H90.5
Congenital malformations of adrenal gland	Q89.1

REFERENCES

Full list of references can be accessed through Springer Publishing Company Connect™ at the following link: http://connect.springerpub.com/content/reference-book/978-0-8261-8843-4/part/part03/toc-part/ch116

117. OXCARBAZEPINE

Carol D. Campbell

PHYSIOLOGY REVIEW

Oxcarbazepine (Trileptal) 10,11-Dihydro-10-oxo-5H-dibenz(b, f)azepine-5-carboxamide was developed to improve the pharmacokinetic profile and decrease medication interactions of its structural analogue carbamazepine.[1,2] It has U.S. Food and Drug Administration (FDA) approval for the treatment of partial seizures in children (ages 4 and older) and adults with epilepsy and can be used as monotherapy or as an adjunct with other anticonvulsants. It acts as a voltage-gated sodium channel blocker and minimally induces the CYP450 system by weakly inducing CYP3A4 and CYP3A5 and inhibiting CYP2C19. It is readily absorbed in the body, then rapidly and almost completely metabolized in the liver to its 10-monohydroxy active metabolite, monohydroxy derivative (MHD). Clearance from the body is primarily through reduction in ketones and O-site conjugation by glucuronic acid. The half-life of oxcarbazepine is approximately 2 hours, while that of MHD is approximately 9 hours.

OVERVIEW OF LABORATORY TEST

Laboratory evaluation of oxcarbazepine can be assessed by oxcarbazepine metabolite, serum (CPT code 80183). Liquid chromatography and tandem mass spectrometry are the techniques used to determine the serum level. An oxcarbazepine metabolite serum level should be ordered to determine the significance of potential or suspected medication interactions when making medication dosage adjustments to assess adherence to treatment and to assess for potential toxicity.[3]

INDICATIONS

Screening
Universal and targeted screenings are not indicated.

Diagnosis and Evaluation
■ Oxcarbazepine therapy should be evaluated in the treatment of partial seizures in epilepsy.[3,4]Additionally, evaluate when oxcarbazepine is used off label for treatment of neuropathic pain and bipolar disorder.[5]
■ Long-term use of oxcarbazepine has been associated with coordination abnormalities, decreased bone mineral density, fatigue, fractures, gait disturbances, osteopenia, osteoporosis, psychomotor slowing, and speech or language problems.[6,7]
■ Signs and symptoms of oxcarbazepine toxicity include anticholinergic effects, drowsiness, hyponatremia, life-threatening arrhythmias, nausea and vomiting, seizures, and coma.[1,8]

Monitoring

- The FDA recommends genetic prescreening for the HLA-B*15:02 allele before prescribing carbamazepine to patients of Asian genetic heritage as those positive for HLA-B*15:02 may be at increased risk for Stevens-Johnson syndrome/toxic epidermal necrolysis (SJS/TEN).[9] The FDA does not recommend prescreening for oxcarbazepine. However, there are warnings and precautions to avoid oxcarbazepine in HLA-B*15:02 positive individuals due to the risk of SJS/TEN unless the benefits clearly outweigh the risks.[1]
- High levels of evidence (systematic reviews) recommend therapeutic drug monitoring (TDM) may be beneficial for patients receiving oxcarbazepine therapy to optimize treatment outcomes, to help in assessing adherence to treatment in the context of breakthrough or uncontrolled seizures, to determine the significance of potential or suspected medication interactions, in diagnosing toxicity, and in renal insufficiency.[3,4]
- Monitor serum levels for achievement of a steady state after initiating oxcarbazepine therapy, changing dosages, switching to another medication formulation, and substituting a generic brand.[3,4]
- Monitoring of trough levels is recommended to maintain consistency.[3]
- TDM may be particularly beneficial with children and adolescents, older adults, in pregnancy, in individuals with intellectual disabilities, and in renal insufficiency.[4]
- Thyroid function tests should be monitored as oxcarbazepine therapy can decrease total and free T4 levels (T3 and TSH are generally unaffected), which has been attributed to increased metabolism of T4 due to liver enzyme induction.[1] These effects would also be consistent with central hypothyroidism, via a disruption of the hypothalamic-pituitary axis.
- Hyponatremia may develop but will likely develop in the first 3 months of therapy so sodium should be monitored.
- Both kidney and hepatic disease can prolong the elimination of oxcarbazepine, which can lead to accumulation and clinical toxicity, affect the protein binding, alter the distribution, and slow the metabolism of oxycarbazepine.
- Review Table 117.1 for additional information and monitoring considerations.

INTERPRETATION

- The generally accepted oxcarbazepine metabolite reference interval is between 10 and 35 mcg/mL. However, response to oxcarbazepine is variable, and reference ranges should be individualized for each patient as they are not always correlated with therapeutic response.[3,4]
- Table 117.2 provides the generally acceptable guidelines for interpretation of oxcarbazepine levels

FOLLOW-UP

- As noted in Table 117.1, CBC, LFTs, renal function, electrolytes (sodium), thyroid function, T_3, T_4, TSH, urinalysis, BUN, height, and weight should be ordered monthly for the first 3 months, then annually.

TABLE 117.1: RECOMMENDED MONITORING FOR OXCARBAZEPINE THERAPY

Initial monitoring	CBC, LFTs, renal function, electrolytes, thyroid function: T_3, T_4, TSH, urinalysis, BUN, height, weight
Monthly monitoring for 3 months then annually	CBC, LFTs, renal function, electrolytes (sodium), thyroid function: T_3, T_4, TSH, urinalysis, BUN, height, weight
Oxcarbazepine monitoring	Check oxcarbazepine level • If initiating therapy, every 2 to 4 weeks when increasing dosage • If changing oxcarbazepine dosages, switching to another medication formulation, or substituting a generic brand • If nonadherence, side effects, or toxicity suspected

BUN, blood urea nitrogen; CBC, complete blood count; LFTs, liver function tests; TSH, thyroid-stimulating hormone.

Sources: Data from Hiemke C, Bergemann N, Clement HW, et al. Consensus guidelines for therapeutic drug monitoring in neuropsychopharmacology: update 2017. *Pharmacopsychiatry.* 2018;51(1–2):9–62. doi:10.1055/s-0043-116492; Schoretsanitis G, Paulzen M, Unterecker S, et al. TDM in psychiatry and neurology: a comprehensive summary of the consensus guidelines for therapeutic drug monitoring in neuropsychopharmacology, update 2017; a tool for clinicians. *World J Biol Psychiatry.* 2018;19(3): 162–174. doi:10.1080/15622975.2018.1439595.

TABLE 117.2: INTERPRETATION FOR OXCARBAZEPINE

TEST	REFERENCE INTERVAL
Oxcarbazepine	10–35 mcg/mL
Metabolite toxicity	>35 mcg/mL

Sources: Data from Hiemke C, Bergemann N, Clement HW, et al. Consensus guidelines for therapeutic drug monitoring in neuropsychopharmacology: update 2017. *Pharmacopsychiatry.* 2018;51(1–2):9–62. doi:10.1055/s-0043-116492; Schoretsanitis G, Paulzen M, Unterecker S, et al. TDM in psychiatry and neurology: a comprehensive summary of the consensus guidelines for therapeutic drug monitoring in neuropsychopharmacology, update 2017; a tool for clinicians. *World J Biol Psychiatry.* 2018;19(3):162– 174. doi:10.1080/15622975.2018.1439595.

PEARLS & PITFALLS

- Warnings and precautions for oxcarbazepine include hyponatremia, anaphylactic reactions and angioedema, cross hypersensitivity reaction to carbamazepine, SJS and TEN, association with HLA-B*1502, suicidal behavior and ideation, withdrawal of anticonvulsants, cognitive and neuropsychiatric adverse reactions, drug reaction with eosinophilia and systemic symptoms (DRESS)/multi-organ hypersensitivity, hematologic events, seizure control during pregnancy, and risk of seizure aggravation.[1]
- The most significant risk with oxcarbazepine is hyponatremia, which will most often occur in the first 3 months of therapy but can occur later.[10]
- The most common side effects of oxcarbazepine are abnormal gait, abnormal vision, ataxia, diplopia, dizziness, fatigue, dizziness, headache, nausea, nystagmus tremor, somnolence, and vomiting.[2]
- Oxcarbazepine should be avoided in the first trimester of pregnancy as it can cause growth deficiencies, fetal malformations, and developmental delays. Although, with its teratogenicity being considered significantly lower than other anticonvulsants, it is a preferred anticonvulsant in pregnancy.[2]

- Folate supplementation should be initiated in females of childbearing age with those on oxcarbazepine therapy receiving at least 0.4 mg per day.[11]
- Oxcarbazepine appears to be well tolerated and safe to use in older adults.[12]

PATIENT EDUCATION

- https://medlineplus.gov/druginfo/meds/a601245.html

RELATED DIAGNOSES AND ICD-10 CODES

Partial seizures   G40.209

REFERENCES

Full list of references can be accessed through Springer Publishing Company Connect™ at the following link: http://connect.springerpub.com/content/reference-book/978-0-8261 -8843-4/part/part03/toc-part/ch117

118. PARATHYROID HORMONE

Jane Faith Kapustin

PHYSIOLOGY/PATHOPHYSIOLOGY REVIEW

Parathyroid hormone (PTH) is polypeptide hormone that is responsible for controlling serum calcium levels within a relatively narrow and constant range.[1,2] PTH is secreted from the four parathyroid glands located adjacent and behind the thyroid gland. The parathyroid glands continuously regulate serum calcium levels via a feedback mechanism. When serum-ionized calcium levels are high, the parathyroid glands secrete less PTH or even stop producing it; when low calcium levels are detected, the parathyroid glands will secrete additional PTH, causing mobilization of calcium from the bone and kidney.[1] PTH also indirectly influences increased absorption of calcium from food by converting vitamin D from an inactive to active form.[3] A figure reviewing this process is found in Chapter 121 (see Figure 121.1). Abnormal calcium levels are often discovered incidentally during routine laboratory monitoring, prompting the clinician to order a PTH level to help determine the cause.[2]

PTH is elevated in most cases of primary hyperparathyroidism (PHPT) that is almost always associated with one or multiple parathyroid adenoma(s) that secrete inappropriately large amounts of PTH, ultimately leading to mobilization of calcium from the bone. If not corrected, this can lead to osteopenia or osteoporosis. Other complications associated with PHPT include nephrolithiasis, fragility bone fractures, cardiac abnormalities, fatigue, and nausea.[4] Definitive treatment for PHPT is surgical removal of the parathyroid adenoma(s).[5,6]

In secondary hyperparathyroidism, PTH becomes elevated in chronic kidney disease as a result of low calcium levels, stimulating the feedback mechanism that will try to regulate calcium levels. Early in the course of kidney disease, PTH and fibroblast growth factor 23 (FGF23) are elevated along with a decrease in 1, 25 dihydroxy vitamin D (calcitriol). In later stages, phosphorus levels rise, and vitamin D will decrease.[7] Another cause of secondary hyperparathyroidism is related to malabsorption following gastric bypass surgery. The resultant hypocalcemia and hypophosphatemia, if long-term, can lead to secondary hyperparathyroidism.[8]

OVERVIEW OF LABORATORY TESTS

PTH (CPT code 83970) is measured through a serum sample. Older assays of PTH measured fragments of PTH and are now regarded as obsolete since second-generation ("intact PTH") and third-generation ("whole PTH") levels are far more accurate and will render more clinically relevant results.[3] Calcium and vitamin D levels are often measured in conjunction with PTH as part of the diagnostic workup for PHPT.

INDICATIONS
Screening
- PTH is not used for screening.

Diagnosis and Evaluation
- PTH is used to diagnose parathyroid disease and determine the cause of calcium abnormalities. PTH is also useful to determine the etiology of hypercalcemia and to diagnose parathyroid gland adenomas or parathyroid hyperplasia.[1]
- PTH is also used to diagnose hypoparathyroidism, a rare condition in which the PTH level is abnormally low and is usually accompanied by hypocalcemia and hypophosphatemia. The majority of cases are associated with damage to or accidental removal of parathyroid glands during thyroidectomy or autoimmune hypoparathyroidism.[9]
- Evaluate PTH when patients are initially diagnosed with osteoporosis to rule out secondary causes of bone loss such as PHPT.[12]
- Evaluate PTH when serum calcium is also elevated to evaluate for PHPT.[3]
- Evaluate PTH in patients with chronic kidney disease to evaluate for secondary HPT. With long-term chronic kidney disease, chronically low calcium levels trigger the overproduction of PTH, leading to secondary hyperparathyroidism.[7,11]
- PTH is used to guide diagnosis of conditions associated with primary and secondary hyperparathyroidism (Table 118.1) as well as hypoparathyroidism.
- PTH is used to monitor a patient's response to treatment when undergoing dialysis.

Monitoring

- Because hypoparathyroidism and resultant hypocalcemia are common complications following surgical thyroidectomy, intraoperative and postoperative PTH measurements are indicated along with calcium and vitamin D levels.[10,11]
- In the case of symptomatic parathyroid adenoma, surgical intervention, minimally invasive parathyroid surgery, is recommended as the standard of care.[12,13] Monitoring intraoperative PTH levels will be performed to guide the surgical team in determining the correct identification and removal of the abnormal parathyroid gland. PTH has a very short half-life of 5 to 10 minutes. Therefore, when the PTH level drops by 50% after a time interval of at least 10 minutes, the team is assured the correct gland with the adenoma has been removed.[3,5,6,14]
- Some patients are not surgical candidates such as in the case of pregnancy or the patient who is a poor surgical risk or refuses surgery. In those cases, monitoring of PTH and calcium levels as well as bone density tests should be assessed annually.[3,14]
- Following surgical correction of PHPT, PTH and calcium level should be monitored periodically. It is extremely rare for PHPT to recur.[5,6]
- To monitor patients on hemodialysis.

INTERPRETATION

- Intact PTH normal range: 15 to 65 pg/mL.[2]
- PTH levels should be interpreted in the context of serum calcium, magnesium, phosphorus, vitamin D, and urine calcium levels in order to determine appropriate related etiology. Consider the general guide shown in Table 118.2.[1,5–9]

TABLE 118.1: COMMON CAUSES OF PRIMARY HPT AND SECONDARY HPT	
PRIMARY HYPERPARATHYROIDISM	**SECONDARY HYPERPARATHYROIDISM**
Parathyroid tumor (s)	Chronic kidney disease (long-term CKD 4, dialysis)
MEN type 1 or 2	Gastric bypass surgery/banding (long-term complication, malabsorption)
Lithium	Celiac disease (severe, decades long)
	Crohn's disease (severe, decades long)
	Vitamin D deficiency (severe)

HPT, hyperparathyroidism; MEN, multiple endocrine neoplasia.

Sources: Data from Drueke TB. Hyperparathyroidism in chronic kidney disease. 2018. https://www.ncbi.nlm.nih.gov/books/NBK278975/; National Institute of Diabetes and Digestive and Kidney Diseases. *Primary Hyperparathyroidism.* https://www.niddk.nih.gov/health-information/endocrine-diseases/primary-hyperparathyroidism; Smit MA, van Kinschot CMJ, van der Linden J, van Noord C, Kos S. Clinical guidelines and PTH measurement: does assay generation matter? *Endocr Rev.* 2019;40(6):1468. doi:10.1210/er2018-00220; Wilhelm SM, Wang TS, Ruan DT, et al. The American Association of Endocrine Surgeons guidelines for definitive management of primary hyperparathyroidism. *JAMA Surg.* 2016;151(10):959–968. doi:10.1001/jamasurg.2016.2310.

TABLE 118.2: PTH AND CALCIUM RELATIONSHIP

PTH LEVEL	SERUM CALCIUM LEVEL	VITAMIN D	PHOSPHORUS	INTERPRETATION
High	High	May be normal or low	Normal or low	Parathyroid gland producing too much PTH. Consider primary hyperparathyroidism
High	Low	Usually low	Usually high (kidney unable to remove)	Secondary hyperparathyroidism due to advanced kidney disease
Low	High	Normal to high	Usually low	Nonparathyroid hypercalcemia. Consider neoplasia
Low	Low	Usually low	High	Hypoparathyroidism
Normal	Low	Usually low	High	Nonparathyroid hypocalcemia. Consider hypoalbuminemia

FOLLOW-UP

- Calcium, phosphorus, vitamin D, and magnesium are helpful follow-up tests to determine the etiology of abnormal PTH levels.
- Urine calcium levels may be evaluated if familial hypocalciuric hypercalcemia (FHH) is suspected.[3]

PEARLS & PITFALLS

- The old mnemonic "bones, stones, abdominal moans, and psychiatric moans" was used to help recall the clinical syndrome of PHPT. However, with increased routine testing of calcium, PHPT is now more commonly diagnosed when patients present with hypercalcemia and are asymptomatic.[3]
- Vitamin D replacement is recommended in PHPT since it will lower PTH levels without raising calcium further.[14]
- Elevated calcium levels can cause vague symptoms for patients such as sense of fogginess, unclear thinking, fatigue, muscle weakness, nausea, and vomiting.[3]
- PTH is adversely affected by high intake of biotin so patients should be cautioned to cease intake at least 72 hours before sample collection.[13]
- Some drugs that may influence the PTH levels include phosphates, anticonvulsants, steroids, rifampin, lithium, isoniazid, and diuretics.
- Parathyroid cancers may be associated with MEN-1 (multiple endocrine neoplasia syndrome 1) and familial hyperparathyroidism.[15]

PATIENT EDUCATION

■ https://www.niddk.nih.gov/health-information/endocrine-diseases/
primary-hyperparathyroidism

RELATED DIAGOSES AND ICD-10 CODES

Hypercalcemia	E83.52	Secondary hyperparathyroidism of renal origin	N25.81
Primary hyperparathyroidism	E21.0	Osteoporosis (without fracture)	M81
Secondary hyperparathyroidism	E21.1	Osteoporosis without pathologic fracture	81.8
Other hyperparathyroidism	E21.2	Osteopenia	M85.8

REFERENCES

Full list of references can be accessed through Springer Publishing Company Connect™ at the following link: http://connect.springerpub.com/content/reference-book/978-0-8261 -8843-4/part/part03/toc-part/ch118

119. PERIPHERAL SMEAR

Kelly Small Casler

PATHOPHYSIOLOGY/PHYSIOLOGY REVIEW

Red blood cells (RBCs), platelets, and white blood cells (WBCs) exist within the blood in an expected quantity, shape, size, and appearance. Some abnormalities in these characteristics can be specific to certain disease states (e.g., Auer rods and leukemia) while others represent nonspecific (anisocytosis) findings. RBCs are the cells occurring in the highest quantity and should appear round and smooth. WBCs are categorized most often by the appearance or absence of granules in the cytoplasm. Those lacking granules are called agranulocytes (lymphocytes and monocytes) and those with granules are called granulocytes (neutrophils, basophils, and eosinophils). Platelets are recognized by their purple hue and absence of a nucleus.

OVERVIEW OF LABORATORY TESTS

The phrase peripheral blood smear may be used interchangeably with other terms such as blood smear scan, platelet scan, platelet estimate, blood smear review, blood smear interpretation, physician (pathologist) review of blood smear, hematomorphology evaluation, or blood smear examination without a differential. Peripheral smears (CPT code 85060) involve microscopic examination of blood components after they are smeared onto a slide and then dipped in dyes and stains to enhance visualization. Usually, 100 total cells (RBCs, WBCs, and platelets) are counted and evaluated for morphology by visual interpretation. Peripheral smears are performed to verify automated differential analyzer results that are outside expectations and can also be specifically requested by clinician order. Some laboratories have developed protocols for automatic reflex to peripheral smear listed in Box 119.1. It may be used in instances such as the first time a patient's platelets are found to be less than 100×10^9 cells/L (10^3 cells/µL) or a patient has a large deviation from their baseline.[1] It is also useful in cases of unexplained anemia, leukopenia, or thrombocytopenia and in cases of suspected inherited hematologic or lymphoproliferative disorders.

INDICATIONS

Screening
- Not used for screening

Diagnosis and Evaluation
- Used to evaluate for underlying cause of cytopenia, lymphoproliferative findings, or hemolytic anemias.[2]
- Used to evaluate suspected malignancy or stem cell disorders.[2]
- Used to evaluate for infection with microorganism that would show up on a peripheral smear (malaria, babesia, borellia, *C. perfringens*, ehrlichiosis).[2]
- Used in the evaluation of patients with a positive International Society on Thrombosis and Hemostasis Bleeding Assessment Tool score.[3]

Monitoring
- Not routinely used

INTERPRETATION

- See Tables 119.1,[4-6] 119.2,[7,8] and 119.3[9] for possible findings reported on peripheral smear and the associated diagnoses.

Box 119.1: Instances When Peripheral Smear Might Be Reflexed From an Automatic Analyzer

WBC <2 or >30 × 10^3 cells/µL	Platelet <100 or >999 × 10^3 cells/µL
HgB <8 g/dL	Lymphocytes >7 × 10^3 cells/µL
RBC >6 × 10^6 cells/µL	Monocytes >3 ×10^3 cells/µL
Eosinophils >2 × 10^3 cells/µL	Basophils >0.5 × 10^3 cells/µL
Immature granulocytes, blasts	Left shift, atypical lymphocytes

HgB, hemoglobin; RBC, red blood cell; WBC, white blood cell.

Source: Data from Gulati G, Song J, Florea AD, Gong J. Purpose and criteria for blood smear scan, blood smear examination, and blood smear review. *Ann Lab Med.* 2013;33(1):1–7. doi:10.3343/alm.2013.33.1.1.

TABLE 119.1: PERIPHERAL SMEAR INTERPRETATION FOR RED BLOOD CELL ABNORMALITIES	
FINDING	**ASSOCIATED DIAGNOSES**
RBC agglutination	Autoimmune hemolysis, cold agglutinins, mycoplasma pneumonia, infectious mononucleosis
Elliptocytes/ovalocytes	Hereditary elliptocytosis, iron deficiency, sickle cell trait, thalassemia, HbC disease, megaloblastic anemia
Rouleaux formations	Plasma cell dyscrasias and hyperproteinemias (myeloma and lymphomas), can also be artifact
Tear drop cells	Myeloproliferative/dysplastic disease, iron deficiency, beta thalassemia major
Burr cells	Uremic syndrome, liver disease, hyposplenism, phosphate or magnesium deficiency, anorexia nervosa
Sickle cells	Sickle cell anemia (only seen in sickle cell trait if exposed to hypoxia)
Fragmented RBC	Microangiopathic hemolysis, megaloblastic anemia
Nucleated RBC	Blood loss anemia, thalassemia, thermal injury, myelodysplastic syndrome, erythroleukemia, asplenia
Basophilic stifling of RBC	Disordered erythropoiesis (lead poisoning or conditions listed under nucleated RBC)
Bite cells (Heinz bodies)	Hemolysis, usually due to medications, G6PD deficiency
Polychromasia, target cells and basophilic stifling	Thalassemia
Anisocytosis and poikilocytosis	Iron deficiency anemia
Target cells	Thalassemia, HbC disease/trait, iron deficiency anemia, liver disease, post splenectomy
Acanthosis (spur cells)	Malabsorption, severe liver failure, postsplenectomy
Schistocytes	Prostatic heart valves, DIC, severe iron deficiency, anemia, burns, snake bites, renal transplant rejection, hemolytic anemias
Spherocytes	Hemolysis
Polychromasia	Hemolysis

DIC, disseminated intravascular coagulation; HbC, hemoglobin C; RBC, red blood cell.

Sources: Data from Peterson P, Blomber DJ, Rabinovitch AJ, et al. Physician review of the peripheral blood smear: when and why an opinion. *Lab Hematol.* 2001;7(4):175–179; Snyder LM, Rao LV, Wallach JB. *Wallach's Interpretation of Diagnostic Tests: Pathways to Arriving at a Clinical Diagnosis.* 2021; Swain F, Bird R. How I approach new onset thrombocytopenia. *Platelets.* 2020;31(3):285–290. doi:10.1080/09537104.2019.1 637835; Tefferi A. Anemia in adults: a contemporary approach to diagnosis. *Mayo Clin Proc.* 2003;78(10):1274–1280. doi:10.4065/78.10.1274.

FOLLOW-UP

■ Follow up testing should be based on differential diagnoses and may include coagulation studies, liver transaminases and bilirubin, iron studies/ferritin, or bone marrow biopsy.

TABLE 119.2: PERIPHERAL SMEAR INTERPRETATION FOR WHITE BLOOD CELL ABNORMALITIES

Dohle bodies	Infection, burns, toxic ingestions, aplastic anemias
Auer rods	Acute myelogenic leukemia
Smudge cell	Chronic lymphocytic leukemia
Toxic granulations, or vacuolization	Infection, leukemoid reactions
Pelger-Huët cells	Myelodysplasia
Blasts with high nuclear to cytoplasmic ratio and bluish cytoplasm or absence of cytoplasmic granules	Acute lymphoblastic leukemia
Neutrophilia with myelocytes and metamyelocytes; basophilia, eosinophilia, anemia, and thrombocytosis	Chronic myelogenous leukemia
Immature cell forms	Acute infection response or malignancies

Sources: Data from Cerny J, Rosmarin AG. Why does my patient have leukocytosis? *Hematol Oncol Clin North Am.* 2012;26(2):303–319. doi:10.1016/j.hoc.2012.01.001; Flanagan B, Keber B, Mumford J, Lam L. Hematologic conditions: leukocytosis and leukemia. *FP Essent.* 2019;485:17–23; Rao LV, Snyder LM, eds. *Wallach's Interpretation of Diagnostic Tests: Pathways to Arriving at a Clinical Diagnosis.* 11th ed. Wolters Kluwer; 2021.

TABLE 119.3: PERIPHERAL SMEAR INTERPRETATION FOR PLATELET ABNORMALITIES

Schistocytes	Thrombotic thrombocytopenic purpura
Giant platelets	Immune thrombocytopenic purpura, congenital thrombocytopenia
Howell-Jolly bodies (can also be seen in RBC)	Asplenia, lead poisoning, thalassemia, megaloblastic anemia

RBC, red blood cells.

Source: Data from Boxer M, Biuso TJ. Etiologies of thrombocytopenia in the community hospital: the experience of 1 hematologist. *Am J Med.* 2020;133(5):e183–e186. doi:10.1016/j.amjmed.2019.10.027.

PEARLS & PITFALLS

■ For timely and accurate diagnosis, consider verbal consultation with the performing facility's pathologist and hematology team regarding the differential diagnoses and rationale for ordering.

PATIENT EDUCATION

■ https://labtestsonline.org/tests/blood-smear

RELATED DIAGNOSES AND ICD-10 CODES

Cytopenia	D75.9
Other pancytopenia	D61.8

REFERENCES

Full list of references can be accessed through Springer Publishing Company Connect™ at the following link: http://connect.springerpub.com/content/reference-book/978-0-8261-8843-4/part/part03/toc-part/ch119

120. PERITONEAL FLUID ANALYSIS

Pam Kibbe and Amanda Chaney

PHYSIOLOGY/PATHOPHYSIOLOGY REVIEW

Ascites is the accumulation of peritoneal fluid in the abdominal cavity from increases in portal hypertension, decreases in colloid osmotic pressure, and increased permeability of the peritoneal capillaries.[1] If portal hypertension is present, excess antidiuretic hormone production results in salt and water retention.[1,2] Although there are many causes of ascites, 80% to 85% of patients have chronic liver disease.[1-3] Other causes include malignancy, liver disease (acute or chronic), cardiac issues (heart failure), nephrotic syndrome, pancreatitis, tuberculosis, or hypoalbuminemia, myxedema, hemoperitoneum, or urologic injury.[3-10]

OVERVIEW OF LABORATORY TESTS

In patients with ascites, performing a paracentesis (or fluid removal of the ascitic fluid) helps determine the etiology, but first an ultrasound is performed to determine the size and depth of a pocket of fluid in the abdomen that is amenable to drainage.[3] Routinely, ascitic fluid should be assessed for gross fluid appearance analysis, cell count with differential, albumin, total protein, and aerobic / anaerobic cultures.[3,11] Fluid is sent for more specific analysis based on the differential diagnosis for underlying etiology since this can assist with etiology diagnosis and guide further management.[3] For example, lactate dehydrogenase and glucose can be used to distinguish spontaneous bacterial peritonitis (SBP).[3] Table 120.1 summarizes parameters that can be assessed from peritoneal fluid.

INDICATIONS

Screening
- Not used

Diagnosis and Evaluation
- Used in the diagnosis and evaluation of suspected ascites. For any patient with new-onset ascites, a diagnostic paracentesis should be performed (guideline).[1]
- Paracentesis with fluid analysis is performed at the time ascites is diagnosed.[3]
- Paracentesis is used anytime SBP is suspected (e.g., cirrhosis + fever, abdominal pain).[3]

Monitoring
- Repeat paracentesis is recommended after 48 to 72 hours of SBP diagnosis to ensure adequate treatment.[1]

INTERPRETATION

- Interpretation is summarized in Table 120.1.

TABLE 120.1: INTERPRETATION OF PARAMETERS THAT CAN BE ASSESSED FROM PERITONEAL FLUID

PARAMETER	ASSOCIATED WITH
Amylase	Pancreatitis (if elevated)
Cytology	Malignancy (peritoneal carcinomatosis)
Bilirubin	Gallbladder perforation or post-transplant bile leak
SAAG	Portal hypertension (if >1.1 g/dL)
Cell count with differential	SBP (if >250 neutrophil/PMN cells/mm³)
Gram stain	SBP, if positive
Protein	Increased risk of SBP
Culture	SBP, if positive

PMN, polymorphonuclear; SAAG, serum-ascites albumin gradient; SBP, spontaneous bacterial peritonitis.

Sources: Data from Runyon BA. Diagnostic and therapeutic abdominal paracentesis. In: Basow D, ed. UpToDate; Runyon BA. Introduction to the revised American Association for the Study of Liver Diseases Practice Guideline management of adult patients with ascites due to cirrhosis 2012. Hepatology. 2013;57(4):1651–1653. doi:10.1002/hep.26359; Runyon BA, Hoefs JC. Culture-negative neutrocytic ascites: a variant of spontaneous bacterial peritonitis. Hepatology. 1984;4(6):1209–1211. doi:10.1002/hep.1840040619; Runyon BA, Montano AA, Akriviadis EA, Antillon MR, Irving MA, McHutchison JG. The serum-ascites albumin gradient is superior to the exudate-transudate concept in the differential diagnosis of ascites. Ann Intern Med. 1992;117(3):215–220. doi:10.7326/0003-4819-117-3-215.

- Neutrocytic ascites is defined as greater than 250 cells/mm³.
- Bacterascites is defined as presence of bacteria in ascitic fluid.
- A serum-ascites albumin gradient (SAAG) greater than 1.1 g/dL is 97% accurate for the diagnosis of portal hypertension and is highly suggestive of chronic liver disease.[1]

FOLLOW-UP

- Perform Gram stain and cultures if there is suspected SBP.[3]
- If tuberculosis infection is suspected, culture peritoneal fluid with an acid-fast bacilli culture.

PEARLS & PITFALLS

- An elevated CA-125 in serum or peritoneal fluid is nonspecific.[3,12]
- Always refer to your local organization's policy and procedure for recommendations on when/how to perform paracentesis.
- History is important in determining whether the ascites is hepatic, renal, or cardiac in origin.
- Physical examination is important in detection of the presence of ascites. Clues to ascites include flank dullness, weight gain, abdominal distention, bulging flanks, dullness to abdominal percussion, or shifting dullness (dullness as patient changes position). Patients may also have underlying signs of chronic liver disease: spider angiomas, palmer erythema, and abdominal wall collateral vein visualization.

■ Ascites associated with heart failure may be associated with jugular venous distention (JVD), peripheral edema, and pulmonary congestion.

PATIENT EDUCATION

■ https://www.niddk.nih.gov/health-information/liver-disease/cirrhosis

RELATED DIAGNOSES AND ICD-10 CODES

Ascites due to cirrhosis, alcoholic	K70.31
Spontaneous bacterial peritonitis	K65.2
Other ascites	R18.8
Ascites due to alcoholic hepatitis	K70.11
Malignant ascites	R18.0

REFERENCES

Full list of references can be accessed through Springer Publishing Company Connect™ at the following link: http://connect.springerpub.com/content/reference-book/978-0-8261 -8843-4/part/part03/toc-part/ch120

121. PHOSPHORUS

Carolyn McClerking

PHYSIOLOGY REVIEW

Phosphorus is an electrolyte that is primarily found in the skeleton where it combines with calcium to form hydroxyapatite, which causes bone hardening. Approximately 1% of phosphorus is extracellular and approximately 14% is intracellular. Low phosphorus levels result from either increased excretion, decreased absorption, or a shift of phosphorus into the cells.[1] High phosphorus levels are often seen in decreased renal function, due to difficulty excreting phosphorus. Two primary influencers of phosphorous homeostasis are parathyroid hormone and vitamin D, which act on the bones, kidneys, and intestines to influence phosphorus levels in the blood (Figure 121.1).[2]

OVERVIEW OF LABORATORY TESTS

Serum phosphorus (CPT code 84100) is evaluated in a serum blood sample. There are two forms of phosphorus in the serum: organic and inorganic. Only inorganic levels can be measured. In the serum, over 50% of phosphorus is free to act physiologically, 33% is bound to small cations, and the remainder is protein bound.[3]

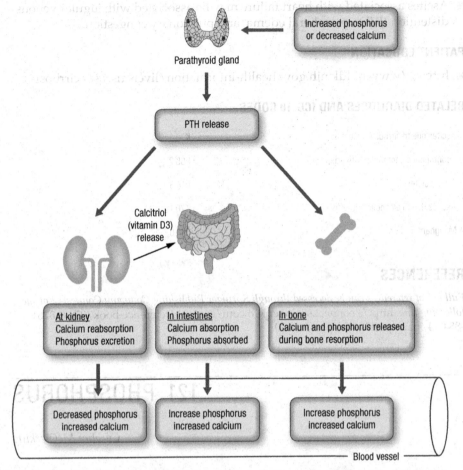

FIGURE 121.1. Parathyroid hormone (PTH) and vitamin D influence on phosphorus and calcium.
In response to increased blood phosphorus levels (or decreased calcium), PTH is released from the parathyroid glands. PTH acts on the kidney, which increases calcium reabsorption and phosphorus excretion while also releasing calcitriol, which increases phosphorus and calcium absorption in the gastrointestinal tract. PTH also acts on the skeletal system, resulting in bone resorption which increases circulating phosphorus and calcium.

INDICATIONS

Screening
- There are no universal screening recommendations for phosphorus.
- Consider targeted screening in those with risk for hypophosphatemia and hyperphosphatemia as per Table 121.1.

Diagnosis and Evaluation
- Signs and symptoms that may warrant evaluation of phosphorous levels include confusion, seizures, paralysis, muscle weakness, and anorexia.[4]

TABLE 121.1: CONDITIONS ASSOCIATED WITH HYPO- AND HYPERPHOSPHATEMIA	
HYPOPHOSPHATEMIA	**HYPERPHOSPHATEMIA**
Intestinal malabsorption	Intravenous (IV) fluids
Diuretics	Magnesium deficiency
Hypovitaminosis D	Malignant hyperthermia
Alcoholic intoxication	Postoperative status
Hyperparathyroidism	Hypoparathyroidism
Diabetic ketoacidosis	Vitamin D toxicity
Trauma	Acidosis
Burn victims	GFR ≤ 45 mL/minute/1.73 m^2
Critical-care/severe stress response	
Use of magnesium/aluminum containing antacids	

Sources: Data from Bollerslev J, Rejnmark L, Marcocci C, et al. European Society of Endocrinology Clinical Guideline: treatment of chronic hypoparathyroidism in adults. *Eur J Endocrinol.* 2015;173(2):G1–G20. doi:10.1530/EJE-15-0628; Kidney Disease: Improving Global Outcomes (KDIGO) CKD-MBD Update Work Group. "KDIGO 2017 clinical practice guideline update for the diagnosis, evaluation, prevention, and treatment of chronic kidney disease-mineral and bone disorder (CKD-MBD)." *Kidney Int Suppl.* 2017;7(1):1–59. doi:10.1016/j.kisu.2017.04.001; Padelli M. Causes, consequences and treatment of hypophasphatemia: a systemic review of the literature. *Press Med.* 2017;46(11):987–999. doi:10.1016/j.lpm.2017.09.002.

Monitoring

- If dietary phosphorus is restricted/limited as part of the management of chronic kidney disease (CKD), monitor serum phosphorus levels monthly and aim for a level in the normal reference interval.[5,6]
- With severe hypo- and hyperphosphatemia, clinicians should correct and monitor phosphorus levels frequently (exact interval not specified), especially in patients in the intensive care unit.[7]
- Patients undergoing treatment for hypo/hyperphosphatemia should have routine monitoring (exact interval not specified) with a goal for a level in the normal reference interval.[8]

INTERPRETATION

- The reference interval for phosphorus is 2.5 to 4.5 mg/dL. Reference intervals are higher in children and may vary depending on the time of blood draw as phosphorus levels fluctuate duirnally.[9]
- The differential diagnosis of levels above or below the reference interval are listed in Boxes 121.1 and 121.2. Conditions listed in Table 121.1 should also be considered.

FOLLOW-UP

Follow-up testing will vary depending on differential diagnosis. Table 121.2 lists common follow-up tests and their rationale.

Box 121.1: Differential Diagnosis of Hypophosphatemia

- Diabetic ketoacidosis with prolonged hyperventilation treatment
- Renal replacement therapy
- Intravenous hyperalimentation without phosphate supplement
- Chronic alcoholism
- Urinary wasting syndrome such as Fanconi syndrome
- Side effect of parenteral iron therapy (depends on preparation)

Sources: Data from Glaspy JA, Lim-Watson MZ, Libre MA, et al. Hypophosphatemia associated with intravenous iron therapies for iron deficiency anemia: a systematic literature review. *Ther Clin Risk Manag.* 2020;16:245–259. doi:10.2147/TCRM.S243462; Kidney Disease: Improving Global Outcomes (KDIGO) CKD-MBD Update Work Group. "KDIGO 2017 clinical practice guideline update for the diagnosis, evaluation, prevention, and treatment of chronic kidney disease-mineral and bone disorder (CKD-MBD)." *Kidney Int Suppl.* 2017;7(1):1–59. doi:10.1016/j.kisu.2017.04.001.

Box 121.2: Differential Diagnosis of Hyperphosphatemia

- Acute or chronic renal failure
- Hyperparathyroidism (will also have elevated PTH and elevated calcium)
- Hypoparathyroidism (will also have decreased PTH and decreased calcium)
- Pseudohypoparathyroidism (will also have elevated PTH and decreased calcium)
- Vitamin D toxicity (will also have elevated calcium)

PTH, parathyroid hormone.

Sources: Data from Blaine J, Chonchol M, Levi M. Renal control of calcium, phosphate, and magnesium homeostasis. *Clin J Am Soc Nephrol.* 2015;10(7):1257–1272. doi:10.2215/CJN.09750913; Kidney Disease: Improving Global Outcomes (KDIGO) CKD-MBD Update Work Group. KDIGO 2017 clinical practice guideline update for the diagnosis, evaluation, prevention, and treatment of chronic kidney disease-mineral and bone disorder (CKD-MBD). *Kidney Int Suppl.* 2017;7(1):1–59. doi:10.1016/j.kisu.2017.04.001; Mantovani G, Bastepe M, Monk D, et al. Diagnosis and management of pseudohypoparathyroidism and related disorders: first international Consensus Statement. *Nat Rev Endocrinol.* 2018;14(8):476–500. doi:10.1038/s41574-018-0042-0; Marcinowska-Suchowierska E, Kupisz-Urbanska M, Łukaszkiewicz J, Płudowski P, Jones G. Vitamin D toxicity–a clinical perspective. *Front Endocrinol.* 2018;9:550. doi:10.3389/fendo.2018.00550.

PEARLS & PITFALLS

- Low levels of phosphate, magnesium, and potassium are major risk factors for development of refeeding syndrome in the frail older adults.[10]
- Severe hypophosphatemia can result in rhabdomyolysis, specifically in children presenting with diabetic ketoacidosis; vigilant monitoring of phosphorus levels is recommended in these situations.[11]
- Hyperphosphatemia causes calcium phosphate to deposit on damaged muscle cells, which leads to hypocalcemia during rhabdomyolysis.[12,13]
- A study found no difference in serum phosphorus levels in patients on hemodialysis, regardless of race or socioeconomic status.[14]
- Hyperphosphatemia is an independent risk factor for mortality in patients presenting to the emergency department.[15]
- High phosphorus levels are associated with all-cause mortality in older adult males with chronic obstructive pulmonary disease (COPD) and cardiovascular disease, raising the question of whether to evaluate levels based on sex.[16]
- Both increased and decreased phosphorus levels are associated with risk of all-cause mortality in dialysis-dependent renal patients.[17]

TABLE 121.2: ADDITIONAL LABORATORY TESTS TO FURTHER EVALUATE CAUSE FOR ABNORMAL PHOSPHORUS LEVELS

LABORATORY TEST	DIFFERENTIAL DIAGNOSIS/RATIONALE
Thyroid-stimulating hormone	Thyroid abnormalities
Creatinine kinase, urine myoglobin	Rhabdomyolysis
Parathyroid hormone-related peptide (PTHrHP)*	Hypercalcemia-related neoplasia
Serum calcium, magnesium, and potassium	Evaluate for other electrolyte abnormalities that are common with hypo/hyperphosphatemia
Blood urea nitrogen (BUN)/creatinine	Chronic or acute kidney problem
Intact PTH	Hyper- or hypoparathyroidism
Vitamin D	Vitamin D deficiency or toxicity

*Not needed unless calcium is also elevated.

Sources: Data from Bollerslev J, Rejnmark L, Marcocci C, et al. European Society of Endocrinology Clinical Guideline: treatment of chronic hypoparathyroidism in adults. *Eur J Endocrinol.* 2015;173(2):G1–G20. doi:10.1530/EJE-15-0628; Kidney Disease: Improving Global Outcomes (KDIGO) CKD-MBD Update Work Group. KDIGO 2017 clinical practice guideline update for the diagnosis, evaluation, prevention, and treatment of chronic kidney disease-mineral and bone disorder (CKD-MBD). *Kidney Int Suppl.* 2017;7(1):1–59. doi:10.1016/j.kisu.2017.04.001; Padelli M. Causes, consequences and treatment of hypophasphatemia: a systemic review of the literature. *Press Med.* 2017;46(11):987–999. doi:10.1016/j.lpm.2017.09.002.

- In the setting of hypophosphatemia, older adults can develop osteomalacia and be at risk for fractures.[18]
- Pseudo hyperphosphatemia is a falsely elevated phosphorus level caused by paraproteinemia, which is related to such conditions as Waldenstrom macroglobulinemia, monoclonal gammopathy of unknown significance (MGUS), or multiple myeloma.[8]
- Failure to take phosphorus binding medications in patients on chronic dialysis can lead to hyperphosphatemia.[19]

PATIENT EDUCATION

- https://www.kidneyfund.org/kidney-disease/chronic-kidney-disease-ckd/complications/high-phosphorus/

RELATED DIAGNOSES AND ICD-10 CODES

Phosphatase deficiency; acid phosphatase, phosphate	E83.39
Disorder of phosphorus metabolism, unspecified	E83.30
Familial hypophosphatemia	E83.31
Hereditary vitamin D-dependent rickets (type 10, type 2)	E83.32

REFERENCES

Full list of references can be accessed through Springer Publishing Company Connect™ at the following link: http://connect.springerpub.com/content/reference-book/978-0-8261-8843-4/part/part03/toc-part/ch121

122. PLATELETS AND MEAN PLATELET VOLUME

Kelly Small Casler

PHYSIOLOGY REVIEW

Platelets, also called thrombocytes, are derived from megakaryocytes in the bone marrow and are produced in response to thrombopoietin, which is produced in the liver.[1] Platelets assist with hemostasis and the coagulation cascade by forming platelet plugs. When released from the bone marrow, immature platelets are initially larger and contain more ribonucleic acid than mature platelets.[2] Excess platelets are stored in the spleen.[3]

OVERVIEW OF LABORATORY TESTS

Platelets are measured through automated laboratory methods. Alternatively, they can be counted manually on a peripheral smear. Mean platelet volumes (MPV) may be reported along with platelet number as part of the complete blood count (CBC) and reflects the mean size of the platelets.[3] Platelet size (and thus, MPV) increases when increased production of platelets is required.[2] The platelet distribution width (PDW) is reported by some laboratories and reflects the amount of variation in platelet size. When elevated, it can signal enlarged or giant platelets.[2] Immature platelet fraction (IPF) can be assessed to evaluate bone marrow function. A low IPF suggests bone marrow dysfunction and a lack of platelet formation/release, while a high IPF suggests functioning bone marrow with an excessive loss of mature platelets.[2]

INDICATIONS

Screening
- Generally not used for screening.

Diagnosis and Evaluation
- Used in the evaluation of fatigue, petechiae, purpura, hemorrhage, or easy/excessive bleeding or bruising.
- Used in the evaluation of anemia to assist in ruling out hemorrhage/bleeding as a cause of anemia.

Monitoring
- Used in routine monitoring in chemotherapy along with white blood cell (WBC) count. Exact monitoring intervals vary.[4]
- Used for monitoring of any platelet disorder.
- Used for monitoring of cirrhosis severity/complications.

INTERPRETATION

- Reference interval, platelets[5]: 150 to 440 × 10^3 cells/µL (or 10^9 cells/L)
- Thrombocytosis refers to an elevated number of platelets and thrombocytopenia refers to decreased platelet numbers. The differential diagnoses for these conditions are listed in Table 122.1
- Reference interval, MPV[5]: 7.8 to 11.0 fL
  - Increased MPV may be seen in cardiovascular disease, diabetes, chronic kidney disease, idiopathic thrombocytic purpura, myeloproliferative disease, hyperthyroidism, preeclampsia, connective tissue disease, or inflammatory bowel disease.[3,5,6]
  - Decreased MPV can be seen in aplastic anemia, viral infections, cytotoxic drugs, autoimmune conditions, and sepsis.[3,5]

FOLLOW-UP

- If reactive thrombocytopenia or thrombocytosis is suspected, confirm counts return to normal after the inciting event has resolved.
- Peripheral smear is useful to help in the differential diagnosis of thrombocytosis or thrombocytopenia. Most laboratories have protocols for automatic confirmation of thrombocytopenia through a peripheral

TABLE 122.1: DIFFERENTIAL DIAGNOSIS OF ABNORMAL NUMBER OF PLATELETS

THROMBOCYTOPENIA	THROMBOCYTOSIS
Pseudo thrombocytopenia: Platelet clumping in EDTA tube (use sodium citrate instead)	Medications, especially prednisone
Splenic sequestration/hypersplenism	Immune disease
Liver disease	Myeloproliferative disorders/malignancy
Sepsis and other critical illness	Trauma
Infection (reactive thrombocytopenia)	Hemolysis or blood loss
Immune thrombocytopenia purpura	Iron deficiency anemia
Thrombotic thrombocytopenic purpura	Functional (sickle-cell disease) or post-operative asplenia
Heparin-induced thrombocytopenia	Polycythemia vera
Leukemia and myelodysplasias	Acute infection/inflammation (sometimes called reactive thrombocytopenia)
Medications	
Alcohol abuse	
Autoimmune disease	
Hemolytic uremic syndrome	
Disseminated intravascular coagulation	
HELLP syndrome	
Systemic lupus erythematosus	
Gestational thrombocytopenia	
Preeclampsia	
Antiphospholipid syndrome	

EDTA, ethylenediaminetetraacetic acid; HELLP, hemolysis, elevated liver enzyme levels, and low platelets.

Sources: Data from ACOG Practice Bulletin No. 207: thrombocytopenia in pregnancy. *Obstetrics & Gynecology.* 2019;133(3):e181–e193. doi:10.1097/AOG.0000000000003100; Boxer M, Biuso TJ. Etiologies of thrombocytopenia in the community hospital: the experience of 1 hematologist. *Am J Med.* 2020;133(5):e183–e186. doi:10.1016/j.amjmed.2019.10.027; Snyder LM, Rao LV, Wallach JB. *Wallach's Interpretation of Diagnostic Tests: Pathways to Arriving at a Clinical Diagnosis.* 2021; Swain F, Bird R. How I approach new onset thrombocytosis. *Platelets.* 2020;31(3):285–290. doi:10.1080/09537104.2019.1637835.

smear and manual evaluation.[7] Table 122.2 summarizes possible findings regarding platelets on peripheral smear.

- Lactate dehydrogenase can assist with evaluation for hemolysis, malignancy, or myelodysplastic syndrome.[7]
- Blood urea nitrogen, creatinine, and glomerular filtration rate are used to evaluate renal function, as renal function impairment is seen with some hereditary thrombocytopenias.[7]
- In suspected hemolysis or hemorrhage, prothrombin time/International Normalized Ratio and partial thromboplastin time should be evaluated.[7]
- In suspected immune thrombocytopenic purpura (ITP), a direct antibody test (Coombs' test) should be ordered to evaluate for co-occurring autoimmune hemolytic anemia.[7]
- In suspected ITP, perform testing for human immunodeficiency virus, hepatitis C virus, and thyroid disorders to rule out these common causes of secondary ITP.[7]
- Bilirubin, albumin, and liver enzymes are helpful to rule out underlying liver disease when thrombocytopenia is noted.[7]
- Platelet antibody studies may be used to evaluate for autoimmune causes of thrombocytopenia.[7,8]
- In rare instances, bone marrow biopsy may be needed to differentiate between decreased platelet production or increased platelet destruction as the cause of thrombocytopenia.[7,9]

PEARLS & PITFALLS

- Remembering that thrombocytopenia is caused by decreased platelet production, increased platelet destruction, dilution, or redistribution (pooling as seen in hypersplenism) will help guide the differential diagnosis.[1,9]
- Platelet count less than 10×10^3 cells/μL is most often used as a trigger for transfusion of platelets.[10]

TABLE 122.2: CLUES TO CAUSE(S) OF THROMBOCYTOPENIA BASED ON PERIPHERAL SMEAR	
DIFFERENTIAL DIAGNOSIS[7]	**CORRESPONDING SIGNS**
ITP, drug-induced thrombocytopenia, liver disease, congenital thrombocytopenia	Peripheral blood smear normal or may have large platelets only
Thrombotic microangiopathies (HUS, DIC, HELLP, TTP)	Red cell fragmentation on smear; other laboratory tests will be suggestive of hemolysis
Reactive thrombocytopenia (bacterial/viral illness or critically ill)	Leukocytosis, sudden platelet drop, toxic granulation
Bone marrow disorder	Blast cells, dysplasia, tear drop cells, nucleated red blood cells

DIC, disseminated intravascular coagulation; HELLP, hemolysis, elevated liver enzyme levels, and low platelets; HUS, hemolytic uremic syndrome; ITP, immune thrombocytic purpura; TTP, thrombotic thrombocytopenic purpura.

■ Pseudothrombocytopenia is not uncommon and occurs when the EDTA used for anticoagulant in hematology tubes causes platelet clumping. This problem can be identified through peripheral smear; for this reason, specimens are often automatically reflexed to peripheral smear in response to thrombocytopenia.[5]

■ MPV results may be inaccurate in the setting of abnormal specimen collection and storage techniques or patient use of anticoagulants.[5]

■ MPV does vary with race, sex, and ethnicity, so clinicians should use reference intervals supplied by their partner laboratory.[3]

■ MPV is helpful in differentiating between genetic platelet disorders and guiding further genetic testing.[7]

■ Elevations/depressions in red blood cells and WBCs along with platelets should prompt consideration of hematologic malignancy.[2]

■ Consider referral to hematology for platelet counts lower than 100 × 103 cells/μL.[7]

■ Platelets may be reported in amounts either ×10^9 cells/L or ×10^3 cells/μL. The conversion between the two measurements is a 1:1 ratio. If the clinician would like to convert this to total number of platelets per cubic millimeter of blood (mm^3), they can add three zeroes to the number. For example, 150 × 10^3 cells/μL (10^9 cells/μL) is 150,000 total platelets per mm^3.

PATIENT EDUCATION

■ https://medlineplus.gov/lab-tests/platelet-tests/

RELATED DIAGNOSES AND ICD-10 CODES

Primary thrombocytosis	D47.3
Qualitative platelet defect	D69.1
Thrombocytopenia, unspecified	D69.9

REFERENCES

Full list of references can be accessed through Springer Publishing Company Connect™ at the following link: http://connect.springerpub.com/content/reference-book/978-0-8261-8843-4/part/part03/toc-part/ch122

123. PLEURAL FLUID ANALYSIS

Olga Amusina, Sarah Fitz, Leah Burt, and Susan Corbridge

PHYSIOLOGY REVIEW

The pleural cavity is a space formed by a double layer of parietal and visceral pleura. Metabolically active cells secrete pleural fluid into the cavity, and the parietal pleura drains it into local lymph nodes, leaving about 10 mL of fluid in the normal pleural space to maintain negative pressure and ensure lubrication.[1] Imbalance between fluid production and reabsorption leads to development of pleural effusions. Pleural effusions can be broadly classified as exudates or transudates. In exudative effusions, protein-rich fluid leaks around the capillaries into the pleural cavity due to a proinflammatory state or pleural hemorrhage when the rate of fluid production overwhelms the lymphatic drainage system.[1] In transudative effusions, low protein fluid is accumulated due to increased capillary permeability, as seen in heart failure or low oncotic pressure states. Overall, more than 50 disorders within the lung, pleura, and other organ systems are associated with pleural effusions (Figure 123.1).[2]

OVERVIEW OF LABORATORY TESTS

Therapeutic interventions for patients with pleural effusions are planned based on fluid etiology. Imaging and pleural fluid analysis including Light's criteria are helpful in establishing the diagnosis. The following tests are performed on pleural fluid: cell count (CPT code 89051); biochemistry (pH [CPT code 83986], glucose [CPT code 82945], total protein [CPT code 84157], LDH [CPT code 83615]); Gram stain with cultures (CPT code 87070); and cytology by direct smear slide analysis (CPT code 88104) (requires 75 mL of fluid) or cell block (CPT code 88305) (requires greater than 150 mL of fluid).[3]

INDICATIONS

Screening

■ There is no recommendation for universal or asymptomatic screening. There are no known recommendations for routine screening of all patients who develop a pleural effusion; however, appropriate cancer screening and recommended age-specific screening laboratory work should be initiated.

Diagnosis and Evaluation

■ Indications to obtain pleural fluid include the presence of new pleural effusion amenable to drainage, provided benefits outweigh the risks of the procedure. The exception is heart failure, which should first be managed with medical therapy, including diuretics.

■ All fluid should be tested at the time of thoracentesis or intrapleural catheter placement unless repeat drainage with known etiology is performed.

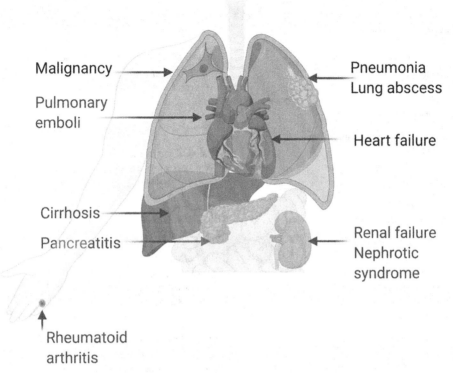

Malignancy

Pulmonary
emboli

Pneumonia
Lung abscess

Heart failure

Cirrhosis

Pancreatitis

Renal failure
Nephrotic
syndrome

Rheumatoid
arthritis

FIGURE 123.1. Common conditions causing pleural effusions and associated body systems.

- Refer to Table 123.1[4–6] for a list of conditions associated with pleural effusions. There are many other potential causes of unspecified fluid collections including injuries: drowning, electrical burn, or those that are drug-induced.
- The patient's symptoms, history, environmental exposures (especially asbestos), medications, and substances, combined with physical examination, inform differential diagnosis.[4]
- Some patients are asymptomatic; however, the most common symptoms include dyspnea, cough, chest pain, fever, weight gain/loss, or fatigue.[5]
- Physical examination consistent with diminished breath sounds with dullness on percussion is concerning for the presence of a pleural effusion. A combination of ultrasound imaging, pleural fluid analysis, and the overall clinical picture will assist in differential diagnosis and help to establish a definitive plan for fluid management.
- The most common cause of right-sided or bilateral pleural effusions is a transudate due to decompensated heart failure. Second most common are malignant pleural effusions,[1] with the most common diagnoses being non-small cell lung cancer and lymphoma.[7]
- One-third of all pleural effusions are exudative effusions due to chest infections and are labeled as noncomplicated, complicated parapneumonic effusions, or an empyema.[5] Empyema can be culture negative. *Streptococcus pneumoniae, Streptococcus intermedius* complex, *Streptococcus anginosus,*

TABLE 123.1: CAUSES OF EXUDATIVE AND TRANSUDATIVE EFFUSIONS FROM MORE TO LESS COMMON WITH LATERALITY

EXUDATE	TRANSUDATE
Malignant effusion: • Primary lung adenocarcinoma • Lymphoma • Metastatic breast and gynecologic malignancies • Mesothelioma	Heart failure (typically bilateral or right side): • Both HFrEF/HFpEF • Less common in right-sided heart failure
Empyema, parapneumonic effusion (typically unilateral): • Bacterial/fungal/viral/parasitic • Tuberculosis	Renal: • Uremia, decompensated renal failure • Peritoneal or hemodialysis patients (up to 20%) • Nephrotic syndrome
Pulmonary emboli (in up to 30% of all patients)	Liver: • Hepatic hydrothorax in liver cirrhosis (typically, right side; can be bilateral)
GI diseases: • Pancreatitis, typically left side • Intraabdominal abscesses • Abdominal surgery • Esophageal perforation	Endocrine/Nutrition: • Hypoalbuminemia • Myxedema coma - bilateral • Ovarian stimulation therapy, right side or bilateral
Inflammatory pleurisy/pleuritis: • Viral • Post MI/CABG/ablation - Dressler syndrome	Pulmonary Hypertension: • Superior vena cava syndrome • Drug-induced when medication causes pulmonary edema
Substance/medication-induced: • Asbestos benign • Drug-induced with or without ILD, unilateral or bilateral	
Connective tissue disorder: rheumatoid arthritis (less than 4%), systemic lupus erythematosus (unilateral or bilateral in up to 40% cases), other types of vasculitis	Trapped lung (unilateral): • Lung no longer fully re-expands with drainage; fluid fills the space
Thoracic duct injury or lymphangioleiomyomatosis (LAM) and chylothorax	

Sources: Data from Bintcliffe OJ, Lee GYC, Rahman NM, Maskell NA. The management of benign non-infective pleural effusions. *Eur Respir Rev.* 2016;25(141):303–316. doi:10.1183/16000617.0026-2016; Camus P. *The Drug-Induced Respiratory Disease Website.* Pneumotox On Line. Updated 2020. https://www.pneumotox.com/drug/index/; Light RW. Pleural effusions. *Med Clin North Am.* 2011;95(6):1055–1070. doi:10.1016/j.mcna.2011.08.005; Noppen M, De Waele M, Li R, et.al. Volume and normal cellular composition of pleural fluid in humans examined by pleural lavage. *Am J Resp Crit Care Medicine.* 2000; 162:1023–1026. doi:10.1183/09031936.04 .00079304.

Staphylococcus aureus, anaerobic infections (Bacteroides/Fusiform), and gram-negative bacilli are the most frequent pathogens.

■ Up to 30% of all effusions are multifactorial, and 12% are idiopathic.[5]

■ Overall, nonmalignant effusions due to other organ failure—such as heart failure, end-stage renal failure, and liver disease—have poor prognoses and may be refractory to therapy.[7]

Monitoring

■ Monitoring does not apply.

INTERPRETATION

Follow a stepwise approach to determine the etiology of pleural fluid (Figure 123.2):

1. Analyze the fluid appearance and cell count (Table 123.2).[8,9] By itself, it is nondiagnostic.
2. Use Light's criteria to classify fluid composition by exudate and transudate (Table 123.3).[2,10] Exudates must meet at least one characteristic, whereas transudates do not meet any. There are exceptions; values well above the cutoff parameters will likely allow for a higher degree of confidence in making an accurate diagnosis.
3. If an exudative effusion is present, determine the cause using common and special characteristics, cultures, and cytology (Table 123.4).
4. Review Gram stain/culture to inform antimicrobial therapy.
5. Positive cytology indicates a malignant effusion. Average cytology and flow cytometry combined has a positivity rate of 60% to 68%.[2,3]
6. Review advanced pleural fluid assays (triglycerides, amylase, cholesterol, creatinine, N-terminal pro-brain natriuretic peptide [NT-BNP], adenosine deaminase [ADA]), Il-27, and IGRA based on clinical index of suspicion.
7. If a transudative effusion, still consider send-off of fluid cytology during initial evaluation.

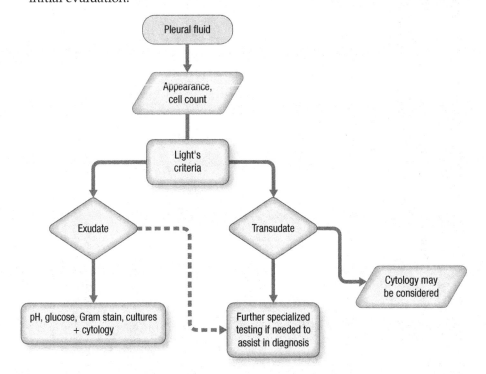

FIGURE 123.2. The decision-making process for basic pleural fluid interpretation.

TABLE 123.2: APPEARANCE/CELL COUNT AND COMMON FLUID ETIOLOGY

PARAMETER	NORMAL	EMPYEMA	HEART FAILURE	MALIGNANCY	HEMOTHORAX	COMMENTS
Appearance	Light, straw-colored	Cloudy, purulent, malodorous, air can be present	Light yellow, straw-colored or bloody	Frankly bloody, brown	Bloody	In chylothorax: cloudy milky, if fasting serosanguinous
Red blood cells	None				>100,000 >50% of serum hematocrit	
Neutrophils	<2%	>1000 (in acute) or low from debris	<1000	Can be high due to inflammation		
Lymphocytes	25%			>50%		Chronic effusions and TB are lymphocyte-predominant
NLR (ANC/ALC) Neutrophil to lymphocyte ratio		>7%		0.4%–9%		Used for prognosis in malignancy
Eosinophils	<2%, high with air in pleural space			None or up to >10%		Drug reaction (IL-2, MTX), repeat thoracentesis
Hematocrit					>50% of serum	
nT-pro-BNP			>1,500 pg/mL			

Sources: Data from Bibby AC, Dorn P, Psallidas I, et al. ERS/EACTS statement on the management of malignant pleural effusions. *Eur Respir J.* 2018;52(1):1800349. doi:10.1183/13993003.00349-2018; Hooper C, Lee Y, Maskell N. Investigation of unilateral pleural effusion in adults: British Thoracic Society pleural disease guideline 2010. *Thorax.* 2010;65: ii18–ii31. doi:10.1136/thx.2010.136986; Light RW. Pleural effusion. *N Engl J Med.* 2002;346(25):1971–1977. doi:10.1056/NEJMcp010731; Light RW. Pleural effusions. *Med Clin North Am.* 2011;95(6):1055–1070. doi:10.1016/j.mcna.2011.08.005; Noppen M, De Waele M, Li R, et al. Volume and normal cellular composition of pleural fluid in humans examined by pleural lavage. *Am J Resp Crit Care Medicine.* 2000; 162:1023–1026. doi:10.1183/09031936.04.00079304.

TABLE 123.3: LIGHT'S CRITERIA: FLUID BIOCHEMISTRY TO DETERMINE TRANSUDATE VS. EXUDATE

	EXUDATE—MUST MEET AT LEAST ONE OF THE CRITERIA	SENSITIVITY (%)	SPECIFICITY (%)
Pleural fluid LDH (U/L)	>200 or >2/3 of the serum upper normal value	78	95
Pleural fluid LDH to serum LDH ratio	>0.6	86	88
Pleural fluid protein to serum protein ratio	>0.5	90	83

LDH, lactate dehydrogenase.

Sources: Data from Light RW. Pleural effusions. *Med Clin North Am.* 2011;95(6):1055–1070. doi:10.1016/j.mcna.2011.08.005; Light RW, MacGregor MI, Ball WC Jr, Luchsinger PC. Pleural fluid lactic acid dehydrogenases and protein content. *Ann Intern Med.* 1972;76:880. doi:10.7326/0003-4819-76-5-880_2

TABLE 123.4: "LIKELY PATHOGNOMONIC" BIOCHEMISTRY FINDINGS IN EXUDATIVE FLUID

	pH	GLUCOSE mg/dL *	LDH	OTHER
Empyema/ parapneumonic	<7.2	<60	Three times upper limit	Malodor, + Gram stain, and cultures
Malignancy	Wide range	Variable	Two to three times upper limit	
Rheumatoid arthritis, connective tissue	<7.2	<30	Two times upper limit	
GI-related			Elevated	High amylase in pancreatitis or esophageal perforation
Chylothorax				Triglycerides >110 mg/dL

*Low pleural fluid glucose is also found in hypoglycemia.

LDH, lactate dehydrogenase.

Sources: Data from Bintcliffe OJ, Lee GYC, Rahman NM, Maskell NA. The management of benign non-infective pleural effusions. *Eur Respir Rev.* 2016;25(141):303–316. doi:10.1183/16000617.0026-2016; Light RW. Pleural effusion. *N Engl J Med.* 2002;346(25): 1971–1977. doi:10.1056/NEJMcp010731; Light RW. Pleural effusions. *Med Clin North Am.* 2011;95(6):1055–1070. doi:10.1016/j. mcna.2011.08.005; Light RW, MacGregor MI, Ball WC Jr, Luchsinger PC. Pleural fluid lactic acid dehydrogenases and protein content. *Ann Intern Med.* 1972;76:880. doi:10.7326/0003-4819-76-5-880_2

FOLLOW-UP

Serum chemistry testing (bloodwork) must accompany pleural fluid analysis, and specific advanced testing may be indicated. Routine serum tests include LDH, total protein, glucose, hematocrit, and BNP. Results are interpreted and compared to corresponding pleural fluid values to assist in diagnosis.

Fluid retesting is typically not recommended unless a new disease process is considered or in suspected malignant effusions to increase the yield of the diagnosis. A second sample sent for cytology may increase yield of a positive diagnosis by up to 27%.[11]

In positive cytology, immune and tumor markers may be added. Advanced testing includes triglycerides, amylase, cholesterol, creatinine, N-terminal pro-brain natriuretic peptide (NT-BNP), IL-27, interferon gamma release assay (IGRA), and adenosine deaminase (ADA) to assist further with diagnosis.[8,11–14]

PEARLS & PITFALLS

- Presence of bilateral, near equal in size pleural effusions in the right clinical setting typically indicate a transudate due to heart failure or another organ dysfunction. Pleural fluid drainage for analysis is only recommended if fluid persists despite medical management.
- In up to 20% of cases, Light's criteria erroneously identified pleural fluid as an exudate, typically due to diuretic therapy.
- If clinical suspicion of heart failure is high, measuring pleural fluid NT-BNP or BNP is suggested. Pleural fluid BNP greater than 1,500 pg/mL is consistent with the diagnosis of transudative effusion due to heart failure.
- A constellation of recent pneumonia, pleuritic pain, fever, and leukocytosis should always lead to evaluation for the presence of pleural effusion. If identified, consider pleural drain placement, fluid analysis, and broad-spectrum antimicrobial therapy without a delay.
- Always send the fluid sample from the existing pleural drain for cultures during the procedure and not later to assure best specimen quality for analysis.
- If the cause of exudative effusion is not determined and the patient is not improving, consider pulmonary embolism (PE). About 20% to 40% patients with PE and pleuritic pain have pleural effusions.[2]
- In areas with endemic TB or in patients with acute febrile illness and lymphocyte-predominant fluid, ADA, IL-27, and IGRA (commercially available as QuantiFERON-TB and T-SPOT) can be sent off (2). TB PCR is considered a gold standard since acid-fast bacilli (AFB) positivity rate is only 10% to 20%. ADA less than 40 U/L suggests against TB diagnosis.[13]
- Large volume effusion, hemorrhagic fluid, NLR scores of 9.0 or higher, and LDH greater than 1,500 are associated with worse prognosis in malignant effusions.[3]

PATIENT EDUCATION

- https://www.nationaljewish.org/conditions/pleural-effusion
- https://patient.info/chest-lungs/pleural-effusion-leaflet

RELATED DIAGNOSES AND ICD-10 CODES

Nonmalignant pleural effusion	J90
Malignant pleural effusion	J91

REFERENCES

Full list of references can be accessed through Springer Publishing Company Connect™ at the following link: http://connect.springerpub.com/content/reference-book/978-0-8261-8843-4/part/part03/toc-part/ch123

124. POTASSIUM TESTING FOR SKIN CONDITIONS

Retha D. Gentry and Lisa E. Ousley

PHYSIOLOGY REVIEW

Fungal Infections of the Skin, Hair, and Nails

Dermatophytosis or tinea is caused by a variety of fungi, and primarily infects the stratum corneum, the outer layer of the epidermis. These fungal infections are named based on the area of the body that is affected. Because infection is generally limited to the outermost skin layer, little inflammation is present. The pattern of infection is visible as outward growth from the center.[1] Infrequently, a deeper dermophyte infection may descend into the dermis via the hair follicles creating inflammatory lesions.[2] Fungi can also infect the outer surface of the hair shaft (ectothrix) or penetrate into the hair shaft (endothrix).[2] Tinea capitis occurs most commonly in childhood and is more common in males before puberty and females after puberty.[1] Tinea capitis is more common in Black children, but Black adults may have a lower incidence of tinea.[5] Dermophytes, yeast, and molds cause *tinea unguium*, or onychomycosis—infection of the nails. The nail infection most commonly begins from the dorsal surface (inside the nail) with a yellow white discoloration created from accumulation of hyperkeratotic debris within the nail plate.[1,3] Onychomycosis is directly correlated with age and may be related to decreased blood flow. Up to 50% of adults in the United States age 75 and older have onychomycosis.[4]

Scabies

Scabies is a contagious infection caused by infestation of the *Sarcoptes scabiei* mite. The female mite, responsible for infestation, burrows into the stratum corneum, laying two to three eggs per day for 1 to 2 months. The burrows appear as light brown streaks. The inflammatory process is caused by the burrowing and the fecal matter left behind.[5] The mites are not visible to the human eye. The skin lesions are either at the site of infestation or secondary to hypersensitivity to the mite.[1] Scabies lesions in infants and young children are more likely on palms, soles, head, back, neck, and face.[3] In older children and adults, scabies lesions appear as tiny vesicles between fingers, on the volar wrist, on the thenar or hypothenar hand, or on the ankles.

OVERVIEW OF LABORATORY TESTS

The potassium hydroxide test, commonly referred to as the KOH mount, is a common office test to determine the presence of fungi. "In experienced hands, a KOH mount is one of the most useful procedures in medical mycology and has been proven more reliable than culture for demonstration of dermatophytes."[6]

KOH microscopy (CPT code 87220) is the easiest, most cost-effective method of examination; it has the highest sensitivity to identify fungal infections of the skin, hair, and nails, and of scabies infestations.[1,7,8] KOH mount is a gold standard for diagnosing onychomycosis.[7]

The direct microscopic examination uses both low power magnification (×10) and low intensity of light or higher magnification (×40) for increased illumination. For fungal infections of the skin, the results are available in minutes.[6] Potassium hydroxide, also known as *lye or caustic potash*, is an inorganic compound used in the wet mount preparation for microscopic visualization of fungal spores or hyphae in skin, hair, nails, and vaginal secretions.[9] KOH (10% to 30%) alkaline solution separates and destroys the stratum corneum cells, thus dissolving keratin that has been scraped from the outer layer of the skin, hair shaft, or nail. This allows the microscopic visibility of dermatophytes or scabies.[2,7,10,11]

INDICATIONS

The KOH mount is indicated for individuals with suspected fungal infection of skin, hair, and nails or scabies infestation.

Screening

Universal and targeted screenings are not recommended or applicable.

Diagnosis and Evaluation

Table 124.1 describes the key clinical practice recommendations for diagnosing fungal infections. Signs and symptoms of fungal infections of the skin depend on the location. If it is on the head (i.e., tinea capitis), there can be hair loss, pruritus, erythema, or dry, scaly areas on the scalp. Tinea found on the body (i.e., tinea corporis, commonly referred to as ringworm) presents as an erythematous, ring-shaped patch with centralized clearing. It is typically found on the trunk, extremities, or buttocks. There may be more than one patch and patches can overlap. They may itch. When these patches are found in the groin area, they are called tinea cruris or jock itch. There is typically a reddened area of skin in the creases of the groin that spreads up the upper thighs. It

TABLE 124.1: KEY RECOMMENDATIONS FOR PRACTICE

CLINICAL RECOMMENDATION	EVIDENCE RATING*
Tinea can be diagnosed based on clinical presentation, but a KOH mount or culture should be performed if appearance is atypical.	C
Onychomycosis should be confirmed with a KOH mount, culture, or periodic acid–Schiff stain before starting treatment.	C

*A, consistent, good-quality patient-oriented evidence; B, inconsistent or limited-quality patient-oriented evidence; C, consensus, disease-oriented evidence, usual practice, expert opinion, or case series. SORT evidence rating system.

Source: Ely JW, Rosenfeld S, Stone MS. Diagnosis and management of tinea infections. *Am Fam Physician*. 2014;90:702–711.

causes pruritus and some dry, flaky skin. Tinea of the feet (i.e., tinea pedis or athlete's foot) causes a scaly, red rash that starts between the toes and itches. It can cause erosions or scales if the rash is more severe or goes untreated. Tinea can also occur on the hands (i.e., tinea manuum) but is less common.[8] Refer to Table 124.2 for common differential diagnoses for fungal skin infections.

Differential Diagnoses for Onychomycosis and Scabies
Onychomycosis (nails)

- Psoriasis
- Lichen planus
- Trauma
- Herpetic whitlow
- Black nail paronychia

Scabies

- Dermatitis herpetiformis
- Dyshidrotic eczema
- Contact dermatitis
- Atopic dermatitis
- Drug-induced rash
- Xerosis

Monitoring
- Superficial fungal skin infections are expected to resolve with topical or oral treatment. Further evaluation is required for unresolved skin lesions. KOH mount is not highly specific for onychomycosis or dermatophytosis and should not be used for monitoring of treatment in these conditions.

TABLE 124.2: DIFFERENTIAL DIAGNOSIS OF FUNGAL INFECTIONS (SKIN)

TINEA CAPITIS (HEAD AND SCALP)	TINEA CORPORIS (BODY)
• Seborrheic dermatitis	• Erythema multiforme
• Alopecia areata	• Nummular eczema
• Atopic dermatitis	• Psoriasis
• Plaque psoriasis	• Urticaria
• Bacterial folliculitis Trichotillomania	• Tinea versicolor
	• Cutaneous candidiasis
	• Lupus erythematosus, subacute cutaneous
	• Cutaneous T-cell lymphoma

MANUUM, PEDIS (HANDS AND FEET)	CRURIS (GROIN)
• Erythrasma	• Erythrasma
• Dyshidrosis	• Cutaneous candidiasis
• Foot eczema	• Intertrigo
• Psoriasis	• Contact dermatitis
• Contact dermatitis	• Inverse psoriasis
• Atopic dermatitis	• Folliculitis

INTERPRETATION

Fungal Infection

■ Microscopic evaluation reveals fungal spores or hyphae which appear cylindrical, 2 to 10 mm, uniform in diameter, and resemble the branches of a tree (Figure 124.1).[6,10,12]

■ Reviewing the slide again in 30 to 60 minutes might reveal hyphae even if the initial examination was negative.[10]

Scabies

■ Microscopic examination will reveal presence of adult mites, eggs, or feces in the burrows.[1]

FOLLOW-UP

■ If the KOH mount is negative but there is clinical evidence of disease, a skin or nail culture should be obtained.[12]

■ To assess resolution of onychomycosis, it is ideal that a nail culture be performed after systemic antifungal treatment. Negative mycology and 100% clearing of the nailbed is the gold standard for resolution of a fungal infection in nails.[13]

■ If the skin or nail fungal infection is not resolved following treatment, a culture should be performed.

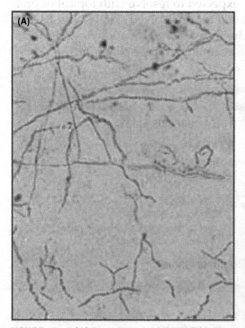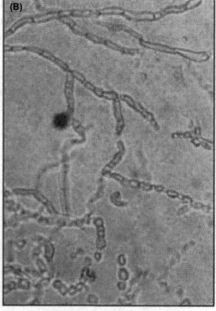

FIGURE 124.1. (A) Fungal hyphae in a KOH preparation of skin scales as seen with the 10x objective. (B) Hyphae and arthroconidia as seen with the 40x objective. *Source:* Reproduced with permission from Mackenzie, D. W. R., Philpot, C. M. (1981). Isolation and Identification of Ringworm Fungi [monograph]. *Journal of Medical Microbiology, 15.* H.M. Stationery Office, London.

- If there is no resolution of disease after treatment and the skin lesion remains, a skin biopsy would be appropriate.

PEARLS & PITFALLS

- The only way to acquire skill in KOH mounts is to repeatedly perform them.
- False-negative KOH preparations often result from inadequate scrapings.[11]
- Shield microscope slides from drafts or apply KOH to the slide before transport.[11]
- If the mount dries, add more KOH solution adjacent to the coverslip.
- The shelf life of a bottle of KOH is at least 5 years.
- KOH can damage microscope lenses.
- Avoid spills and excess KOH on the slide.[11]
- Misinterpretation of hair shafts and clothing fibers can result in false positives. The hair shafts and fibers are typically larger than hyphae without segmentation or branching. The edges between squamous cells are also mistaken for hyphae.[11]
- The KOH solution should not be applied on skin surfaces, the face, or mucous membranes.[6]
- Applying the coverslip with a little pressure to express the excess KOH evens the specimen for microscopic examination.[6]
- To avoid distortion and loss of texture for a hair mount, do not press the coverslip.[6]
- Skin and hair samples can be immediately examined under the microscope. Toenail specimens require a minimum of 10 minutes to several hours in KOH solution before examination.[11]
- Allow 30 minutes to 2 hours for KOH to penetrate thick, hyperkeratotic specimens. Hair and nail specimens may require 24 to 48 hours.[6]
- Malassezia furfur are thick-walled spherical yeast in clusters, often with short filaments resembling 'spaghetti and meatballs', characteristic of pityriasis versicolor scales.[6]
- In CLIA-approved labs, a KOH mount can generate a charge.[10]
- There is concern about spreading the infection to nearby areas while collecting a specimen.
- Collecting the specimen may be painful to patients.

PATIENT EDUCATION

- https://familydoctor.org/familydoctor/en/diseases-conditions/tinea-infections/treatment.html
- https://www.cdc.gov/fungal/diseases/ringworm/definition.html

RELATED DIAGNOSES AND ICD-10 CODES

Dermatophytosis, unspecified	B35.9	Tinea pedis	B35.3
Superficial fungal infection	B36.0	Tinea corporis	B35.4
Tinea cruris	B35.6	Tinea capitis	B35.0

| Tinea manuum | B35.2 | Onychomycosis | B35.1 |
| Tinea versicolor | B36.0 | Scabies | B86 |

REFERENCES

Full list of references can be accessed through Springer Publishing Company Connect™ at the following link: http://connect.springerpub.com/content/reference-book/978-0-8261 -8843-4/part/part03/toc-part/ch124

125. PREALBUMIN AND ALBUMIN

Janyce Cagan Agruss and Kate Sustersic Gawlik

PHYSIOLOGY REVIEW

Albumin is a water-soluble, globular protein that is produced in the liver and represents more than half of all proteins found in the blood plasma. Albumin is a transport protein that helps to carry vitamins, enzymes, and other important substances like free fatty acids and hormones.[1] It is also used as a mechanism for drug delivery.[2] In addition, it sets the plasma oncotic pressure and helps to prevent fluids from leaking out of the bloodstream and into the tissues. If the albumin level is too low, as often seen in liver and kidney diseases, fluid will go into the tissue and edema will result. This edema is often seen in the feet, ankles, hands, around the eyes, lower back, and other parts of the body. Since albumin also acts as a transport protein, when serum levels are decreased, important substances cannot get where they are needed in the body.[1]

Prealbumin, or transthyretin (TTA), is the precursor to albumin. Similar to albumin, prealbumin is also a serum transport protein that is produced in the liver. However, it is much smaller than albumin and has a shorter half-life (2 to 4 days versus 20 to 22 days). Prealbumin plays a small role in binding thyroxine and a central role in binding retinol binding protein (RBP). RBP transports vitamin A throughout the body and would be cleared through the kidney if it were not attached to prealbumin.[3] Acute illness, infection, and injury create inflammation, which causes a cytokine-mediated response, leading to increased vascular permeability. This causes a decrease in serum albumin and prealbumin, making them negative acute phase reactants (i.e., inversely associated with acute phase reactants like C-reactive protein [CRP]).[4]

Although used in the past to assess nutritional status, current evidence suggests there is a weak relationship between these serum protein levels and nutritional status. Poor nutritional intake does not consistently correlate with a decrease in albumin and prealbumin and increased nutritional intake does not necessarily increase these levels, rendering albumin and prealbumin as neither specific, nor sensitive indicators of nutritional status.[4]

OVERVIEW OF LABORATORY TESTS

Prealbumin (CPT code 84134) and albumin (CPT code 82040) are serum blood tests. The tests measure the total amount of the albumin or prealbumin in the blood. Prealbumin is an immunoturbidimetric assay and albumin uses spectrophotometry. They are often included in other laboratory panels including the comprehensive metabolic panel (CMP). Total protein (CPT code 84155) can also be ordered, which measures the total amount of proteins in the serum.

There is also a test for detecting albumin in the urine, called the urine albumin test, formerly called the microalbumin test. This test measures the amount of albumin in the urine as an early indicator of kidney damage. See Chapter 152 for more information on this test.

INDICATIONS

Screening

- Universal screenings are not currently recommended.
- Albumin and prealbumin have historically been utilized as nutrition-related serum biomarkers. As previously noted, current evidence does not support their validity in adults, older adults, or children and they are not useful in the routine evaluation of nutritional screening or nutritional status.[5–10]

Diagnosis and Evaluation

- Albumin and prealbumin are not diagnostic markers.
- They have been used as independent prognostic indicators for a number of conditions.
  - Low serum prealbumin levels were significantly associated with COVID-19 severity and poor outcomes including mortality.[11,12]
  - Low serum prealbumin levels were associated with poor prognosis in certain cancers including liver and gastric cancers.[13–15]
  - Low serum albumin has prognostic value for predicting mortality and morbidity in older adults both in the hospital and in the community dwelling setting.[16]
  - Low serum albumin in patients with pulmonary arterial hypertension is associated with disease severity and higher mortality.[17]
  - Low serum albumin levels are strongly and independently associated with kidney function decline and a poorer renal prognosis in a variety of populations.[18,19]

Monitoring

- Monitoring of albumin or prealbumin is not recommended.

INTERPRETATION

Albumin

- Normal albumin level is between 3.5 to 5.5 g/dL. This may vary based on the laboratory (Table 125.1).

Prealbumin

■ There are numerous reasons for an increase or decrease in levels of albumin or prealbumin. See Table 125.2 for some common etiologies.

TABLE 125.1: PREALBUMIN REFERENCE INTERVAL BY AGE

AGE RANGE	REFERENCE INTERVAL mg/dL*
0 to <15 days	2–12
15 days to <1 year	5–24
1 to <5 years	12–23
5 to <13 years	14–26
13 to <16 years	18–31
16 to <19 years	17–33 (females)
	20–35 (males)
Adult males	21–43
Adult females	17–34

*Will vary based on laboratory and population.

Pediatric reference values from Caliper database (https://caliperproject.ca)

TABLE 125.2: FACTORS THAT AFFECT PREALBUMIN AND ALBUMIN

FACTORS THAT INCREASE PREALBUMIN LEVELS[2,3]	FACTORS THAT DECREASE PREALBUMIN LEVELS[2,3]
• Renal dysfunction • Corticosteroid therapy • NSAIDS • Dehydration	• Times of physiological stress • Infection • Liver disease • Thyroid disease • Overhydration • Nephrotic syndrome • Acute blood loss • Malnutrition • Inflammation

FACTORS THAT INCREASE ALBUMIN LEVELS	FACTORS THAT DECREASE ALBUMIN LEVELS
• Dehydration • High protein diet • Steroids, insulin, or hormones • Severe diarrhea	• Hepatic diseases • Chronic kidney disease or nephrotic syndrome • Following weight loss surgery • Protein-losing enteropathies (crohn disease, ulcerative colitis, celiac disease) • Sepsis • Stress • Poor nutrition / low protein diets • Cardiac failure • Burns • Cachexia

FOLLOW-UP

■ Follow-up testing will vary based on the underlying condition.

PEARLS & PITFALLS

■ The focus of the nutritional assessment should be on risk factors like unintended weight loss, undernutrition, declining food/fluid intake, and slow wound healing. Body mass index, hemoglobin, and total cholesterol are useful biomarkers of malnutrition in older adults.[7,8]

PATIENT EDUCATION

■ https://medlineplus.gov/lab-tests/prealbumin-blood-test/

RELATED DIAGNOSES AND ICD-10 CODES

Other disorders of plasma-protein metabolism, not elsewhere classified	E88.09
Other disorders of glycoprotein metabolism	E77.8
Abnormality of plasma protein, unspecified	R77.9
Abnormality of albumin	R77.0

REFERENCES

Full list of references can be accessed through Springer Publishing Company Connect™ at the following link: http://connect.springerpub.com/content/reference-book/978-0-8261 -8843-4/part/part03/toc-part/ch125

126. PROGESTERONE

Brooke Rengers

PHYSIOLOGY REVIEW

Progesterone is a sex steroid essential for reproduction in females. It is primarily produced in the ovaries by the corpus luteum following ovulation in the luteal phase of the menstrual cycle. Progesterone levels peak approximately 6 to 8 days following ovulation and return to basal levels if the ovum is not fertilized. In the presence of pregnancy and once established, the placenta serves as the main source of progesterone. It is essential for maintaining the endometrium of the uterus, preventing uterine contraction, and preparing the breasts for lactation. Progesterone levels fluctuate throughout the female life course. In postmenopausal women, progesterone is no longer supplied by the ovaries, but small amounts are produced by the adrenal glands. For males, the adrenal glands and testes are responsible for the production of progesterone.[1-3]

OVERVIEW OF LABORATORY TESTS

Progesterone testing is primarily used for the detection of ovulation in females.[1] Laboratory evaluation of progesterone status can be assessed by a serum progesterone level (CPT code 84144). Serum progesterone may be measured by a variety of immunoassays and the specificity of the assay can vary.[1,4–6]

INDICATIONS

Screening

- Universal screening of serum progesterone is not supported by evidence.
- Ovulatory dysfunction may occur secondary to infertility. Collect serum progesterone during the mid-luteal phase of the menstrual cycle, or approximately day 21 of a 28-day cycle, or 1 week before anticipated menses.[7–9]
- Check serum progesterone levels in the presence of threatened miscarriage, ectopic pregnancy, or molar pregnancy.

Diagnosis and Evaluation

- Evaluate progesterone in the setting of suspected infertility, secondary amenorrhea, unexplained abnormal uterine bleeding, threatened miscarriage, ectopic pregnancy, molar pregnancy, or pregnancy of unknown origin.[1,4–6,8–12] Repeat testing may be necessary. A meta-analysis found a single serum progesterone measurement was insufficient for establishing a diagnosis.[4–6,7,11]

Monitoring

- In the case of infertility, monitoring serum progesterone coupled with other tests (e.g., cervical mucous) can indicate timing of ovulation.[7,9,13]
- May be used for ovulation assessment following ovulation induction in assisted reproduction.[1,2]

INTERPRETATION

- Normal values of serum progesterone vary between laboratories and references.[1,5,6] One set of reference intervals is provided in Table 126.1. Testing is not routinely performed on males.
- Increased levels of serum progesterone may indicate pregnancy, ovulation, progesterone-secreting ovarian tumor or cyst, congenital adrenal hyperplasia, or molar pregnancy.[14]
- Decreased levels of serum progesterone may indicate primary or secondary hypogonadism, threatened miscarriage, fetal demise, preeclampsia, or short luteal phase syndrome.[14]

FOLLOW-UP

- Consider testing of 17-hydroxyprogesterone in the presence of infertility and recurrent high serum progesterone levels. This could be a possible sign of adrenal tumor.[15]

TABLE 126.1: REFERENCE VALUES OF SERUM PROGESTERONE

MAYO CLINIC LABORATORIES[5,6]

AGE	VALUE
Males	
<4 weeks	Not established
4 weeks to < 12 months	≤0.66 ng/mL (confidence interval 0.63–0.94 ng/mL)
12 months to 9 years	≤0.35 ng/mL
≥18 years	<0.20 ng/mL
Females	
<4 days old	Not established
4 days to <12 months	≤1.3 ng/mL (confidence interval 0.88–2.3 ng/mL)
12 months to 9 years	≤0.35 ng/mL

MENSTRUAL CYCLE	VALUE
Follicular phase	≤0.89 g/mL
Luteal phase	1.8–24 ng/mL

PREGNANCY	VALUE
First trimester	11–44 ng/mL
Second trimester	25–83 ng/mL
Third trimester	58–214 ng/mL
Post-menopause	≤0.20 ng/mL

REPRODUCTIVE ENDOCRINOLOGY[1]

MENSTRUAL CYCLE	VALUE
Follicular phase	<1.5 ng/mL
Luteal phase	>7 ng/mL

PREGNANCY	VALUE
First trimester	≥40 ng/mL
Third trimester	≥150 ng/mL
Post-menopause	<0.5 ng/mL

Sources: Data from Carmina E, Stanczyk F, Lobo R. Evaluation of hormonal status. In: Strauss JF 3rd, Barbieri RL, eds. *Yen and Jaffe's Reproductive Endocrinology.* 8th ed. Elsevier; 2018:887–915; Mayo Clinic Laboratories. *Progesterone, Serum.* Mayo Clinic laboratories endocrinology catalog. https://endocrinology.testcatalog.org/show/PGSN; Piette P. The history of natural progesterone, the never-ending story. *Climacteric.* 2018;21(4):308–314. doi:10.1080/13697137.2018.1462792.

■ Serum progesterone below 10 ng/mL at 6 to 8 weeks of pregnancy may indicate a miscarriage or ectopic pregnancy. Repeat serum progesterone levels.[1]

PEARLS & PITFALLS

■ Due to the pulsatile nature of progesterone production following ovulation, a single low serum progesterone level during the mid-luteal phase is not indicative of ovulatory dysfunction.[2,7,9]
■ In one study, serum progesterone of less than 14 ng/dL in threatened miscarriage prior to 16 weeks of gestation demonstrated accuracy and reproducibility prognostic of spontaneous miscarriage.[10] However, one systematic review and meta-analysis found that serum progesterone was not useful in predicting fetal viability in patients with threatened miscarriage.[12]
■ Committee opinion from the American College of Obstetricians and Gynecologists suggests a single serum progesterone level greater than 3 ng/mL is confirmatory of ovulation.[7] Others suggest levels of 5 ng/mL or greater indicate ovulation.[8]
■ Low levels of evidence exist for serum progesterone screening and diagnostic evaluation.

PATIENT EDUCATION

■ https://www.hormone.org/your-health-and-hormones/glands-and -hormones-a-to-z/hormones/progesterone
■ https://medlineplus.gov/lab-tests/progesterone-test/

RELATED DIAGNOSES AND ICD-10 CODES

Female infertility, unspecified[5,6]	N97.9
Recurrent pregnancy loss[5,6]	N96
Amenorrhea, unspecified[5,6]	N91.2

REFERENCES

Full list of references can be accessed through Springer Publishing Company Connect™ at the following link: http://connect.springerpub.com/content/reference-book/978-0-8261 -8843-4/part/part03/toc-part/ch126

127. PROLACTIN

Jane Faith Kapustin

PHYSIOLOGY/PATHOPHYSIOLOGY REVIEW

Prolactin (PRL) is a human peptide hormone synthesized in the anterior pituitary by the lactotrophs. Secretion of PRL is inhibited by dopamine in the hypothalamus in a negative feedback loop.[1] PRL is responsible for breast epithelial cell proliferation and milk production during pregnancy and after delivery. During pregnancy, the PRL level is normally elevated to support those functions in pregnant and lactating females; the PRL level can become 10 times the normal level in pre-pregnancy. Otherwise, the PRL level is low in males and nonpregnant or lactating females.[2]

Other hormones, estrogen, and dopamine regulate the production and release of PRL. Dopamine inhibits the secretion of PRL.[3] Elevated PRL levels are needed to prepare and maintain breast milk supply in pregnancy and following birth. Suckling by the infant during lactation will cause the release of PRL from the pituitary in a feedback mechanism via a neuroendocrine reflex pathway.[1]

PRL suppresses gonadotropin-releasing hormone (GnRH) which will in turn suppress ovulation and reduce testosterone levels. When PRL is elevated (hyperprolactinemia) in a nonpregnant or nonlactating state, problems with infertility and gonadal dysfunction often result.[4]

OVERVIEW OF LABORATORY TESTS

Prolactin (CPT code 84146) can be measured from a serum sample that should be drawn after fasting. It is necessary to note the time of laboratory testing since PRL varies by Circadian cycle and is released in a pulsatile fashion. The ideal time to draw PRL is mid-morning.[2]

INDICATIONS

Screening

- There is no recommendation for routine universal screening of PRL level.
- The American Society for Reproductive Medicine does not recommend routine screening of PRL for infertility unless menstrual cycles are abnormal or galactorrhea is present.[5]

Diagnosis and Evaluation

- PRL may be used to evaluate signs/symptoms suspicious for hypo- or hyperprolactinemia (Box 127.1).

Box 127.1: Signs and Symptoms That Warrant Testing

- Adenoma detected via CT or MRI
- Amenorrhea/oligomenorrhea
- Cranial nerve palsies-especially with invasive tumors or with pituitary apoplexy
- Erectile dysfunction
- Galactorrhea in non-pregnant/lactating men or women
- Gynecomastia in men
- Headache
- Hydrocephalus
- Hypogonadism
- Hypopituitarism
- Hypothalamic/pituitary dysfunction
- Infertility
- Infiltrative disease of hypothalamus or pituitary
- Loss of libido
- Pituitary damage or resection
- Seizures
- Unilateral exophthalmos
- Visual field deficit, blurred vision, decreased visual acuity

Sources: Data from Al-Chalabi M, Bass AN, Alsalman I. *Physiology,* Prolactin. 2020. https://www.ncbi.nlm.nih.gov/books/NBK507829/; Melmed S, Casanueva FF, Hoffman AR, et al. Diagnosis and treatment of hyperprolactinemia: an endocrine society clinical practice guideline. *J Clin Endocrinol Metab.* 2011;96(2):273–288. doi:10.1210/jc.2010-1692; Nelson L. *Hyperprolactinaemia: Diagnosis and Management.* 2017. https://www.gponline.com/hyperprolactinaemia-diagnosis-management/neurology/neurology/article/937857; O'Shea P, Kavanagh-Wright L, Bell, M. *National Laboratory Handbook. Laboratory Testing for Hyperprolactinaemia.* 2019. https://www.hse.ie/eng/about/who/cspd/ncps/pathology/resources/lab-testing-for-hyperprolactinaemia.pdf.

Monitoring

- During treatment of prolactinoma, PRL levels are monitored every 3 to 6 months.[3,4,7]
- Some antipsychotic medications cause hyperprolactinemia, so it is recommended to monitor PRL levels at initiation. During treatment, if the patient develops symptoms of hyperprolactinemia (galactorrhea, amenorrhea, low sexual desire, or erectile dysfunction), the drug should be discontinued and an antipsychotic agent less often associated with elevated prolactin can be substituted.[8] The older antipsychotics such as olanzapine, haloperidol, and risperidone are most often associated with hyperprolactenemia.[3,9]
- Guidelines recommend PRL monitoring (at baseline and every 6 to 12 months thereafter) during gender affirming hormone therapy (male to female) to monitor for prolactinoma formation.[7]

INTERPRETATION

Reference intervals for PRL are[10]:

- Male: 4.0 to 15.2 ng/mL
- Nonpregnant female: 4.8 to 25 ng/mL
- Pregnant female: 80 to 400 ng/mL

- Hyperprolactinemia levels should be interpreted within the clinical context. Prolactin levels greater than the upper limit level of 200 ng/mL most likely are associated with the effects of psychoactive medications or excess estrogen but could also be due to macroprolactinoma. Macroprolactinomas are benign lesions that are larger than 10 mm in diameter and can cause compressive symptoms such as headache and visual field deficits.[6,11]
- Levels over 300 to 500 ng/mL are typically associated with macroadenomas. Levels can be as high as 20,000 ng/mL.[1]
- Hypoprolactinemia or PRL deficiency is usually related to pathology of the anterior pituitary such as tumor, head trauma, or infection. The most common cause is postpartum pituitary necrosis (Sheehan Syndrome).[12]
- The differential diagnoses for elevated or decreased prolactin levels are summarized in Table 127.1.

FOLLOW-UP

- Follow-up testing and imaging should help confirm the diagnosis. The gold standard for prolactinoma diagnosis confirmation is MRI of the pituitary with gadolinium enhancement.[13]
- When the PRL level is elevated, other pituitary hormones such as adrenocorticotropic hormone (ACTH), luteinizing hormone (LH), follicle-stimulating hormone (FSH), and estrogen or testosterone should be obtained to rule out other pituitary conditions.[11]

PEARLS & PITFALLS

- Macroprolactinemia, a large PRL-IgG antibody complex that is inactive biologically, can interfere with most immunoassays that measure PRL levels and can create a false elevation of PRL. Therefore, clinical evaluation is recommended to support a proper diagnosis. People with systemic lupus erythematosus are particularly susceptible to this effect.[11]

TABLE 127.1: DIFFERENTIAL DIAGNOSIS OF DECREASED OR ELEVATED PROLACTIN LEVELS

HYPERPROLACTINEMIA	HYPOPROLACTINEMIA
Pituitary adenoma or other pituitary tumors	Familial puerperal alactogenesis
Hypothalamic disease	Head injury
Cirrhosis	Hemochromatosis
Acromegaly	Idiopathic hypogonadotropic hypogonadism
Pregnancy	Parasellar diseases
Primary hypothyroidism	Pituitary tumor or treatment of tumor
Renal failure	Pituitary macroadenomas
Cushing disease	Pituitary infection—histoplasmosis, TB
Parasellar mass	Pituitary infiltrative diseases (lymphocytic hypophysitis, sarcoidosis)
Dopamine antagonist medications	
Estrogen/psychotropic agents	Postpartum pituitary necrosis (Sheehan syndrome)

Sources: Data from Pekic S, Popovic V. Diagnosis of endocrine disease: expanding the cause of hypopituitarism. *Eur J Endocrinol.* 2017;176:R269–R282. doi:10.1530/EJE-16-1065; Thapa S, Bhusal K. *Hyperprolactinemia.* StatPearls Publishing; 2020. https://www.ncbi.nlm.nih.gov/books/NBK537331/.

- When abnormally low levels of PRL are obtained in the case of a large macroprolactinoma (greater than 3 cm), dilution of the sample may be necessary to overcome interference with the "hook effect." A large prolactinoma should produce a very large PRL, but the antigen–antibody binding effect creates a false low PRL. In these cases of macroprolactinoma, the pituitary mass may be missed.[10,13-15]
- Because exercise increases PRL, levels should be obtained at least 30 minutes following exercise.[13,15]
- Many pharmacologic agents can lead to elevated levels of PRL such as benzodiazepines, estrogen, antipsychotics, antiemetics, dopamine receptor blocking agents, some antidepressants, and neuroleptics.[9]
- Often, prolactinomas and PRL levels increase during pregnancy.[16,17]
- For women with prolactinomas, serum PRL measurements are not recommended during pregnancy since test results are uninterpretable.[16,17]
- Prolactinoma is more common among women. It is often found incidentally in men as a result of a head scan for another problem.[4]
- It is recommended to avoid PRL measurement in a pregnant female with a prolactinoma.[6]

PATIENT EDUCATION

- https://medlineplus.gov/lab-tests/prolactin-levels/
- https://www.webmd.com/a-to-z-guides/prolactin-test#2

RELATED DIAGNOSES AND ICD-10 CODES

Prolactinoma, benign neoplasm of pituitary gland	D35.2
Galactorrhea 092.6, galactorrhea not associated with childbirth	N64.3
Gynecomastia, hypertrophy of the breast	N62
Hypogonadism, testicular hypofunction	E29.1

REFERENCES

Full list of references can be accessed through Springer Publishing Company Connect™ at the following link: http://connect.springerpub.com/content/reference-book/978-0-8261 -8843-4/part/part03/toc-part/ch127

128. PROSTATE-SPECIFIC ANTIGEN

Sean M. Tafuri and Susanne A. Quallich

PHYSIOLOGY REVIEW

Prostate-specific antigen (PSA) is an enzyme that is produced by the prostate and aids in seminal fluid function and fertility. Typically, it is produced as a proenzyme, proPSA, which is later cleaved into PSA.

PSA can be produced and secreted by either benign or malignant prostate tissue. Once secreted, it either remains free (unbound) or binds to proteins (complexed) circulating in the blood. Because elevations in PSA can be seen in both benign and cancerous prostate tissue, PSA should be considered prostate-specific, not prostate cancer specific.[1,2]

OVERVIEW OF LABORATORY TESTS

Laboratory evaluation of PSA is assessed using a serum blood sample and can be assessed through the following tests, with the more specific tests usually ordered by urology or oncology providers:

- Total PSA (CPT code 84153) includes both free PSA (fPSA) and complexed PSA (cPSA).[3]
- Free PSA (CPT code 84154), also known as percent-free PSA, is the measure of the percentage of PSA that circulates in the blood unbound to proteins. This test is helpful to look at if the total PSA is within the borderline range of 4 to 10 ng/mL. There is no agreed upon cutoff percentage for when to biopsy, but most sources recommend biopsy if the fPSA is less than 10%.[2,3]
- Complexed PSA (cPSA) (CPT code 84152) is also known as bound PSA. cPSA provides the same information that may be gathered from checking both total and free PSA, but with the benefit of using a single analyte. Use of cPSA for screening and diagnosis is unclear and is not used in routine practice.[2,3]

INDICATIONS

Screening
- Screening is summarized in Table 128.1 and discussed in the text that follows. Men with risk factors (Box 128.1) may benefit most from screening.

Who Should Be Screened and When?
- The American Academy of Family Physicians (AAFP) recommends against PSA screening for prostate cancer.[4]
- The American Urological Association (AUA) recommends against screening men younger than 40 years of age or men 40 to 54 years of age who are at average risk for the development of prostate cancer.[5]

TABLE 128.1: COMPARISON OF SCREENING RECOMMENDATIONS

ORGANIZATION	WHEN TO INITIATE SHARED DECISION-MAKING	INTERVAL
American Cancer Society (ACS)	≥45 years old and high risk*	No recommendation
	40 years old and 2+ first degree relative diagnosed with prostate ca ≤ 65 years of age	
	≥50 years old at average risk and will live another 10 years	
American Academy of Family Physicians (AAFP)	Do not screen	If used, 2–4 years
American Urological Association (AUA)	40–55 years old if high risk	2 years
	55–59 years old if average risk	
US Preventive Services Task Force (U.S.PSTF)	55–59 years old if average risk	No recommendation

*For definition of high risk see Box 128.1.

Note: Discontinue screening after age 70 or with life expectancy fewer than 10–15 years.

Box 128.1: Risk Factors for Prostate Cancer

- Men aged 65 to 74 years of age
- Black men
- Men with positive family history of prostate cancer, especially if they are a first-degree relative and/or were diagnosed at younger than 65 years of age
- Men with positive family history of other heritable cancers (breast, colorectal, ovarian, pancreatic, melanoma)
- Male patients who have germline mutations in genes involved in DNA repair pathways (e.g., BRCA1 or BRCA2)

Source: Data from Sartor AO, Vogelzang N, Lee W, Richie JP, Savarese D. Risk factors for prostate cancer. https://www.uptodate.com/contents/risk-factors-for-prostate-cancer?topicRef=7567&source=related_link#H2.

- The AUA, United States Preventive Services Task Force (USPTF), and the AAFP recommend that for men 55 to 59 years of age, the risks and benefits of PSA screening should be discussed with patients to aid them in making an informed decision. Screening can provide a small potential benefit of detecting prostate cancer early and preventing possible death. However, many men who undergo this screening will experience the harms of testing. Possible harms include false positives that lead to more testing (prostate biopsy), overdiagnosis, overtreatment, and complications from treatment. The choice to undergo screening must be made on an individual basis by each patient using shared decision-making.[4-7]
- The AUA, USPSTF, and the AAFP recommend against PSA screening in men 70+ years of age or older.[4-6]

- The AUA recommends against screening in men who have a life expectancy of fewer than 10 to 15 years.[5]
- The American Cancer Society (ACS) recommends discussing PSA screening with patients who are 50+ years of age who are at average risk of prostate cancer and are anticipated to live for at least another 10 years.[3]
- The ACS recommends discussing PSA screening with patients who are 45 years of age and are at high risk of developing prostate cancer. They define high-risk groups to be Black men and/or men who have a first-degree relative that has been diagnosed with prostate cancer at 65 years of age or younger.[3]
- The ACS recommends discussing PSA screening with patients who are 40 years of age and have 2+ first-degree relatives who were diagnosed with prostate cancer at 65 years of age of younger.[3]

How Often to Screen
- The AUA recommends a screening interval of 2+ years.[3]
- The AAFP recommends a screening interval of 2 to 4 years.[4]

Diagnosis and Evaluation

- In men who are symptomatic for prostate symptoms, the National Institute for Health and Care Excellence (NICE) recommends that general practitioners consider performing a PSA test and digital rectal exam (DRE) to evaluate for suspected prostate cancer. Presenting symptoms include erectile dysfunction, gross hematuria, or any lower urinary tract symptoms, such as nocturia, increased urgency or frequency, incomplete bladder emptying, intermittency, dribbling, hesitancy, straining, and weak or split stream. However, research suggests that this would put men at risk of overdiagnosis.[8]

Monitoring

- Monitoring of complexed (bound) PSA is appropriate for detecting recurrence in men with prostatic carcinoma.[2]
- PSA should be monitored 6 to 8 weeks after any treatment for prostate cancer, with follow-up testing once or twice per year thereafter.
- PSA can also offer providers a method for estimation of treatment success after acute prostatitis management.

INTERPRETATION

- Less than 4 ng/mL is generally thought of as a "normal" value for PSA.[1] Table 128.2 highlights the age-specific reference intervals for PSA.
- Although the specific number used to mark abnormality is highly contested, it has been widely accepted than any value greater than 4 ng/mL warrants further investigation.[9,10] But this is a very general guide, and the provider should place an individual PSA in the context of ethnicity, personal history, family history, and current medications.
- Using lower cutoff points (2.5 to 4.0 ng/mL) would result in about 80% false-positive PSA tests.[11,12]

TABLE 128.2: AGE-ADJUSTED REFERENCE RANGES OF TOTAL PROSTATE-SPECIFIC ANTIGEN

AGE (YEARS)	PSA (ng/mL)
40–49	0–2.5
50–59	0–3.5
60–69	0–4.5
70–79	0–6.5

Note: These should be seen as a general guide for possible referral to a urologist for additional evaluation; if the PSA value is above the reference range for a patient's age, referral should be initiated.

Sources: Data from Coley CM, Barry MJ, Fleming C, Mulley AG. Early detection of prostate cancer. Part I: prior probability and effectiveness of tests. The American College of Physicians. Ann Intern Med. 1997;126(5):394–406. doi:10.7326/0003-4819-126 -5-199703010-00010; Freedland S, O'Leary MP, Givens J. Measurement of prostate-specific antigen. UpToDate. https://www .uptodate.com/contents/measurement-of-prostate-specific-antigen?search=measurement%20of%20prostate&source=search_ result&selectedTitle=1~150&usage_type=default&display_rank=1.

- PSA is used as a screening tool for prostate cancer and has a high sensitivity but low specificity, leading to many false positives.[9,10]
- The free PSA level is generally used to determine whether further evaluation is warranted.[9,10]
- There is no specific cutoff point that allows PSA to differentiate between benign prostatic disease or malignant tumors.[9,10]
- Stamey et al.'s 1987 study showed that PSA was found to be elevated in 86% of men who were diagnosed with benign prostatic hyperplasia, proving that it is not a specific marker of cancer.[9]
- 5-alpha reductase inhibitors have been found to decrease PSA levels by approximately 50% within the first year of use. This decrease should be taken into consideration when determining the significance of the PSA level in a patient. No exact cutoff point or amount of change in PSA level has been determined.[13,14]
- Box 128.2 reviews causes of PSA elevation other than prostate cancer.

FOLLOW-UP

The following tests may be used by the urology specialist to clarify the clinical picture.

- **PSA density** is estimated by dividing the PSA level (ng/mL) by the weight of the patient's prostate (g). As the PSA density increases, the probability of cancer increases. This test may be used in patients with larger prostates who are found to have elevated PSA, in order to adjust for size.[1,4,15]
- **PSA velocity (PSAV)** is not its own test. It is a measure of the rate of change of PSA. It has been thought to improve the screening and management of prostate cancer, as rapidly rising levels may be indicative of cancer. However, it has been found that its calculation does not provide much benefit clinically. Rapid elevations in PSAV may be more indicative of prostatitis than prostate cancer. The ACS guidelines do not recommend including PSAV in prostate screening.[1,4,16]

Box 128.2: Other Causes of Elevated Prostate-Specific Antigen

- Benign prostatic hyperplasia (BPH)
- Cystoscopy
- Ejaculation
- Epididymitis
- Perineal trauma
- Prostate biopsy
- Prostatic infarction
- Prostatitis
- Transurethral resection of the prostate (TURP)
- Urinary tract infections (UTIs)
- Urinary retention

Sources: Data from Bichler K-H, Naber KG. Elevated PSA as differential diagnostic error-source in prostate cancer with consequences in medical law. In: *Prostatitis and Its Management.* 2016:131–140. doi:10.1007/978-3-319-25175-2_14; Freedland S, O'Leary MP, Givens J. Measurement of prostate-specific antigen. *UpToDate.* https://www.uptodate.com/contents/measurement-of-prostate-specific-antigen?search=measurement%20of%20prostate&source=search_result&selectedTitle=1~150&usage_type=default&display_rank=1.

- **Prostate health index (PHI)** is a combined measurement of three forms of PSA: total PSA, free PSA, and proPSA. It is found to be more specific than free or total PSA for detecting prostate cancer.[17]
- **PCA3** is a novel urinary biomarker. It is a prostate-specific gene that is found to be overexpressed in many malignant prostate cancers. Elevated levels are strongly associated with prostate cancer.[1,18,19]
- **4Kscore test** is a combination of total PSA, free PSA, complexed PSA, and human kallikrein 2 (hK2). Like PHI, using the combination of PSA measurements is found to be more specific than free or total PSA alone. 4K may be helpful in men with slightly elevated PSA to help determine if they should undergo further intervention.[3]

PEARLS & PITFALLS

- PSA circulates in the blood in two forms: free/unbound or bound to protein.[2]
- Early prostate cancers are typically found in asymptomatic patients, often via elevated PSA.
- When interpreting PSA test results, the provider must be mindful of the clinical evaluation and provide patient education.
- The DRE is often used to screen for prostate cancer, but there is limited evidence supporting its efficacy for screening. DRE is not as effective as measuring PSA levels but, in some cases, it may detect cancers in men with normal PSA levels. Therefore, it should be done as part of the overall prostate cancer screen since the sensitivity of PSA screening can be increased with inclusion of DRE.[4,20]
- Men can have both prostate enlargement benign prostatic hypertrophy and occult prostate cancer, both of which can increase the PSA level.
- Prostate size does not necessarily predict PSA level.

- PSA level and subsequent rises must always be placed in the context of patient age, race, family history, and individual risk factors, such as body mass index (BMI).
- PSA can be artificially elevated in men who have ejaculated within the last 2 to 3 days, are constipated, and who potentially engaged in activities that put pressure on the prostate (e.g., cycling).[5]
- It is prudent to repeat a newly elevated PSA in 2 to 3 months to assess for spurious elevations.
- Black men remain at highest risk for prostate cancer, and this should guide targeted screening for this group of patients.
- Debate still exists about the utility of the PSA alone due to its high sensitivity but low specificity.
- Do not refer for prostate biopsy based solely on PSA velocity in the absence of other indications, such as established risk factors. Clinicians may wish to refer for urology evaluation and risk factor discussion, as treatment is rarely determined on a single value.
- Contemporary screening involves appropriate patient selection, shared decision-making, and risk stratification for individual patients.
- Know when to stop screening an individual patient.
- PSA can detect a large amount of prostate cancers, but the majority of these cancers are low risk and not clinically significant, potentially leading to overdiagnosis and overtreatment. This is where the value of shared decision-making is evident. Historically, widespread prostate cancer screening has resulted in a pattern of overtreatment, which in turn resulted in a rise in treatment complications such as sexual function challenges and urinary incontinence issues.
- A normal PSA result should not discourage further evaluation if prostate cancer is suspected due to an individual's presentation or history. While a PSA of 2.5 ng/mL or less is technically normal, the range of PSA levels represents a continuum of risk, and prostate cancer can be present at low or normal PSA levels. If there is any doubt, refer to a urology clinician. Many large academic centers have clinicians that specialize in prostate cancer risk discussion and evaluation.
- A higher PSA can indicate a higher risk for prostate cancer, but it can also indicate a large prostate.
- PSA screening recommendations in transgender females post-gender affirmation hormone treatment have not been firmly established.[21] The prostate is not removed, so the prediction is that the overall risk is much less than that for cis-males but may not be zero. The World Professional Association of Transgender Health (WPATH) and the Endocrine Society recommend transfeminine patients follow established risk screening recommendations for their pre-transition risk categorization (e.g., Black individuals remain at higher risk). Note that 1 ng/mL should be considered the upper threshold of normal in this group of patients.[22]

PATIENT EDUCATION

- https://www.auanet.org/guidelines/prostate-cancer-early-detection
  -guideline
- https://www.auanet.org/guidelines/prostate-specific-antigen-(psa)-best
  -practice-statement
- https://www.choosingwisely.org/patient-resources/psa-test-for-prostate
  -cancer/

RELATED DIAGNOSES AND ICD-10 CODES

Benign prostatic hyperplasia	N40.1
Prostatitis	N41.0
Urinary tract infection	N39.0
Epididymitis	N45.1
Perineal trauma	071.82

REFERENCES

Full list of references can be accessed through Springer Publishing Company Connect™ at the following link: http://connect.springerpub.com/content/reference-book/978-0-8261-8843-4/part/part03/toc-part/ch128

129. PROTEIN C

John Prickett

PHYSIOLOGY REVIEW

Protein C is an integral part of the endogenous anticoagulation system and has coordinated activity with protein S. It is synthesized by the liver and circulates as a zymogen, requiring vitamin K for activation into a serine protease.[1] Its primary function in regulating the clotting process is to deactivate activated factor V (FVa) and activated factor VIII (FVIIIa). Additionally, activated protein C has anti-inflammatory and anti-apoptotic properties. A synthetic activated protein C (drotrecogin alfa) has been developed and is utilized in treating sepsis, but with limited success.[2]

Deficiencies in protein C contribute to a hypercoagulable state and are primarily due to mutations. More than 200 mutations have been identified that fall into two categories.[3,4] Type I mutations cause a decrease in the amount of protein C, while Type II mutations lead to diminished function of protein C.[5-7] Transient decreases of protein C also occur and are often associated with liver disease, medications (particularly vitamin K antagonists), disseminated intra-vascular coagulation (DIC), infections, uremia, and autoantibodies. Testing should be performed outside of an active clotting event and when patients are off medications that could interfere with testing.[8,9]

OVERVIEW OF LABORATORY TESTS

Protein C is evaluated using either a functional assay or an immunoassay. Functional assays (CPT code 85303) are based on partial thromboplastin time (PTT), activated factor X (FXa), or enzymatic activity using a chromogenic sub-stance. They are more clinically relevant as they report the amount of protein C. However, they are affected by acute state and some medications. This needs to be taken into consideration when interpreting results.[6,7,10] Immunoassays (CPT code 85302) are helpful to determine whether a Type I and Type II defect exists, but are not commonly performed in clinical practice.

INDICATIONS

Screening

Universal screenings are not recommended.

Targeted screenings should be considered in individuals with the following:

■ Strong family history of pathologic thromboses (more than two other symptomatic family members), and/or
■ Known family history of protein C deficiency in a first-degree relative.
■ Testing for protein C in unselected patients presenting with their first episode of venous thromboembolism (VTE) is not indicated as it does not reduce recurrence of VTE.[11]

Diagnosis and Evaluation

As with other hypercoagulable laboratory tests, consider testing for protein C deficiency in the following patients[11,12]:

■ First VTE at younger than 40 years old,
■ VTE in an unusual location (portal, mesenteric, or cerebral vein),
■ Recurrent VTE,
■ Pregnant individuals with a previous VTE due to a minor provoking factor (e.g., travel),
■ Asymptomatic pregnant individuals with a family history of venous thrombosis in a first-degree relative that was unprovoked, or provoked by pregnancy, oral contraceptive use, or a minor provoking factor,
■ Infants/children presenting with purpura fulminans, and/or
■ Individuals who develop skin necrosis in association with oral vitamin K antagonists (VKA) after VKA treatment is completed.

Monitoring

■ No routine monitoring of the protein C is recommended.

In individuals who have indeterminate levels or levels felt to be the result of transient state, serial testing may be indicated until a baseline level is obtained. If mutation is suspected, repeating once to verify is a common practice.

INTERPRETATION

- See Tables 129.1 and 129.2 for test result interpretation.
- Clinical significance of elevated levels of protein C are unknown, but generally thought to not impose thrombophilic risk.[13]
- Choosing Wisely guidelines suggest that protein C should not be tested in the setting of an active clotting event or other acute illness, and should not be tested within 4 to 6 weeks of taking an anticoagulant medication (particularly anti-vitamin K antagonists).[14]

FOLLOW-UP

- No routine follow-up testing is typically indicated.
- Depending on the patient presentation, risk factors, and diagnosis, protein C is typically ordered with other tests for hypercoagulation including but

TABLE 129.1: PROTEIN C REFERENCE INTERVAL

	PROTEIN C VALUES*
Mean concentration (IU/dL)	
Adults	65 to 135 IU/dL
Infants (full term)	40 IU/dL
Infants (6 months)**	60 IU/dL
Normal intervals (% activity)	70% to 140%

* Normal values may vary by laboratory.

** Activity increases with age until normal adult levels are obtained.

Sources: Data from Gupta A, Patibandla S. Protein C deficiency. In: *StatPearls.* StatPearls Publishing; 2020. https://www.ncbi.nlm.nih.gov/books/NBK542222/; Chalmers E, Cooper P, Forman K, et al. Purpura fulminans: recognition, diagnosis and management. *Arch Dis Child.* 2011;96(11):1066–1071. doi:10.1136/adc.2010.199919; Miletich J, Sherman L, Broze G Jr. Absence of thrombosis in subjects with heterozygous protein C deficiency. *N Engl J Med.* 1987;317(16):991–996. doi:10.1056/NEJM198710153171604

TABLE 129.2: ABNORMAL LEVELS OF PROTEIN C

PROTEIN C LEVEL	INTERPRETATION
Less than 1% activity	Inherited homozygous mutation
	Typically diagnosed early in neonatal life
	Often leads to purpura fulminans
50% to 55% activity	Inherited heterozygous mutation
55% to 70% activity	Suspicious for secondary decrease due to acute state or medication

Sources: Data from Chalmers E, Cooper P, Forman K, et al. Purpura fulminans: recognition, diagnosis and management. *Arch Dis Child.* 2011;96(11):1066–1071. doi:10.1136/adc.2010.199919; Miletich J, Sherman L, Broze G Jr. Absence of thrombosis in subjects with heterozygous protein C deficiency. *N Engl J Med.* 1987;317(16):991–996. doi:10.1056/NEJM198710153171604

not limited to: prothrombin time (PT), aPTT (partial thromboplastin time), homocysteine, protein S, Factor V Leiden, prothrombin gene mutation, lupus anticoagulant, antiphospholipid antibodies, and antithrombin.
- A variety of functional methods may be required to identify specific severe Type 2 functional defects when levels of protein C are not less than 5%.[11]

PEARLS & PITFALLS

- The incidence of a protein C mutation in the general population is 0.02% to 0.5%, but as high as 2% to 5% in patients with VTE.[3,15,16]
- The presence of a heterozygous mutation connotes a 5- to 7-fold increased risk of first time VTE but does not help predict likelihood of secondary thromboses.[1]
- Full anticoagulation is generally not an acceptable practice in individuals with a protein C mutation in the absence of a personal history of venous thrombosis.
- It is speculated that protein C deficiency represents a risk for arterial thrombosis, but there has been a paucity of quality data to support this. Its effect seems to be related to an increased risk of venous thrombosis,[17] though this is a controversial topic and warrants further investigation.[7]
- The gene that encodes protein C is called the *PROC* gene and is located on chromosome 2 (2q13-14).[18]
- There is an increased risk of thrombosis with the combination of protein C deficiency and the use of oral contraceptives.[19,20]
- Neonates and children presenting with purpura fulminans need urgent testing for both protein S and C deficiency.[4,11,19,20]
- Pregnant individuals with protein C deficiency should consider antepartum and postpartum thrombosis prophylaxis.[21]

PATIENT EDUCATION

- https://rarediseases.org/rare-diseases/protein-c-deficiency/
- https://rarediseases.info.nih.gov/diseases/4521/protein-c-deficiency
- https://labtestsonline.org/tests/protein-c-and-protein-s

RELATED DIAGNOSES AND ICD-10 CODES

Activated protein C resistance	D68.51
Hypercoagulable state	D68.59

REFERENCES

Full list of references can be accessed through Springer Publishing Company Connect™ at the following link: http://connect.springerpub.com/content/reference-book/978-0-8261 -8843-4/part/part03/toc-part/ch129

130. PROTEIN ELECTROPHORESIS

Nicole Peters Kroll

PHYSIOLOGY REVIEW

Proteins make up a significant part of the body's cells and they are integral in forming tissues and organs. The two main types of proteins in the body are albumin and globulin. When these proteins are measured together, they are considered total protein. Albumin is generated in the liver and measures hepatic function. It also encompasses approximately 60% of the total protein in blood and maintains colloidal osmotic pressure in the vascular space. Another critical role albumin plays is it carries hormones, enzymes, and medications throughout the body. All non-albumin proteins in the body are grouped together and called globulins. Many globulins are also created in the liver excluding antibodies (immunoglobulins) and some complement proteins. Globulins also function to transport ions, hormones, and lipids in the blood.[1,2] Globulins can be monoclonal, produced by one type of cell, or polyclonal, which is an inflammatory response. Monoclonal and polyclonal globulins are secreted in blood, and at times in urine and other body fluids.[2]

Proteins are characterized by the way they move in an electric field (electrophoresis). There are five defined bands in electrophoresis: albumin, $alpha_1$, $alpha_2$, beta, and gamma.[3] Albumin is the largest and quickest moving protein. Globulins are then categorized by how they compare to albumin. Alpha (α_1 & α_2) globulins, which include haptoglobins (attach to hemoglobin), ceruloplasmin (transports copper), prothrombin, and cholinesterase, have comparable movement to albumin. Beta (β_1 and β_2) globulins are composed of lipoproteins, transferrin, plasminogen, and complement proteins, as well as fibrinogen and gamma (γ) globulins or immunoglobulins; all have minimum movement with electrophoresis.[1,2]

OVERVIEW OF LABORATORY TESTS

Protein electrophoresis (CPT code 84165) is a common laboratory test that can be performed on any body fluid.[3,4] This test detects and quantifies the existence of atypical proteins and the lack of normal proteins and identifies the pattern of migration across the electrical field linked with selected states of health.[5] Negatively charged proteins move toward the positively charged anode in a medium and the proteins separate based on their charge.[3] While this test alone will not provide a conclusive diagnosis, it assists clinicians with evidence to suggest that a disease or health disorder is impacting protein production in the body.[3,6] Protein electrophoresis is a vital group of blood, urine, and cerebral spinal fluid tests used for many indications to evaluate the extent of and determine changes in certain disease processes.[3]

Quantitative immunoglobulin analysis also is a laboratory test that will measure monoclonal immunoglobulins. Serum protein electrophoresis (SPEP) was found to have a higher sensitivity and be less likely to have bias.[6] The advantage to SPEP is it differentiates between the monoclonal and the polyclonal proteins.[3] SPEP is also preferred over urine protein electrophoresis (UPEP) as protein is not always found in urine and UPEP is the least sensitive of the two tests. Even with the low sensitivity, UPEP does provide important guidance in patients with kidney disease.[7] Multiple studies also compared electrophoresis completed on different types of mediums. Immunofixation (IFE) and capillary electrophoresis-based immunosubtraction are the two types of mediums to choose from and the decision is generally made based on the type of equipment a laboratory possesses to perform the test. IFE was found to be the gold standard with an increased sensitivity.[6]

INDICATIONS

Screening

- Universal screenings for protein electrophoresis are not recommended.[8]
- Targeted screenings should be considered in the following populations:
  - Suspected or known multiple myeloma including the presence of the following symptoms[1,8–10]:
    - Bone fractures or pain
    - Carpal tunnel syndrome
    - Hypercalcemia
    - Anorexia
    - Lethargy
    - Anemia
    - Renal insufficiency with associated serum protein elevation
  - Signs or symptoms of immunocompromised conditions[8]
  - Suspected or known Waldenström macroglobulinemia[10]
  - Suspected or known amyloidosis[10]
  - Suspected or known monoclonal gammopathy of undetermined significance (MGUS)[10]

Diagnosis and Evaluation

- Consider testing for the following physical examination and/or laboratory findings
  - Unexplained neurologic symptoms such as peripheral neuropathy[8]
  - Night or unexplained sweating[8]
  - Splenomegaly[8]
  - Proteinuria[3]
- Table 130.1 provides a summary of differential diagnoses that can be related to changes in SPEP.[1,3,11]

Monitoring

- Once the diagnosis of a disorder has been established, protein electrophoresis may be ordered to monitor for relapse or medication efficacy.[1]

PROTEIN	ELECTROPHORESIS INCREASED (ELEVATED BAND)	ELECTROPHORESIS DECREASED (FAINT OR ABSENT BAND)
Albumin	Dehydration	Malnutrition, malabsorption, nephrotic syndrome, hepatic disease, inflammation, kidney disease, pregnancy, hemodilution
Alpha 1 globulins	Acute and chronic inflammation, cancer, liver tumor, germ cell tumor	Nephrosis, hepatic disease, alpha 1 antitrypsin deficiency
Alpha 2 globulins	Nephrotic syndrome, acute and chronic inflammation, adrenal insufficiency, severe diabetes mellitus	Malnutrition, hepatic disease, hemolysis, Wilson's disease, hemolysis
Beta 1 and 2 globulins	Hypercholesterolemia, iron deficiency anemia, multiple myeloma, pregnancy, inflammation	Malnutrition, autoimmune disorder, LDL—abnormally low, C3 consumption
Gamma globulins	Lupus, cirrhosis, polyclonal immunoglobulins–infection or inflammation; monoclonal band– multiple myeloma, lymphoma, Waldenström's	Agammaglobulinemia, hypogammaglobulinemia, inherited humoral immunodeficiency, kidney disease, sepsis, malnutrition, viral infections, amyloidosis, leukemias

TABLE 130.1: DIFFERENTIAL DIAGNOSIS USING SERUM PROTEIN ELECTROPHORESIS

*Diagnosis should not be based solely on serum protein electrophoresis.

- Immediate to high-risk patients with monoclonal gammopathy should be monitored yearly.[3]

INTERPRETATION

- Protein electrophoresis is a commonly run laboratory test; however, consensus on reporting varies greatly.[4,6,12]
- Table 130.2 provides a summary of normal laboratory values for SPEP.[10]
- Normal reference range for UPEP is the lack of atypical monoclonal protein (M Protein, M Spike). Twenty percent of multiple myeloma patients will have proteins in their urine with the most common finding being a gamma band elevation.[12]

FOLLOW-UP

- Follow-up will be determined by the disease or health condition suspected.[13]

PEARLS & PITFALLS

- SPEP can be used to measure the amount of heavy chain monoclonal protein produced by myeloma cells.[5]
- Protein electrophoresis is most commonly performed on serum.[3]
- Steroids, hormones, immunizations, and insulin can increase protein levels.[1,13]
- Oral contraceptives, ammonium ions, and those that are hepatoxic can decrease protein levels.[13]

TABLE 130.2: REFERENCE INTERVALS FOR SERUM PROTEIN ELECTROPHORESIS

PROTEIN	INTERVAL
Albumin fraction*	Adult: 3.5–5.5 gm/dL Children • Premature Infant: 3.0–3.9 g/dL • Infant: 2.2–4.8 g/dL • Child: 3.6–5.2 g/dL • Adolescent: 3.9–5.1 g/dL
Alpha 1 globulin fraction*	Adult: 0.2–0.4 gm/dL Children • Premature Infant: 0.1–0.3 g/dL • Infant: 0.1–0.3 g/dL • Child: 0.1–0.4 g/dL • Adolescent: 0.2–0.4 g/dL
Alpha 2 globulin fraction*	Adult: 0.5–0.9 gm/dL Children • Premature Infant: 0.3–0.6 g/dL • Infant: 0.5–0.9 g/dL • Child: 0.5–1.2 g/dL • Adolescent: 0.4–0.8 g/dL
Beta 1 & 2 globulin fraction*	Adult: 0.6–1.1 gm/dL Children • Premature Infant: 0.6–1.1 g/dL • Infant: 0.4–0.6 g/dL • Child: 0.5–0.9 g/dL • Adolescent: 0.5–1.1 g/dL
Gama globulin fraction*	Adult: 0.7–1.7 gm/dL Children • Premature Infant: 0.7–1.4 g/dL • Infant: 0.5–1.3 g/dL • Child: 0.5–1.7 g/dL • Adolescent: 0.6–1.2 g/dL
Globulin fraction*	Adult: 2–3.5 g/dL

*The above reference intervals may very slightly from between laboratories.

- Aspirin, bicarbonates, chlorpromazine, corticosteroids, and neomycin can affect protein electrophoresis results.[1,13]
- To be utilized to its full potential, SPEP should be used in conjunction with other laboratory tests and clinical presentations.[3]

PATIENT EDUCATION

- https://johnshopkinshealthcare.staywellsolutionsonline.com/RelatedItems/167,protein_electrophoresis_serum
- https://www.urmc.rochester.edu/encyclopedia/content.aspx?contenttypeid=167&contentid=protein_electrophoresis_serum
- https://www.uofmhealth.org/health-library/hw43650

RELATED DIAGNOSES AND ICD-10 CODES

Multiple myeloma	C90.0
Chronic lymphocytic leukemia	C91.10
Monoclonal gammopathy	D47.2
Amyloidosis	E85
Waldenström macroglobulinemia	C88.0

REFERENCES

Full list of references can be accessed through Springer Publishing Company Connect™ at the following link: http://connect.springerpub.com/content/reference-book/978-0-8261-8843-4/part/part03/toc-part/ch130

131. PROTEIN S

John Prickett

PHYSIOLOGY REVIEW

Protein S is a naturally occurring vitamin K-dependent anticoagulant factor. It is predominantly synthesized in the liver, though there is data to support some endothelial cell and megakaryocyte production. It exists in circulation, bound to C4b-binding protein (C4BP) and as a free protein.[1] Free protein S is the active portion of the protein and represents about 30% to 40% of total circulating protein S antigen. Though its primary function is to act as an anticoagulant, it is thought to have some regulatory function of the complement system.[1,2] Deficiency of protein S causes an increased risk for hypercoagulation.

True protein S deficiencies are due to an autosomal dominant heredity and there are three different types of deficiencies.[3] Type I represents decreased total (~50% normal) and free levels of protein S (as low as 15%).[4,5] Type II represents a qualitative defect and is associated with normal measured levels of protein S, but diminished function.[6,7] Type III defects typically have normal total levels, but selectively decreased free levels and diminished function.[8,9] Other causes of transient nonhereditary deficiencies are found in pregnancy, oral hormonal contraception use, disseminated intravascular coagulation (DIC), acute thrombosis, HIV, various infections (e.g., varicella-zoster), nephrotic syndrome, liver disease, and with some chemotherapies (e.g., L-asparaginase).[10,11] As C4BP can act as an acute phase reactant, elevations of C4BP have been described as causing temporary reduced levels of protein S. These nonhereditary, transient drops in protein S have not been routinely shown to cause hypercoagulability.[12] Its prevalence has been difficult to determine but may be present in about 0.03% to 0.13% of the general population and in between 3% to 5% of patients with venous thromboembolism (VTE).[13–15]

OVERVIEW OF LABORATORY TESTS

Testing for free protein S (CPT code 85306) is the most accurate serum test as it represents the active form of protein S. It is done by immunoassay, utilizing either monoclonal antibody-based or ligand-based (C4BP) methods.[16,17] Testing for total protein S antigen (CPT code 85305) is done utilizing polyclonal antibody-based methods.[18] Functional assays assess by utilizing coagulation-based assays in which clot formation is proportionate to plasma protein S activity, but are largely inaccurate due to a large number of potential interfering conditions, and should be interpreted in the context of other factors.[19]

INDICATIONS

Screening

Universal screenings are not recommended.

Targeted screenings should be considered in individuals with the following:

- Strong family history of pathologic thromboses (more than two other symptomatic family members), and/or
- Known family history of protein S deficiency in a first-degree relative.
- Testing for protein S in unselected patients presenting with their first episode of VTE is not indicated as it does not reduce recurrence of VTE.[20]

Diagnosis and Evaluation

As with other hypercoagulable laboratory tests, consider testing for protein S deficiency in the following patients[20,21]:

- First VTE at younger than 40 years old,
- VTE in an unusual location (portal, mesenteric, or cerebral vein),
- Recurrent VTE,
- Pregnant individuals with a previous VTE due to a minor provoking factor (e.g., travel),
- Asymptomatic pregnant individuals with a family history of venous thrombosis in a first-degree relative that was unprovoked, or provoked by pregnancy, oral contraceptive use, or a minor provoking factor,
- Infants/children presenting with purpura fulminans, and/or
- Individuals who develop skin necrosis in association with oral vitamin K antagonists (VKA) after VKA treatment is completed.

Monitoring

- No routine monitoring of the protein S free or total tests is recommended.
- In individuals who have indeterminate levels or levels felt to be the result of transient state, serial testing may be indicated until baseline level is obtained. If mutation is suspected, repeating once to verify is a common practice.

INTERPRETATION

■ Table 131.1 reviews the values and ranges generally accepted when interpreting test results for protein S.[22–26]

■ There has been substantial difficulty in establishing normal values, which complicates determination of "normal" protein S concentrations. Values and ranges are generally accepted when interpreting test results.[22–26]

■ Determining the type of protein S deficiency should be in consultation with a hematologist. Based on the type of protein S deficiency, levels of free protein S, total protein S antigen, and total protein S activity will vary. Refer to Table 131.2[28] for guidance on distinguishing protein S deficiency type I, II, and III.

■ For individuals with VTE and a strong family history, levels of less than 60 to 65 units/dL are considered low.[26]

■ For individuals who are asymptomatic or have their first VTE in the absence of any family history, levels of free protein S lower than 33 units/dL are more consistent with a true deficiency.[26]

■ Results need to be interpreted in the context of a patient's other medical conditions and medications since protein S deficiency can be acquired or transient (Box 131.1).

■ Choosing Wisely guidelines suggest that protein S should not be tested in the setting of an active clotting event or other acute illness, and should not be tested within 4 to 6 weeks of taking an anticoagulant medication (particularly anti-vitamin K antagonists).[22,27]

● Elevated levels of protein S are typically not clinically significant.

TABLE 131.1: PROTEIN S REFERENCE INTERVAL

	PROTEIN S VALUES*
Mean concentration (mcg/dL)	25
Normal intervals (% activity)	70–140 (Males)
	60–130 (Females)

*There has been substantial difficulty in establishing normal values, which complicates the determination of protein S deficiency. Normal values may vary by laboratory.

TABLE 131.2: INTERPRETATION OF TYPES OF PROTEIN S DEFICIENCY

TYPE OF DEFICIENCY	FREE PROTEIN S	TOTAL PROTEIN S ANTIGEN	TOTAL PROTEIN S ACTIVITY
1	Decreased	Decreased	Decreased
2	Normal	Normal	Decreased
3	Decreased	Normal	Decreased

Source: Data from Protein C and Protein S |Lab Tests Online, https://labtestsonline.org/tests/protein-c-and-protein-s.

Box 131.1: Causes of Acquired Protein S Deficiencies

- Cancer
- Disseminated intravascular coagulation
- HIV
- Inflammation
- Kidney disease
- Liver disease
- Medications (chemotherapy, warfarin, oral contraceptives)
- Myeloproliferative disorders
- Nephrotic syndrome
- Pregnancy
- Severe infections
- Vitamin K deficiency

Sources: Data from D'Angelo A, Vigano-D'Angelo S, Esmon CT, Comp PC. Acquired deficiencies of protein S. Protein S activity during oral anticoagulation, in liver disease, and in disseminated intravascular coagulation. *J Clin Invest.* 1988;81(5):1445–1454. doi:10.1172/JCI113475; Lijfering WM, Mulder R, ten Kate MK, Veeger NJ, Mulder AB, van der Meer J. Clinical relevance of decreased free protein S levels: results from a retrospective family cohort study involving 1143 relatives. *Blood.* 2009;113(6):1225–1230. doi:10.1182/blood-2008-08-174128.

FOLLOW-UP

Follow-up, repeat testing of protein S may be appropriate to confirm deficiency, especially if findings of initial testing were felt to be compromised due to the patient having an active clotting event or other acute illness.

Depending on the patient presentation and risk factors, protein S is typically ordered with other tests for hypercoagulation including but not limited to pro-thrombin time (PT), aPTT (partial thromboplastin time), homocysteine, protein C, Factor V Leiden, prothrombin gene mutation, lupus anticoagulant, antiphospholipid antibodies, and antithrombin.

A variety of functional methods may be required to identify specific severe type II functional defects when levels of protein S are not lower than 5%.[20]

PEARLS & PITFALLS

- Of the inherited hypercoagulable tests, protein S has been more difficult to assess due to variation in levels in different populations and fluctuations in free levels within individuals.[22]
- Protein S may be sufficient on its own to inactivate FVa, but it acts as cofactor along with protein C to inactivate FVIIIa.[1]
- As with other inherited thrombophilic risks, protein S deficiency increases the risk of VTE and has been postulated to increase the risk of arterial thromboses; however, this has not been elaborated in the literature.[24,29]
- Pregnant individuals with protein S deficiency should consider antepartum and postpartum thrombosis prophylaxis.[30]
- Neonates and children presenting with purpura fulminans need urgent testing for both protein S and C deficiency.[20]

PATIENT EDUCATION

- https://rarediseases.org/rare-diseases/protein-s-deficiency/
- https://rarediseases.info.nih.gov/diseases/4524/protein-s-deficiency/cases/21328
- https://labtestsonline.org/tests/protein-c-and-protein-s

RELATED DIAGNOSES AND ICD-10 CODES

Other primary thrombophilia (antithrombin III deficiency, hypercoagulable state NOS, primary hypercoagulable state NEC, primary thrombophilia NEC, protein C deficiency, protein S deficiency, thrombophilia NOS)   D68.5

REFERENCES

Full list of references can be accessed through Springer Publishing Company Connect™ at the following link: http://connect.springerpub.com/content/reference-book/978-0-8261-8843-4/part/part03/toc-part/ch131

---

132. PROTHROMBIN GENE MUTATION (G20210A)

John Prickett

PHYSIOLOGY REVIEW

Prothrombin (Factor II) is a liver-synthesized, vitamin K-dependent factor that is critical in the coagulation pathway. When catalyzed by prothrombinase (FVa, FXa, phospholipid, Ca2+), it is cleaved into thrombin (FIIa), which is central to the conversion of fibrinogen to fibrin. Additionally, when bound to thrombomodulin, it is responsible for activation of the antithrombotic protein C.[1] It is coded by the F2 gene located on chromosome 1. A mutation that codes for prothrombin, termed "prothrombin G20210," causes an increase in the amount of prothrombin, which leads to abnormal clotting and a greater risk of blood clots.

The most common recognized mutation, G20210A, is the second most commonly inherited cause of thrombophilia after Factor V Leiden (FVL). It is transmitted in an autosomal dominant pattern and the mutation leads to approximately a 30% greater generation of thrombin.[2,3] Despite this, its role in thrombophilia is poorly understood. The prevalence in the general population is estimated to be about 2% in Caucasians and appears infrequently in other populations.[4] Presence of the mutation seems to be a risk for venous thrombosis while its contribution to arterial thromboses and pregnancy demise seems to be low. The increased risk for venous thromboses for individuals who are heterozygous for the mutation is estimated to be about 3- to 4-fold over the general population. Homozygosity is felt to likely impart a greater thrombophilic risk though this has been difficult to quantify. Thrombophilic risk is further increased in the presence of other thrombophilic factors (OCP use, pregnancy, cancer, and other inherited or acquired factors).[5-9]

OVERVIEW OF LABORATORY TEST

Testing for prothrombin gene mutation (CPT code 81240) is done by utilizing molecular techniques to identify the mutated G20210A gene, primarily by polymerase chain reaction (PCR). While other mutated genes have been identified, their prevalence is too low to recommend routine testing as part of thrombophilia evaluation. The test is able to detect the presence of one mutated allele (heterozygous) or two mutated alleles (homozygous).[10,11]

INDICATIONS

Screening

- Universal or targeted screenings are not recommended.
- It is recommended that asymptomatic adults with a family history of prothrombin mutation G20210A should not be tested.[12]

Diagnosis and Evaluation

Prothrombin gene mutation testing is often ordered as part of a thrombophilia workup. Testing should also be considered in the following[13]:

- First venous thromboembolism (VTE) or deep venous thrombosis (DVT) at younger than 50 years old,
- Personal or family history of unprovoked recurrent DVT or VTE,
- First VTE with oral contraceptive use, pregnancy, or hormone replacement therapy,
- Unexplained miscarriages, especially in the second or third trimester
- VTE in an unusual location (portal, renal, mesenteric, eye, or cerebral vein), and/or
- Recurrent VTE

Monitoring

- No routine monitoring of the prothrombin gene mutation test is recommended.

INTERPRETATION

- Testing is reported of the presence or absence of one or more alleles of the G20210A prothrombin gene mutation.[10,11]
- Attempts to determine normal prothrombin levels have been unsuccessful as the range varies with age and in certain physiologic conditions.

FOLLOW-UP

- This test is often ordered along with testing for FVL[10,11] and as part of a thrombophilia workup.

■ Depending on the patient presentation and risk factors, prothrombin gene mutation testing is typically ordered with other tests for hypercoagulation including but not limited to prothrombin time (PT), aPTT (partial thromboplastin time), homocysteine, protein C, protein S, and antithrombin III.

PEARLS & PITFALLS

■ Results of prothrombin gene mutation testing may not be beneficial in determining treatment of VTE.[12,14]
■ The coexistence of prothrombin gene mutation and FVL in individuals with VTE is not uncommon.[8]
■ The prothrombin G20210A single-nucleotide polymorphism was shown in a meta-analysis to be associated with an increased risk of preeclampsia.[15]
■ Prothrombin G20210A polymorphism may represent a risk factor for myocardial infarction.[16]

PATIENT EDUCATION

■ https://www.stoptheclot.org/learn_more/prothrombin-g20210a-factor-ii -mutation/

RELATED DIAGNOSES AND ICD-10 CODES

Prothrombin gene mutation	D68.52

REFERENCES

Full list of references can be accessed through Springer Publishing Company Connect™ at the following link: http://connect.springerpub.com/content/reference-book/978-0-8261 -8843-4/part/part03/toc-part/ch132

133. PROTHROMBIN, PARTIAL THROMBOPLASTIN TIME, AND INTERNATIONAL NORMALIZED RATIO

Samara Linnell and Kate Sustersic Gawlik

PHYSIOLOGY REVIEW

There are various proteins and cell fragments found in the blood. These proteins and cell fragments react with one another to form a clot in order to stop bleeding, and work to achieve a balance between clotting and bleeding. There are various factors found in the clotting cascade that come together to promote optimal functioning. This process, known as hemostasis, is crucial for human survival.[1] Primary hemostasis is when platelets aggregate and form a plug (clot) at the damaged site. Secondary hemostasis involves the two main coagulation pathways, the intrinsic and extrinsic pathways, that join together to form the common pathway.[1] The intrinsic pathway is one that is initiated by trauma inside the vascular system, involving platelets, chemical mediators, collagen, and factors XII, XI, IX, and VIII. The extrinsic pathway is the activation of tissue factor following trauma from outside the vascular system. The common pathway involves factors I, II, V, VII, and X and happens when the intrinsic and extrinsic pathways join together to form the fibrin network for clot formation.[1]

There are congenital genetic mutations (e.g., von Willebrand disease [VWD] or hemophilia) that can occur, where individuals do not have enough of the needed clotting components and are at increased risk for uncontrolled bleeding.[2,3] Nutritional deficits can also affect clotting factors. And rarely, acquired conditions can occur where these factors are made insufficient for clotting.[4]

While there are specific factors found in the blood that can be measured, the prothrombin (PT), partial thromboplastin time (PTT), also known as activated partial thromboplastin time (aPTT), and International Normalized Ratio (INR) values are commonly used to assess whether there is a problem in one of the pathways involving the clotting cascade and to alert the clinician that further testing may be indicated. If something is abnormal with these values, it should prompt a clinician to order more specific laboratory values. These laboratory values are also used when monitoring patients on warfarin anticoagulation to keep tight control in lessening a hypercoagulable state.[5]

OVERVIEW OF LABORATORY TESTS

PT (CPT code 85610) is a measurement of both the extrinsic and common pathways of coagulation, based on the amount of time which is required for a fibrin clot to occur after adding other elements to the blood, such as tissue factor, phospholipid, and calcium.[1,5] The PT level relies on the following components: Factors VII, X, V, II, and fibrinogen.[1,5] The PT level is calculated by seeing how long it takes for the specimen to clot once calcium is added to this mixture. The aPTT (CPT code 85730) level evaluates the intrinsic and common pathways of coagulation. The PT and aPTT tests are often both needed to evaluate different hematologic states. aPTT is the amount of time it takes the blood to form a clot in seconds.[1,5,6] All factors except factor VII and factor XIII are tested in the aPTT. The INR (CPT code 85610) is a standardized number that is determined using PT in the following calculation:

$$INR = Patient\ PT \div Control\ PT$$

The information jointly derived from the PT, aPTT, and INR provide a more holistic picture of how the blood is maintaining hemostasis. Individually, the PT and aPTT give more information about the specific possible missing factors in the clotting cascade, medication issues, or nutritional deficiencies contributing to bleeding or clotting issues.

INDICATIONS
Screening
There is no universal screening for PT/aPTT levels.

Targeted screening with PT/aPTT levels should be considered in the following populations:

- Preoperative screening to evaluate bleeding or thrombosis risk in patients with a known history of increased risk of bleeding or thrombosis[6]
  - In children with no personal or family history of bleeding, routine preoperative screening for PT/aPTT levels is not indicated.[7]
  - In adults, obtaining a PT/aPTT level for low-risk surgeries without a clinical indication is not warranted. These tests are not reliable predictors of perioperative bleeding.[8]
- Family history of VWD, including any extended family members[2]
- Prior diagnosis of VWD and currently pregnant (screen in third trimester to determine delivery plan)[2,3]
- To determine liver synthesis function and to calculate the Model for End-stage Liver Disease (MELD) score or the Child-Pugh score for cirrhosis mortality[4]
- To provide a baseline level prior to initiation of anticoagulants[7-9]

Diagnosis and Evaluation
Consider drawing PT/aPTT levels in the following circumstances:

- Often used in initial hemostasis and hemophilic testing when there is a clinical suspicion for a bleeding or clotting disorder.[5,9,10]
- Individual has signs or symptoms of excessive unexplained bleeding or thrombosis.[10-14]
  - Unexplained bruising/bleeding
  - Hemorrhage
  - Hematoma
  - Petechiae or petechial rash
  - Signs of disseminated intravascular coagulation (DIC)
  - Swollen extremity with or without prior trauma
  - A consistent menorrhagia history in a patient who is not taking oral contraceptives[13]
  - Patients with an unprovoked deep venous thrombosis (DVT) or pulmonary embolism (PE) where there is no family history (where lupus anticoagulant positivity is in question)
- Any individual with International Society on Thrombosis and Hemostasis (ISTH) bleeding assessment tool (BAT) score of six or greater
- Patients with severe liver disease
- To determine severity of congenital factor deficiencies such as hemophilia and VWD
- To determine what type of dysfibrinogenemia diagnoses

■ COVID-19 can cause moderate elevations of PT/aPTT. There is current discussion that this may be more likely with the presence of a lupus anticoagulant.

Monitoring

■ PT/aPTT/INR is most frequently used to monitor anticoagulation (e.g., warfarin, heparin, direct oral anticoagulants).[11,15-19]
  ● Warfarin
    ■ Patients initiated on warfarin are monitored at least two times per week at the start of therapy, then weekly, then every 2 to 3 weeks until they are stable enough to be checked monthly. Patients with stable INR levels can be checked at longer intervals (6 to 12 weeks).
    "The American College of Chest Physicians guidelines recommend short-term warfarin therapy, with the goal of maintaining an INR of 2.5 +/− 0.5, after major surgery. Therapy for venous thromboembolism (VTE) includes an INR of 2.5 +/− 0.5, with the length of therapy determined by associated conditions."
    ■ INR should be indefinitely maintained between 2 and 3 for atrial fibrillation.
    ■ INR should be maintained between 2.5 and 3.5 for patients with mechanical heart valves.
      ● One mechanical aortic valve replacement has Food and Drug Administration (FDA)-approved recommendations of an INR of 1.5 to 2.0 when used with aspirin.
    ■ INR needs to be raised to a therapeutic level to discontinue the initial daily low molecular weight heparin injections that are needed when beginning warfarin.
    ■ The Clinical Pharmacogenetics Implementation Consortium (CPIC) has specific guidelines for warfarin dosing for individuals with common genetic variants. *CYP2C9, VKORC1, CYP4F2,* and the *CYP2C* cluster, plus known nongenetic factors, account for ~50% of warfarin dose variability. Testing and associated dosing adjustments should be considered in patients with suspected genetic variants.
    ■ See Table 133.1 for factors that may alter the INR levels for patients taking warfarin.
    ■ See Table 133.2 for adjusting maintenance warfarin dosing based on INR level.
  ● Unfractionated heparin[20]
    ■ The aPTT should not be used to monitor children under the age of 12. The anti-factor Xa assay for heparin must be used.
    ■ Individuals over the age of 12 should have their aPTT levels kept in the heparin therapeutic range as determined by the ex vivo method; however, aPTT is not the most accurate method for monitoring heparin therapy. The anti-factor Xa assay is more accurate and does not rely on aPTT monitoring.
■ Oral factor Xa inhibitors do not require routine monitoring.[21]
■ Monitor PT levels to see improvements in vitamin K deficiencies, liver disease, or other states of malnutrition.

TABLE 133.1: FACTORS THAT MAY ALTER THE INTERNATIONAL NORMALIZED RATIO WHILE ON WARFARIN

Medications	Antacids, antibiotics, antifungals, aspirin, acetaminophen, cold/allergy medications, ibuprofen, amiodarone
OTC supplements	Ginkgo, garlic, ginseng, green tea, vitamin E, St. John's wort
Conditions	CHF, thyroid problems, malnutrition/skipping meals
Foods	• Foods high in vitamin K such as kale, mustard greens, Brussels sprouts, spinach, broccoli, asparagus, collard greens. May eat in moderation to avoid labile levels of INR because too little will increase bleeding risk, and too much vitamin K will decrease warfarin's effectiveness • Grapefruit, garlic, alcohol, cranberries/juice

CHF, congestive heart failure; INR, International Normalized Ratio; OTC, over the counter.

Source: Kamal AH, Tefferi A, Pruthi RK. How to interpret and pursue an abnormal prothrombin time, activated partial thromboplastin time, and bleeding time in adults. *May Clin Proc.* 2007;82(7):864–873. doi:10.4065/82.7.864

TABLE 133.2: ADJUSTING MAINTENANCE DOSE OF WARFARIN BASED ON INTERNATIONAL NORMALIZED RATIO LEVEL

INR LEVEL	DOSE ADJUSTMENT	RETEST
Less than 2	Increase weekly dose by 5%–20%	1 week
2–3* • 2.5 +/– 0.5 VTE* • 2–3 for atrial fibrillation • 2.5–3.5 for patients with mechanical heart valves • 2.5 +/– 0.5 after major surgery	Continue same dose	1 month
3.0–3.5	Decrease weekly dose by 5%–15%	1 week
INR of 3.6–4	Withhold no dose to one dose Decrease weekly dose by 10%–15%	1 week
INR greater than 4	Withhold no dose to one dose Decrease weekly dose by 10%–20%	3–7 days

*Can vary based on the underlying etiology.

INR, International Normalized Ratio; VTE, venous thromboembolism.

■ Monitor levels postoperatively for treatment needs, especially after major surgery and with a prior history of a coagulation problem.
■ The Choosing Wisely recommendation advises that clinicians should not routinely monitor coagulation tests during a course of therapeutic plasma exchange, unless the procedure is performed daily.[22]

INTERPRETATION

See Tables 133.3 and 133.4 for interpretation of results.

TABLE 133.3: REFERENCE VALUE FOR PROTHROMBIN, ACTIVATED PARTIAL THROMBOPLASTIN TIME, AND INTERNATIONAL NORMALIZED RATIO

COAGULATION TEST	NORMAL RANGE
PT	13–15 seconds
aPTT	25–35 seconds
INR	≤ 1.1

aPTT, activated partial thromboplastin time; INR, International Normalized Ratio; PT, prothrombin.

TABLE 133.4: INTERPRETATION CONSIDERATIONS WITH ABNORMAL PROTHROMBIN/ ACTIVATED PARTIAL THROMBOPLASTIN TIME LEVELS

PT LEVEL	aPTT LEVEL	PATHWAY AFFECTED	NEXT STEPS AND DIFFERENTIAL DIAGNOSES
Normal	Normal	Both intrinsic and extrinsic pathways are intact	Could be a mild factor deficiency; evaluation should focus on platelet function activity. Consider mild von Willebrand disease or platelet function disorders
Normal	Prolonged	Intrinsic	Mixing study to distinguish abnormalities in the clotting factors (VIII, IX, and XI) vs. clotting factor inhibitors (mostly factor VIII inhibitor and lupus anticoagulant)
Prolonged	Normal	Extrinsic	Warfarin therapy *Uncommon Consider evaluation for vitamin K deficiency or factor VII deficiency
Prolonged	Prolonged	Both intrinsic and extrinsic pathways are affected	Could be liver failure, acute DIC, defects in the common pathway, or warfarin overdose. Consider liver function tests, fibrinogen levels, and factor assays

aPTT, activated partial thromboplastin time; DIC, disseminated intravascular coagulation; PT, prothrombin.

Source: Kamal AH, Tefferi A, Pruthi RK. How to interpret and pursue an abnormal prothrombin time, activated partial thromboplastin time, and bleeding time in adults. *May Clin Proc.* 2007;82(7):864–873. doi:10.4065/82.7.864

FOLLOW-UP

Once the initial PT/PTT (INR) panel is drawn, additional testing may be needed based on these results. Depending on the patient presentation and risk factors, follow-up tests can include but are not limited to liver function tests, fibrinogen, thrombin time, mixing studies, homocysteine, protein C, protein S, factor assays, prothrombin gene mutation, lupus anticoagulant, antiphospholipid antibodies, and antithrombin (Figure 133.1).

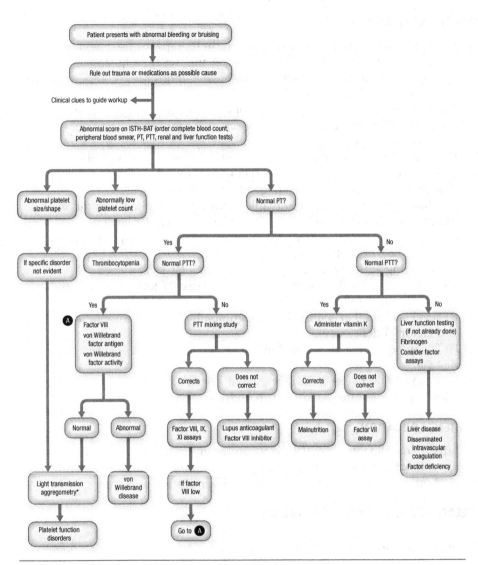

*—This test should be ordered only by a hematologist.

FIGURE 133.1. Laboratory evaluation for abnormal bruising and bleeding. PT, prothrombin; PTT, partial thromboplastin time.

- Indiscriminate testing for heritable thrombophilias in unselected patients presenting with a first episode of venous thrombosis is not indicated.[13]
- Consider obtaining antiphospholipid antibodies to evaluate for antiphospholipid antibody syndrome (APS) with both an elevated PT and history or strong family history of thrombosis. Presence of these antibodies decreases prothrombin and simultaneously causes increased thrombin, causing PT level to possibly prolong.[23]

PEARLS & PITFALLS

- For patients receiving maintenance warfarin therapy for treatment of VTE, home point-of-care INR patient self-testing and dosage adjustment is recommended in suitable patients who have demonstrated competency and who can afford this option.[19]
- The ISTH has a BAT that can screen for a possible bleeding disorder.[12]
- Consider referral to hematology after screening for consultation on abnormal findings.
- Vitamin K levels should not be tested unless the patient has an abnormal INR and has not responded to vitamin K therapy.[24,25]
- Ask about a family history of congenital factor deficiencies.[2]
- Specimen tubes that are not fully filled may have a limited amount of plasma and factors present, causing false elevation in PT level.[26]
- Consider PT level when there is evidence of malnutrition, prolonged antibiotic use, or problems with fat digestion.[26]
- Direct acting anticoagulants (DOAC's) prolong PT level.[26]
- High cholesterol and triglyceride levels decrease PT level due to more fibrinogen and factor VII levels.[26]
- PT level is normal in some severe coagulopathy issues (hemophilia A, B, and factor XI deficiency).[26]
- PTT may be normal or elevated in VWD, depending on the severity of the disease.[2,3]
- PTT can be falsely elevated if the patient has APS.[23]
- Alert for liver failure workup when both the PT and PTT are elevated.[26]

PATIENT EDUCATION

- https://medlineplus.gov/lab-tests/prothrombin-time-test-and-inr-ptinr/
- www.heart.org/en/health-topics/arrhythmia/prevention--treatment-of -arrhythmia/a-patients-guide-to-taking-warfarin

RELATED DIAGNOSES AND ICD-10 CODES

Von Willebrand disease	D68.0	Pulmonary embolism	126.9
Menorrhagia	N92.0	Venous thrombotic event	Z86.718
Epistaxis	R04.0	Hemophilia A	D68.311
Coagulation defect, unspecified	D68.9	Hemophilia B	D67
Antiphospholipid antibody syndrome	D68.61	Hypercoagulable disorder	289.81
Deep vein thrombosis	182.40	Bruising easily	459.89

REFERENCES

Full list of references can be accessed through Springer Publishing Company Connect™ at the following link: http://connect.springerpub.com/content/reference-book/978-0-8261 -8843-4/part/part03/toc-part/ch133

134. QUAD SCREEN/SECOND TRIMESTER ANEUPLOIDY SCREENING

Cara A. Busenhart

PHYSIOLOGY/PATHOPHYSIOLOGY REVIEW

Chromosomal abnormalities affect approximately 1/250 births, including live births, fetal deaths, and pregnancy terminations.[1] The most common aneuploidy, trisomy 21, accounts for more than 50% of fetal chromosomal abnormalities.[1] As maternal age increases, the risk of Down syndrome increases (Table 134.1). Trisomy 18 occurs in approximately one in 2,000 recognized pregnancies and one in 6,600 live births. This accounts for about 15% of fetal chromosomal abnormalities.[1]

OVERVIEW OF LABORATORY TESTS

The quad screen is a measurement of four markers in the serum of a pregnant patient to inform the patient and provider about the likelihood that the fetus will have certain aneuploidies (trisomy 21 or trisomy 18) or neural tube defects.[2,3] The four markers measure levels of alpha feto-protein (AFP), human chorionic gonadotropin (hCG), unconjugated estriol (ue3), and dimeric inhibin A (inhibin).[4,5] The test is typically performed between 15- and 20-weeks' gestation (and occasionally up to 22 weeks, depending on laboratory) and is one of multiple screening options that should be offered to all pregnant patients regardless of age.[1,3,4,6]

The overall screen positive (abnormal) rate for the quad screen is 5% and the screen negative (normal) rate is 95%.[1,4] The detection rate for Down syndrome (trisomy 21) is 80% to 81%.[4,7] Trisomy 18 detection is similar to that for Down syndrome (~80%), with a false-positive rate of only 0.5%.[7] The detection rate for neural tube defect is at least 90% for anencephaly and 80% for spina bifida.[7]

TABLE 134.1: DOWN SYNDROME RISK RELATED TO MATERNAL AGE	
MATERNAL AGE (YEARS)	**RISK OF DOWN SYNDROME**
20	1 in 1,500
30	1 in 800
35	1 in 270
45	In excess of 1 in 50

INDICATIONS

Screening

■ The American College of Obstetricians and Gynecologists recommend that the quad test be made available as one option for prenatal screening or diagnosis of genetic disorders in pregnancy.[1,4] If the pregnant patient presents after the first trimester (up to 25% of pregnancies), the quad screen may be the only viable screening option for aneuploidy.[1,4,5,7]

■ If the pregnant patient has undergone noninvasive first trimester screening via cell-free fetal DNA (cfDNA), the patient should not be offered the quad screen since there is little clinical value in additional testing.[7,8] However, a single test for alpha-fetoprotein (AFP) may be offered to screen for neural tube structural defects in the pregnancy since cfDNA would not screen for this defect.

Diagnosis and Evaluation

■ Not used for diagnosis; it is only used for screening.

Monitoring

■ Not used in monitoring.

INTERPRETATION

Overall Risk Interpretation

■ Likelihood ratios are computed for each marker within the quad screen and are combined with the patient's age, race, and weight, as well as the number of fetuses in the current gestation, diabetes status, and gestational age to provide a risk estimate for Down syndrome, trisomy 18, and neural tube defects.[1,2,7,9]

■ If abnormal values are noted, gestational age should be confirmed as this is vitally important to interpretation of the results.[1]

■ Multiple gestation, unsure pregnancy dating (gestational age), maternal weight, presence of maternal diabetes, and maternal age can all influence the interpretation of results.[4,7,9]

Serum Marker Values and Fetal Risk

■ Decreased levels of AFP are associated with chromosomal abnormalities (i.e., low levels = increased risk); elevated levels are associated with neural tube defects, such as anencephaly and spina bifida (i.e., increased levels = increased risk).[2]

■ Abnormal values of hCG have been implicated in increased miscarriage risk, which is often related to chromosomal abnormalities.[2]

■ A risk of Down syndrome (trisomy 21) is indicated by decreased AFP and uE3 and elevated hCG and inhibin.[7,9]

■ A risk of trisomy 18 is indicated by decreased AFP, uE3, and hCG (inhibin levels are not used in this aneuploidy assessment).[7,9]

■ In general, elevation of either hCG or inhibin levels in the second trimester has significant association with adverse pregnancy outcomes overall.[7]

When several markers are elevated, the likelihood of an adverse pregnancy outcome is higher.
■ Sensitivity and false-positive rate
  ● Quad screen: sensitivity of 80% to 82%; false-positive rate of 5%.[1,5]
  ● Quad screen false-positive rate is much higher than with alternative first trimester screening with cfDNA, which has a false-positive rate of 0.1% and sensitivity of 99%.[1,10]
  ● False-positive rate increases with maternal age.[10]
■ While a negative test result cannot guarantee an unaffected fetus, a negative result is quite reassuring as the negative predictive value is greater than 99%.[1]

FOLLOW-UP

■ With any positive result:
  ● Pregnant patients should be offered genetic counseling, a comprehensive ultrasound evaluation, and diagnostic testing to confirm results.[4,9] Diagnostic testing includes either amniocentesis or chorionic villus sampling (CVS), depending on the gestational age of the pregnancy.[2] Many patients, though, elect not to have diagnostic testing.[1]
■ With any negative result:
  ● Pregnant patients should be made aware that their risk of a fetus with any of the conditions screened by the test are low, but the screening test cannot guarantee that the fetus is unaffected.
  ● Pregnant patients should be informed that there is potential for a fetus to be affected by genetic disorders that are not evaluated by the screening test.
  ● Even if the pregnant patient has a negative screening test result for Down syndrome, trisomy 18, or neural tube defect, they still have the option to choose diagnostic testing later in pregnancy.[4]
■ Alternatives to quad screening include:
  ● First trimester ultrasound and/or maternal serum marker testing (PAPP-A)[6]; triple screen (does not include inhibin) and penta screen (adds hyperglycosylated hCG)—these tests do not offer any benefit or improved test characteristics.[5]
  ● cfDNA screening is offered in the first trimester and is expensive but may be more cost-effective than the quad screen related to its improved sensitivity and specificity.[10]
  ● Diagnostic tests: amniocentesis or CVS[4]—these tests are more invasive, yet provide greater certainty of risk and/or confirmation of diagnosis.
  ● For neural tube defects, second trimester ultrasound often identifies most abnormalities and is a routine part of all pregnancy care.[7]

PEARLS & PITFALLS

■ Test results are difficult to interpret in multiple gestation pregnancies, where most serum markers will be altered by the presence of multiple fetuses.[2]
■ Advantages to quad testing include that it is a test at a single point in time and does not require specialized equipment and/or personnel to

administer. Therefore, it is very useful in low resource settings.[4,5] Another advantage is the ability to screen for open neural tube defects, which differentiates this test from other maternal serum testing and/or diagnostic tests which screen for aneuploidy alone.[5]

■ Disadvantages to quad screening include the lower detection rate for aneuploidy compared to other available tests (first trimester and second trimester combined screening tests).[4]

■ Patients should not undergo more than one screening test for aneuploidy during the pregnancy, as rates of detection are not improved, and the cost of multiple tests may be burdensome.[5]

■ A wide variety of prenatal screening and diagnostic tests is available, and each test offers varying levels of performance and information to the pregnant patient and her clinician. Therefore[4,7,9]:
  ● There is a need for nuanced, patient-centered counseling.
  ● Each patient should be counseled in each pregnancy about options for testing, including the risk of fetal chromosomal/structural abnormalities, basic information about each condition, and the relative benefits and limitations of the available screening and diagnostic tests.

■ Informed decision-making can only occur if the patient has appropriate health literacy and is able to engage with their clinician.[11]

■ All patients should be instructed that they have the right to accept or decline testing.[1,4]

■ Decisions about screening and possible results carry significant anxiety for expectant parents.[1,2]

■ Parents should understand that the results of screening may aid them in determining next steps and/or progression of the pregnancy.[1,6,9]

PATIENT EDUCATION

■ https://www.acog.org/womens-health/infographics/prenatal-genetic -testing-chart
■ https://www.acog.org/womens-health/faqs/prenatal-genetic-screening -tests
■ https://americanpregnancy.org/prenatal-testing/quad-screen-742/

RELATED DIAGNOSES AND ICD-10 CODES

Maternal care for (suspected) chromosomal abnormality in fetus, not specified	O35.2XX0
Maternal care for other (suspected) fetal abnormality and damage, not applicable or not specified	O35.8XX0
Maternal care for (suspected) central nervous system malformation in fetus, not applicable or specified	O35.0XX0
Abnormal chromosomal and genetic finding on antenatal screening of mother	O28.3
Encounter for antenatal screening for chromosomal anomalies	Z36.0
Down syndrome, unspecified	Q90.9

Trisonomy 18	Q91.3
Neural tube defect	
• Anencephaly	Q00
• Spina bifida	Q05.9

REFERENCES

Full list of references can be accessed through Springer Publishing Company Connect™ at the following link: http://connect.springerpub.com/content/reference-book/978-0-8261-8843-4/part/part03/toc-part/ch134

135. RED BLOOD CELL COUNT AND INDICES

Kelly Small Casler

PHYSIOLOGY REVIEW

Red blood cells (RBCs), also called erythrocytes, are the most abundant type of blood cell arising from hematopoietic stem cells in the bone marrow. One RBC carries multiple Hgb molecules, each comprised of two pairs of globin chains. A heme-iron dyad is present on each globin chain to bind oxygen, delivering it to the tissues. RBCs account for approximately 45% of the whole blood volume, with the other 55% of whole blood being plasma. Decreased numbers of RBCs are termed anemia. Anemia can occur from faulty RBC production or loss of RBC to hemolysis or hemorrhage. In pregnancy, blood volume expansion leads to anemia in some patients.[1] Elevations in RBC numbers is termed erythrocytosis.

OVERVIEW OF LABORATORY TESTS

An RBC count is often the first item reported on a complete blood count (CBC) and reflects the number of RBCs present per microliter or liter of blood. Hemoglobin (Hgb) concentration reflects the amount of Hgb present in a specified volume of blood. Hematocrit (Hct) (also called packed cell volume) reflects the percentage of the whole blood volume that is composed of RBCs. Traditionally, Hct was measured by measuring the quantity of RBCs that collected at the bottom of the test tube after centrifuging; currently, it is measured through computer analysis.

RBC indices are reported with RBC counts to describe the relationship of Hgb to the RBC count and volume. Mean corpuscular volume (MCV) reflects the average volume, or size, of one RBC. It is usually estimated by dividing the Hct by the RBC count. Small cells have a low MCV (referred to as microcytic) and large cells have a high MCV (macrocytic). Normal size cells are called normocytic. It is common for there to be variations in the size/volume of the cells, but excessive variation of RBC size is called anisocytosis, and is reflected as an elevation of the red cell distribution width (RDW). Mean corpuscular hemoglobin, or MCH, is the mass or average amount of Hgb per each RBC. It can be calculated by dividing the Hgb content by the RBC count. Mean corpuscular hemoglobin concentration (MCHC) is the average content of Hgb in the entire volume of RBCs and is calculated by dividing the Hgb by the Hct. An elevated MCHC is termed hyperchromia while decreased MCHC is termed hypochromia.

Point-of-care tests are available to test Hgb or Hct levels. Capillary whole blood samples are used but tend to produce slightly higher Hgb results compared to venous blood samples used for laboratory-based tests. Proper technique per manufacturer instructions is crucial in getting an accurate result.[2]

INDICATIONS
Screening
- For anemia, universal screening with a CBC or Hgb/Hct has not been shown to reduce mortality or lead to detection of serious disease and is therefore not recommended in adults.[1,3] However, targeted screening in patients with a glomerular filtration rate lower than 60 mL/min/1.73 m^2 is recommended.[4,5]
- Screening for anemia is recommended by some authorities in pregnant individuals and not recommended by others:
  - The United States Preventive Services Task Force (USPSTF) notes there is insufficient evidence, especially regarding mortality/morbidity reduction, to recommend screening for anemia in pregnant individuals.[6]
  - The American College of Obstetricians and Gynecologists recommends for screening, though recommendations for frequency or method of screening (CBC versus Hgb versus ferritin) are not made.[1] This recommendation is mostly based in expert consensus/opinion.
  - United Kingdom guidelines recommend anemia screening once in the first trimester and once again in the third trimester, but the guidelines acknowledge the limited impact screening has on morbidity/mortality.[7]
- Screening for anemia with Hgb is recommended by some authorities for children. While the USPSTF concludes the evidence is insufficient to support screening children ages 6 to 24 months,[8] the American Academy of Pediatrics (AAP) does recommend universal screening for children ages 9 to 12 months.[9,10]
  - Re-screening for anemia with Hgb again at age 24 months is suggested by the AAP since iron deficiency may not be severe enough to lead to anemia (and thus, picked up on screening with Hg) by age 12 months.[10] Children with risk factors for iron deficiency anemia (low socioeconomic status, premature infants, low birth weight infants, poor nutrition) should especially be re-screened.[9] These high-risk children can be re-screened yearly as needed.[11]

- The Centers for Disease Control and Prevention recommends screening for anemia in nonpregnant adolescents every 5 to 10 years.[11]
- Patients with traumatic injuries or menorrhagia can also be screened for anemia using RBC/Hgb/Hct.

Diagnosis and Evaluation

- See Box 135.1[9,12] for signs and symptoms that warrant evaluation of RBC/Hgb/Hct for the detection of anemia.

Monitoring

- Hgb is used to monitor response to iron therapy: Hgb should increase by 1 g/dL within 2 to 4 weeks of treatment initiation. If it does not, then patients should have evaluation for alternate diagnoses or occult bleeding. They may also need referral for intravenous iron treatment.[9,13]
- Hgb and RBCs are monitored at initiation and during certain drug therapies, such as chemotherapy.
- Frequent monitoring of RBC and RBC indices at varying intervals is common for hospitalized patients.[14]

Box 135.1: Signs/Symptoms Associated With Anemia

- Angina
- Angular cheilitis/glossitis
- Behavior changes
- Cardiac murmur
- Cold sensitivity
- Dry/rough skin
- Easy bleeding/bruising
- Fatigue
- Hair loss
- Headaches
- Heart failure
- Hemodynamic instability
- Malaise
- Pallor
- Pica
- Restless legs syndrome
- Shortness of breath
- Sleep disorders
- Spoon nails (koilonychia)
- Syncope-presyncope
- Tachycardia

Sources: Data from Baker RD, Greer FR, The Committee on Nutrition. Diagnosis and prevention of iron deficiency and iron-deficiency anemia in infants and young children (0–3 years of age). *Pediatrics.* 2010;126(5):1040–1050. doi:10.1542/peds.2010-2576; on behalf of the SPOG Pediatric Hematology Working Group, Mattiello V, Schmugge M, et al. Diagnosis and management of iron deficiency in children with or without anemia: consensus recommendations of the SPOG Pediatric Hematology Working Group. *Eur J Pediatr.* 2020;179(4):527–545. doi:10.1007/s00431-020-03597-5

- Hgb and Hct are monitored every 3 months in transgender males receiving gender-affirming therapy with testoterone.[15] Levels are also monitored in cisgender males requiring testosterone therapy.[16]

INTERPRETATION: ANEMIA

- Reference intervals for Hgb levels and reference limits for diagnosing anemia are listed in Tables 135.1 and 135.2 with the following caveats to be noted.
  - Normal ranges can vary significantly by race, ethnicity, age, and sex, making it difficult to include just one set of reference ranges.[17]
  - On average, Hgb levels in males with Caucasian genetic heritage are 1 to 2 g/dL higher than in women with Caucasian genetic heritage or males of other genetic heritage.[17,18]
  - World Health Organization cutoffs for anemia based on Hgb are the most widely accepted reference limit for anemia and are listed in Table 135.2, but do not account for racial, ethnic, or gender differences.[19]

TABLE 135.1: NORMAL HEMOGLOBIN CONTENT BY AGE ACCORDING TO NHANES DATA

12 months	11.1–14.1 g/dL
4 years	11.2–14.3 g/dL
6 years	11.4–14.5 g/dL
10 years	11.8–15 g/dL
21 years and older	12–15.6 g/dL

NHANES, National Health and Nutrition Examination Survey

Source: Data from Fulgoni VL, Agarwal S, Kellogg MD, Lieberman HR. Establishing pediatric and adult RBC reference intervals with NHANES data using piecewise regression. *Am J Clin Pathol.* 2019;151(2):128–142. doi:10.1093/ajcp/aqy116

TABLE 135.2: ANEMIA DEFINITIONS

POPULATION	DEFINITION OF ANEMIA
Pregnancy (ACOG): first & third trimester[1]	HgB <11 g/dL or Hct <33%
Pregnancy (ACOG): second trimester	HgB <10.5 g/dL or Hct <32%
Children 6–59 months of age (WHO)	HgB <11.0 g/dL
Children 5–11 years (WHO)	HgB <11.5 g/dL
Children 12–14 years old & non-pregnant females age 15 and older (WHO)	HgB <12.0 g/dL
Pregnancy (all trimesters) (WHO)	HgB <11.0 g/dL
Males age 15 and above (WHO)	HgB <13 g/dL

ACOG, American College of Obstetricians and Gynecologists; Hct, hematocrit; HgB, hemoglobin; WHO, World Health Organization.

Sources: Data from American College of Obstetricians and Gynecologists. ACOG Practice Bulletin No. 95: Anemia in Pregnancy. *Obstet Gynecol.* 2008;112(1):201–207. doi:10.1097/AOG.0b013e3181809c0d; McLean E, Cogswell M, Egli I, Wojdyla D, de Benoist B. Worldwide prevalence of anaemia, WHO vitamin and mineral nutrition information system, 1993–2005. *Public Health Nutr.* 2009;12(4):444–454. doi:10.1017/S1368980008002401

- Up to 5% of the population may have a result outside of the listed reference intervals, but be completely absent of disease (this concept is reviewed in Chapter 3).[18,20,21]

INTERPRETATION: ERYTHROCYTOSIS

- The terms "erythrocytosis" and "polycythemia" are used interchangeably by some individuals; however, erythrocytosis should only be used to refer to increases in the RBC count alone, while polycythemia is used to describe elevations in the RBC count in addition to elevations in white blood cell (WBC) count and platelets.[22]
- Erythrocytosis is diagnosed after a persistent elevation in the Hgb/Hct for 2 months or longer.[23]
- Relative erythrocytosis is seen in dehydration, burns, or diuretic use and resolves after correction of the underlying abnormality.[22]
- Primary erythrocytosis involves a defective bone marrow that causes myeloproliferation. Erythropoietin (EPO) levels are usually low. The most common cause of primary erythrocytosis is polycythemia vera.[22,24] Box 135.2[22,25–29] summarizes findings that should alert the clinician to possible polycythemia vera.
- Secondary erythrocytosis occurs in conditions associated with hypoxia. Hypoxia triggers release of EPO (smoking, chronic obstructive pulmonary disease, obstructive sleep apnea, congenital heart disease, residing at high altitudes). Secondary erythrocytosis can also occur as a result of hepatologic and renal carcinomas or other neoplasms.[22,24]

FOLLOW-UP: ANEMIA

- Identifying anemia through a low Hgb, Hct, or RBC count is perhaps the easiest step of interpreting RBC counts and their indices. The next step is

---

Box 135.2: When to Consider Referral for Polycythemia Vera Evaluation

- Splenomegaly
- Severe or aquagenic pruritis
- Budd-Chiari syndrome/portal vein thrombosis
- Hgb >16.5 g/dL in males and >16 g/dL in females
- Hct >48%-50% in males and ≥45%-47% in females. Hct >60% in males and >53% in females makes PV extremely likely
- The presence of leukocytosis and thrombocytopenia*

*Does not always occur, but when present usually associated with worse outcomes

Sources: Data from Ayalew Tefferi. Clinical manifestations and diagnosis of polycythemia vera. In: *UpTo Date.* 2020; Barbui T, Masciulli A, Marfisi MR, et al. White blood cell counts and thrombosis in polycythemia vera: a subanalysis of the CYTO-PV study. *Blood.* 2015;126(4):560–561. doi:10.1182/blood-2015-04-638593; Lamy T, Devillers A, Bernard M, et al. Inapparent polycythemia vera: an unrecognized diagnosis. *Am J Med.* 1997;102(1):14–20. doi:10.1016/S0002-9343(96)00351-8; Maffioli M, Mora B, Passamonti F. Polycythemia vera: from new, modified diagnostic criteria to new therapeutic approaches. *Clin Adv Hematol Oncol.* 2017;15(9):700–707; Prchal JT. Primary and secondary erythrocytoses. In: Kaushansky K, Lichtman MA, Prchal JT, et al., eds. *Williams Hematology, 9th ed.* McGraw-Hill Education; 2015. http:accessmedicine.mhmedical.com/content.aspx?aid=1121095073; Tefferi A. Polycythemia vera: a comprehensive review and clinical recommendations. *Mayo Clin Proc.* 2003;78(2):174–194. doi:10.4065/78.2.174;

to identify the type of anemia and its etiology. This is usually approached in one of two ways: either through a morphologic approach using MCV to guide differential diagnosis of anemia type (see Table 135.3)[30-32] or the kinetic approach (Table 135.4).[32] The kinetic approach requires evaluation of the reticulocyte production index (RPI), an additional laboratory test.

- In anemia, if hemolysis is suspected, evaluate a peripheral blood smear, lactate dehydrogenase (LDH), haptoglobin, bilirubin, and/or direct coombs' to assess for clues to hemolysis or blood loss. Haptoglobin levels will be decreased in hemolysis, while LDH and bilirubin will be increased.
- Always consider evaluation for occult gastrointestinal bleeding in patients with iron deficiency anemia.
- Consider all RBC indices to get a full clinical picture (Table 135.5).[34,35]
- Differentiating iron deficiency anemia (IDA), anemia of chronic disease/anemia of inflammation (ACD/AI), and thalassemia from one another is not always straightforward. Clues to thalassemia are present on the RBC indices and include a MCV lower than 75 fL and RBC count greater than 4.5×10^6 cells/μL.[33] Other clues to differentiate thalassemia from IDA and ACD/AI are summarized in Table 135.6.[34-37] Differentiation of ACD/AI from IDA may also require ferritin and iron studies.

TABLE 135.3: DIFFERENTIAL DIAGNOSIS OF ANEMIA USING MEAN CORPUSCULAR VALUE (MORPHOLOGIC APPROACH)

MICROCYTIC (MCV <80)		NORMOCYTIC (MCV 80 TO 100)	MACROCYTIC (MCV >100)*	
Differential Diagnosis	Parameters used to evaluate for the diagnosis	Proceed to kinetic approach—order RPI: RPI <2 (no reticulocytosis): consider ACD^ or early IDA. RPI >3 (reticulocytosis present): consider blood loss/hemolysis	Differential Diagnosis	Parameters used to evaluate for the diagnosis
IDA	Ferritin, iron studies		Vitamin B12 deficiency	Vitamin B12 level
ACD/AI	CRP, sTfR, iron studies		Folate deficiency	Serum folate
Thalassemia	Hgb electrophoresis, genetic testing		Medication side effects	History
Plumbism (lead poisoning)	Serum lead level			
Sideroblastic anemia	Peripheral blood smear, liver transaminases, bone marrow biopsy			

(Continued)

TABLE 135.3: DIFFERENTIAL DIAGNOSIS OF ANEMIA USING MEAN CORPUSCULAR VALUE (MORPHOLOGIC APPROACH) (*CONTINUED*)

MICROCYTIC (MCV <80)		NORMOCYTIC (MCV 80 TO 100)	MACROCYTIC (MCV >100)*
Hereditary spherocytosis	Family history		
G6PD deficiency	Family history/ genetic tests		

*Alcohol overuse also causes macrocytosis and can be identified through history. Gamma-glutamyl transferase and liver transaminases can also assist with diagnosis.

^Check CRP to evaluate for inflammation or a blood urea nitrogen/creatinine to evaluate for chronic kidney disease.

ACD/AI, anemia of chronic disease/anemia of inflammation; CRP, C-reactive protein; IDA, iron deficiency anemia; MCV, mean corpusclar volume; RPI, reticulocyte production index; sTfR, serum transferrin receptor.

Sources: Data from Auerbach M, James SE, Nicoletti M, et al. Results of the first American prospective study of intravenous iron in oral iron-intolerant iron-deficient gravidas. *Am J Med.* 2017;130(12):1402–1407. doi:10.1016/j.amjmed.2017.06.025; Ho JC, Chan AKC, Lau KK, Chan HHW. Iron deficiency as a common treatable cause of chronic normocytic anemia. *Blood.* 2014;124(21):4032–4032. doi:10.1182/blood.V124.21.4032.4032; Piva E, Brugnara C, Spolaore F, Plebani M. Clinical utility of reticulocyte parameters. *Clin Lab Med.* 2015;35(1):133–163. doi:10.1016/j.cll.2014.10.004

TABLE 135.4: KINETIC APPROACH TO DIFFERENTIAL DIAGNOSIS

UNDERPRODUCTION/NO RETICULOCYTOSIS (RPI <2)	ADEQUATE BONE MARROW RESPONSE (RPI >3)
Nutritional anemias, anemia of inflammation, thalassemia, sideroblastic anemia, plubism, medication side effects, aplastic anemia	Blood loss/hemolysis, G6PD deficiency, response to therapy for micro- or macrocytic anemia

Source: Data from Piva E, Brugnara C, Spolaore F, Plebani M. Clinical utility of reticulocyte parameters. *Clin Lab Med.* 2015;35(1): 133–163. doi:10.1016/j.cll.2014.10.004

TABLE 135.5: OTHER INFORMATION FROM RED BLOOD CELL INDICES THAT MAY BE HELPFUL DURING MORPHOLOGIC APPROACH

MCH DECREASED	MCH INCREASED	HYPOCHROMIA (LOW MCHC)	HYPERCHROMIA (HIGH MCHC)	ANISOCYTOSIS (ELEVATED RDW)
Differential Diagnoses	Differential Diagnoses	Differential Diagnoses	Diifferential Diagnoses	Differential Diagnoses
Lead poisoning, sideroblastic anemia, ACD, thalassemia, IDA	Alcoholism, folate deficiency, B12 deficiency, hemochromatosis, liver disease	IDA, sideroblastic anemia, lead, ACD, thalassemia	Spherocytosis, hemolysis, sickle cell disease	Sideroblastic anemia, IDA, hemolytic anemia, folate deficiency, vitamin B12 deficiency, liver disease

ACD, anemia of chronic disease; MCH, mean corpuscular hemoglobin; MCHC, mean corpuscular hemoglobin concentration; RBC, red blood cell; RDW, red cell distribution width.

Sources: Data from Aydogan G, Keskin S, Akici F, et al. Causes of hypochromic microcytic anemia in children and evaluation of laboratory parameters in the differentiation. *J Pediatr Hematol Oncol.* 2019;41(4):e221–e223. doi:10.1097/MPH.0000000000001382; Hoffmann JJML, Urrechaga E, Aguirre U. Discriminant indices for distinguishing thalassemia and iron deficiency in patients with microcytic anemia: a meta-analysis. *Clin Chem Lab Med (CCLM).* 2015;53(12). doi:10.1515/cclm-2015-0179

TABLE 135.6: DIFFERENTIATING THALASSEMIA VERSUS IRON DEFICIENCY ANEMIA

PARAMETER	THALASSEMIA	IDA
MCHC	Normal (low in some instances)	Low
RDW	Normal	Elevated
Mentzer index* (MCV/RBC)	<13	>13

*89–95% AUROC[35]; 97% to 100% sensitivity in children[34,37]

AUROC, area under the receiver operating characteristic; IDA, iron deficiency anemia; MCHC, mean corpuscular hemoglobin concentration; MCV, mean corpuscular volume; RBC, red blood cell; RDW, red blood cell distribution width.

Source: Data from Hanna M, Fogarty M, Loughrey C, et al. How to use… iron studies. *Arch Dis Child Educ Pract Ed.* 2019;104(6): 321–327. doi:10.1136/archdischild-2018-315234

- Failure for RBC count and RBC indices to improve in response to iron therapy is termed "iron refractory iron deficiency anemia" (IRIDA) and warrants referral to hematology.

FOLLOW-UP: ERYTHROCYTOSIS

- EPO levels are sometimes used in the follow-up of erythrocytosis.[25,26]
  - An elevated EPO level is seen with secondary erythrocytosis.[25]
  - A normal EPO level is sometimes seen with PV.
  - A decreased EPO level is seen with PV, familial polycythemia, renal disorders, and neoplasms.[25]
- If there is high suspicion for PV (Box 135.2), genetic analysis for *JAK2 V617F* mutation can be performed.[25,26]

PEARLS & PITFALLS

- Individuals can be iron deficient without signs of anemia. Therefore, if using Hgb to screen for iron deficiency, consider checking Hgb yearly to pick up on iron deficiency as it progresses to anemia over time.[10]
- Elevations in RDW can be used to identify uncontrolled inflammatory bowel disease.[38]
- Up to 85% of patients with AI/ACD have concurrent iron deficiency.[39]
- Hepcidin is being investigated to differentiate AI/ACD from iron deficiency.[40]
- Due to volume expansion, pregnancy often results in a pseudoanemia.
- In a recent large retrospective study, anemia was found to be associated with poorer maternal and neonatal outcomes such as premature birth, small for gestational age, and longer hospitalization,[41] the study has been critiqued for weaknesses.[42]
- Testosterone therapy can cause erythrocytosis, but whether the erythrocytosis can lead to health risks is still a matter of debate.[16]
- Consideration of the patient's age helps prioritize the differential diagnosis of anemia. For example, a neonate with anemia would first need to be evaluated for congenital hemolytic conditions or isoimmunization while a newly menstruating adolescent may first need to be evaluated for iron deficiency.[43–45]

- In the absence of other signs and symptoms suggestive of PV, it is appropriate to recheck an elevated RBC count in 1 to 2 months to evaluate for a spurious result.
- The female lower reference limit and male upper reference limit for Hct/Hgb should be used when interpreting values in transgender women. In transgender men, the reference range for males should be used unless the patient is still menstruating.[15]

PATIENT EDUCATION

- https://labtestsonline.org/tests/complete-blood-count-cbc

RELATED DIAGNOSES AND ICD-10 CODES

Anemia, unspecified	D46.9
Polycythemia vera	D45

REFERENCES

Full list of references can be accessed through Springer Publishing Company Connect™ at the following link: http://connect.springerpub.com/content/reference-book/978-0-8261-8843-4/part/part03/toc-part/ch135

---

136. RESPIRATORY SYNCYTIAL VIRUS

Courtney Sexton and Rosie Zeno

PHYSIOLOGY REVIEW

Respiratory syncytial virus (RSV) is a single, negative-strand RNA virus transmitted from person to person via direct contact with contaminated fomites or the aerosolized respiratory droplets of infected persons and commonly results in upper respiratory tract infections (URI) in people of all ages.[1] RSV is highly restricted to the respiratory epithelium of the infected host. Once inoculated, viral replication occurs in the nasopharynx with an average incubation period of 4 to 6 days before the onset of URI symptoms.[2]

The onset of subsequent lower respiratory tract (LRT) symptoms occurs approximately 1 to 3 days after the start of URI symptoms. Viral invasion of the bronchiolar epithelium causes epithelial necrosis and inflammation of the bronchi and bronchioles. Resultant edema and mucus production obstructs the small airways causing alveolar air trapping and expiratory wheezing. Infected and necrotic epithelial cells are shed into the airway lumen causing further obstruction and inflammation of the small airways.

Seasonal outbreaks in the United States occur in late fall (October) to early spring (May) with a peak incidence in late January to early February.[3] RSV-related morbidity and mortality are primarily attributed to severe lower respiratory tract infections (LRTI) in young children, older adults, and individuals who are immunocompromised, have a functional disability, or who have chronic cardiopulmonary disease.[4-13]

OVERVIEW OF LABORATORY TESTS

- Molecular testing by real-time, reverse transcription polymerase chain reaction (rRT-PCR) (CPT code 87634) is the gold standard for RSV detection due to its superior sensitivity and specificity in all age groups and its quick specimen-to-result time (hours) compared to viral culture (days).[14,15] Multiplex rRT-PCR arrays can detect multiple respiratory pathogens with comparable sensitivity and specificity (97.9% and 100%, respectively) compared to laboratory-based PCR tests.[16-18] The availability of respiratory viral panels and number of analyses detected vary by institution and the specific testing platform.[19]
- Rapid antigen detection test (RADT) (CPT code 87807) is a reasonable alternative for RSV testing in infants and young children due to its rapid turnaround time (fewer than 30 minutes), its acceptable sensitivity and specificity, and its relatively low cost.[14] However, RADT is significantly less sensitive in adults (29%) compared to young children (81%), which is attributed to higher viral loads in the respiratory secretions of young children.[14,20] Some RADTs are available for use at the point of care with comparable diagnostic accuracy to laboratory-based RADT.[18]
- Serologic testing for RSV IgG antibodies (CPT code 86756) is not recommended for use diagnostically but instead for research and viral surveillance as seroprevalence is high and presence of IgG antibodies typically indicates past exposure and immunity.[14] Viral respiratory culture (CPT code 87254) is highly specific (100%) but its specimen-to-result time (3–5 days) and low sensitivity (17%–39%) make it less useful for diagnosis and clinical decision-making.[19,21]

INDICATIONS

Screening

- There are no recommendations for universal screening.
- Viral URIs are self-limiting, management is supportive, and the diagnosis can be made clinically without laboratory confirmation of the viral etiology.
- The American Academy of Pediatrics recommends the following for the diagnosis of bronchiolitis in young children (younger than age 2 years)[22]:
  - Diagnose bronchiolitis and assess severity on the basis of the history and physical examination findings (Evidence Quality: B; Recommendation Strength: Strong).
  - Assess risk factors for severe RSV disease (younger than 12 weeks of age, history of prematurity, underlying cardiopulmonary disease, or immunodeficiency) to guide evaluation and management (Evidence Quality: B; Recommendation Strength: Moderate).

- When bronchiolitis is diagnosed clinically, laboratory studies should not be routinely obtained. (Evidence Quality: B; Recommendation Strength: Moderate).
- Consider RSV testing only when laboratory confirmation will affect clinical management decisions regarding antibiotic stewardship, infection control measures, continued palivizumab (Synagis®) immunoprophylaxis, or further clinical evaluation for those at higher risk for RSV-related morbidity and mortality[14,15,19,22]:
  - Immunocompromised individuals, and/or
  - Young children (younger than age 2 years) and older adults (older than 50 years) requiring hospitalization for acute LTRI (see Table 136.1)

Diagnosis and Evaluation

- RSV symptoms are nonspecific and often overlap with other viral and bacterial etiologies of upper and lower respiratory tract infections.
  - Common viral pathogens: influenza A and B, human metapneumovirus, parainfluenza viruses, coronaviruses, adenoviruses, rhinovirus
  - Common bacterial pathogens: *M. pneumoniae*, *S. pneumoniae*, or *B. pertussis*
- The American Society for Clinical Pathology recommends the following in their Choosing Wisely statement[16,23]:
  - Use rapid point of care or molecular tests for commonly suspected pathogens according to seasonality (RSV and/or influenza A and B) in place of broad respiratory pathogen panels to expedite diagnoses and management decisions.
  - Testing with broad respiratory pathogen panels should be considered when the results will affect patient management such as altering/discontinuing empiric antimicrobial therapy or changing infection control measures.
- In young children (younger than 2 years of age), RSV is the most commonly identified pathogen in cases of bronchiolitis and pneumonia.[4–8] RSV infection in most healthy adults is limited to the upper respiratory tract, but older adults (older than 50 years of age) with comorbidities or immunocompromise are also at greater risk for severe LRTI.[9–13]

TABLE 136.1: INDIVIDUALS AT HIGHER RISK FOR RSV-RELATED MORBIDITY AND MORTALITY	
Infants and children[4–8]	Younger than 6 months old, especially those born prior to 35 weeks' gestation, and those born during the first half of Respiratory Syncytial Virus season
	Chronic lung disease like bronchopulmonary dysplasia, cystic fibrosis, persistent asthma
	Down syndrome, congenital heart disease, or medical complexity
Adults[9–13]	Older than 65 years of age
	Chronic pulmonary disease like persistent asthma, chronic obstructive pulmonary disease (COPD)
	Chronic cardiovascular disease or functional disability

Monitoring

■ Testing is not indicated for monitoring purposes.

INTERPRETATION

■ RSV tests should be interpreted carefully in clinical context.
■ A negative result indicates that either:
  ● RSV is not the etiology of the LTRI.
  ● There was not adequate viral load in the specimen for detection.
■ PCR-based tests are the gold standard for their superior sensitivity and specificity; thus, a positive result confirms the presence of RSV in the respiratory secretions.
  ● Not all positive results indicate *active* infection. Molecular testing is able to detect viral DNA even after symptoms clinically resolve. While viral yields are highest early in the infectious process, the average duration the virus can be detected by PCR is 11 days but may persist for weeks in immunocompromised individuals.[24]
  ● A negative RSV result in the context of high clinical suspicion either eliminates RSV in favor of another causative organism, or the result may be attributed to an insufficient viral specimen collection.[24]
■ RADTs for RSV are less sensitive (29%) in adults compared to children (81%) but specificity is consistently high (97%). Therefore, a positive result can rule in RSV but a negative result in the context of high clinical suspicion should prompt confirmation testing by PCR if the results will influence patient management.[14,15,17]
■ Passive immunity to RSV secondary to maternal–infant transfer or palivizumab (Synagis) prophylaxis does not affect the results of PCR tests but may interfere with RADTs causing false-negative results.[25]

FOLLOW-UP

■ There are no recommendations for follow-up testing to monitor the clinical course or resolution of disease.
■ A negative result on RADT for RSV may warrant follow-up testing with rRT-PCR testing if clinical suspicion is high and a positive result will influence patient management.
■ A negative rRT-PCR test result may warrant repeat testing if an insufficient collection of the respiratory specimen is suspected, and if the results will influence patient management.

PEARLS & PITFALLS

■ Although prior immunity is insufficient to prevent reinfection, the poor sensitivity of antigen detection testing in older adults is attributed to prior RSV immune responses that subsequently diminish the viral burden in respiratory secretions and the duration of viral shedding.[14] Age is inversely associated with viral shedding, which may explain the higher sensitivity of antigen detection tests in young children compared to adults.

- Optimal respiratory specimens are obtained via nasopharyngeal (NP) swab, NP wash or aspirate, or a lower respiratory specimen (endotracheal aspirate, bronchoalveolar lavage).
- Specimen collection, handling, and transport are essential components of obtaining reliable test results. Consult the laboratory if uncertain to decrease specimen-to-result time and to avoid unnecessary costs and repeated specimen collection from the patient.[19]
- Symptoms of viral respiratory infections overlap, yet only few rapid tests are available that detect multiple viral antigens. Most rapid tests exclusively detect RSV and influenza viruses.[15]
- Palivizumab (Synagis) immunoprophylaxis is recommended for high-risk infants that meet specific criteria in the first year of life. A maximum of five monthly doses are given during RSV season. If these infants are hospitalized with bronchiolitis, testing should be performed to identify whether RSV is the etiologic pathogen of the infection. If so, monthly palivizumab injections should be discontinued due to the low likelihood of a second RSV infection in the same season.[22]

PATIENT EDUCATION

- https://www.healthychildren.org/English/health-issues/conditions/chest-lungs/pages/RSV-When-Its-More-Than-Just-a-Cold.aspx
- https://www.cdc.gov/rsv/index.html

RELATED DIAGNOSES AND ICD-10 CODES

Respiratory Syncytial Virus Diagnoses[26]

Respiratory syncytial virus as the cause of diseases classified elsewhere	B97.4
● May use independently but best used as a secondary infectious agent code to identify a specific condition or disease (e.g., coded secondary to acute respiratory tract infection, J06)	
Acute bronchiolitis due to respiratory syncytial virus	J21.0
Acute bronchitis due to respiratory syncytial virus bronchitis	J21.5
Respiratory syncytial virus pneumonia	J21.1

REFERENCES

Full list of references can be accessed through Springer Publishing Company Connect™ at the ollowing link: http://connect.springerpub.com/content/reference-book/978-0-8261-8843-4/part/part03/toc-part/ch136

137. RESPIRATORY VIRAL PANELS

Sarah Fitz, Leah Burt, Olga Amusina, and Susan Corbridge

PATHOPHYSIOLOGY REVIEW

The most common constellation of respiratory complaints adult patients present with are cough and dyspnea accompanied by fevers, myalgia, and fatigue. In most acute upper respiratory infections and in some cases of community-acquired pneumonia (CAP) and bronchiolitis (lower tract infections), causative agents are viral pathogens. Syndromes of viral and bacterial infections often overlap and can be nearly impossible to distinguish clinically without testing. Cost-effective rapid multiplexed molecular tests for viral illnesses and some bacterial illnesses can provide results during outpatient or emergency department (ED) visits, inform clinical practice, decrease the number of unnecessary antibiotic prescriptions, guide isolation practices, and be used in contact tracing. These measures also transform our understanding of respiratory pathogen epidemiology.[1,2]

Recent CDC data suggest that, out of all infected patients presenting to clinicians in the United States, there are an estimated 18 million annual cases of seasonal influenza viruses, with a 0.1% mortality rate.[3] The exception to successful broad viral testing is targeted testing for the large outbreak of SARS-CoV-2 virus causing the COVID-19 pandemic, with 38.9 million total cases worldwide at the time of this writing and 8% to 10% rate of hospitalizations accounting for a 7% mortality rate.[1,4] Rates of CAP in the United States are estimated at 24.8 cases per 10,000 persons annually prior to the COVID-19 pandemic, with a 25% rate of hospitalization and a 10% overall mortality rate, making CAP the second most common cause of hospitalizations.[5] Common CAP pathogens are listed in Table 137.1. The gold standard for diagnosis is an abnormal radiographic finding; however, chest x-ray is not always indicated. The most common etiology of lower respiratory tract infections (LRTI)

TABLE 137.1: COMMUNITY-ACQUIRED PNEUMONIA (CAP) PATHOGENS	
TYPICAL	**ATYPICAL**
Strep pneumoniae	Mycoplasma
Staph pneumoniae (MSSA/rarely community-acquired MRSA)	Chlamydia
Haemophilus influenzae	Legionella
Moraxella catarrhalis	
Pseudomonas aeruginosa (consider in chronic lung disease patients)	

MRSA, methicillin-resistant staphylococcus aureus; MSSA, methicillin-sensitive staphylococcus aureus; staph, staphylococcus.

in the community (pneumonia and bronchiolitis) includes viruses and *Streptococcus pneumoniae*—a potentially highly invasive disease—and CAP is the sixth leading cause of death in all age groups.[6] For hospitalized patients with LRTI diagnosis, using specimens from bronchial secretions or serum for molecular and conventional culture testing, identification is commonly performed. The Infectious Diseases Society of America does not recommend respiratory pathogen panel (RPP) testing unless the patient is immunocompromised, has severe viral illness, or if RPP testing would influence the decision regarding antiviral or antibiotic prescribing.[7] The Choosing Wisely initiative, created by the American Board of Internal Medicine Foundation, includes a similar recommendation that broad or panel testing only be pursued if it is likely to change management or prevent spread of infection.[8]

Hospital-acquired pneumonia (HAP), including ventilator-associated pneumonia (VAP), has mortality rates up to 30%.[9] Common pathogens are listed in Box 137.1. Risk factors for high mortality and resistant microorganisms include length of hospital stay greater than 5 days prior to the event, antibiotic use within previous 90 days, development of severe sepsis and septic shock, acute kidney injury requiring initiation of renal replacement therapy, or acute respiratory distress syndrome (ARDS). Although several studies have demonstrated an increased rate of diagnosing bacterial pathogens in HAP and VAP using molecular studies,[10] current guidelines recommend noninvasive sputum or endotracheal tube sputum aspirates for quantitative cultures, with the exception of MRSA PCR testing.[2] Faster testing for bacterial organisms can be performed using nucleic acid amplification tests (NAATs), but it is often difficult to distinguish between colonization and invasive disease. Empiric therapy should be guided by institutional antibiograms. The overall cost associated with treating respiratory infections is extremely high, and multiplex viral testing during seasonal outbreaks, along with targeted testing for influenza and SARS-CoV-2 during the pandemic, are well justified, leading to a decrease in hospitalization, decreased use of antibiotics, and decreased costs associated with conventional testing.

Box 137.1: Hospital-Associated Pneumonia (HAP)/Ventilator-Associated Pneumonia (VAP) Pathogens

- Acinetobacter
- Enterobacter
- Escherichia coli
- Klebsiella pneumoniae
- Pseudomonas aeruginosa
- Morganella
- Staphylococcus aureus (MSSA and MRSA)
- Streptococcus species

MRSA, methicillin-resistant staphylococcus aureus; MSSA, methicillin-sensitive staphylococcus aureus; staph, staphylococcus.

OVERVIEW OF LABORATORY TEST

Viral Respiratory Polymerase Chain Reaction or Respiratory Pathogen Panel (CPT Codes 87632 and 87633)

The term "respiratory pathogen panel" most commonly refers to the viral respiratory polymerase chain reaction (PCR). A PCR test is a type of NAAT. This test is used to "amplify" or copy small segments of DNA to evaluate it.[11] Without this amplification process, a large amount of DNA would be necessary to understand the genetic material being studied. For respiratory PCR testing, usually a nasal or nasopharyngeal swab is used to gather secretions from the nasal passages or nasopharynx. Alternatively, a sample of nasal secretions may be aspirated using a syringe. The laboratory sample is then placed in a liquid transport medium. The sample is heated, and the DNA strands separate. Enzymes are used to build templates of the original DNA, and this process is replicated many times and uses equipment that takes only a few hours to complete this process. For a respiratory panel, technology known as the multiplex PCR allows testing for many different pathogens and can be kept up to date by adding more novel pathogens as they are discovered.[12] PCR testing for the pathogens commonly found in the respiratory panel is ideal due to the sensitivity and short turnaround time as compared with other testing methods. PCR testing of this nature has been done in a laboratory but is increasingly available as point-of-care testing, which can yield faster results as there is no transport time to and from the laboratory; additionally, it provides for testing availability regardless of weekends or holidays when the laboratory may be closed.[13]

Pathogens commonly tested for using the RPP or respiratory PCR are mostly viruses, but sometimes bacteria are included as well. Common viruses tested include influenza A, influenza B, adenovirus, parainfluenza, respiratory syncytial virus (RSV), human metapneumovirus (HPMV), coronaviruses, rhinovirus, and enterovirus.[7] Also on some respiratory panels, mycoplasma pneumonia, *Bordetella pertussis*, and *Chlamydia pneumoniae* may be tested for. Please note that COVID-19 is not included on a RPP and is tested for separately. Additionally, sputum culture is a separate laboratory test and is discussed in Chapter 82. Test types are listed in Table 137.2.

Myriad RPPs are available on the market. Panels vary by how many strains of bacteria and viruses they test for, including antibiotic resistance genes.[14,17] Panels also vary by performance characteristics, levels of complexity, and turnaround times.[14] While sensitivity varies by both pathogen and specific test branding, technology is advanced to the point where most tests are considered highly accurate.[14,18,19] To accurately interpret results, providers must be familiar with the scope of the RPP test offered by their specific laboratory. Judgment on involvement of specific pathogens cannot be made if the test used does not test for them.[14,20] Table 137.3[14,21] shows pathogens commonly, sometimes, or rarely evaluated on RPP.[14,21]

INDICATIONS

Screening

■ There is no recommendation for universal or asymptomatic screening.

TABLE 137.2: TEST TYPES, ORGANISMS TESTED FOR, CURRENT PROCEDURAL TERMINOLOGY CODES, AND TESTING NOTES

TEST	ORGANISM(S)	CPT CODE(S)	LAB TURNAROUND TIME	NOTES
Viral respiratory PCR (respiratory pathogen panel)	influenza A, influenza B, adenovirus, parainfluenza, RSV, human metapneumovirus, coronaviruses, rhinovirus, and enterovirus[7]	87632 87633[13]	1–8 hrs[14]	Clinicians must note the acceptable specimen and collection techniques, as well as which organisms are detected on the PCR at their respective institutions.
	Bordetella pertussis and parapertussis	87798		This is sometimes covered in the respiratory pathogen panel (as previously noted) or may be tested for separately.
	Chlamydophila pneumoniae	87486		This is sometimes covered in the respiratory pathogen panel (as previously noted) or may be tested for separately.
	Mycoplasma pneumoniae	87581		This is sometimes covered in the respiratory pathogen panel (as previously noted) or may be tested for separately.
Viral culture, respiratory	RSV, rhinovirus, adenovirus, coronavirus, HPMV, enterovirus, parainfluenza virus, human bocavirus[7]	87254	3–5 days[15]	Viral cultures can be sent from a variety of sources, which makes them advantageous if other testing sites may be used, such as pleural fluid or bronchoalveolar lavage. However, the time required to yield results has made viral cultures less desirable from a clinical treatment standpoint.
Rapid antigen detection	Influenza RSV	87807	1–3 days	
Direct fluorescent antibody test	Influenza A and B, RSV, parainfluenzas, adenovirus, HPMV	87275 87276 87279 87280 87299	2–3 days[16]	Direct fluorescent antibody testing can be used for many viruses found in the respiratory virus PCR. This test evaluates the fluorescent staining characteristic of certain organisms in the patient specimen. Specificity is about 80% to 90%[18]

CPT, current procedural terminoloy; HPMV, human metapneumovirus; PCR, polymerase chain reaction; RSV, respiratory syncytial virus.

TABLE 137.3: PATHOGENS COMMONLY, SOMETIMES, OR RARELY EVALUATED ON RESPIRATORY PATHOGEN PANEL

EXAMPLES OF PATHOGENS COMMONLY TESTED FOR	EXAMPLES OF PATHOGENS SOMETIMES TESTED FOR	EXAMPLES OF PATHOGENS UNCOMMONLY TESTED FOR
• Influenza • Respiratory syncytial virus (RSV) • Adenovirus • Parainfluenza virus • Coronavirus • Rhinovirus • Enterovirus • Human metapneumovirus	• Bocavirus • Influenza subtyping • Parainfluenza subtyping • Respiratory syncytial virus (RSV) subtyping • Bordetella pertussis and parapertussis • Chlamydophila pneumoniae • Mycoplasma pneumoniae	• Cytomegalovirus (CMV) • Middle East respiratory syndrome coronavirus (MERS-CoV) • Severe acute respiratory syndrome-associated coronavirus (SARS-CoV) • Respiratory fungi • Hantavirus

Sources: Data from Ramanan P, Bryson AL, Binnicker MJ, Pritt BS, Patel R. Syndromic panel-based testing in clinical microbiology. *Clin Microbiol Rev.* 2017;31(1). doi:10.1128/cmr.00024-17; CMS.gov. Medicare Coverage Database. Proposed local coverage determination (LCD): respiratory pathogen panel testing (DL38916). https://www.cms.gov/medicare-coverage-database/details/lcd-details.aspx?LCDId=38915&name=331*1&UpdatePeriod=920#0

- Targeted RPP screenings should be used in clinical instances where positive results have the potential to change treatment courses.[20,22]
- RPP screening will likely not change treatment among ambulatory patients being supported for self-limiting respiratory infections.
- RPP screening will likely not change treatment among patients successfully receiving empiric antibiotic treatment for CAP.
- Appropriate use of RPP screening varies based on the patient treatment setting.[17]
- Outpatient screening: Ambulatory patients with specific characteristics increasing their risk of respiratory infections not covered by standard, empiric therapy should receive diagnostic testing. These include patients with travel histories, specific infectious exposures, immunocompromised states or pulmonary risk factors, or those whose misdiagnoses could lead to public health outbreaks.[7,22]
- Insurance or Medicare coverage of RPP testing may depend on the reason for ordering the test; be aware that a panel with greater than five organisms covered may not be considered reasonable unless it will have a clinically significant impact on the patient's care.[18]
- Targeted screening is recommended for patients requiring inpatient treatment of respiratory infections. This includes patients who have failed outpatient antibiotic therapy, as well as patients requiring intensive care unit admission.[22]
- In more severe illness, the likelihood of an infectious etiology not responsive to standard, empiric therapy increases. Therefore, inpatient RPP screening facilitates narrowed, more targeted treatment. Antibiotic therapy can be deescalated or avoided in viral infections. Bacterial infections can be treated according to resistance patterns earlier. In addition, the use of invasive sample collection procedures may be avoided.[14]
- Table 137.4 shows the patient characteristics clinicians should consider when determining if RPP targeted screening is necessary.

TABLE 137.4: PATIENT CHARACTERISTICS CLINICIANS SHOULD CONSIDER WHEN DETERMINING IF RESPIRATORY PATHOGEN PANEL TESTING IS NECESSARY

Exposure history	• Recent travel (within 2 weeks) • Infectious disease exposures • Exposure to animals that transmit zoonotic pathogens (rodent exposure OR Yersinia pestis exposure, endemic in the western United States)
Immunocompromised	• Leukopenia • Active alcohol abuse • Chronic, severe liver disease • Asplenia
Pulmonary risk factors	• Severe obstructive or structural lung disease
Public health concerns	• Possible infection with influenza, legionella, or bioterrorism agents

Sources: Data from Chesnutt AN, Chesnutt MS, Prendergast NT, Prendergast TJ. Pneumonia. In: Papadakis M, McPhee S, Rabow M, eds. *Current Medical Diagnosis & Treatment 2021*. McGraw-Hill; 2021.; Metlay JP, Waterer GW, Long AC, et al. Diagnosis and treatment of adults with community-acquired pneumonia. An official clinical practice guideline of the American Thoracic Society and Infectious Diseases Society of America. *Am J Respir Crit Care Med*. 2019;200(7):e45–e67. doi:10.1164/rccm.201908-1581ST; Miller JM, Binnicker MJ, Campbell S, Carroll KC, Chapin KC, Gilligan PH, et al. A guide to utilization of the microbiology laboratory for diagnosis of infectious diseases: 2018 update by the Infectious Diseases Society of America and the American Society for Microbiology. *Clin Infect Dis*. 2018;67(6):e1–e94. doi:10.1093/cid/ciy381.

Diagnosis and Evaluation

The differential diagnosis of respiratory infections is broad and includes both upper respiratory tract infections (URTI) and LRTI.[20] RPP may be used to assist in this differential diagnosis process. When RPP testing is negative, differential diagnosis includes (but is not limited to) reactive airway diseases, bronchiectasis, heart failure, lung cancer, pulmonary vasculitis, atelectasis, or pulmonary thromboembolic disease.

Monitoring

■ Not used for monitoring.

INTERPRETATION

■ To make an accurate diagnosis, results must be interpreted within each individual patient's clinical context. The presence of a positive pathogen does not necessarily equate with a clinically significant episode. On the other hand, a negative RPP does not absolutely exclude the involvement of a respiratory pathogen.[21]

■ **Positive result**: A positive result does not necessarily equal a clinically significant infection. Clinicians should ask themselves: *Are my patient's symptoms adequately explained by the presence of the identified pathogen?*

■ Many RPP tests are extremely sensitive and are able to detect viruses in asymptomatic patients.[23] Furthermore, positive results do not distinguish between colonization and active infection.[14]

■ Along these same lines, sensitive RPP tests may continue to detect the presence of viruses after the clinically significant infection has resolved.[14,24,25]

- If not specifically tested for, RPPs may fail to detect clinically significant co-infections such as fungal pneumonia.[14]
- The likelihood of a false positive increases in panels that test for many targets.[26]
- **Negative result**: A negative result does not necessarily exclude respiratory pathogen involvement. Clinicians should ask themselves: *Was the RPP test performed by a skilled clinician able to obtain a quality sample?*
- Test results are dependent on optimal sampling procedures.[27] If an inadequate sample was obtained, the test may be falsely negative.[21]
- Viral titer concentration does not necessarily correspond to symptom severity. If a patient has low viral titers at the time of testing, the patient may test negative despite having clinically significant disease.[17]

FOLLOW-UP

- There is no recommendation in the literature for re-testing with RPP due to the variable duration of viral shedding. If a patient has ongoing symptoms and initial RPP was negative, the clinician should consider other causes of respiratory illness.

PEARLS & PITFALLS

- While RPP testing is not generally recommended for a patient presenting with symptoms of respiratory tract infection, it may be helpful in specific situations to limit unnecessary antibiotic use.
- Each clinician should review the specific testing techniques and organisms included on the RPP at their laboratory. If there is a concern for a specific organism, the clinician may need to test for it separately if it is not included on the RPP.
- Clinicians should educate patients on the procedure for obtaining the nasopharyngeal sample, as it may cause anxiety and brief discomfort.
- Patients should receive information about why antibiotics are usually not indicated for outpatient respiratory illness. Patients should be offered follow-up options and specific parameters to prompt them to call back if they are not improving.

PATIENT EDUCATION

- https://labtestsonline.org/tests/respiratory-pathogens-panel
- https://www.choosingwisely.org/patient-resources/colds-flu-and-other -respiratory-illnesses-in-adults

RELATED DIAGNOSES AND ICD-10 CODES

Acute upper respiratory infection	J06.9[28]
Acute lower respiratory infection	J22
Community-acquired pneumonia	J18.9
Influenza due to unidentified influenza virus with other respiratory manifestations	J11.1
Cough	R05

REFERENCES

Full list of references can be accessed through Springer Publishing Company Connect™ at the following link: http://connect.springerpub.com/content/reference-book/ 978-0-8261-8843-4/part/part03/toc-part/ch137

138. RETICULOCYTE INDICES

Kelly Small Casler

PHYSIOLOGY/PATHOPHYSIOLOGY REVIEW

Reticulocytes are immature erythrocytes (red blood cells) that are produced from erythroblasts during bone marrow erythropoiesis. They normally constitute 1.0% to 1.5% of RBC volume and have a life span of 4 days.[1-3] After obtaining hemoglobin, reticulocytes remain in the bone marrow for 3 days before being released into the bloodstream.[3] Over the span of the next 24 hours, they mature into erythrocytes (RBCs).[3] In the presence of acute blood loss, hemolysis, or nutrient deficiencies (iron, folate, or vitamin B12), the body will initiate reticulocytosis through the release of erythropoietin (EPO). EPO triggers bone marrow to not only release reticulocytes into the circulation earlier than usual, but to also increase reticulocyte production. Reticulocytosis usually occurs 3 to 4 days after EPO release; absence of reticulocytosis in response to EPO release may signal an impairment in the bone marrow.[1,4]

OVERVIEW OF LABORATORY TESTS

Absolute Reticulocyte Count and Reticulocyte Count

Reticulocytes can be counted automatically by a laboratory analyzer (most accurate) or manually by technicians or pathologists using a blood smear. After counting, the total number of reticulocytes (absolute reticulocyte count) are divided by the total number of RBCs, providing the percentage of reticulocytes per all red blood cells, called the reticulocyte count (CPT code 85045).

Reticulocyte Index and Reticulocyte Production Index

In an anemic patient, the absolute reticulocyte count (ARC) and reticulocyte count do not usually provide useful information on their own since they do not consider the severity of the patient's anemia. Therefore, the patient's reticulocyte count can be adjusted for the severity of anemia with the reticulocyte index (RI). Table 138.1 summarizes how the RI is calculated. An elevated RI is used to assure clinicians that the bone marrow is responding appropriately to the anemia. However, in response to anemia, reticulocytes are released into circulation earlier. This early release may make it look like the reticulocyte count increased when the bone marrow may or may not truly have increased production. To

TABLE 138.1: RETICULOCYTE PARAMETERS AND NORMAL VALUES			
PARAMETER	**NORMAL VALUE**	**DEFINITION**	**INTERPRETATION**
Absolute reticulocyte count (ARC)	$50-150 \times 10^9$ /L	Total number of reticulocytes	
Reticulocyte count	0.5%–2.5%	Percent of RBCs that are reticulocytes (ARC/RBC)	
Reticulocyte index (RI)	1.1%–5%	Retic count × (pt Hct/ normal Hct)	<1–2 inadequate reticulocytosis; >2 adequate reticulocytosis
Reticulocyte production index (RPI) Corrected reticulocyte count	1%*	RI/maturation time correction factor**	<2 inadequate response to anemia; >3 adequate response to anemia

*If the Hct/Hgb is normal, RPI of 1 is considered normal.

**The maturation time correction factor is the time in days required for RBCs to mature depending on the severity of anemia. For an Hct 36% to 45% the time is 1.0; for Hct 26% to 35% the time is 1.5; for Hct 16% to 25% the time is 2.0, and for an Hct of 15% or lower the time is 2.5[14]

Hct, hematocrit; HgB, hemoglobin; RBC, red blood cells.

Sources: Data from Mais DD. Diseases of red blood cells. In: *Laposata's Laboratory Medicine (M. Laposata, Ed)*. 3rd ed. Lange; 2019:247–280; Hoffbrand AV, Moss PAH. *Essential Haematology*. 6th ed. Wiley-Blackwell; 2011:15–32; Mathur S, Hutchison R, Mohi G. Hematopoiesis. In: McPherson RA, Pincus MR, eds. *Henry's Clinical Diagnosis and Management by Laboratory Methods*. 23rd ed. Elsevier; 2017

account for this and to see if the bone marrow is producing enough new erythrocytes to respond to the anemia, the reticulocyte production index (RPI), also called the corrected reticulocyte count, is calculated. The RPI is calculated by dividing the RI by reticulocyte maturation time in the blood. For a patient with a hematocrit of 45%, reticulocyte maturation time is 1.0 day (normal); for 35% it is 1.5 days, for 25% it is 2.0 days, and for 15% it is 2.5 days.[2] An elevated RPI reflects an appropriate bone marrow response and is seen with hemolytic anemia, hemorrhage, or response to nutritional deficiency replacement (B12, folate, iron). A decreased RPI is associated with ineffective erythropoiesis and is seen in iron deficiency anemia (IDA) or vitamin B12/folate deficiencies prior to treatment (since the bone marrow does not yet have adequate nutrients to construct new reticulocytes). A decreased RPI can also occur in dysfunction in the bone marrow (e.g., aplastic anemia).[3]

Other Reticulocyte Values

Three reticulocyte parameters reflect erythropoiesis at its earliest stages. Reticulocyte mean cell volume (MCVr) reflects the size and volume of reticulocytes and is a similar measurement to the MCV that is reported with RBC indices. MCVr is used to detect early treatment response to vitamin B12, folate, or iron supplementation.[3,5] The immature reticulocyte fraction (IRF), also called the reticulocyte maturity index, identifies the youngest reticulocytes in circulation. It measures the RNA content of reticulocytes and, since immature reticulocytes have higher RNA content compared to more mature reticulocytes, IRF can identify erythropoiesis very early. Therefore, it is often used as the first marker of bone marrow regeneration after chemotherapy or stem cell transplant.[3,5] It is also used to identify adequate response to erythropoiesis stimulating therapy or iron, vitamin B12, or folate replacement.[3] Reticulocyte mean cell hemoglobin content (RET-He or CHr) reflects the hemoglobin (Hgb) content (pg/cell) of reticulocytes. Since the average life span of a reticulocyte is 4 days, CHr values increase within 2 to 3 days of iron therapy initiation, much sooner than Hgb. CHr values will also be one of the first parameters to decrease in nutritional deficiencies or bone marrow depression.

INDICATIONS

Screening

- Guidelines regarding pediatric iron deficiency screening[6] and anemia screening in chronic kidney disease (CKD)[7] both support the use of CHr as an alternative to Hgb measurement.

Diagnosis and Evaluation

- Reticulocyte indices are used along with a complete blood count and iron studies to classify and investigate states of anemia in a variety of chronic diseases.[8]

Monitoring

- Reticulocyte count is used in sickle cell disease to determine the cause of different sickle cell complications. The count will be low in aplastic crisis, normal in splenic sequestration, and high in hyper-hemolytic crisis.[9]
- Reticulocyte count is monitored every 4 to 12 weeks during hydroxyurea therapy in sickle cell disease.[10]
- IRF is used for monitoring response to erythropoiesis-stimulating agents (ESA) since IRF will rise prior to reticulocyte count.[3]
- IRF is used to monitor response to blood transfusions and condition status in aplastic anemias and neonatal anemia.[3]
- IRF is used to monitor responses to nutritional replacements.[3]

INTERPRETATION

- Table 138.1 reviews the interpretation of reticulocyte parameters.
- A normal CHr is 27.5 to 29 pg or more.[11-13]

FOLLOW-UP

- If the clinical picture is unclear, a complete blood count, ferritin, and iron studies are often used along with reticulocyte indices.

PEARLS & PITFALLS

- A reticulocyte count may be able to help differentiate thalassemia from IDA. It is typically higher in thalassemia than in IDA.[15]
- One study suggested RPI may not be an accurate predictor of bone marrow erythropoiesis in pediatrics. Consider using other parameters in this population.[16]

■ IRF performs better than ARC or reticulocyte count for monitoring response to bone marrow transplant and is also used in determining timing for stem cell harvesting in donors.[3]

■ IRF and RPI provide similar information, so IRF could be used in lieu of calculating RPI.[3]

■ Related to its ability to pick up iron deficiency prior to progression to anemia, CHr (lower than 27.5 pg) is more accurate for iron deficiency screening in 9 to 12 months old compared to Hgb (lower than 11 g/dL).[12,17]

■ CHr is not helpful at differentiating anemia of chronic disease and iron deficiency anemia (IDA).[18]

■ CHr is less expensive, requires less blood for testing, and seems less affected by inflammation compared to iron studies and Hgb testing.[15,18,19]

■ A reticulocyte count/IRF ratio greater than 7.7 has been proposed as an indicator of possible hereditary spherocytosis.[20]

■ CHr appears more accurate than ferritin or transferrin saturation in identifying iron deficiency in hemodialysis patients.[21]

PATIENT EDUCATION

■ https://medlineplus.gov/lab-tests/reticulocyte-count/

RELATED DIAGNOSES AND ICD-10 CODES

Screening for iron deficiency	Z13.0
Anemia, unspecified	D64.9

REFERENCES

Full list of references can be accessed through Springer Publishing Company Connect™ at the following link: http://connect.springerpub.com/content/reference-book/978-0-8261-8843-4/part/part03/toc-part/ch138

---

139. SEMEN AND SPERM ANALYSIS

Danielle A. Quallich and Susanne A. Quallich

PHYSIOLOGY/PATHOPHYSIOLOGY REVIEW

With the onset of puberty, spermatogenesis is initiated by testosterone production in the Leydig cells of the testes. Due to the influence of luteinizing hormone (LH) and follicle-stimulating hormone (FSH), which are released from the anterior pituitary, the testes begin to produce sperm in a four-step process of development: spermatogonia, spermatocyte, spermatid, and spermatozoon.

Spermatogenesis occurs in the Sertoli cells of the testes, which are found within the seminiferous tubules. Spermatozoa, or sperm, are transported to the epididymis through the rete testis and efferent ducts. This production cycle takes approximately 74 days to complete, with an additional 12 days for final maturation as the sperm traverse the length of the epididymis.[1] The duration of this cycle is important, as any changes in the semen analysis following medical or surgical intervention will not be reflected for at least 3 months, and is the reason that appointments are scheduled in 3-month intervals.

Sertoli cells are responsive to FSH excretion and secrete inhibin, which exerts negative feedback on FSH production in males. This production process is governed by a negative feedback loop, with testosterone acting as the primary negative feedback component that slows LH and FSH secretion (Figure 139.1). Pulsatile secretion of LH is controlled by gonadotropin-releasing hormone (GnRH) from the hypothalamus. Inhibin, released during spermatogenesis, also specifically inhibits activity, or downregulates FSH. This feedback system can be overridden by the administration of exogenous testosterone, or medications such as luteinizing hormone-releasing hormone (LHRH) antagonists, both of which will stop the body's own production of testosterone (and halt spermatogenesis as a result). Testicular volume offers a preliminary estimate of function, and in particular sperm production.

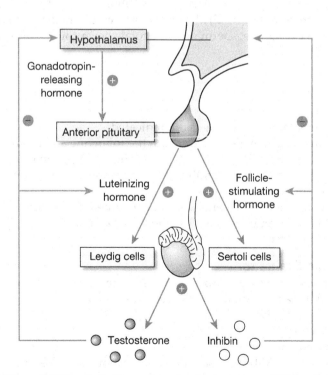

FIGURE 139.1. The male HPG axis. GnRH, gonadotropin-releasing hormone; HPG, hypothalamic-pituitary-gonadal. *Source: Yedinak C, Hurtado CR, Leung AM, et al. Endocrine system. In: Tkacs NC, Herrmann LL, Johnson RL, eds. Advanced Physiology and Pathophysiology. Springer Publishing Company; 2021. Fig. 17.39.*

Infertility is defined as "the failure to achieve a clinical pregnancy after 12 months or more of regular unprotected intercourse."[2] A male factor alone is the cause of infertility in up to 20% of infertile couples and a contributing factor in another 30% to 40% of all couples presenting for infertility evaluations.[3] Males continue to produce sperm until death; there is not a parallel condition to menopause in females that results in the cessation of male reproductive potential. Sperm quality and production can decline with age, certain comorbidities, and the effects of some medications.

OVERVIEW OF LABORATORY TESTS

Laboratory evaluation of semen production and function is completed with a semen analysis(CPT code 89320). This test is frequently accompanied by a total testosterone and LH and FSH testing as well, to establish the sensitivity of the gonadal system to the hormonal signals. Other tests can be added based on clinical presentation for other contributors, such as prolactin, estradiol, or a karyotype. Males are advised in advance that they will need to provide a semen sample after a period of abstinence of 2 to 5 days. The sample is collected through masturbation and must be collected into a container that is not toxic to sperm, or by using a special condom designed for semen collection (latex condoms alter sperm viability, especially if they are lubricated). If the sample is collected at home, it should arrive to the laboratory within 60 minutes to ensure the accuracy of the results.[4] The primary values that are evaluated are the volume of the ejaculate, sperm motility, total sperm count, and sperm morphology (shape).

INDICATIONS

Screening
- Universal population screening is not indicated.
- Targeted screening may be considered in the following situations[3]:
  - In males with established primary or secondary hypogonadism who wish to start or add to their family prior to beginning any treatment for hypogonadism.
  - Before and after chemotherapy and/or treatment for malignancy.
  - Adolescent or prepubertal males who have been diagnosed with Klinefelter's syndrome

Diagnosis and Evaluation
- Semen analysis may be used for diagnostic purposes (in addition to a referral to a fertility specialist) with the following signs/symptoms that can predispose to infertility:
  - Varicocele(s)
  - Hypogonadism +/- obesity
  - Genetic causes: cystic fibrosis, Klinefelter's syndrome, Kallman's syndrome, Y-chromosome microdeletions, various neuromuscular conditions

- History of treatment with chemotherapeutic agents
- Obstructive azoospermia: previous vasectomy or inguinal hernia repair (as infant, child, or adult)
- Anabolic steroid use (current or historical)
- Hypogonadotropic hypogonadism
- Normal spermatogenesis, with recent ejaculation making count lower
- Partial androgen resistance
- Testicular failure
- Ejaculatory and/or sexual dysfunction

- Fertility specialists follow a "rule of 3" when considering a diagnosis based on the semen analysis: three samples, each 3 weeks apart, collected after 3 days of abstinence.

Monitoring

- Because sperm take approximately 90 days to mature, monitoring is not needed for at least 3 months after any intervention.
- Subsequent semen analyses will be needed depending on the intervention and treatment; intervals for the timing of samples varies. Subsequent semen analyses may be accompanied by a total testosterone level.

INTERPRETATION

- Interpretation is summarized in Table 139.1.

FOLLOW-UP

- There are several additional tests that can be performed on a semen sample, including a sperm penetration assay, peroxidase staining, direct immunobead testing, sperm DNA fragmentation, and computer-aided semen analysis. The clinical usefulness of specialized sperm testing remains controversial and should be pursued with the direction of a fertility specialist.
- Follow-up should include referral when the conditions in Box 139.1 are identified.

TABLE 139.1: NORMAL SEMEN ANALYSIS	
SEMEN PARAMETERS	**NORMAL VALUES**
Morphology (strict criteria)	≥4% normal forms
Motility	≥32%
Sperm concentration	≥15 million
Sperm count	≥39 million
Volume	1.5–5.0 mL

Source: Adapted from Cooper TG, Noonan E, von Eckardstein S, et al. World Health Organization reference values for human semen characteristics. *Hum Reprod Update.* 2010;16:231–245. doi:10.1093/humupd/dmp048

Box 139.1: When to Consider Referral to a Fertility Specialist[8,10]

- A patient or partner request
- An abnormal semen analysis
- Azoospermia (no sperm in ejaculate)
- A male with a spinal cord injury or other neurologic issue (including previous surgery) that compromises ejaculation)
- Fertility evaluation before and after chemotherapy and/or treatment for malignancy
- A couple with a female partner age 40 or older
- A partner who has had a previous vasectomy
- A couple that has timed intercourse, and without a positive pregnancy test for >12 months
- Genetically male patients who are considering gender affirmation treatment, before hormone therapy or early after beginning treatment.

Note: Ideally, both partners should undergo evaluation at the same time, in order to address any potential male factor diagnoses in a less invasive, and possible more cost-effective, manner.

PEARLS & PITFALLS

- Many areas of the United States do not have easy access to a male fertility specialist; in addition, there are clear knowledge gaps among providers and patients about what a male infertility evaluation can yield or its utility.[5]
- Male infertility may be linked with higher risk for other health issues such as hypogonadism, certain malignancies, and decreased longevity.[6]
- Use and type of lubricants are important to know as some commercial lubricants such as Vaseline, Surgilube, and KY jelly can be spermatotoxic.
- The Affordable Care Act (2010) does not mandate infertility evaluation and treatment, leaving the issue to the individual states. Currently only 16 states address coverage for infertility, and only six of these mandate *male factor* evaluation and treatment. So, patients may wish to evaluate insurance coverage prior to proceeding with evaluation and testing.[9]
- Not all laboratories process semen samples in a manner that includes standardized methods and quality control procedures according to World Health Organization (WHO) standards.[7]

PATIENT EDUCATION

- https://www.urologyhealth.org
- https://www.resolve.org
- https://www.reproductivefacts.org

RELATED DIAGNOSES AND ICD-10 CODES

Left varicocele	I86.1
Bilateral varicoceles	I86.8
Hypogonadotropic hypogonadism	E23.0
Cystic fibrosis	E84.9

Klinefelter's syndrome	Q98.4
Cryptorchidism	Q53.9
History of vasectomy	Z98.52
Oligospermia	N46.1
Erectile dysfunction	N52.9

REFERENCES

Full list of references can be accessed through Springer Publishing Company Connect™ at the following link: http://connect.springerpub.com/content/reference-book/978-0-8261-8843-4/part/part03/toc-part/ch139

140. SERUM OR PLASMA OSMOLALITY

Carolyn McClerking

PHYSIOLOGY REVIEW

Identifying and understanding how osmolarity and osmolality impact fluid status and body homeostasis is important in the prevention of life-threating disorders in all patients, especially those who are most sensitive to changes, such as older adults.[1] The terms "osmolality" and "osmolarity" are sometimes used interchangeably; however, there are important differences. Both measure the amount (in units of concentration, called osmoles) of a substance present in a solution. Osmolarity describes the amount in terms of volume (per liter), while osmolality describes the amount in terms of weight (per kilogram).[2] Typically, only osmolality is measured in clinical practice and it is useful in evaluating patients with alterations of fluid homeostasis, such as dehydration, hyper- or hypotension, intracranial pressure, and seizures. Disturbances in osmolality provide rationale for the use of intravenous fluids, which can quickly change plasma osmolality.[3]

OVERVIEW OF LABORATORY TESTS

Osmolality (CPT code 83930) is measured in plasma and serum, by osmometry using an osmometer. Osmolality levels can also be estimated by mathematical equations using electrolyte, urea, and glucose parameters if osmometry is not available and if calculation of an osmol gap (difference between measured osmolality and calculated osmolality) is needed.[4,5] A calculator is available online for these equations at https://www.mdcalc.com/serum-osmolality-osmolarity#use-cases

Plasma and serum osmolality measurements are most commonly used to evaluate and treat fluid imbalances. However, whole blood measurements can be used in cases of emergency, since plasma/serum measurements require a longer length of time to determine results.[6] Whole blood and plasma results cannot be used interchangeably, however.[6]

INDICATIONS

Screening

- Not used for universal screening.
- May be used for patients with critical illness or in older adults who are at risk for developing electrolyte or fluid disorders.[7]
- Increased osmolality may help identify patients at risk of chronic kidney disease.[8]

Diagnosis and Evaluation

- Used to evaluate fluid and electrolyte disorders.
- Serum/plasma osmolality is particularly useful in the acute care setting to differentiate true hyponatremia from pseudohyponatremia. True hyponatremia is associated with a serum osmolality lower than 275 mOsm/kg. Pseudohyponatremia is associated with normal osmolality.[9]
- Used to evaluate signs/symptoms that could be due to altered osmolality levels (Table 140.1)[10–13]
- Serum osmolal gap is evaluated to assess for toxic alcohol (i.e., methanol, ethylene glycol, isopropanol) ingestion.

Monitoring

- Routine monitoring of serum osmolality may be used for patients with acute metabolic disorders and in patients who are critically ill.[14,15]
- Routine monitoring may be used for patients undergoing dialysis.[16]
- Routine monitoring is used in patients receiving mannitol to avoid adverse reactions of a hyperosmolar state/renal failure.[17]

TABLE 140.1: SIGNS/SYMPTOMS OF HYPO-/HYPEROSMOLALITY

HYPEROSMOLALITY	HYPOOSMOLALITY
Coma	Coma
Cramping	Diarrhea
Excessive thirst	Fatigue
Orthostatic hypotension	Headache
Lethargy	Irritability
Muscle weakness	Mental confusion
Urinary frequency	Nausea
	Seizure activity
	Vomiting

Sources: Data from Argyropoulos C, Rondon-Berrios H, Raj DS, et al. Hypertonicity: pathophysiologic concept and experimental studies. Cureus. 2016;8(5):e596. doi:10.7759/cureus.596; Ball SG, Iqbal Z. Diagnosis and treatment of hyponatraemia. Best Pract Res Clin Endocrinol Metab. 2016;30(2):161–173. doi:10.1016/j.beem.2015.12.001; Braun MM, Barstow CH, Pyzocha NJ. Diagnosis and management of sodium disorders: hyponatremia and hypernatremia. Am Fam Physician. 2015;91(5):299–307; Muhsin SA, Mount DB. Diagnosis and treatment of hypernatremia. Best Pract Res Clin Endocrinol Metab. 2016;30(2):189–203. doi:10.1016/j.beem.2016.02.014

INTERPRETATION

■ Reference interval for serum/plasma osmolality is 275 to 295 mOsm/kg.[3,18]

■ The differential diagnosis for levels above or below the reference intervals is found in Table 140.2.[19–23]

■ Normal osmolal gap is less than 10 mOsm/kg.[24] Serum osmolal gap is increased in toxic alcohol ingestion.[25] Serum osmolal gap can also be elevated in chronic renal failure, ketoacidosis, and lactic acidosis.[26]

FOLLOW-UP

■ After identifying hypo- and hyperosmolality, evaluate for hypo- and hypernatremia as sodium is the primary extracellular solute and main contributor to serum osmolality.[27]

■ Urine osmolality may help clarify the clinical picture. The ratio of serum to urine osmolality may even help differentiate between glomerular versus tubular causes of acute renal failure.[28] In hyponatremic patients with decreased plasma/serum osmolality, urine osmolality assists in identification of inadequate water excretion.[7]

TABLE 140.2: CONDITIONS PREDISPOSING TO HYPO- OR HYPEROSMOLALITY

	POSSIBLE CAUSE
Elevated osmolality	Diabetes insipidus
	Ethanol, methanol, or ethylene glycol ingestion
	Hyperglycemia
	Mannitol therapy
	Sepsis
	Uremia
Decreased osmolality	Hyponatremia
	Increased hydration
	SIADH

SIADH, syndrome of inappropriate antidiuretic hormone.

Sources: Data from Farhan S, Vogel B, Baber U, et al. Calculated serum osmolality, acute kidney injury, and relationship to mortality after percutaneous coronary intervention. *Cardiorenal Med.* 2019;9(3):160–167. doi:10.1159/000494807; Moen V, Brudin L, Rundgren M, Irestedt L. Osmolality and respiratory regulation in humans: respiratory compensation for hyperchloremic metabolic acidosis is absent after infusion of hypertonic saline in healthy volunteers. *Anesth Analg.* 2014;119(4):956–964. doi:10.1213/ANE.0000000000000404; Muneer M, Akbar I. Acute metabolic emergencies in diabetes: DKA, HHS, and EDKA. In: Islam MS, ed. *Diabetes: From Research to Clinical Practice.* Vol 4. Springer International Publishing; 2021:85–114; Spasovski G, Vanholder R, Allolio B, et al. Clinical practice guideline on diagnosis and treatment of hyponatraemia. *Eur J Endocrinol.* 2014;170(3):G1–G47. doi:10.1530/EJE-13-1020; Tabibzadeh N, Wagner S, Metzger M, et al. Fasting urinary osmolality, CKD progression, and mortality: a prospective observational study. *Am J Kidney Dis.* 2019;73(5):596–604. doi:10.1053/j.ajkd.2018.12.024

PEARLS & PITFALLS

- In patients with traumatic brain injury, elevated plasma osmolality may prolong QTC interval and increase the possibility of developing atrial fibrillation.[2]
- Hyperosmolality was found to be correlated with worse outcomes in critically ill patients admitted with gastrointestinal, neurologic, cardiovascular, and vascular disorders; there was no association noted in patients with respiratory disease, however.[30]
- The sample volume can have a dramatic effect on the result of plasma osmolality; a smaller volume may elicit a higher result.[31]
- A study evaluating patients with heart failure post discharge found that lower serum osmolality levels were associated with an increased incidence of mortality and readmission rate.[18,32]
- A study suggests an elevated osmolality/osmolarity (by calculation) can help diagnose dehydration in older adults.[5]

PATIENT EDUCATION

- https://www.healthline.com/health/osmolality-blood#uses

RELATED DIAGNOSES AND ICD-10 CODES

Other specified abnormal findings of blood chemistry	R79.89

REFERENCES

Full list of references can be accessed through Springer Publishing Company Connect™ at the following link: http://connect.springerpub.com/content/reference-book/ 978-0-8261-8843-4/part/part03/toc-part/ch140

---

141. SKIN BIOPSY

Retha D. Gentry and Lisa E. Ousley

PHYSIOLOGY REVIEW

Skin, the body's largest organ, together with hair, nails, and glands form the integumentary system. The role of the integumentary system includes temperature and water regulation, immunity, and waste secretion. Human skin consists of three layers: the hypodermis (subcutaneous tissue), the dermis, and the epidermis. Skin cells proliferate from the hypodermis and push upward to the epidermis. The epidermis, the outmost layer, holds the greatest potential for skin cell pathology.

As part of the diagnostic process, a skin biopsy is sometimes necessary to ensure a definitive diagnosis. They can be used to diagnosis a variety of inflammatory, vascular, melanocytic, and nonmelanocytic skin disorders. Inflammatory skin diseases include an extensive group of conditions that range from mild pruritis to severe inflammatory lesions. These noncontagious conditions may occur in isolation or in combination with other systemic disorders.[1] Melanocytic lesions are pigmented and develop from proliferation of melanocytes.[2] Although the least common, melanomas are malignant and the most serious type of melanocytic lesions.[1] Nonmelanocytic lesions may also be pigmented, especially in skin of color. Nonmelanocytic lesions are keratinocytic, vascular, or reactive.

OVERVIEW OF LABORATORY TESTS

Histopathologic examination of tissue is often necessary to make a dermatology diagnosis.[2] Skin biopsies are performed after assessment of the visible lesion(s) and selection of the biopsy site and technique.[3] These biopsies result in a specimen for diagnostic evaluation of neoplastic disorders, nonneoplastic disorders, cutaneous infections, cutaneous manifestations of systemic disease, and drug reactions.[2,4] There are three main types of skin biopsies performed in the primary care office: shave biopsy, incisional (punch), and excisional (full punch or elliptical).

Shave biopsy (CPT codes 11102 and 11103) utilizes a scalpel to remove a small section of the epidermis and a portion of the dermis. A shave biopsy is used when a full-thickness specimen is not required for diagnosis.[5] The difference between a shave and saucerization biopsy is the excision depth of the specimen, with saucerization excising below the skin's surface into the subcutaneous fat.[2]

During a punch biopsy (CPT codes 11104 and 11105), the clinician uses a small circular cutting instrument (trephine) or punch tool to remove a portion of the skin including the epidermis, dermis, and superficial fat. The tools commonly range in size from 2 mm to 10 mm.[5] Depending on the size of the lesion and instrument used, the punch results in incisional (partial removal of the lesion together with a section of normal skin) or excisional (removal of entire lesion).

Excisional biopsies (CPT codes 11400-11471, 11600-11646) use a scalpel to remove an entire area or mass of abnormal skin, including a portion of normal skin down to or through the fatty layer of skin.[7] Excisional biopsy results in removal of the entire lesion. Incisional results in partial removal of the lesion together with a section of normal skin.

Scissor excisions (CPT codes 11200 and 11201) are performed on pedunculated lesions (skin tags). Anesthesia is rarely used for removal of these lesions.

INDICATIONS

The purpose of a skin biopsy is to obtain a specimen for histopathologic evaluation. Skin biopsy is necessary when the lesion or dermatitis diagnosis is uncertain, when clinical examination fails to provide a useful diagnosis, or when the patient has not responded to the initial treatment.[3,5,6] Key evidence-based practice recommendations for determining the most appropriate biopsy type are listed in Table 141.1.[7]

Screening

- No universal or targeted screenings are recommended.
- The United States Preventive Services Task Force found there was insufficient evidence to recommend that visual skin cancer screenings be conducted by trained clinicians.[8]

Diagnosis and Evaluation

- Diagnoses for skin lesions are extensive. See Tables 141.2 and 141.3 for common differential diagnoses based on lesion type and disease examples correlated with biopsy type.

Monitoring

- Biopsy can be used to monitor resolution of disease or effectiveness of treatment.

TABLE 141.1: KEY RECOMMENDATIONS FOR PRACTICE

CLINICAL RECOMMENDATION	EVIDENCE RATING	REFERENCES	COMMENTS
For diagnostic purposes, lesions should be excised using narrow margins.	C	7	Consensus Guidelines
For large lesions with low malignant suspicion, punch and shave biopsies may be more appropriate related to staging and prognosis.	C	7	Consensus Guidelines
If melanoma is suspected, excise the lesion using a 1- to 3- mm margin.	C	7	Consensus Guidelines
Survival rates in patients with melanoma are not affected by biopsy type.	B	7	

Note: A = consistent, good-quality patient-oriented evidence; B = inconsistent or limited-quality patient-oriented evidence; C = consensus, disease-oriented evidence, usual practice, expert opinion, or case series. SORT evidence rating system.

Source: Data from Lyons F, Ousley, L. Dermatology for the Advanced Practice Nurse. Springer Publishing Company; 2015.

TABLE 141.2: DISEASE EXAMPLES CORRELATED WITH BIOPSY TYPE

DISEASE EXAMPLES CORRELATED WITH BIOPSY TYPE			
TYPES OF LESIONS	PUNCH	SHAVE	EXCISIONAL
Melanocytic lesions (e.g., melanoma, nevus, and atypical pigmented lesions)	*Yes	No	Yes
Inflammatory lesions (e.g., psoriasis, dermatitis, lichen planus, erythema multiforme, urticaria, pemphigus, lupus SLE, etc.)	Yes	No	Yes
Nonmelanocytic epidermal lesions (e.g., cysts, keratosis, scar, wart, papilloma, skin tags, superficial basal or squamous cell carcinoma, etc.)	Yes	**Yes	Yes

*Suspected melanoma should not be punch biopsied.

**Shave biopsy would only be used for superficial lesions.

Source: Data from Lyons F, Ousley, L. Dermatology for the Advanced Practice Nurse. Springer Publishing Company; 2015.

TABLE 141.3: COMMON DIFFERENTIAL DIAGNOSES BASED ON LESION TYPE	
INFLAMMATORY	**MELANOCYTIC**
Atopic dermatitis	Café au lait spots
Contact dermatitis	Lentigo
Drug reaction	Melanoma
Erythema multiforme	Moles
Folliculitis	Mongolian spots
Lichen planus	Nevi
Psoriasis	
Urticaria	
NONMELANOCYTIC	
Actinic keratosis	
Carcinomas	
Cysts	
Dermatofibromas	
Seborrheic keratosis	
Scar	
Warts	

Source: Data from Lyons F, Ousley, L. *Dermatology for the Advanced Practice Nurse.* Springer Publishing Company; 2015.

INTERPRETATION

- The selection of biopsy site and technique, performing the procedure, and handling the specimen all assist the pathologist in interpretation.[9]
- Interpretation is dependent on the completeness of the requisition form sent with specimen.[10]
- Many skin conditions have nonspecific histopathology. Skin biopsy cannot substitute for competent clinical skill.[3]

FOLLOW-UP

- Biopsy results will guide referral to a surgeon or dermatologist.
- Follow-up testing may not be warranted if entire lesion was excised.

PEARLS & PITFALLS

- The majority of skin biopsies performed are benign.[9]
- Accurate diagnosis is dependent on the selection of the appropriate biopsy technique and site selection.[3]
- The patient should be notified of the results as quickly as possible.[3]
- The goal of a shave biopsy is to produce a saucer-shaped skin defect that has smooth edges.[5]
- Skin biopsies are considered relatively harmless procedures; however, scarring, bleeding, and infection are risks.[9]
- Patients may experience allergic reactions to injections, topical medications, dressings, and tape.[4]

- Punch biopsy of the face, palms, and soles should be avoided if there is another choice for a biopsy site.[4]
- Infected lesions and older lesions should be avoided as biopsy sites.[3]
- Infection rates are higher if biopsy is obtained in the groin and axilla. Only biopsy these areas if other sites are unavailable.[3]
- If infection occurs, it is usually within 3 days. Treatment includes removal of sutures and/or antibiotics.[6]
- For a generalized rash, the trunk, arms, and upper legs are the more favorable biopsy site.[2]
- Elbows and knees should be avoided.[2]
- Biopsy sites in lower legs, even in young individuals, are slower to heal.[2]
- Interpretation of inflammatory skin disorders is limited without knowledge of clinical context.[4]
- Children with anemia may have impaired healing.[3]
- Skin of color is more prone to developing keloids.
- Pigmented and oily skin tend to have more scar formation than pale dry skin.[3]
- Aging skin repairs itself more slowly; wound healing may take as much as four times longer to complete.[1]

PATIENT EDUCATION

- https://www.mayoclinic.org/tests-procedures/skin-biopsy/about/pac-20384634
- https://www.hopkinsmedicine.org/neurology_neurosurgery/centers_clinics/cutaneous_nerve_lab/physicians/patient_instructions_biopsy_site_care.html

RELATED DIAGNOSES AND ICD-10 CODES

Inflammatory		Blue nevus	D22.9
Dermatitis	L30.9	Spitz nevus	D22.9
Urticaria	L50.9	Nonmelanocytic	
Psoriasis	L40.9	Basal cell carcinoma	C44.91
Folliculitis	L66.2	Squamous cell carcinoma	C44.92
Drug reaction	L27.0	Warts	B07.9
Melanocytic		Seborrheic keratosis	L21.9
Melanoma	C43.9	Actinic keratosis	L57.0
Dysplastic nevi	D22.9	Epidermal cyst	L72.0

REFERENCES

Full list of references can be accessed through Springer Publishing Company Connect™
at the following link: http://connect.springerpub.com/content/reference-book/978-0-8261-8843-4/part/part03/toc-part/ch141

142. STOOL STUDIES FOR INFECTION

Christine Colella and Kelly Small Casler

PATHOPHYSIOLOGY REVIEW

Stool studies are most often used to evaluate prolonged cases of diarrhea. Diarrhea, which most commonly occurs acutely, is defined as the passage of watery or loose stool at least three times in a 24-hour period or more frequently than is usual for an individual.[1] When lasting longer than 14 days, diarrhea is referred to as chronic.[2] Visible blood or mucus in the diarrhea is characterized as dysentery, which is often accompanied by weight loss.[2]

OVERVIEW OF LABORATORY TESTS

For short-lived cases of acute diarrhea, laboratory tests are rarely needed. For longer duration of symptoms, identification of etiology is important not only for treatment, but for public health prevention and control.[2] Testing options for investigation of diarrhea are noted in the list that follows.

- **Stool/fecal leukocyte examination (CPT code 89055).** This test uses microscopy to identify white blood cells in the feces, which usually results from inflammation. Inflammation can be due to infectious or noninfectious causes (inflammatory bowel disease) and is not disease specific. There are many drawbacks to the fecal leukocyte examination, including poor sensitivity (less than 70%) and specificity (50%),[3,4] which have led several expert groups to discourage its use in clinical practice.[5,6] For this test to be useful, specimens have to be evaluated quickly, since leukocytes can degenerate within 15 minutes after specimen collection.[3]
- **Comprehensive ova and parasite (O & P) stool examination (CPT codes 87177 and 87209).** Parasitic infection is more common in areas of poor sanitation. The most common parasites in the United States include giardia and cryptosporidium, which are often ingested through the ingestion of contaminated water. The O & P examination uses microscopy to look for specific parasites and their eggs (ova). Three samples are recommended to achieve adequate test sensitivity.[7,8] Consequently, stool O & P tests are being replaced by more accurate molecular tests that can be performed on a single stool sample. Therefore, stool O & P tests are primarily reserved for testing when molecular tests are negative, but suspicion of parasitic infection remains high.[7]
- **Comprehensive stool culture (CPT codes 87045, 87046, 87427).** A comprehensive stool culture can be ordered to look for a range of pathogens or for specific pathogens. There are many possible causes of infectious diarrhea such as *Campylobacter* species, *Salmonella*, *Shigella*, *Escherichia coli*, *Vibrio* species, and *Yersinia* (Table 142.1).[9,10]

(continued)

TABLE 142.1: MOST COMMON DIFFERENTIAL DIAGNOSES FOR DIARRHEA

POSSIBLE PATHOGEN	INCUBATION	SYMPTOMS IN ADDITION TO DIARRHEA	SOURCES OF INFECTION	DIAGNOSTIC TEST
Norovirus	6–48 hours	Abdominal pain, possible fever, vomiting/nausea	Shellfish, prepared foods, vegetables, fruits	Molecular test
Rotavirus	1–3 days	Abdominal pain, possible fever, vomiting/nausea	Vegetables, fruits, daycare	Molecular testing; EIA latex agglutination
Giardia lamblia (parasite)	3–25 days	Abd pain, N/V	Fecal contaminated food/water	Stool ova and parasite microscopic examination & stain; Molecular testing
Cryptosporidium parvum (parasite)	1–14 days	N/V may have abdominal pain and fever.	Vegetables, fruits, unpasteurized milk, water, unpasteurized milk	Stool ova and parasite microscopic examination & stain; Cryptosporidium molecular testing
Listeria monocytogenes	1 day–2 months	Fever, N/V	Processed meats, hot dogs, soft cheese, pates, fruit/vegetables	Stool culture; molecular testing
Vibrio cholerae	1–5 days	Symptoms very variable. May or may not have abdominal pain, fever, mucus, N/V, blood in stool	Salty or brackish waters exposure, travel to cholera-endemic regions or raw or undercooked shellfish ingestion	Stool culture; molecular testing
Clostridium perfringens	6–24 hours	Abdominal pain,	Seafood, contaminated beef/poultry	Stool culture; enterotoxin test
Non-EHEC	8–72 hours	N/V, abdominal pain	Ground beef and other meat, fresh produce, unpasteurized milk and juice	Stool culture; molecular testing

TABLE 142.1: MOST COMMON DIFFERENTIAL DIAGNOSES FOR DIARRHEA (CONTINUED)

POSSIBLE PATHOGEN	INCUBATION	SYMPTOMS IN ADDITION TO DIARRHEA	SOURCES OF INFECTION	DIAGNOSTIC TEST
EHEC	0.5–12 days	Bloody diarrhea, N/V, abdominal pain, may or may not have fever	Ground beef and other meat, fresh produce, unpasteurized milk and juice	Culture and sensitivity or molecular test for strain typing; shiga toxin test; tests for non-O157 strains are more difficult to perform
Yersinia spp	3–7 days	Abdominal pain (mimicking appendicitis), fever, school-age children; Fever, mucus, vomiting/nausea (possible)	Undercooked pork; Unpasteurized milk	Stool culture (will need special medium) and sensitivity with serotyping; molecular testing
Salmonella	8–24 hours	Bloody diarrhea (not always), fever, mucus, abdominal pain, vomiting/nausea (possible)	Poultry, eggs, egg products, fresh produce, meat, fish, unpasteurized milk, juice, nut butter, vegetables/fruits	Stool culture and sensitivity with serotyping; Molecular testing
Campylobacter jejuni	1–7 days	Bloody diarrhea, fever, mucus, abdominal pain, vomiting/nausea (possible)	Poultry; Unpasteurized milk	Stool culture and sensitivity with serotyping; molecular testing
Shigella spp	1–7 days	Bloody diarrhea, fever, mucus, abdominal pain, vomiting/nausea	Raw vegetables, undercooked eggs	Culture and sensitivity with serotyping; molecular testing

EHEC, enterohemorrhagic Escherichia coli (also called shiga-toxin producing Escherichia coli or STEC); EIA, enzyme immunoassay; PCR, polymerase chain reaction; spp, species).

Sources: Data from Bellido-Blasco JB, Arnedo-Pena A. Epidemiology of infectious diarrhea. In: Nraigu JO, ed. Encyclopedia of Environmental Health. Elsevier; 2011:659–671. doi:10.1016/B978-0-444-63951-6.00689-6; Farthing M, Salam MA, Lindberg G, et al. Acute diarrhea in adults and children: a global perspective. J Clin Gastroenterol. 2013;47(1):12–20. doi:10.1097/MCG.0b013e31826df662; Shane AL, Mody RK, Crump JA, et al. 2017 Infectious Diseases Society of America clinical practice guidelines for the diagnosis and management of infectious diarrhea. Clin Infect Dis. 2017;65(12):e45–e80. doi:10.1093/cid/cix669; Siddiqi HA, Salwen MJ, Shaikh MF, Bowne WB. Laboratory diagnosis of gastrointestinal and pancreatic disorders. In: McPherson RA, Pincus MR, eds. Henry's Clinical Diagnosis and Management by Laboratory Methods. 23rd ed. Elsevier; 2017:306–323.

- **Other tests.** Antigen tests and toxin tests are also used to look for antibodies or toxins produced by specific organisms. Molecular tests are becoming more common due to increased accuracy compared to the older tests that were previously described. Over time, molecular tests have also proven to be cost-effective and can test for the presence of up to 23 different pathogens (combination of viral, bacterial, and parasitic) from one sample.[11]

INDICATIONS

Screening
- Not used for screening.

Diagnosis and Evaluation
- The decision to test and which test to use should be influenced by the differential diagnosis (Tables 142.1 and 142.2). Pretest probability for bacterial infection is highest for patients with five or more diarrhea episodes per day, elevated CRP greater than 50 mg/dL, fever, bloody stools, and/or abdominal tenderness.[6,9,12]
- In immunocompetent persons, most episodes of gastrointestinal (GI) infection in the United States resolve on their own without treatment, so testing may not be needed.[7] Therefore, stool cultures or molecular tests are primarily used when the individual patient is at high risk of complications, of spreading disease to others, and during known or suspected outbreaks.[5]
- Stool cultures or molecular tests are used to evaluate inpatients with diarrhea that develops in the first 3 days of hospitalization (suspected acquisition of infection prior to hospitalization).[13]
- Parasitic molecular antigen testing is used if diarrhea is present for 7 or more days (sooner if the patient is immunocompromised or has recent international travel).[5,7]

Monitoring
- Repeat testing can be done to prove eradication, but is not usually needed.[6]

TABLE 142.2: TESTING IN PRESENCE OF HISTORICAL CLUES

HISTORY	CONSIDER TESTING FOR
Travelers's diarrhea for 14 days or more	Cryptosporidium parvum, Giardia lamblia, and other Intestinal parasitic infections endemic to area of travel
Treated with antibiotics in last 8 to 12 weeks	Clostridioides difficile testing
Childcare center attendee	EHEC, rotavirus, cryptosporidium, giardia, shigella

EHEC, enterohemorrhagic *Escherichia coli*/shiga toxin producing *E. coli*.

Sources: Data from Bellido-Blasco JB, Arnedo-Pena A. Epidemiology of infectious diarrhea. In: Nraigu JO, ed. *Encyclopedia of Environmental Health.* Elsevier; 2011:659–671. doi:10.1016/B978-0-444-63951-6.00689-6; Farthing M, Salam MA, Lindberg G, et al. Acute diarrhea in adults and children: a global perspective. *J Clin Gastroenterol.* 2013;47(1):12–20. doi:10.1097/MCG.0b013e31826df662; Shane AL, Mody RK, Crump JA, et al. 2017 Infectious Diseases Society of America clinical practice guidelines for the diagnosis and management of infectious diarrhea. Clin Infect Dis. 2017;65(12):e45–e80. doi:10.1093/cid/cix669; Siddiqi HA, Salwen MJ, Shaikh MF, Bowne WB. Laboratory diagnosis of gastrointestinal and pancreatic disorders. In: *McPherson RA, Pincus MR, eds. Henry's Clinical Diagnosis and Management by Laboratory Methods.* 23rd ed. Elsevier; 2017:306–323.

INTERPRETATION

- Reported as positive or negative by pathogen.

FOLLOW-UP

- If testing for infectious causes of diarrhea is negative, consider alternate differential diagnoses of diarrhea (Table 142.3).[3,10]
- Consider blood cultures for history suggestive of or at risk for sepsis or enteric fever: age younger than 3 months, enteric fever exposures, immunocompromise, or high-risk comorbidities.[6]
- Serologic testing for *E. coli* is available to evaluate for post-diarrheal hemolytic-uremic syndrome (HUS).[6]
- Consider referral for endoscopy in patients with persistent diarrhea, especially those with immunocompromise.[6]
- If enteric fever is suspected, consider cultures of duodenal fluid, urine, and/or bone marrow (higher sensitivity than blood culture).[6]
- Electrolyte evaluation may help influence the treatment plan if patient is dehydrated.[9]
- A complete blood count may be useful since eosinophilia may be seen in the presence of a parasite[8] and signs of hemolysis, including fragmented red blood cells on a peripheral blood smear, may be present with HUS.[6]
- With bloody diarrhea, co-order Shiga toxin tests to evaluate for the presence of O157:H7 and non-O157:H7 Shiga toxin-producing *E. coli* strains.[8]

TABLE 142.3: FOLLOW-UP TESTING CONSIDERATIONS FOR NEGATIVE INFECTION TESTS

DIFFERENTIAL DIAGNOSIS	INDICATED TESTING
Celiac disease	Tissue transglutaminase
Hepatitis A	Hepatitis antibody testing
Human immunodeficiency virus	HIV
Hyperthyroidism	Thyroid-stimulating hormone or thyroxine (T4)
Inflammatory bowel disease	Fecal calprotectin
Lactase deficiency	Lactose tolerance test
Lipid malabsorption	Fecal fat stain
Pancreatic insufficiency	Fecal elastase
Small bowel bacterial overgrowth	Bacterial small bowel aspirate count
Zollinger-Ellison syndrome	Gastrin

Sources: Data from Gupta A, Johnson DH, Agrawal D. Devolution and devaluation of fecal leukocyte testing: a 100-year history. JAMA Intern Med. 2018;178(9):1155. doi:10.1001/jamainternmed.2018.3150; Siddiqi HA, Salwen MJ, Shaikh MF, Bowne WB. Laboratory Diagnosis of Gastrointestinal and Pancreatic Disorders. In: McPherson RA, Pincus MR, eds. Henry's Clinical Diagnosis and Management by Laboratory Methods. 23rd ed. Elsevier; 2017:306–323.

PEARLS & PITFALLS

■ Clinicians should communicate suspected pathogens and travel history to the laboratory personnel to help guide testing.

■ Fresh stool samples offer the greatest accuracy, but rectal swabs can be used if stool samples are not obtainable.[6]

■ Collaboration with public health officials is essential, especially during suspected outbreaks.

■ Tests for bacterial infection are more likely to be positive in the presence of fever, bloody stools, and/or abdominal tenderness.[6]

■ Combination nucleic acid amplification tests are available that test for multiple pathogens from one sample, but these tests could overdetect, identifying agents that are normal flora. Research continues to be done on the cost-effectiveness of these types of tests.[6,11,14]

■ If antibiotic resistance is prevalent in an area, bacterial sensitivity testing can be ordered with stool culture. This test is rarely needed, however.[5]

■ Order testing is based on the pathogen(s) suspected from the differential diagnoses after a thorough history and physical.[9,12]

■ Identification of a pathogen does not always equate to infection—consider colonization and normal flora, only order tests in the presence of suspicious symptoms, and correlate testing with clinical symptoms.[9]

PATIENT EDUCATION

■ https://www.webmd.com/a-to-z-guides/what-is-a-stool-culture
■ http://www.pathgroup.com/wp-content/uploads/2012/08/Stool-Collecting-and-Handling-Instructions-7-6-09.pdf

RELATED DIAGNOSES AND ICD-10 CODES

Other fecal abnormalities such as blood or mucous	R19.5
Diarrhea, unspecified	R19.7
Abdominal pain, cramping	R10.9
Nausea, vomiting, unspecified	R11.2
Melena (blood in stool)	K92.1

REFERENCES

Full list of references can be accessed through Springer Publishing Company Connect™ at the following link: http://connect.springerpub.com/content/reference-book/978-0-8261-8843-4/part/part03/toc-part/ch142

143. STREPTOCOCCAL SORE THROAT TESTING

Kimberly R. Joo

PHYSIOLOGY REVIEW

Strep throat is a type of pharyngitis that is caused by a bacterial infection of the oropharynx.[1] Strep throat acquired its name from the causative pathogen, *Streptococcus pyogenes*, or *S. pyogenes*. This bacterium produces complete hemolysis of red blood cells when placed on sheep blood culture agar and consequently is referred to as beta-hemolytic streptococcus. The Lancefield streptococcus classification places *S. pyogenes* in Group A beta-hemolytic strep (GABHS). *S. pyogen*es is considered to be the most pathogenic bacterium in the genus *Streptococcus*.[2]

GABHS pharyngitis can be responsible for both suppurative and nonsuppurative complications if left untreated. Suppurative complications can include bacteremia, endocarditis, meningitis, otitis media, pneumonia, peritonsillar abscess, retropharyngeal abscess, cervical lymphadenitis, and mastoiditis. These can occur when a *S. pyogenes* infection transfers from the oropharynx to other nearby structures. Nonsuppurative complications include acute rheumatic fever and post streptococcal glomerulonephritis.[1,3] Identification and treatment of GAS pharyngitis is paramount to the prevention of these severe complications.

OVERVIEW OF LABORATORY TESTS

Throat Culture

The throat culture (TC; CPT code 87081) has been the long-established "gold standard" for diagnosing strep throat in patients of all ages. However, its use in the outpatient setting is limited due to the length of time involved between the collection of the specimen and the results, which can be up to 48 to 72 hours.[4] Throat cultures are currently recommended only as a backup method for strep throat diagnosis in children who have received negative results with rapid antigen detection tests (RADT) due to the higher prevalence of strep throat in this population and the higher risk of complications from strep throat.[5]

Rapid Antigen Detection Tests

Rapid antigen detection tests (RADT; CPT code 87880) were introduced in the early 1980s. These tests detect antigens to *S. pyogenes* at the point of care and they have evolved over the years to include latex agglutination tests, color immunochromatographic assays, enzyme immunoassays, and optical immunoassays.[4] These tests work by acid extraction of GAS cell wall antigen from a throat swab. An immunologicl reaction detects the absence or presence of the GAS cell wall antigen, which is a carbohydrate.[6] Since their inception, RADTs have been the standard method of strep throat diagnosis at the point of care for patients of all ages.[7] They are widely used due to their quick results, low cost, and ease of use.[6] The sensitivity for RADTs is usually lower than the specificity and can vary somewhat depending on the manufacturer of the test.[8] A Cochrane systematic review of the literature that included 98 research studies on RADT for strep throat in children determined the overall sensitivity for these tests to be 85.6% and overall specificity to be 95.4%.[9] Another Cochrane systematic review of the literature determined that RADTs most likely reduce the number of antibiotic prescriptions for pharyngitis by 25%.[10]

Nucleic Acid Amplification Test

The newest point of care laboratory testing for GAS includes nucleic acid amplification tests (NAAT), also known as molecular assays (CPT code 87651). These assays test for specific genetic material of *S. pyogenes*, such as nucleic acids, using real-time polymerase chain reaction (PCR) or helicase-dependent amplification (HDA)-based methodology.[11] In 2017, the U.S. Food and Drug Administration (FDA) gave clearance to three NAATs for GAS: the cobias Liat, the Luminex Aries, and the Cepheid Xpert Xpress.[12] Since then, other NAAT tests have received clearance, including the Revogene Strep A and the Alere i Strep A. These NAAT assays for GAS have shown improved sensitivity over the RADT (95.5%–100%) and specificities (95.5%–100%). Positive predictive values (PPV) range from 86.3% to 100% and negative predictive values range from 95.5% to 100% for these tests.[12-19] Due to the high sensitivity for this type of testing, throat cultures are not recommended for negative test results in children or adults.[12]

The advantages of NAAT for GAS include the increased sensitivity, eliminated need for backup throat culture with negative results, reduction in empiric use of antibiotics, and detection of group C streptococcus (GCS) and group G streptococcus (GGS) with some assays.[11] The disadvantages of NAAT for GAS include the higher cost of testing, the larger and possible multiple instruments, inability to distinguish between active GAS infection and GAS colonization, and possible unnecessary antibiotics prescribed when GBS or GGS is detected.[11]

INDICATIONS

Distinguishing between viral pharyngitis and strep throat is difficult due to the similarity of symptoms.[1] The most common symptoms of strep throat are odynophagia (painful swallowing), sore throat, and fever. Other symptoms can include headache, abdominal pain, nausea, and vomiting. Clinical symptoms of strep throat are pharyngeal and tonsillar erythema, tonsillar hypertrophy with or without exudate, palatial petechiae, and anterior cervical lymphadenopathy. Patients with strep throat may also present with a raised, red, sandpaper-feeling rash on their torso, known as scarlatiniform rash.[1] It is important to note that strep throat does not typically cause rhinorrhea, cough, conjunctivitis, hoarseness, or oral ulcers. These symptoms are more likely to indicate viral pharyngitis.[1]

The Modified Centor Criteria is commonly used in clinical practice to estimate the likelihood that the pharyngitis is streptococcal. Patients are given a score based on criteria that include the patient's age, and management recommendations are given based on the criteria score.[20,21] A score of greater than or equal to 2 recommends testing for GAS. Another pharyngitis decision-making tree was created in 2006 to assist with the management of strep throat.[22]

Children under the age of 3 are unlikely to develop strep throat and they are also not at risk to develop severe complications from strep pharyngitis such as rheumatic fever. As a result, children under 3 years of age should not be routinely tested for strep throat.[23] A clinician may choose to test a child under the age of 3 for strep throat if there is a close member of the household who has strep throat or if they attend daycare.

Screening
There are no universal or targeted screenings for strep throat.

Diagnosis and Evaluation
These tests (throat culture, RADT, and NAAT) are used to rule in or rule out the following diagnoses:

- Strep pharyngitis
- Scarlet fever
- Scarlatiniform rash

These tests can also be used to rule out streptococcal pharyngitis when the following diagnoses are suspected: viral pharyngitis; upper respiratory infection; mononucleosis; hand, foot, and mouth disease; influenza; rubella; measles; cytomegalovirus; respiratory syncytial virus; Vincent's angina; Lemierre's syndrome; Group C *streptococcus*; Group G *streptococcus*; *N. gonorrhoeae*; *Mycoplasma pneumonia*; and *Chlamydophila pneumonia*.[7]

Monitoring
- Patients receiving antibiotics for a positive strep test should be monitored for improvement of symptoms within 24 to 48 hours.
- Patients with a negative strep test who are diagnosed with viral pharyngitis should be monitored for symptom improvement in 7 to 10 days.
- Backup throat culture results should be monitored for pediatric patients who have a negative RADT and throat culture ordered.

INTERPRETATION
- Positive RADT or NAAT: Diagnosis is strep throat.
- Negative RADT or NAAT: Sore throat is most likely due to a virus (see differential diagnoses noted previously).

FOLLOW-UP
- Positive RADT or NAAT: No follow-up testing recommended.
- Negative NAAT: No follow-up testing recommended.
- Negative RADT: Follow-up testing includes a throat culture for pediatric patients aged 18 and under.

PEARLS & PITFALLS

- Children under the age of 3 should not routinely be tested for strep throat.[23]
- The Centor Criteria and clinician judgment are controversial for diagnosing strep throat.[24]
- One study found that it is reasonable to consider re-testing with NAAT for GAS as early as 1 week following a positive test result by RADT or NAAT for GAS that was treated with antibiotics.[25]
- Antistreptococcal antibody titers are not recommended in the routine diagnosis of acute pharyngitis.[21]

PATIENT EDUCATION

- https://www.cdc.gov/groupastrep/diseases-public/strep-throat.html

RELATED DIAGNOSES AND ICD-10 CODES

Streptococcal pharyngitis	J02.0
Acute pharyngitis, unspecified	J02.9
Scarlet fever with otitis media	A38.0
Scarlet fever with myocarditis	A38.1
Scarlet fever with other complications	A38.8
Rheumatic chorea with heart involvement	I02.0
Rheumatic chorea without heart involvement	I02.9
Other specified rheumatic heart disease	I09.89
Rheumatic heart disease, unspecified	I09.9
Acute pharyngitis due to other specified organisms	J02.8
Pain in the throat	R07.0

REFERENCES

Full list of references can be accessed through Springer Publishing Company Connect™ at the following link: http://connect.springerpub.com/content/reference-book/978-0-8261-8843-4/part/part03/toc-part/ch143

144. SYPHILIS TESTS (RAPID PLASMA REAGIN AND *TREPONEMA PALLIDUM*)

Courtney DuBois Shihabuddin and Stephanie L. Marrs

PHYSIOLOGY REVIEW

Syphilis is an infection caused by the spirochete bacterium *Treponema pallidum*. Most new cases of syphilis are sexually acquired. The clinical manifestations depend upon the stage of disease.[1] Transmission of *T. pallidum* usually occurs via direct physical contact with an infectious lesion, most commonly during sexual intercourse. In addition, *T. pallidum* readily crosses the placenta, and can easily result in fetal infection.[2] *T. pallidum* can initiate infection wherever disease inoculation occurs. Therefore, any type of contact with infected secretions can lead to a primary syphilis lesion at the site of contact. This means that syphilis can be spread by kissing or touching a person who has active lesions on the lips, oral cavity, breasts, or genitals.[3]

Patients may seek evaluation for symptoms or signs of primary infection (e.g., chancre), secondary infection (e.g., diffuse rash), or tertiary infection (e.g., symptoms of aortic insufficiency). Alternatively, patients may be completely asymptomatic and infection is identified during screening. Asymptomatic infection may be more common in re-infected individuals.

OVERVIEW OF LABORATORY TESTS

Serologic tests provide a presumptive diagnosis of syphilis. There are two types of serologic tests for syphilis: nontreponemal tests and treponemal-specific tests. The use of only one test is insufficient for diagnosis since serologic testing (especially nontreponemal tests) can be associated with false-positive results.[4] False-negative results can often occur in patients with advanced immunosuppression and or/early disease as serologic testing relies upon a humoral immune response to infection.[5]

Nontreponemal tests (also known as tests for reagin antibodies) are based upon the reactivity of serum from infected patients to a cardiolipin-cholesterol-lecithin antigen.[6] Despite the nonspecific nature of these screening tests, they have traditionally been used for initial syphilis screening due to their low cost, ease of performance, and ability to be quantified for the purpose of following response to therapy. The exception is the Venereal Disease Research Laboratory (VDRL) test, which is tested on cerebral spinal fluid and used to test for neurosyphilis.[7]

Nontremponal tests include:

- Rapid plasma reagin (RPR) (CPT code 86593)
- Toluidine red unheated serum test (TRUST)
- Venereal Disease Research Laboratory (VDRL, CSF) (CPT code 86592)

Treponemal tests are historically more complex and expensive to perform than nontreponemal tests and therefore are often only used as confirmatory tests for syphilis when the nontreponemal tests are reactive.[7] Specific treponemal tests include:

- Fluorescent treponemal antibody absorption (FTA-ABS) (CPT code 86780)
- Microhemagglutination test for antibodies to *T. pallidum* (MHA-TP) (CPT code 86781)
- *T. pallidum* particle agglutination assay (TPPA) (CPT code 86780)
- *T. pallidum* enzyme immunoassay (TP-EIA) (CPT code 86592)
- Chemiluminescence immunoassay (CIA) (CPT code 86780)

INDICATIONS

Screening

Asymptomatic patients should be screened for syphilis if they are at high risk for having acquired disease, a risk for transmitting disease to others, or are pregnant. The United States Preventive Services Task Force (USPSTF) recommends against routine screening for asymptomatic individuals who are not at high risk for syphilis infection.[8] All pregnant women should be screened for syphilis as part of routine prenatal care to reduce risk of stillbirth and severe birth defects.[8,9]

Asymptomatic patients who are at increased risk of infection should also be routinely screened. This includes:

- Known sexual contact with a partner who has early (i.e., primary, secondary, or early latent) syphilis[4]
- All sexually active men who have sex with men (MSM)[2]
- All people living with human immunodeficiency virus (PLWH)[2]
- Individuals engaging in high-risk sexual activity[4]
- All commercial sex workers[4]
- Individuals with a history of incarceration[4]
- Individuals living in local areas with high prevalence[8]

Diagnosis and Evaluation

Syphilis can present with a wide range of symptoms, or may present with no symptoms at all. Therefore, the threshold for screening should be low. The following groups of patients should be screened regardless of their risk behaviors:

- Patients who present with "classic" syphilis symptoms, including but not limited to a painless genital ulcer (primary syphilis); a diffuse, symmetric macular or papular eruption involving the trunk and extremities (secondary syphilis); general paresis; tabes dorsalis (tertiary syphilis)[10]
- Any sexually active individual with an undiagnosed genital ulcer or a rash that involves the palms of the hands and soles of the feet[11]
- Patients who present with less-specific signs and symptoms (e.g., cranial nerve dysfunction, chronic headache, aortic insufficiency, meningitis, other signs of meningovascular disease, including cerebrovascular accidents), particularly if no other etiology is identified[12]

The differential diagnosis for syphilis is famously broad and varies by stage. Testing for syphilis should be performed on all patients who present with signs and/or symptoms of infection. Refer to Table 144.1 for a list of signs and symptoms by stage.

Monitoring

Initial serologic testing for syphilis is traditionally a nontreponemal test (e.g., RPR). Asymptomatic patients with a negative nontreponemal test require no further testing. A reactive nontreponemal test is then confirmed with a treponemal test, such as FTA-ABS. Patients who present early after discovery of a rash or ulcer may have negative serologic testing. If the clinician has a high suspicion of syphilis, repeat serologic testing should be performed in 2 to 4 weeks.[4]

Positive nontreponemal tests are reported as a titer of antibody (e.g., 1:32, which represents the detection of antibody in serum diluted 32-fold). Titers tend to wane over time even without treatment, but successful therapy accelerates the pace of antibody decline. Changes in titer are followed after treatment to detect a therapeutic response. Successful treatment of syphilis requires a four-fold decline in the nontreponemal titer. This decline is equivalent to a change of two dilutions (e.g., from 1:16 to 1:4 or from 1:32 to 1:8), and is considered to be an acceptable response to syphilis therapy.[14]

INTERPRETATION

A patient must have both a positive screening nontreponemal test *and* a positive treponemal confirmatory test to support a diagnosis of syphilis. If a patient does not have a history of previously treated syphilis, these results are consistent with a new infection that must be treated.

Patients who have a history of previously treated syphilis are more complicated. The need for additional treatment depends upon the patient's clinical presentation and their nontreponemal titer. Treponemal tests often remain

TABLE 144.1: SIGNS AND SYMPTOMS OF SYPHILIS BY STAGE			
PRIMARY SYPHILIS	**SECONDARY SYPHILIS**[13]	**TERTIARY SYPHILIS**	**NEUROSYPHILIS (CAN OCCUR AT ANY STAGE)**
Chancroid	Dermatophytosis	Congestive heart failure	Brain tumors
Condyloma acuminata	Erythema annulare centrifugum	HIV infection	CNS infection (e.g., meningitis, encephalitis)
Herpes simplex 1 and 2	Granuloma annulare	Lymphoma	Ophthalmologicdisorders
HIV infection	Herpes zoster	Sarcoidosis	Stroke
Lymphogranuloma super-infection of lesion	HIV infection	Trauma	Uveitis
Trauma	Lichen planus		
Venereum	Mycobacterial infection		
	Sarcoidosis		
	Subacute lupus erythematosus		

positive long after infection. Titers of nontreponemal assays decline following successful therapy, and usually will revert to nonreactive over time. If a patient has a history of previously treated syphilis, the presence of a positive nontreponemal test indicates a new infection, an evolving response to recent treatment, treatment failure, or the presence of a serofast state. Individuals are considered to be serofast if they have a persistently reactive nontreponemal test despite adequate treatment, generally (but not always) at a low titer (e.g., 1:8).

Successful interpretation of the serologic test requires comparing the current titer to the patient's prior post-treatment titer. Comparison is only possible when using the same nontreponemal test method (e.g., RPR). A new syphilis infection is diagnosed when quantitative testing using a nontreponemal test reveals a *four-fold or greater increase* in titer from the patient's previous post-treatment test, provided the same type of test was completed (Table 144.2).

FOLLOW-UP

Patients who have had greater than or equal to a four-fold decline in titers, but whose nontreponemal titers do not serorevert, or continue to fall after 24 months of monitoring, are considered serofast. Patients who remain serofast should be tested for HIV, as the serofast state can result from immunodysregulation of antibody production.[4]

Consider testing for other sexually transmitted infections including chlamydia, gonorrhea, HIV, and trichomonas.

TABLE 144.2: INTERPRETATION OF SYPHILIS TEST RESULTS				
TYPE OF TEST	NO INFECTION	PAST TREATMENT OR POSSIBLE EARLY INFECTION	SYPHILIS DIAGNOSIS	FALSE POSITIVE
Treponemal (Objective, inexpensive, automated)	Nonreactive	Reactive	Reactive	Nonreactive
Nontreponemal (RPR, Rapid Plasma Reagin; VDRL, Venereal Disease Research Laboratory; Subjective, variable by 1 dilution up or down, used to monitor treatment outcomes)	Nonreactive	Nonreactive	Reactive because pt. has syphilis Reactive if previously treated—assess for increase or decrease by fourfold dilution	Reactive with a low titer (e.g., 1:1)

PEARLS & PITFALLS

- A patient who is positive for syphilis is at high risk for other sexually transmitted diseases (STIs).
- Latex condoms can provide some protection from syphilis but if the chancre is exposed, transmission can still occur.
- Syphilis is a reportable disease.
- Males account for most cases of syphilis with gay, bisexual, and MSM occurring at disproportionally higher incidence. Females only account for about 16.7% of cases.

PATIENT EDUCATION

- https://www.cdc.gov/std/syphilis/stdfact-syphilis.htm
- https://www.cdc.gov/std/syphilis/facts-brochures.htm

RELATED DIAGNOSES AND ICD-10 CODES

Primary genital syphilis	A51.0
Early syphilis	A51.9
Early syphilis, latent	A51.5
Secondary syphilis	A51.49
Late syphilis (tertiary)	A52.9
Latent syphilis	A53.0
Neurosyphilis	A52.3
Congenital syphilis	A50.9
Maternal syphilis complicating pregnancy	A53.9
Contact with and (suspected) exposure to infections with a predominantly sexual mode of transmission	Z20.2

REFERENCES

Full list of references can be accessed through Springer Publishing Company Connect™ at the following link: http://connect.springerpub.com/content/reference-book/978-0-8261-8843-4/part/part03/toc-part/ch144

145. TESTOSTERONE AND SEX HORMONE BINDING GLOBULIN

Danielle A. Quallich, Lisa Ward, Susanne A. Quallich, and Kelly Small Casler

PHYSIOLOGY REVIEW

Testosterone is the main sex hormone (androgen) in both males and females and is derived from cholesterol and regulated by a negative feedback loop called the hypothalamic-pituitary-gonadal (HPG) axis (see Chapter 139, Figure 139.1). When testosterone levels are low, the hypothalamus stimulates the pituitary gland to secrete FSH and LH. In males, FSH stimulates spermatogenesis, while LH stimulates the testicles to produce testosterone. Small amounts of testosterone are also produced by the adrenal glands. Testosterone helps to regulate fertility, muscle mass, fat distribution, libido, red blood cell production, and bone density in all sexes, but its effects are more easily recognized in males.[1]

Testosterone secretion occurs in a circadian rhythm with peak levels between 4 a.m. and 8 a.m. and trough levels between 4 p.m. and 8 p.m.[2] In males, testosterone levels increase dramatically during puberty and remain high into adulthood. In females, testosterone levels peak during early adulthood. In all sexes, testosterone levels can increase after exercise and steadily decline after mid-adulthood.[2-4]

Sex hormone binding globulin (SHBG) is a transport protein produced by the liver that binds estrogens and testosterone, making them inactive. Approximately 65% of testosterone is bound to SHBG and approximately 30% is bound to albumin.[2] Albumin binds to testosterone loosely, in contrast to SHBG which binds testosterone tightly, resulting in albumin-bound testosterone (but not SHBG-bound) being available to act on target tissues (referred to as bioavailability).

OVERVIEW OF LABORATORY TESTS

Testosterone circulates in the blood in several forms and is most assessed by serum total testosterone (CPT code 84403) and free testosterone (CPT code 84402). Total testosterone (TT) refers to the total testosterone within the body, both testosterone that is bound to proteins (SHBG and albumin) and un-bound (free). Free testosterone (FT) refers to the testosterone within the bloodstream that is not bound to proteins. It is considered the active form of testosterone, can act on target tissues, and makes up less than 5% of total testosterone.[2] It can be directly measured, but is most often calculated from measured TT, albumin, and SHBG.[5] Bioavailable testosterone (free testosterone plus testosterone bound to albumin) is often of interest to clinicians since it is the portion of testosterone that is available to act on target tissues. This measurement is calculated (also using TT, albumin, and SHBG), rather than measured in the laboratory.[6] There is some controversy about the accuracy of the calculation methods, however.[7,8] SHBG (CPT code 84270) is measured in the serum. Its measurement is primarily used to help estimate bioavailable and/or free testosterone levels.

In most cases, measuring TT provides clinicians adequate information for assessment.[2,9,10] If need be, more detailed assessments of testosterone levels can be made by testing for FT or bioavailable testosterone. FT measurements are more appropriate in females and children where the TT present is very small.[2] FT and bioavailable testosterone are also used to clarify when TT is near the lower limit of normal or if TT is normal and clinical conditions that can alter SHBG (Table 145.1)[11,12] are suspected to be influencing the free or bioavailable testoterone.[10,11]

INDICATIONS
Screening
- The United States and Australian Endocrine Societies as well as the American Urological Association recommend against general population routine screening because it is not cost effective.[9,11,13,14]
- Targeted screening can be considered for individuals who are at an increased risk of sequelae related to abnormal testosterone levels. This includes patients with obesity, diabetes, low-trauma fractures, premature osteoporosis, HIV, weight loss, rheumatoid arthritis, advanced renal disease, advanced COPD, thyroid disease, hyperlipidemia, chronic glucocorticoid or opioid use, or polycystic ovary syndrome (PCOS).[11,13-16]

TABLE 145.1: CONDITIONS THAT CAN INFLUENCE SEX HORMONE BINDING GLOBULIN LEVELS

CONDITIONS THAT CAN DECREASE SHBG AND RESULT IN MORE BIOAVAILABLE TESTOSTERONE	CONDITIONS THAT CAN INCREASE SHBG AND RESULT IN LESS BIOAVAILABLE TESTOSTERONE
Acromegaly	Aging
Androgen steroid use	Anticonvulsant use
Glucocorticoid use	Cirrhosis
Hypothyroidism	Estrogen use
Insulin resistance/metabolic syndrome	Hepatitis
Nephrotic syndrome	HIV
Obesity	Hyperthyroidism
PCOS	
Progesterone	
T2DM	

HIV, human immunodeficiency virus; PCOS, polycystic ovary syndrome; SHBG, sex hormone binding globulin; T2DM, type 2 diabetes mellitus.

Sources: Data from Bhasin S, Cunningham GR, Hayes FJ, et al. Testosterone therapy in men with androgen deficiency syndromes: an Endocrine Society clinical practice guideline. *J Clin Endocrinol Metab.* 2010;95(6):2536–2559. doi:10.1210/jc.2009-2354; Luo X, Yang X-M, Cai W-Y, et al. Decreased sex hormone-binding globulin indicated worse biometric, lipid, liver, and renal function parameters in women with polycystic ovary syndrome. *Int J Endocrinol.* 2020;2020:1–6. doi:10.1155/2020/7580218

Diagnosis and Evaluation

- TT is used to evaluate clinical symptoms of hypogonadism (Table 145.2).[2,11,13–17] Two abnormally low morning testosterone levels are needed to confirm a diagnosis of hypogonadism/testosterone deficiency.[11,18,19]
- Used to evaluate congenital hypogonadism in the presence of ambiguous genitalia.
- If abnormal SHBG is suspected or noted (Table 145.1), evaluating a FT level (in addition to TT) may be useful.[9,14,18]
- TT is used to assist in diagnosing conditions such as Klinefelter syndrome, hypogonadotropic hypogonadism, or congenital adrenal hyperplasia.[15]

Monitoring

- For males on testosterone therapy for hypogonadism/deficiency, TT is monitored at 3 to 4 months after therapy initiation, and then every 6 to 12 months once target levels (mid-range of reference intervals) and symptom improvement are achieved. The exact monitoring interval of TT varies with replacement product.[11,14,20,21]
- To monitor levels in transgender individuals undergoing hormone therapy for gender transition, measure TT and SHBG every 3 months in the first year of therapy and then every 6 to 12 months and as needed.[22,23] Exact intervals vary with type of therapy (Table 145.3).[24]

TABLE 145.2: INDICATIONS FOR TOTAL TESTOSTERONE TESTING BASED ON SIGNS/SYMPTOMS

MALES	FEMALES
Changes in bone mineral density	Baldness
Decreases in energy and muscle mass	Changes in fat distribution
Decreased libido	Decreases in energy
Depression	Decreased libido
Early/delayed puberty	Depression
Erectile dysfunction	Early/delayed puberty
Gynecomastia	Hirsutism
Hypogonadic testes	Infertility
Infertility	Menstrual irregularities
Loss of body and facial hair	Premature osteoporosis
Sexual dysfunction	Sleep disturbances
	Virilization

Sources: Data from Bhasin S, Cunningham GR, Hayes FJ, et al. Testosterone therapy in men with androgen deficiency syndromes: an Endocrine Society clinical practice guideline. *J Clin Endocrinol Metab.* 2010;95(6):2536–2559. doi:10.1210/jc.2009-2354; Lexicomp Online. *Lab Tests and Diagnostic Procedures*; Mitchell KA. Testosterone deficiency evaluation, management, and treatment considerations. In: Quallich SA, Lajiness MJ, eds. *The Nurse Practitioner in Urology.* Springer International Publishing; 2020:15–36. doi:10.1007/978-3-030-45267-4_2; Mulhall JP, Trost LW, Brannigan RE, et al. Evaluation and management of testosterone deficiency: AUA guideline. *J Urol.* 2018;200(2):423–432. doi:10.1016/j.juro.2018.03.115; Paduch DA, Brannigan RE, Fuchs EF, et al. *White Paper: The Laboratory Diagnosis of Testosterone Deficiency.* Published November 24, 2020. http://university .auanet.org/common/pdf/education/clinical-guidance/Testosterone-Deficiency-WhitePaper.pdf; Qaseem A, Horwitch CA, Vijan S, Etxeandia-Ikobaltzeta I, Kansagara D, for the Clinical Guidelines Committee of the American College of Physicians. Testosterone treatment in adult men with age-related low testosterone: a clinical guideline from the American College of Physicians. *Ann Intern Med.* 2020;172(2):126. doi:10.7326/M19-0882; Washington State Healthcare Authority. Testosterone Testing. https://www.hca.wa.gov/about-hca/health-technology-assessment/testosterone-testing.-table

TABLE 145.3: GENDER-AFFIRMING HORMONE THERAPY MONITORING

TYPE OF MEDICATION	WHEN TT TYPICALLY MEASURED*	USUAL TARGET LEVEL*
Parenteral testosterone enanthate/cypionate	Measured midway of injection intervals or measure a peak and trough	Mid-range of reference interval (i.e., 400–700 ng/dL)
Parenteral testosterone undecanoate	At 6 weeks, 16 weeks, and 54 weeks of therapy	Mid-range of reference interval (i.e., 400–700 ng/dL); if less than this may need to adjust dosing interval*
Transdermal testosterone	At least 1 week after use and at least 2 hours after patch change	Mid-range of reference interval (i.e., 400–700 ng/dL)

*Dosing interval adjustments considered FDA off-label use of medication.

Source: Data from Hembree WC, Cohen-Kettenis PT, Gooren L, et al. Endocrine treatment of gender-dysphoric/gender-incongruent persons: an Endocrine Society clinical practice guideline. *J Clin Endocrinol Metab*. 2017;102(11):3869–3903. doi:10.1210/jc.2017-01658

- The usual target TT goal for hormone therapy in transitioning males is determined along with clinical history. Usual TT targets approximate usual reference intervals of 300 to 1,000 ng/dL, though some experts advocate higher levels up to 1,200 ng/dL may be needed if clinical history suggests undertreatment. This is somewhat controversial as supraphysiologic levels increase risk of adverse events.
- For individuals using injectable testosterone, peak (24 to 48 h after injection) and trough (immediately before injection) levels may also be used to guide treatment decisions.[23,25]
- The usual TT target in transitioning females is a TT of 30 to 100 ng/dL.[23]
- SHBG may be monitored in individuals receiving gender-affirming hormone therapy, so that bioavailable T can be calculated.

INTERPRETATION

- Reference intervals are listed in Table 145.4.[26–28]
- A TT level of less than 300 to 320 ng/dL is usually used as a cutoff of testosterone deficiency for males.[14–16]
- Differential diagnosis of TT levels is reflected in Tables 145.5 and 145.6.

FOLLOW-UP

- See Table 145.6 and Figure 145.1 for further testing recommendations based on differential diagnosis.
- If TT is decreased, complete a repeat fasting morning level to confirm abnormality along with a serum LH and FSH to distinguish primary versus secondary hypogonadism (Table 145.6).[9,14,29,30]
- Males presenting with low testosterone levels in addition to breast symptoms (gynecomastia) should have evaluation of serum estradiol levels.[14]
- Males and females interested in conceiving, who also have low levels (males) of testosterone or elevated levels (females), should undergo a

TABLE 145.4: REFERENCE INTERVALS

	TOTAL TESTOSTERONE	FREE TESTOSTERONE	BIOAVAILABLE TESTOSTERONE
Female ≥ 18 years	15–70 ng/dL	0.8–9.2 pg/mL	2.2–25.5 ng/dL
Female, prepubertal	<17 pg/mL	<2.2 pg/mL	0.3–5.5 ng/dL
Male ≥ 18 years	280–1,100 ng/dL	47–244 pg/mL	130–680 ng/dL
Male, prepubertal	<20 ng/dL	<3.7 pg/mL	0.3–13.0 ng/dL

Note: These reference intervals are guides. Best practice is to follow reference intervals provided by the laboratory since intervals vary based on age, sex, and stage of puberty (Tanner stage).

Sources: Data from Mayo Clinic Laboratories. *Testosterone, Total and Bioavailable, Serum*. Test ID:TTBS. Accessed December 6, 2020. https://www.mayocliniclabs.com/test-catalog/Clinical+and+Interpretive/80065; Snyder LM, Rao LV, Wallach JB. *Wallach's Interpretation of Diagnostic Tests: Pathways to Arriving at a Clinical Diagnosis*. 2021; University of Rochester Medical Center. *Free Testosterone*. Health Encyclopedia. htps://www.urmc.rochester.edu/encyclopedia/content .aspx?contenttypeid=167&contentid=testosterone_free.

TABLE 145.5: DIFFERENTIAL DIAGNOSIS OF ABNORMAL TESTOSTERONE LEVELS

DECREASED TESTOSTERONE (MALE)		INCREASED TESTOSTERONE LEVEL (MALE)
Primary hypogonadism	Secondary hypogonadism	
Castration/trauma	Hypothalamic/pituitary dysfunction/pituitary tumors	Adrenal tumors
Aging	Hemochromatosis	Exogenous testosterone use
Klinefelter syndrome/Prader-Willi syndrome	Kallman syndrome	Exercise
Autoimmune conditions/infections	HIV infection	Hyperthyroidism
Drugs (alcohol, ketoconazole, antidepressants)	Chemotherapy/Radiation therapy	Congenital adrenal hyperplasia
Infection	Drugs (opioids, estrogens, steroids, GNRH agonists)	Androgen resistance Testicular tumors
DECREASED TESTOSTERONE (FEMALE)		INCREASED TESTOSTERONE (FEMALE)
Primary hypogonadism	Secondary hypogonadism	Ovarian or adrenal tumor
Primary ovarian failure/ oophorectomy	Secondary ovarian failure	CAH
		PCOS

CAH, congenital adrenal hyperplasia; GNRH, gonadotropin-releasing hormone; HIV, human immunodeficiency virus; PCOS, polycystic ovary syndrome.

TABLE 145.6: INTERPRETATION OF TOTAL TESTOSTERONE AIDED BY LUTEINIZING HORMONE/FOLLICLE-STIMULATING HORMONE LEVELS

TOTAL TESTOSTERONE	LH	FSH	POSSIBLE CAUSE	FOLLOW-UP TESTING
Low	High	High	Primary hypogonadism or oophorectomy	Karyotype if suspected genetic disorder
Low	Low/normal	Low/normal	Secondary hypogonadism	Check prolactin (r/o pituitary dysfunction) iron (r/o hemochromotosis) MRI if TT -150 mg/dL
High	High	High	Hyperthyroidism	Check TSH, T4
High	Low	Low	Ovarian tumor, adrenal tumor, or CAH	
High	High/normal	Normal	PCOS	
Normal	Normal	High	Spermatogenesis impairment	Check semen analysis

CAH, congenital adrenal hyperplasia; FSH, follice-stimulating hormone; LH, luteinizing hormone; MRI, magnetic resonance imaging; PCOS, polycystic ovarian syndrome; TSH, thyroid-stimulating hormone; TT, total testosterone.

comprehensive reproductive health examination in order to further assess reproductive status.[9,11,14,21,31] If fertility issues are suspected in a male, follow-up testing often includes a semen analysis and referral to a male fertility specialist.[26]

■ In cases of suspected pituitary abnormality, imaging of the pituitary gland may be done in addition to measurement of prolactin, TSH, and FSH.[14,26]

■ If SHBG is abnormal, check a free testosterone (FT) as TT may be inaccurate.[9,14,18]

PEARLS & PITFALLS

■ TT is more accurate in the fasting state as food ingestion (especially high fat/high carbohydrate) can temporarily decrease TT levels.[32,33]

■ Acute illness can cause artificially decreased testosterone measurements.[11,14]

■ Diagnosis of low testosterone should be made after two measurements taken on separate occasions both drawn in the morning, ideally before 10:00 a.m.[10,11,14] Circadian fluctuations in testosterone levels may cause variations in test results if the levels are tested at any other time.[15]

■ In males, serum testosterone levels show steady decline after age 40 at about 0.5% per year.[3]

■ TT levels are influenced by age, alcohol consumption, triglyceride levels, and some medications. Differential diagnosis of low testosterone starts with consideration of obesity, normal age-related decline, and medication side effects.[3,17–19]

■ Individuals with low testosterone levels are at an increased risk to develop cardiovascular or cardiometabolic diseases.[14]

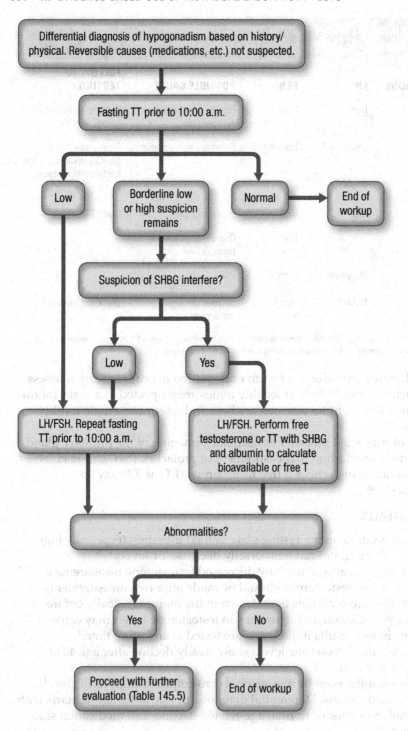

FIGURE 145.1. Workup of suspected hypogonadism. FSH, follicle-stimulating hormone; LH, luteinizing hormone; SHBG, sex hormone binding globulin; T, testosterone; TT, total testosterone.

■ Conditions that increase or decrease SHBG can affect the levels of bioavailable/free testosterone; in these instances, FT measurement may be used in addition to TT to guide clinical decision-making.[2,17] However, guidelines for testosterone therapy are based on TT levels.

■ Individuals with 21-hydroxylase deficiencies are known to have problems producing sufficient androgen levels. Individuals at high risk (e.g., Ashkenazi Jews) should be considered for testing.[26]

■ Older men with concomitant chronic diseases can be treated with testosterone replacement or supplementation therapy, but there is limited data justifying meaningful outcomes in this population without confirmation of true hypogonadism.[9,18,29]

■ Only perform testosterone testing in patients exhibiting signs/symptoms of androgen deficiency or requiring monitoring for pharmaceutical therapy.[34]

■ In transgender individuals, prioritize gender-affirming designations in electronic health records to communicate to the laboratory the reference intervals that should be reported for testosterone levels.[25]

■ Do not interpret testosterone levels as abnormal without correlating to signs/symptoms.[11,13–17,26]

■ Due to the day-to-day fluctuations in the testosterone levels, individuals should have their laboratory testosterone values repeated at least twice to confirm interpretation, and at least one level must be before 10 am.[14–16]

■ When SHBG is low, it increases bioavailable testosterone (and sometimes androgenic symptoms such as hair growth), although TT would not usually be elevated.[35]

■ Physical examination of the testes helps clarify the clinical picture, especially in younger patients.

■ Insurance approval for testosterone replacement products will typically require two low levels of testosterone.

PATIENT EDUCATION

■ https://www.mayocliniclabs.com/test-catalog/Clinical+and+Interpretive/83686

■ https://www.urologyhealth.org

RELATED DIAGNOSES AND ICD-10 CODES

Testicular hypofunction	E29.01
Hypopituitarism	E23.0
Ambiguous genitalia	Q56.4
Erectile dysfunction	N52.9
Delayed puberty	E30.0
Precocious puberty	E30.1
Hypogonadism, male	E29.1

| Hypogonadism, female | E28.39 |
| Endocrine disorder, decreased testosterone level | E34.9 |

REFERENCES

Full list of references can be accessed through Springer Publishing Company Connect™ at the following link: http://connect.springerpub.com/content/reference-book/ 978-0-8261-8843-4/part/part03/toc-part/ch145

---

146. THYROID ANTIBODIES

Jane Faith Kapustin

PHYSIOLOGY/PATHOPHYSIOLOGY REVIEW

The thyroid gland produces and secretes two hormones, thyroxine (T4) and triiodothyronine (T3), which play important roles in metabolism, growth and development, and body homeostasis. The proteins thyroglobulin (Tg) and enzyme thyroid peroxidase (TPO) are critical elements in T4 and T3 production. Thyroid-stimulating hormone (TSH) from the pituitary gland initiates production of thyroid hormone when it attaches to thyrotropin (also called TSH receptor).[1,2]

Autoimmune thyroid diseases, such as Hashimoto's disease and Graves' disease, are characterized by lymphocytic infiltration and antibody production against either TSH receptors or the thyroid itself.[1,2] In Hashimoto's thyroiditis, antibodies target the thyroid, resulting in hypothyroidism and TPO antibodies being released into general circulation, a characteristic sign of Hashimoto's thyroiditis.[2,3] In Graves' disease, thyrotropin receptor antibodies (TR-Abs) (sometimes called TSH receptor antibody, abbreviated TSHR-Ab) attack and overstimulate receptors, resulting in thyroid enlargement and overproduction and release of T4 and T3. Hyperthyroidism results.[4] Thyroid-stimulating immunoglobulin antibodies (TSI-Ab) and thyroid-stimulating hormone receptor binding inhibitor immunoglobulin (TBII) are two types of thyrotropin receptor antibodies (TR-Abs).

OVERVIEW OF LABORATORY TESTS

With suspicion of autoimmune thyroid disease, there are four main antibodies that can be tested (CPT codes 86376 and 86800); the first two are antibodies to the thyroid gland itself, while the latter two are antibodies to thyrotropin (TSH) receptors. (1) Thyroglobulin antibodies (Tg-Ab) serve as an overall marker of autoimmune thyroid disease yet are not sensitive or specific for any one autoimmune thyroid disease. The main use for Tg-Ab is to monitor for the return of thyroid cancer following treatment; in one systematic review, an elevated Tg-Ab had an odds ratio of 1.93 for thyroid cancer.[5] (2) TPO-Ab is most sensitive for Hashimoto's thyroiditis. (3) Thyroid-stimulating immunoglobulin antibody (TSI-Ab) is most sensitive for Graves' disease. (4) TBII-Ab is associated with both Graves' disease and Hashimoto's disease, but has a weaker association to the latter.

TPO-Ab, TSI, and TBII are usually detectable early in the immune process but may dissipate as the disease progresses.[1] Approximately 10% to 15% of patients with autoimmune disease will have negative antibodies. In some cases, antibodies may be present without evidence of hypo- or hyperthyroidism, which signals a potential for later development and merits monitoring over time.[6] Further, some people with signs/symptoms of autoimmune thyroid disease may initially test negative for antibodies and will require periodic monitoring since they may develop antibodies over time.

INDICATIONS

Autoimmune thyroid antibodies are indicated for presentation of goiter, abnormal thyroid function tests, or specific constellation of signs and symptoms suggestive of an autoimmune thyroid disorder (Table 146.1).

TABLE 146.1: SIGNS OR SYMPTOMS SUGGESTIVE OF AUTOIMMUNE THYROID CONDITIONS

GRAVES' DISEASE	HASHIMOTO'S DISEASE
Cardiac dysrhythmias	Cold intolerance
Eye irritation	Dry skin
Eyelid retraction	Exhaustion
Exophthalmos	Fatigue
Extraocular muscle dysfunction	Full sensation in the throat
Hair loss	Painless thyroid enlargement
Hyperactive deep tendon reflexes	Sore throat
Increased metabolic rate	Transient neck pain
Increased sweating	Weight gain
Insomnia	
Osteoporosis	
Palpable nodules	
Proptosis	
Psychiatric disorders	
Thyroid bruits	
Thyroid enlargement	
Tremor	
Weight loss	

Sources: Data from Mincer DL, Jialal I. Hashimoto thyroiditis. 2020. https://www.ncbi.nlm.nih.gov/books/NBK459262/; Ross DS, Burch HB, Cooper DS, et al. 2016 American Thyroid Association Guidelines for Diagnosis and Management of Hyperthyroidism and Other Causes of Thyrotoxicosis. *Thyroid.* 2016;26(10):1343–1421. doi:10.1089/thy.2016.0229

Screening

■ Although one systematic review showed screening pregnant patients with TPO-Ab, TSH, and T4 resulted in more diagnosis but did not improve outcomes,[7] the American College of Obstetricians and Gynecologists (ACOG) and the American Thyroid Association (ATA) support using thyroid antibodies for screening high-risk patients (abnormal TSH, preexisting thyroid disease, family history of thyroid disease, or overt signs of thyroid disease) prior to conception or early in pregnancy.[8,9]

Diagnosis and Evaluation

■ Thyroid antibodies are tested in the presence of abnormal thyroid function tests, or a specific constellation of signs and symptoms suggestive of an autoimmune thyroid disorder (Table 146.1).[1,3]

■ TPO-Ab can be used to confirm Hashimoto's thyroiditis, but there are no recommendations for routine antibody tests in the case of uncomplicated hypothyroidism (elevated TSH, low T4) that responds appropriately to treatment.[1,3]

■ In cases of subclinical hypothyroidism (TSH 5 to 10 mIU/L, normal free T4), testing for TPO-Ab and Tg-ab may give insight about the likelihood of autoimmune thyroid disease and the need for thyroid hormone replacement.[3,6]

■ TSI and other TR-Abs are used to evaluate individuals with signs/symptoms suspicious for Grave's disease and to determine the extent of disease activity.[8,10]

Monitoring

■ Thyroid antibodies (and TSH) should be monitored in those with a history of head and neck radiation before and after radiation treatment.[2,11] Damage to the thyroid following radiation can cause reduced blood supply and a localized immune response, leading to overexpression of thyroid antibodies (TPO and Tg-Ab).

■ In hyperthyroidism, TSI and other TR-Abs levels can be monitored periodically to assess when it is appropriate to stop antithyroid medication.[12] The American Thyroid Association recommends laboratory monitoring every 3 to 6 months during medical management for Grave's disease.[4]

■ TSI and TR-Ab are used to detect relapse of Graves' disease following treatment with antithyroid medication.[12]

■ TgAb and Tg levels are used to monitor for the recurrence of thyroid cancer. Monitoring depends on the individual patient but should be tested at 3, 6, and 12 months and annually thereafter.[1,13]

■ Patients with positive antibodies, but normal thyroid function tests during pregnancy, should be monitored at 6- to 12-month intervals for the development of future hypo/hyperthyroidism.[7,10]

■ TPO-Ab are used in pregnancy to monitor hypothyroidism.

■ Neonates of mothers that have taken thyroid medication during the pregnancy should be monitored for symptoms as well as be tested at birth, 3 days, and 7 to 10 days.[14]

INTERPRETATION

Reference intervals/limits are included in the list that follows[15,16]:

- Tg-Ab (lower than 20 IU/mL)
- TSI (less than 140% of basal activity)
- TPO-Ab (less than 35 IU/mL)
- TR-Ab (TSII), (1.75 IU/L or less)
- When thyroid antibodies are negative, signs and symptoms are most likely not related to autoimmune thyroid disease.
- When TPO-Ab and/or Tg-Ab are positive, it is most likely Hashimoto's disease, particularly if the antibody levels are high.[2]
- Mildly elevated thyroid antibodies (TPO, TR-Ab) can be found in other conditions such as type 1 diabetes, rheumatoid arthritis, thyroid cancer, and pernicious anemia.
- Positive TSI and/or TR-Ab indicate Grave's disease.[4]
- Table 146.2 further explains interpretation of thyroid antibody laboratory results

FOLLOW-UP

- In the presence of abnormal thyroid antibody tests and unclear clinical picture, follow-up testing and referral may also be needed to evaluate for thyroid cancer or other autoimmune disorders (type 1 diabetes, celiac disease, rheumatoid arthritis, pernicious anemia, and other collagen disorders).
- In the presence of hyperthyroidism without presence of thyroid antibodies, endocrinology referral and follow-up testing with scintigraphy may be needed to evaluate for toxic multinodular goiter. Other differential diagnosis considerations include iodine excess, thyroid cancer, toxic adenomas, TSH-producing pituitary tumors, and germ cell tumors.[13,17]

PEARLS & PITFALLS

- A small percentage of people with autoimmune thyroid disease will have negative thyroid antibody levels. Anti-TPO antibodies can vary over time and may not always be present, so lack of positivity does not exclude the diagnosis of Hashimoto's thyroiditis.[3]
- Significantly elevated antibody levels are more indicative of Graves' disease and Hashimoto's thyroiditis.
- Graves' disease is the most common cause of thyrotoxicosis and can lead to life-threatening conditions if not treated.
- For patients with type 1 diabetes, expect that about 40% will experience concomitant autoimmune thyroid disease. Other autoimmune disorders that may occur with Hashimoto's disease include pernicious anemia, adrenal insufficiency, and celiac disease.[1,2]
- First-degree relatives of people with Hashimoto's disease have a nine-fold greater risk of developing the condition.[3]
- Thyroid function tests may appear abnormal under certain circumstances such as pregnancy and critical illness. Therefore, the clinical context must be considered when interpreting results.[18]

	TABLE 146.2: THYROID FUNCTION TESTS AND AUTOIMMUNE DISORDERS OF THE THYROID	
LABORATORY TEST	**RESULT WITH HYPERTHYROID AUTOIMMUNE THYROID DISEASE (GRAVES' DISEASE)**	**RESULT WITH HYPOTHYROID AUTOIMMUNE THYROID DISEASE (HASHIMOTO'S DISEASE)**
Tg-Ab*	Present in 50%–70% of cases	Present in 80%–90% of cases
TPO-Ab*	Present in 85% of cases	Present
TSI	Present in 80%–90% of cases	Present in 15% of cases
TBII/TR-Ab	Present	May be present

*TPO-Ab and Tg-Ab are both highly sensitive but are not as specific. Instead, the concentration of the antibody levels must be considered along with signs/symptoms over time.

TBII, TSH receptor binding inhibitor immunoglobulin; Tg-Ab, thyroglobulin antibody; TPO, thyroid peroxidase antibody; TR-Ab, thyrotropin/thyroid-stimulating hormone receptor antibody; TSI, thyroid-stimulating immunoglobulin.

Sources: Data from American Thyroid Association. *Thyroid Antibody Tests*. https://www.thyroid.org/thyroid-function-tests/; Frohlich E, Wahl R. Thyroid autoimmunity: role of anti-thyroid antibodies in thyroid and extra-thyroidal diseases. *Front Immunol.* 2017;8:521. doi:10.3389/fimmu.2017.00521; Mincer DL, Jialal I. Hashimoto thyroiditis. 2020. https://www.ncbi.nlm.nih.gov/books/NBK459262/; Ross DS, Burch HB, Cooper DS, et al. 2016 American Thyroid Association Guidelines for Diagnosis and Management of Hyperthyroidism and Other Causes of Thyrotoxicosis. *Thyroid.* 2016;26(10):1343–1421. doi:10.1089/thy.2016.0229

- The postpartum period is a common time for women to manifest hypothyroidism associated with Hashimoto's thyroiditis.[7,10]
- Approximately 10% of pregnant patients can develop postpartum thyroiditis; those with type 1 diabetes are at highest risk (25%). Therefore, they have a low threshold for testing postpartum patients with signs/symptoms.[7,10]
- Because thyroid antibodies cross the placenta, neonates of pregnant patients with autoimmune thyroid conditions need to be closely monitored for development of thyrotoxicosis and/or hypo- or hyperthyroidism.[7–10]

PATIENT EDUCATION

- https://medlineplus.gov/lab-tests/thyroid-antibodies/

RELATED DIAGOSES AND ICD-10 CODES

Autoimmune thyroiditis	E06.3
Thyrotoxicosis with diffuse goiter	E05.0
Thyrotoxicosis with diffuse goiter without thyrotoxic crisis or storm	E05.00
Thyrotoxicosis with diffuse goiter with thyrotoxic crisis or storm	E05.01
Malignant neoplasm of thyroid gland	C73
Benign neoplasm of thyroid gland	D34
Thyroid goiter, non-toxic	E04

Non-toxic multimodal goiter	E04.2
Hypothyroidism	E03, E03.9, E03.8
Hyperthyroidism, thyrotoxicosis	E05, E05.9
Transitory neonatal hyperthyroidism	P72.1

REFERENCES

*Full list of references can be accessed through Springer Publishing Company Connect™
at the following link:* http://connect.springerpub.com/content/reference-book/
978-0-8261-8843-4/part/part03/toc-part/ch146

147. THYROID FUNCTION TESTS

Kate Sustersic Gawlik and Kelly Small Casler

PHYSIOLOGY REVIEW

The thyroid is an endocrine gland that is located in the anterior middle portion of the neck between the cricoid cartilage and suprasternal notch. It is a highly vascular organ that consists of two lobes that are connected by an isthmus. These lobes are composed of a large number of tiny saclike structures called follicles. Follicles are the functional unit of the thyroid. Each follicle is formed by a single layer of epithelial (follicular) cells and is filled with a secretory substance called colloid, which consists largely of a glycoprotein–iodine complex called thyroglobulin.[1] Thyroglobulin is a protein that is used to synthesize the two major hormones made by the thyroid: thyroxine (T4) and triiodothyronine (T3). Iodine is necessary for production of these hormones. Without adequate dietary iodine intake, these hormones cannot be synthesized. Once produced, T4 is secreted into the blood and is transported to every tissue in the body. T4 serves as a prohormone and is partially converted peripherally to triiodothyronine (T3) at the cellular level in virtually all organs.[1] Some of the major functions of the thyroid hormones include:

- Regulate the rate of metabolism (basal metabolic rate).
- Affect heat production and body temperature.
- Affect oxygen consumption, cardiac output, and blood volume.
- Affect enzyme system activity.
- Affect metabolism of carbohydrates, fats, and proteins.
- Regulate growth and development.

The amount of T4 and T3 that is made is regulated by a negative feedback loop called the hypothalamic-pituitary-thyroid (HPT) axis.[1,2] When the body senses that it needs more thyroid hormone, the hypothalamus releases thyrotropin-releasing hormone (TRH) that stimulates the anterior pituitary to release thyroid-stimulating hormone (TSH). The TSH then stimulates the thyroid to make more T4. When the T4 reaches a stable level in the serum, the pituitary's production of TSH ceases. This is illustrated in Figure 147.1.[1,2]

Over 99% of T4 and 98% of T3 are bound to specific transport proteins. It is important to note that if the levels of transport proteins change, this can alter the level(s) of serum total T4 available, but does not necessarily indicate thyroid disease.[1,3] Some disorders or medications that can alter the binding proteins include estrogen use, androgen use, pregnancy, genetic disorders, and disorders of thyroid function.

The three major thyroid-binding proteins are T4–binding globulin (TBG), which carries ≈ 70% of T4 and T3; T4-binding prealbumin (TBPA), which binds ≈ 10% of circulating T4 and lesser amounts of T3; and albumin, which binds ≈ 15% of circulating T4 and T3. The thyroid hormones that are not protein-bound (free T4 and free T3) are able to enter the tissues and target organs and exert their effects. These are the biologically active form of the hormones.[1-3]

OVERVIEW OF LABORATORY TESTS

The TSH (CPT code 84443) is the single best initial test for measuring thyroid function. Only a TSH should be ordered in the initial evaluation of a patient with suspected thyroid dysfunction.[4] If the TSH is abnormal, the free T4 (CPT code 84439) should be ordered to confirm diagnosis.[5] Occasionally, a free T3 (CPT code 84481) is ordered. If a TSH is abnormal, some laboratories automatically do reflex testing to include free T4 and T3, although a total T3 or free T3 should not be done to diagnose hypothyroidism (Grade A evidence).[6] Free thyroid hormone assays directly determine the amounts of unbound, bioactive thyroid hormone circulating in the blood. T3 measurement, whether total or free, has limited utility in diagnosing hypothyroidism because levels are often normal due to hyperstimulation of the remaining functioning thyroid tissue due to the elevated TSH.

Total T4 and T3 assays can be ordered, and these tests measure the total concentration of T4 and/or T3 circulating in the blood. Measurement of total T4 (CPT code 84436) gives a reliable reflection of clinical thyroid status in the absence of protein-binding abnormalities and non-thyroidal illness. In the hyperthyroid patient, total T3 is rarely helpful since it is the last test to become abnormal.[7]

In certain circumstances, a laboratory evaluation of the thyroid can be assessed by ordering a thyroid panel (CPT code 80091) which usually includes a TSH, a free T4, and a free T3 or total T3. Occasionally, a T3 resin uptake test is included. Along with the T4 value, the free thyroxine index (FTI) can be calculated. FTI corrects for changes in certain proteins that can affect total T4 levels.

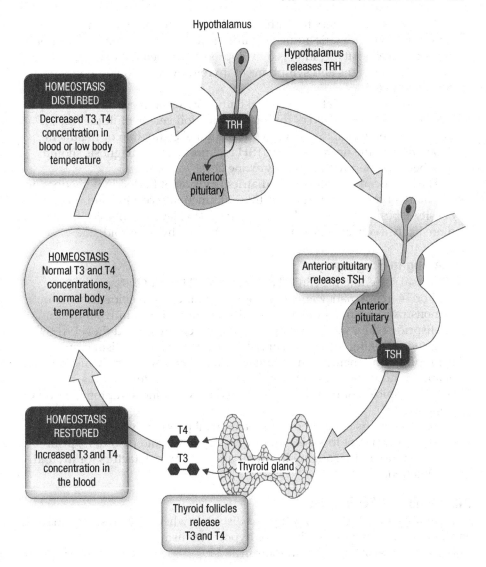

FIGURE 147.1. The hypothalamic-pituitary-thyroid axis. TSH, thyroid-stimulatig hormone.

INDICATIONS

Screening

- The United States Preventive Services Task Force determined there is insufficient evidence to universally screen asymptomatic, nonpregnant adults for thyroid dysfunction.[5]
- The Choosing Wisely initiative has the following recommendations for thyroid screening:

- The American Society for Clinical Pathology does not recommend screening asymptomatic adults, regardless of age, for thyroid dysfunction at routine well visits. Testing is only appropriate when patients are demonstrating signs and symptoms of thyroid dysfunction or are considered at-risk.[8]
- The American Society for Clinical Pathology recommends only ordering TSH for initial evaluation of thyroid dysfunction versus multiple tests. If the TSH is abnormal, follow-up with additional evaluation or treatment depending on the findings. If the TSH is abnormal, the diagnosis should then be confirmed with a free thyroxine (T4).[5]
- The American Academy of Pediatrics Division of Endocrinology does not recommend routinely measuring thyroid function levels in children with obesity. Obesity can cause slightly elevated TSH levels in obesity, but this is more likely a consequence of obesity versus true hypothyroidism.[9]

Screening in Pregnancy

- Universal screening for clinical and subclinical thyroid disease using a TSH or T4 in pregnancy are not recommended. Current evidence does not demonstrate improved pregnancy outcomes or neurocognitive function in offspring when subclinical hypothyroid levels are treated (Level A).[10–12] Targeted screening for women at risk for overt hypothyroidism is still appropriate and includes individuals with a personal or family history of autoimmune diseases, thyroid disease, type 1 diabetes mellitus, or clinical suspicion of thyroid disease based on signs and symptoms (Level C evidence).[6,10]
- Verbal screenings should be completed on all pregnant women at the initial prenatal visit to assess for any history of thyroid disorders, prior or current use of thyroid medications, and/or any risk factors for thyroid dysfunction.

Diagnosis and Evaluation

Individuals should be tested for thyroid disorders when they present with signs and symptoms of hyperthyroidism or hypothyroidism.

Hyperthyroidism signs/symptoms include:

- Unintentional weight loss
- Tachycardia
- Arrhythmia or palpitations
- New onset of nervousness, irritability, anxiety
- Fine tremor usually in hands and fingers
- Diaphoresis
- Fatigue
- Muscle weakness
- Insomnia
- Goiter
- More frequent bowel movements or diarrhea

Hypothyroidism signs/symptoms include:

- Fatigue
- Constipation
- Weight gain
- Hoarseness
- Muscle weakness
- Arthralgias
- Depression
- Menorrhagia
- Puffy face
- Impaired memory or mild cognitive slowing
- Goiter

Serum TSH measurement has the highest sensitivity and specificity of any single blood test used in the evaluation of suspected hyperthyroidism, and hypothyroidism should be used for initial testing.

If hyperthyroidism is strongly suspected, a serum TSH, free T4, and total T3 should be assessed at the initial evaluation to increase diagnostic accuracy.[13]

Monitoring

- Monitoring of TSH is typically done every 4 to 6 weeks when adjusting dosage of levothyroxine (Level A).[10]
- Assessment of serum free T4, in addition to TSH, should be considered when monitoring levothyroxine therapy (Grade B evidence), although in most patients, a normal TSH indicates a correct dose of T4.[6,10]
- A total or free T3 level should not be ordered when monitoring levothyroxine dose in hypothyroid patients. Blood level of total or free T3 does not correlate with a patient's clinical response.[6,14]
- For patients taking levothyroxine, TSH levels should be maintained in the recommended reference range stated in the guidelines (0.4 to 4 mIU/L). When TSH levels were noted to be outside this reference range, the risk of heart disease, stroke, broken bones, and death was higher.[15]
- The wide reference range of 0.4 to 4 mIU/L range offers flexibility to treat to the patient preference since many patients may feel better at different TSH levels.[15]
- In monitoring patients with hypothyroidism on levothyroxine replacement, blood for assessment of serum free T4 should be collected before dosing because the level will be transiently increased by up to 20% after levothyroxine administration.[6]
- In pregnant persons with hypothyroidism, the TSH level should be monitored, and the levothyroxine dose should be adjusted until the TSH is between the lower limit of the reference range and 2.5 mU/L. (Level A).[5]
- In pregnant persons with hyperthyroidism, free T4 should be monitored, and the antithyroid drug (thioamide) dose should be adjusted until the

free T4 is at the upper end of the normal pregnancy range. In the event of T3 thyrotoxicosis, monitor total T3 with a goal level at the upper end of the normal pregnancy range (Level A).[5]

INTERPRETATION

- See Tables 147.1, 147.2, 147.3, and 147.4 for reference values.
- Refer to Figure 147.2 for an interpretation algorithm.
- Serum TSH during pregnancy varies by population and trimester. Laboratories and institutions should provide reference ranges that represent the typical population for whom care is provided. These reference ranges should be derived from healthy TPOAb-negative pregnant women, who have adequate iodine intake and who do not have any form of thyroid disease.[16] Different TSH cutoffs should be used for thyroid peroxidase (TPO) antibody–positive women versus TPO antibody-negative women. A systematic review and meta-analysis concluded that the association of subclinical hypothyroidism with preterm birth was no longer apparent after adjusting for TPO antibody positivity. These results support getting a reflex TPO antibody measurement for women with a TSH concentration higher than 4.0 mIU/L, and gestational TSH monitoring for TPO antibody-positive women prior to conception.[17]

TABLE 147.1: REFERENCE VALUES FOR THYROID-STIMULATING HORMONE

AGE RANGE	NORMAL TSH REFERENCE RANGE*
4 days old to <6 months**	0.73–4.77 mIU/L
6 months to <14 years old**	0.7–4.17 mIU/L
14 to <19 years old**	0.47–3.41 mIU/L
Adult	0.5–4.5 mIU/L

*Will vary based on laboratory and population.

** Pediatric reference values from Caliper database (https://caliperproject.ca).

TSH, thyroid-stimulating hormone.

TABLE 147.2: REFERENCE VALUES FOR FREE T4

AGE RANGE	NORMAL FREE T4 REFERENCE RANGE*
5 to 14 days**	1.05–3.21 ng/dL
15 to 29 days**	0.68–2.53 ng/dL
30 days to <1 year**	0.47–3.41 ng/dL
1 to <19 years**	0.5–4.5 ng/dL
Adult ≥20	0.9–1.7 ng/dL

*Will vary based on laboratory and population.

** Pediatric reference values from Caliper database (https://caliperproject.ca).

TABLE 147.3: REFERENCE VALUES FOR TOTAL T4		
AGE RANGE	**NORMAL TOTAL T4 REFERENCE RANGE***	
	Female	**Male**
7 days to <1 year**	5.87–13.7 mcg/dL	5.87–13.7 mcg/dL
1 to <9 years**	6.16–10.3 mcg/dL	6.16–10.3 mcg/dL
9 to <12 years**	5.48–9.31 mcg/dL	5.48–9.31 mcg/dL
12 to <14 years**	5.08–8.34 mcg/dL	5.01–8.28 mcg/dL
14 to <19 years	5.46–13 mcg/dL	4.68–8.62
Adult ≥20	4.5–11.7 mcg/dL	

*Will vary based on laboratory and population.

**Pediatric reference values from Caliper database (https://caliperproject.ca).

TABLE 147.4: REFERENCE VALUES FOR TOTAL T3		
AGE RANGE	**NORMAL TOTAL T3 REFERENCE RANGE***	
	Female	**Male**
4 days to <1 year**	84.6–234 ng/dL	84.6–234 ng/dL
1 to <12 years**	113–189 ng/dL	113–189 ng/dL
12 to <15 years**	97.7–176 ng/dL	97.7–176 ng/dL
15 to <17 years**	92.5–142 ng/dL	93.8–156 ng/dL
17 to <19 years	89.8–168 ng/dL	89.8–168 ng/dL
Adult ≥20	80–200 ng/dL	

*Will vary based on laboratory and population.

**Pediatric reference values from Caliper database (https://caliperproject.ca).

FOLLOW-UP

- Once an adequate replacement dosage has been determined, repeat TSH testing at 6-month and then 12-month intervals are appropriate (expert opinion).[6]
- If chronic or recent severe hyperthyroidism or hypothyroidism is present, both TSH and free T4 should be monitored for 1 year until their condition becomes stable (expert opinion).[6]
- If there is no palpable abnormality of the thyroid but the patient has abnormal thyroid function tests, a routine ultrasound is not necessary and should not be ordered.[18]
- The cause of thyrotoxicosis should be determined and additional tests including TRAb, radioactive iodine uptake, and thyroidal blood flow via ultrasound should be completed.[13]

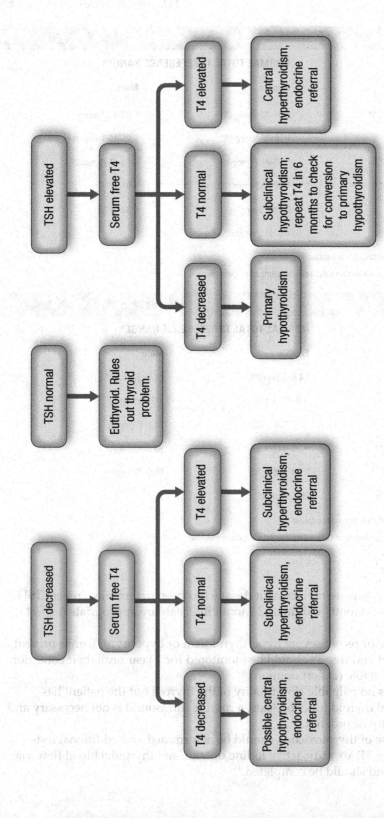

FIGURE 147.2. Interpretation of thyroid-stimulating hormone (TSH) results in patients not currently on thyroid hormone supplementation.

PEARLS & PITFALLS

■ For pregnant women or women with thyroid conditions who are planning to conceive, the recommendations for screening, diagnosis, and ongoing management are different and vary by trimester. Consultation with a specialist is recommended. Women who are lactating can also have special considerations.[16]

■ In patients with unstable thyroid states, such as those recently treated for hyperthyroidism or those who have been receiving excess thyroid hormone replacement, serum thyroxine (T4) measurement more accurately indicates the thyroid status than does serum TSH.[13]

■ Thyroid dysfunction can be associated with infertility and should be considered when a woman is having difficulty conceiving.[16]

■ Patients diagnosed with autoimmune thyroiditis have higher rates of depression and anxiety.[19]

■ There are many factors including medications and disease states that alter T4 and T3 binding capability. These should be considered prior to making a diagnosis.[6]

PATIENT EDUCATION

■ http://www.thyroid.org/wp-content/uploads/patients/brochures/ata -hypothyroidism-brochure.pdf

■ https://www.thyroid.org/thyroid-information/thyroid-information-files

RELATED DIAGNOSES AND ICD-10 CODES

Hypothyroidism, unspecified	E03.9
Thyrotoxicosis, unspecified without thyrotoxic crisis or storm	E05.9
Thyrotoxicosis, unspecified with thyrotoxic crisis or storm	E05.91

REFERENCES

Full list of references can be accessed through Springer Publishing Company Connect™ at the following link: http://connect.springerpub.com/content/reference-book/ 978-0-8261-8843-4/part/part03/toc-part/ch147

148. TRICHOMONIASIS

Deanna Hunt

PATHOPHYSIOLOGY REVIEW

Trichomoniasis is a common, curable, sexually transmitted infection caused by a protozoan parasite, *Trichomonas vaginalis*. Trichomoniasis is the most common nonviral sexually transmitted infection (STI), transmitted almost exclusively through sexual contact.[1] Trichomoniasis can present similarly to chlamydia and gonorrhea, but is more prevalent among people aged 40 to 49, whereas chlamydia and gonorrhea more commonly affects people aged 19 to 24 years.[2,3] Signs and symptoms of trichomoniasis are listed in Box 148.1, although approximately 70% of those who have trichomoniasis do not have symptoms.[4] Trichomoniasis most often infects the vulva, vagina, cervix, and/or urethra.[2]

OVERVIEW OF LABORATORY TESTS

There are several options for testing of trichomoniasis. Clinical guidelines from the American College of Obstetricians and Gynecologists (ACOG), Centers for Disease Control and Prevention (CDC), and Infectious Disease Society of America (IDSA) emphasize that molecular testing is the preferred testing option, when available, due to its stronger sensitivity and specificity.[2,5,6]

Microscopy

Wet-mount microscopy (CPT code 87210) (also called hanging drop) evaluates genital secretions under the microscope and is commonly used due to low cost and convenience. However, a drawback is that wet mounts are only 40% to 60%

Box 148.1: Signs and Symptoms Associated With T. Vaginalis

- Clear or mucopurulent urethral discharge
- Green or yellow malodorous vaginal discharge
- Lower abdominal pain
- Painful intercourse or ejaculation
- Punctate hemorrhages on cervix (strawberry cervix)
- Thin, purulent, malodorous vaginal discharge
- Urinary dysuria and frequency
- Urethral itching or burning
- Vaginal pruritus and burning
- Vaginal erythema

Sources: Data from Edwards T, Burke P, Smalley H, Hobbs G. *Trichomonas vaginalis:* clinical relevance, pathogenicity and diagnosis. *Crit Rev Microbiol.* 2016;42(3):406–417. doi:10.3109/1040841X.2014.958050; Sobel JD, Mitchell C. Trichomoniasis. In: Barbieri RL, ed. *UpToDate.* UpToDate; 2022. https://www.uptodate.com/contents/trichomoniasis

sensitive, which is much lower than molecular testing and cultures.[3,7,8] Because of the low sensitivity, wet mounts are not recommended as a screening method for asymptomatic individuals.[9] To enhance sensitivity, clinicians should look at the slides immediately following collection of a wet mount, as the organisms will only remain mobile for 10 to 20 minutes after the sample is collected.[1,9] Concurrent to the wet mount, the clinician can also test the pH of the specimen and conduct a "whiff test." Vaginal pH greater than 4.5 is consistent with trichomoniasis as is a positive whiff test.[1,10]

Molecular Tests

Molecular nucleic acid amplification tests (NAATs) for *T. vaginalis* (CPT code 87661) offer high detection rates and sensitivity, resulting in enhanced treatment and care. NAATs have greater than 90% sensitivity and specificity, and as a result are now considered the gold standard for detection.[3] NAATs samples can be obtained from a vaginal or endocervical cells sample, a urethral swab, or a first-catch urine. There are multiple brands of NAATs for *T. vaginalis* and ideal sample selection will vary between product.[7,8,11,12] While some NAATs have similar performance between urine or vaginal sampling, others may not; therefore, clinicians should reference the product insert at their clinical site.[13] Of note, NAATs for *T. vaginalis* are typically bundled as part of multiplex panels that can test for bacterial vaginosis, candida, and, sometimes, chlamydia and gonorrhea with one swab or urine sample. An overview of the characteristic of the diagnostic assays for *Trichomoniasis* can be found in Table 148.1. *T. vaginalis* NAATs can sometimes be conducted with a Pap test sample, but this practice is not usually recommended due to the possibility of false negatives and false positives.[2,4] Additionally, the presence of the parasite may be an incidental finding on Pap smear cytology.[12]

Cultures

Trichomoniasis cultures (CPT codes 87070, 87140, 87147 or 87149) were once considered the gold standard with a specificity near 100% and a sensitivity around 70% to 85%, but are now considered outdated due to advancements in testing technology and slow turnaround time (7 days).[10] Currently, cultures are only used if there is a need for antimicrobial susceptibility testing.[8]

TABLE 148.1: OVERVIEW OF TRICHOMONIASIS TESTING	
TYPE OF TEST	**RESULT TIME**
Microscopy	Immediate
Culture	1–5 days
Enzyme immunoassay	10 minutes
Nucleic DNA probe test or NAAT	1-3 days

Source: Data from Advances in laboratory detection of trichomonas vaginalis (Updated). Published 2016. https://www.aphl.org/aboutAPHL/publications/Documents/ID_2016November-Laboratory-Detection-of-Trichomonas-update.pdf.

Rapid Antigen Test

There is one rapid antigen test (CPT code 87808) commercially available in the United States with sensitivities between 83% and 90%. Vaginal mucosa samples are collected and tested at the point of care, with results available within 10 minutes.[7,11,12] An advantage to this test is that the sample can be self-collected, resulting in higher acceptability among adolescents and accurate results.[11] The drawback to the test is it is only approved for use with patients with a vagina and it is unable to be bundled with other point-of-care tests including chlamydia or gonorrhea testing.[8]

INDICATIONS

Screening

- Screening is recommended in patients listed in Box 148.2.
- There are no recommendations for universal screening for other populations, including pregnant individuals.[2]

Diagnosis and Evaluation

- Testing should be performed if any patient is experiencing any systems concerning for trichomoniasis (Box 148.1).

Monitoring

- Test of cure is recommended in patients with a vagina within 3 months of treatment. They can be retested as early as 2 weeks if using NAATs.[2]

INTERPRETATION

- Wet mounts are considered positive if motile trichomonads are noted (Figure 148.1). The trichomonads will both spin and shake.[1] Multiple white blood cells will also be noted.
- NAATs, culture, and rapid antigen tests are either positive or negative.

FOLLOW-UP

- Infection with *T. vaginalis* should prompt consideration of infection with other sexually transmitted diseases. Consider testing patients with a positive test for human immunodeficiency virus, syphilis, gonorrhea, chlamydia, and hepatitis.[1,2]

Box 148.2: Screening Recommendation for T. Vaginalsis

- HIV-positive persons with a vagina
- Incarcerated persons
- Past history of STIs
- Persons not in a mutually monogamous relationship
- Persons who exchange sex for money or drugs
- Persons who report inconsistent condom use
- Persons whose sexual partner has other concurrent partners
- Persons with a new or multiple partner

Source: Data from Centers for Disease Control and Prevention. *Disease Characterized by Vaginal Discharge. 2015 Sexually Transmitted Diseases Treatment Guidelines.* Published 2015. https://www.cdc.gov/std/tg2015/default.htm.

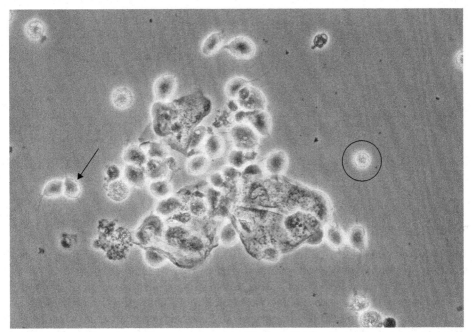

FIGURE 148.1. Positive wet mount microscopy. Microscopy of trichomoniasis. The arrow depicts trichomonads. The circle depicts a white blood cell. The larger cells that are also seen are epithelial cells. *Source: https://phil.cdc.gov/Details.aspx?pid=14500.*

PEARLS & PITFALLS

- Trichomoniasis is not required to be reported to public health departments; therefore, prevalence is difficult to accurately determine.[1]
- There is a strong correlation between HIV infection and trichomoniasis. Up to 53% of patients with a vagina who are infected with HIV are also infected with trichomoniasis. Additionally, the treatment of trichomoniasis is associated with a significant decrease in HIV viral load and shedding within the genital tract.[2,14,15]

PATIENT EDUCATION

- https://www.cdc.gov/std/trichomonas/default.htm

RELATED DIAGNOSES AND ICD-10 CODES

Trichomoniasis	A59.9
Vaginal itching	L29.8
Vaginal discharge	N89.8

REFERENCES

Full list of references can be accessed through Springer Publishing Company Connect™ at the following link: http://connect.springerpub.com/content/reference-book/978-0-8261-8843-4/part/part03/toc-part/ch148

149. TROPONIN

Audra Hanners and Kelly Small Casler

PHYSIOLOGY/PATHOPHYSIOLOGY REVIEW

Troponins are muscle proteins that assist muscle contraction regulation. There are two troponins that exist primarily in cardiac muscle: cardiac troponin T (cTnT) and cardiac troponin I (cTnI). Cardiac troponin I is myocardium specific, whereas cTnT has some small expression in skeletal muscle in addition to cardiac muscle. During acute coronary syndromes, reduced blood flow results in myocyte and muscle ischemia, injury, and/or infarction which results in troponin release into the bloodstream.[1] Because of the high specificity of cTnI and cTnT to cardiac muscle injury, cardiac troponins are used to clinically evaluate for myocardial infarctions in patients with chest pain.[1] However, several other pathologic conditions (cardiac and noncardiac) result in troponin release (Box 149.1).[2–10]

OVERVIEW OF LABORATORY TESTS

Cardiac troponins are detected in serum using monoclonal antibodies or enzyme-linked immunosorbent assays (ELISAs) that are specific for cardiac troponins and do not react with skeletal muscle troponins.[11] Troponin testing options include cTnI, cTnT, and high-sensitivity troponin (hs-Tn) (CPT code 84484). The latter are newer troponin assays and offer more precision in the evaluation for acute coronary syndrome (ACS).[12] Compared to traditional cardiac troponins, hsTn reduces the need for stress testing, allows earlier rule out of ACS (decreased time to discharge), and lowered cost in evaluation.[13,14]

Point-of-care (POC) troponin testing is also available with conflicting reports of quality and usefulness. The benefit of POCT troponin is the 15 to 20 minutes turnaround compared to 60 minutes.[15] However, low clinical sensitivity of traditional POC troponin tests have been associated with patients being underdiagnosed, undertreated, or prematurely discharged from the acute care. Many experts argue that POC troponin testing lacks high-quality evidence to support its accuracy to rule out AMI diagnosis.[16,17] However, more recent studies with hs-Tn POC has shown accuracy that is equal to laboratory.[18]

INDICATIONS

Screening

- Not indicated/used.

Box 149.1: Causes of Troponin Release and Elevation Other Than Myocardial Infarction

- Aortic dissection
- Cardiac arrhythmias
- Cardiac myopathy
- Cardiac trauma
- Cardiopulmonary resuscitation
- Chemotherapy
- Defibrillator use
- End-stage renal disease
- Extreme burns
- Extreme exertion
- Heart failure
- Myocarditis
- Myopericarditis
- Neurologic events
- Pulmonary embolus
- Rhabdomyolysis
- Sepsis

Sources: Data from Allan JJ, Feld RD, Russell AA, et al. Cardiac troponin I levels are normal or minimally elevated after transthoracic cardioversion. *J Am Coll Cardiol.* 1997;30(4):1052–1056. doi:10.1016/s0735-1097(97)00260-x; Aroney CN, Cullen L. Appropriate use of serum troponin testing in general practice: a narrative review. *Med J Aust.* 2016;205(2):91–94. doi:10.5694/mja16.00263; Eggers KM, Jernberg T, Lindahl B. Cardiac troponin elevation in patients without a specific diagnosis. *J Am Coll Cardiol.* 2019;73(1):1–9. doi:10.1016/j.jacc.2018.09.082; Franz WM, Remppis A, Kandolf R, Kübler W, Katus HA. Serum troponin T: diagnostic marker for acute myocarditis. *Clin Chem.* 1996;42(2):340–341; Horwich TB, Patel J, MacLellan WR, Fonarow GC. Cardiac troponin I is associated with impaired hemodynamics, progressive left ventricular dysfunction, and increased mortality rates in advanced heart failure. *Circulation.* 2003;108(7):833–838. doi:10.1161/01.CIR.0000084543.79097.34; Müller-Bardorff M, Weidtmann B, Giannitsis E, Kurowski V, Katus HA. Release kinetics of cardiac troponin T in survivors of confirmed severe pulmonary embolism. *Clin Chem.* 2002;48(4):673–675; Ramezani F, Ahmadi S, Faridaalee G, Baratloo A, Yousefifard M. Value of Manchester acute coronary syndromes decision rule in the detection of acute coronary syndrome: a systematic review and meta-analysis. *Emerg (Tehran).* 2018;6(1):e61. https://www.ncbi.nlm.nih.gov/pmc/articles/PMC6368935; Reynolds HR, Srichai MB, Iqbal SN, et al. Mechanisms of myocardial infarction in women without angiographically obstructive coronary artery disease. *Circulation.* 2011;124(13):1414–1425. doi:10.1161/CIRCULATIONAHA.111.026542; Villata G, Bollati M, Gambino A, Biondi-Zoccai G, Sheiban I. Comment on the "pilot" GRACIA-2 randomized trial. *Eur Heart J.* 2007;28(19):2417–2418; author reply 2418–2419. doi:10.1093/eurheartj/ehm329

Diagnosis and Evaluation
- Indicated in patients with chest pain and/or suspected acute coronary syndrome.[4]
- Troponin is sometimes used to evaluate for non-MI causes of chest pain (PE, aortic dissection, pericarditis).[19]

Monitoring
- After the first measurement, troponin is usually monitored in a serial fashion. Traditional Tns are monitored and redrawn at 3 and 6 hours after the first (baseline measurement), but hs-Tn can be repeated as early as 1 or 2 hours after a baseline troponin.[19]
- cTn may also be used for prognosis in some conditions like heart failure and amyloidosis.[19]

INTERPRETATION

- Troponins are considered positive if the result is greater than the 99th percentile of the reference limit.[20]
- Interpretation of troponin elevations must be conducted within the clinical context. Consensus from the Fourth Universal Definition of Myocardial Infarction (MI) recommends that an elevated cardiac troponin, without clinical evidence of ischemia (Box 149.2), requires an alternative search for the cause of myocardial necrosis/injury.[22]
- Hs-Tn has largely replaced traditional cardiac troponin levels since they detect much lower levels of Tn with much higher precision and sensitivity. However, interpretation and accuracy of hs-Tn varies on the length of time since onset of symptoms, baseline Tn level, intervals between samples, and amount of change between samples (called delta).[21] Usually, a delta of 20% is considered characteristic of an acute myocardial infarction.[19,22]
- Although interpretation of troponin generally relies on observation of levels over time, in some instances, when combined with a clinical risk score, a single measurement of hs-Tn negates the need for serial troponins and allows quicker diagnosis and discharge.[23] One such clinical risk score is the History, EKG, Age, Risk factors, and Troponin (HEART) score.[24,25] A link to this calculator can be found at https://www.mdcalc.com/heart-score-major-cardiac-events.
- A single measurement may be relied upon if a patient has been symptom free for 3 hours or longer and if it has been several hours since symptom onset.[19,26]
- The use of troponin is limited in critically ill patients since critical illness causes elevations in troponin.[19]
- The sensitivity of hs-Tn ranges from 92% to 95% and the specificity ranges from 68% to 84%.[23] In one study, hs-Tn less than the 99th percentile ruled out acute myocardial infarction with a 99% NPV.[27] False positives are more common than false negatives.

FOLLOW-UP

- Electrocardiograms (ECG) are used in follow-up of and in addition to troponin to clarify the clinical picture.[11]

Box 149.2: Fourth Universal Definition of Myocardial Infarction Clinical Evidence of Ischemia

Clinical evidence of ischemia can be met by one of the following:

- History of present illness consistent with myocardial ischemia symptoms
- Acute, ischemic electrocardiogram changes
- Imaging consistent with ischemic abnormalities (heart wall motion abnormality)
- Pathologic Q waves on electrocardiogram
- Coronary thrombus on angiogram

- Echocardiography, angiography, stress testing, and/or coronary imaging may be used in follow-up of elevated troponin levels if there is a high suspicion of acute myocardial infarction.[2]

PEARLS & PITFALLS

- Dialogue and research continue regarding the relationship of troponin to age, race, and sex. Men tend to have higher levels of troponin than women.[2–7,28–32] Older adults often have troponin levels that are higher than percentile cutoffs, so serial troponin monitoring for rise/fall is very important.[33]
- Exact recommendations for serial troponins will vary based on clinical context, laboratory test, and organization policies/algorithms. COMPASS MI (https://compass-mi.com/) is one algorithm available to clinicians to interpret troponins within the clinical context that considers length of time between measurements.[34]
- Cardiac troponin elevation can be due to cardiac or noncardiac conditions and is a good predictor of major adverse events, especially in the context of hospitalization.[2]
- Stress testing (exercise and pharmacologic) may inconsistently cause a small rise in hs-Tn which has not been correlated with inducible myocardial ischemia.[35]
- Troponin testing has replaced historical use of myoglobin and CK-MB in the evaluation of chest pain.[36]
- In pediatrics, troponin testing is not recommended unless there is concerning history or electrocardiogram (ECG) abnormalities.[37]
- In MI related to percutaneous coronary intervention or coronary artery bypass graft, troponin usually peaks in 1 to 6 hours after symptom onset, but can peak as late as 72 hours.[38]

PATIENT EDUCATION

- https://medlineplus.gov/lab-tests/troponin-test/

RELATED DIAGNOSES AND ICD-10 CODES

Acute ischemic heart disease	I24.9
Chest pain	R07.9
Other specified abnormal findings of blood chemistry (high troponin I level or elevated troponin I measurement)	R79.89

REFERENCES

Full list of references can be accessed through Springer Publishing Company Connect™ at the following link: http://connect.springerpub.com/content/reference-book/ 978-0-8261-8843-4/part/part03/toc-part/ch149

150. URIC ACID

Danielle Hebert

PHYSIOLOGY REVIEW

Uric acid is considered to be a weak organic acid as well as a natural oxidant in the human body.[1] It is the end product of purine metabolism by the body, occurring through the liver which produces urate by breaking down dietary or endogenously produced purine compounds.[1-3] Dietary intake accounts for one-third of uric acid development with the remaining two-thirds being produced endogenously.[2,4]

Approximately 65% to 75% of the uric acid produced daily is excreted renally while the remaining 25% to 35% will be excreted through the intestines.[2,4] Renal clearance levels in women of reproductive age are enhanced by estrogenic compounds, leading to lower normal reference values.[5] The decrease of estrogen in menopause leads to an equalization of normal reference values for both men and women.[5]

OVERVIEW OF LABORATORY TESTS

Laboratory evaluation of uric acid levels is primarily assessed through the serum uric acid test (CPT code 84550).[1-15] It is recommended that the patient not eat or drink for 4 hours prior to the serum test.[9,10] Uric acid may also be evaluated through a urinary uric acid test (CPT code 84560) that requires a 24-hour collection of the sample.[11,12] However, it is not a recommended test as the results can be impacted by dietary intake.[12]

INDICATIONS

Screening

- There are no universal screenings recommended for uric acid.[7]
- There is a lack of specified symptoms associated with hyperuricemia or hypouricemia and often the abnormal uric acid level is found as part of the workup for symptomatology of other diagnoses.
- Consider targeted screening for those at risk of developing hyperuricemia: angiotensin-converting enzyme inhibitors, acidosis, alcoholism, antitubercular drugs, beta blockers, chemotherapy-related side effects, dehydration, diabetes, diuretics (thiazide or loop), excessive exercise, hypertension, hypoparathyroidism, immunosuppressants, lead poisoning, leukemia, levodopa, low dose aspirin, medullary cystic kidney disease, nicotinic acid, non-losartan angiotensin II receptor blockers, obesity, polycythemia vera, purine-rich diet, renal failure, testosterone, and toxemia of pregnancy.[5,7,8,10,14]
- Consider targeted screening for those at risk of developing hypouricemia: amanita phalloides poisoning, diabetes, Fanconi syndrome, fluid

volume excess, hereditary diseases of metabolism, HIV infection, high dose salicylates, liver disease, low purine diet, malignancies such as Hodgkin lymphoma, medicines (fenofibrate, losartan, trimethoprim-sulfamethoxazole), syndrome of inappropriate antidiuretic hormone (SIADH) secretion, and patients on total parenteral nutrition.[8,9]

Diagnosis and Evaluation

- Evaluate uric acid in the presence of kidney or ureteral injury, nephrolithiasis, cardiovascular disease, and metabolic syndrome.[3,7,10]
- Consider obtaining levels of uric acid for those patients who present with sudden onset of monoarticular joint pain with a history of gout or tophi.[7] Gout is considered to be a chronic disease that manifests with symptomatic flares.[13] Approximately 10% to 25% of patients with hyperuricemia will develop gout with diagnosis often based upon history, risk factors (age, comorbidities), and clinical signs: erythema, monoarticular joint pain (often foot), swelling, redness, and sensitivity to touch.[13,14]

Monitoring

- In the presence of new asymptomatic hyperuricemia, recheck the uric acid level after 1 week; if it remains above 8 mg/dL complete the workup to determine the cause.[5] If the uric acid level is between 7 and 8 mg/dL, repeat the laboratory test in 6 to 12 months.[5] If the uric acid level is less than 7 mg/dL, no further testing is indicated.[5]
- It is recommended that the serum uric acid level be kept lower than 6 mg/dL when treating long-term for gout and lower than 5 mg/dL when tophi is present.[12,14,15]

INTERPRETATION

Tables 150.1 and 150.2 provide general reference ranges for normal, hypouricemia, and hyperuricemia. Individual laboratory tests may have differing ranges. Women of childbearing age will have lower reference ranges and rates of gout; however, following menopause, rates and references will be equal to those for men.[5,13]

TABLE 150.1: INTERPRETATION OF SERUM URIC ACID LEVELS

Normal Adult Range	3.5–7.2 mg/dL
Hypouricemia	<2 mg/dL
Hyperuricemia	Male >/= 7 mg/dL
	Female >/= 6 mg/dL

Sources: Data from Li Q, Li X, Kwong JS-W, et al. Diagnosis and treatment for hyperuricaemia and gout: a protocol for a systematic review of clinical practice guidelines and consensus statements. *BMJ Open.* 2017;7(6):e014928. doi:10.1136/bmjopen-2016-014928; Mount Sinai Health System. *Uric acid-blood.* https://www.mountsinai.org/health-library/tests/uric-acid-blood; Uric acid. Published October 6, 2020. https://www.ucsfhealth.org/medical-tests/003476; Valsaraj R, Singh AK, Gangopadhyay KK, et al. Management of asymptomatic hyperuricemia: Integrated Diabetes & Endocrine Academy (IDEA) consensus statement. *Diabetes & Metab Syndr.* 2020;14(2): 93–100. doi:10.1016/j.dsx.2020.01.007; Yu K-H, Chen D-Y, Chen J-H, et al. Management of gout and hyperuricemia: multidisciplinary consensus in Taiwan. *Int J Rheum Dis.* 2018;21(4):772–787. doi:10.1111/1756-185x.13266

TABLE 150.2: INTERPRETATION OF URINARY URIC ACID LEVELS	
Normal	250–750 mg/24 hr

Source: Data from Mount Sinai Health System. Uric Acid Urine Test. https://www.mountsinai.org/health-library/tests/uric-acid-urine-test

FOLLOW-UP

■ Check complete blood count with differential, chemistry profile, liver chemistries, and urinalysis for new diagnosis of asymptomatic hyperuricemia.[5]

PEARLS & PITFALLS

■ Hyperuricemia has been identified as an independent risk factor associated with cardiovascular disease, hypertension, and metabolic syndrome.[1,6,7,13,14]
■ Uric acid may be seen in up to 10% to 15% of presenting kidney stones.[2]
■ Examples of dietary resources that can contribute to hyperuricemia include animal protein, seafood, beer, and alcohol.[5,7,12]

PATIENT EDUCATION

■ https://www.mayoclinic.org/healthy-lifestyle/nutrition-and-healthy-eating/in-depth/gout-diet/art-20048524[16]
■ https://www.ucsfhealth.org/medical-tests/003476[9]

RELATED DIAGNOSES AND ICD-10 CODES

Gout, unspecified	M10.9[17]
Hyperuricemia without signs of inflammatory arthritis and tophaceous disease	E79.0[18]
Other disorders of purine and pyrimidine metabolism (may be used for hypouricemia)	E79.8[19]
Calculus of kidney (may be used for uric acid renal calculus or uric acid nephrolithiasis)	N20.0[20]

REFERENCES

Full list of references can be accessed through Springer Publishing Company Connect™ at the following link: http://connect.springerpub.com/content/reference-book/978-0-8261-8843-4/part/part03/toc-part/ch150

151. URINALYSIS

Sara Revelle and Kelly Small Casler

PHYSIOLOGY REVIEW

The kidneys are responsible for filtration, reabsorption, and secretion of waste materials from the blood. Ureters carry urine to the bladder, where it is stored until it is able to be released through the urethra during urination. A variety of conditions can alter kidney function allowing substances not normally found in urine to be excreted. Abnormalities of the bladder, ureters, and urethra can cause abnormal substances to be found in the urine as well.

OVERVIEW OF LABORATORY TEST

Urinalysis is one of the oldest and most widely used laboratory tests for both screening and diagnostic purposes.[1] The test includes gross visual analysis (for clarity and turbidity), chemical analysis using dipstick, and, sometimes, microscopic examination. The chemical analysis can be interpreted using an automated analyzer (sometimes done at the point of care) or by visual analysis (Figure 151.1A/B).[2] Microscopic examination is labor and time intensive, requiring sample preparation (centrifuging of urine and removal of supernatant) and

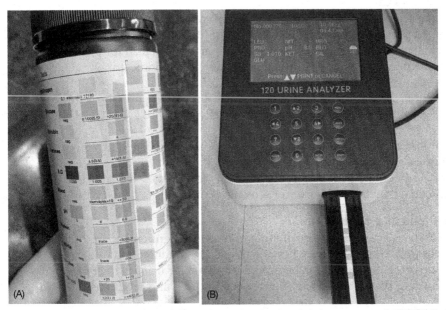

FIGURE 151.1. Urinalysis by dipstick. **(A)** Urinalysis using visual analysis (non-automated). **(B)** Urinalysis using automated analyzer (dipstick is placed on analyzer stage which is inserted into analyzer to be read).

TABLE 151.1: URINALYSIS OPTIONS WITH CURRENT PROCEDURAL TERMINOLOGY CODES	
OPTION	**CPT CODE**
Urinalysis by dipstick; non-automated, but with microscopy	81000
Urinalysis by dipstick; automated and with microscopy	81001
Urinalysis by dipstick; non-automated and no microscopy	81002
Urinalysis by dipstick; automated, but no microscopy	81003
Urinalysis as microscopy only	81005

evaluation by the clinician or laboratory personnel. Newer methods to replace microscopic examination with digital-imaging techniques are being explored.[2-4] Urinalysis can provide clues to problems within the urinary tract or liver, as well as problems with metabolism, such as diabetes.[5] As summarized in Table 151.1, current procedural terminology (CPT) codes for urinalysis vary based on whether the dipstick is interpreted using an automated flowmeter or non-automated methods (visual inspection) and whether microscopy is performed.

INDICATIONS

Screening

- The American Academy of Pediatrics (AAP) recommends against ordering urinalysis for healthy, asymptomatic pediatric patients as part of routine well child care.[6]
- There are insufficient levels of evidence to recommend urinalysis to screen for the presence of bladder cancer in asymptomatic adults.[7]
- Evidence does not support the use of urinalysis to screen for preeclampsia in pregnancy, since proteinuria alone is not a good indicator of preeclampsia outcomes.[8,9]
- Multiple organizations recommend against screening urinalysis due to lack of evidence of net benefits and a small amount of evidence of potential harms.[10-16]
- Routine preoperative testing with urinalysis is not needed for low-risk surgeries.[17,18]
- A 2015 Cochrane review found too little evidence was available to evaluate potential benefits and harms of screening urinalysis.[19]

Diagnosis and Evaluation

- Urinalysis is used in the evaluation of multiple signs and symptoms including dysuria, urinary frequency, urinary urgency, polyuria, and urine color changes. It can be used to evaluate for urinary tract problems including suspected urinary tract infection (UTI) and urolithiasis.

Monitoring

- Urinalysis is not typically used for monitoring/prognosis. Follow-up urinalysis for those diagnosed with simple acute cystitis whose symptoms resolve with use of antimicrobials is usually not necessary.[20,21]

INTERPRETATION AND FOLLOW-UP

Gross Analysis

Color

- Normal color is pale to dark yellow.
- Hydration status, dietary intake, medications, and pathophysiology can impact color. Dark yellow color typically indicates a concentrated specimen which can result from dehydration and exercise. Other variations in color and their etiology are listed in Table 151.2[22-28]

TABLE 151.2: COLOR VARIATION ETIOLOGY

COLOR	POTENTIAL CAUSE		
	DIETARY	MEDICATION	PATHOLOGY
Red	Beets	Phenytoin	Hemoglobinopathies
	Rhubarb	Sennosides (Ex-Lax)	Rhabdomyolysis
	Blackberries		Urinary tract infection
Orange	Carrots	Coumadin	Bile pigments
		Nitrofurantoin	
		Phenothiazines	
		Phenazopyridine	
		Rifampin	
		Vitamin C	
Green/Blue	Dye in enteral feeds	Amitriptyline	Pseudomonas infection
	Asparagus	Indomethacin	
		Propofol	
		Triamterene	
Brown/Black (tea colored)	Fava beans	Cascara	Jaundice
	Rhubarb	Chloroquine	Hepatobiliary disease
		Metronidazole	Methemoglobin
		Nitrofurantoin	Myoglobin
		Riboflavin	
		Senna	
White			Pyuria
			Chyluria
			Phosphate crystals

Sources: Data from Cavanaugh C, Perazella MA. Urine sediment examination in the diagnosis and management of kidney disease: core curriculum 2019. *Am J Kidney Dis.* 2019;73(2):258–272. doi:10.1053/j.ajkd.2018.07.012; Fogazzi GB, Verdesca S, Garigali G. Urinalysis: core curriculum 2008. *Am J Kidney Dis.* 2008;51(6):1052–1067. doi:10.1053/j.ajkd.2007.11.039; Lexicomp Online. *Propofol;* Meyrier A. Sampling and evaluation of voided urine in the diagnosis or urinary tract infection in adults. In: Calderwood SB, ed. *UpToDate.* UpToDate; 2022. https://www.uptodate.com/contents/sampling-and-evaluation-of-voided-urine-in-the-diagnosis -of-urinary-tract-infection-in-adults; Rao LV, Snyder LM, eds. *Wallach's Interpretation of Diagnostic Tests: Pathways to Arriving at a Clinical Diagnosis.* 11th ed. Wolters Kluwer; 2021; Queremel Milani DA, Jialal I. Urinalysis. In: *StatPearls.* StatPearls Publishing; 2021. http://www.ncbi.nlm.nih.gov/books/NBK557685/; Wad R. Urinalysis in the diagnosis of kidney disease. In: Curhan GC, ed. *UpToDate.* UpToDate; 2022. https://www.uptodate.com/contents/urinalysis-in-the-diagnosis-of-kidney-disease

Turbidity

- Normal urine is transparent. However, lack of turbidity cannot rule out UTI on its own.[29]
- Common causes of turbid urine include contamination by genital secretions, as well as presence of cellular debris including erythrocytes, leukocytes, bacteria, crystals, squamous epithelial cells, or casts.[22,26,28,30]
- Refrigerated urine can become cloudy due to the presence of phosphates or urates, making adequate examination difficult.

Odor

- Not typically reported but may serve as a helpful indicator of underlying issues. Normal urine odor is referred to as *urinoid*.[26] Table 151.3 lists interpretation considerations based on odor.
- Foul-smelling urine is not specific to UTI. Odor often depends on hydration status and amount of urea in the urine.[31]

Chemical Analysis by Dipstick

Leukocyte Esterase

- The leukocyte esterase (LE) test pad detects an esterase (enzyme) released by white blood cells (WBCs), specifically neutrophils and macrophages.[26–28,30,32] WBCs, and thus leukocyte esterase, are normally absent in the urine. Positive results are usually referred to as pyuria, and are reported as trace, small (1+), moderate (2+), or large (3+) amounts.
- LE is most frequently used with nitrite testing to evaluate for the presence/absence of UTI. However, positive results reflect the presence of WBCs from inflammation of the urinary tract, which could be due to infectious or noninfectious causes.
- In the pediatric population, LE sensitivity for UTI ranges from 64% to 97.6% and specificity ranges from 71% to 95%.[33,34] In adults, the sensitivity for UTI ranges from 62% to 86% and specificity ranges from 70% to 93%.[35]

TABLE 151.3: ODOR CONSIDERATIONS

ODOR	POTENTIALLY ASSOCIATED CONDITION
Strong, pungent	Infection (ammonia smell produced by bacteria)
Sweet, fruity, acetone	Ketones associated with diabetic ketoacidosis
Honey	Diabetes
Burnt sugar	Maple urine disease
Mousy, musty	Phenylketonuria
Sweaty feet	Isovaleric acidemia
Rancid butter, fishy	Hypermethioninemia

Sources: Data from Echeverry G, Hortin GL, Rai AJ. Introduction to urinalysis: historical perspectives and clinical application. In: Rai AJ, ed. *The Urinary Proteome*. Vol 641. Methods in Molecular Biology. Humana Press; 2010:1–12. doi:10.1007/978-1-60761-711-2_1; Fogazzi GB, Verdesca S, Garigali G. Urinalysis: core curriculum 2008. *Am J Kidney Dis*. 2008;51(6):1052–1067. doi:10.1053/j.ajkd.2007.11.039; Queremel Milani DA, Jialal I. Urinalysis. In: *StatPearls*. StatPearls Publishing; 2021. http://www.ncbi.nlm.nih.gov/books/NBK557685/.

- Other causes of a positive LE test besides UTI include nephrolithiasis, bladder/renal malignancy, glomerulonephritis, pelvic inflammation, corticosteroid use, cyclophosphamide, balanitis, acute renal failure, sexually transmitted infections (STIs), noninfectious cystitis, and exercise.[26-28,30-32]
- False-positive results are seen in contaminated specimens with multiple squamous epithelial cells.
- False-negative results are seen with dilute urine (decreased specific gravity), glycosuria, ketonuria, proteinuria, vitamin C, and certain oxidizing drugs including nitrofurantoin, cephalexin, tetracycline, and gentamicin.[26-28,30,32,36-38]

Nitrite

- Nitrite is formed when urinary nitrates (a component of dietary metabolites) are broken down by certain bacteria. Normally, nitrites are not present in the urine. Results are reported as positive or negative.[26-28,30,32]
- Positive nitrite on urine dipstick is highly specific for UTI but is not highly sensitive since only nitrate-reducing bacteria (e.g., *E. coli*, *Proteus*, *Enterobacter*, or *Klebsiella*) produce positive results. In the pediatric population, the specificity for UTI is 95% to 100%, but sensitivity is only 28% to 84%,[34] with the worst performance in children younger than 2 years of age.[39] In the adult population, specificity is similar to pediatric populations[35,40] while sensitivity is lower (46% to 55%).[35] For this reason, positive nitrite results are generally considered more useful to confirm UTI than negative nitrite results are to exclude UTI. The positive likelihood ratio (LR) of UTI when nitrites are positive was 29.3 in one metanalysis.[36]
- False-positive results occur in the presence of phenazopyridine (Pyridium) or excess exposure of the test strip to air.[26,28,32]
- Absence of nitrite does not exclude the diagnosis of UTI. False-negative results occur if there is lack of nitrates in the diet, dilute urine, acidic urine, elevated urobilinogen, or the UTI causing organism is not a nitrate-reducing bacteria. Recent voiding can also cause a false negative since it takes 4 hours for nitrates to be converted to nitrite.[26-28,30,32]
- The use of urinary dipstick to exclude or confirm the diagnosis of UTI is most accurate when LE and nitrite results are considered together.[34,41-43] The presence of both are highly specific (96% to 100%) for UTI[35] and the combined absence of both has a negative LR of 0.22.[40]

Urobilinogen

- Urobilinogen reflects the level of bilirubin since bilirubin is converted to urobilinogen in the intestine. Urobilinogen can either be excreted in the feces or reabsorbed into circulation and later excreted by the kidney.[24,28,32] Reference intervals are 0.2 to 1 mg/dL.
- The presence of excess urobilinogen in the urine is called urobilinogenuria. Differential diagnosis includes sickle cell disease, thalassemia, hemolysis, and liver/biliary disease.[24,28,32] Clinical history and physical examination as well as a complete blood count and liver enzymes with bilirubin help clarify the clinical picture.
- False positives can occur in the presence of phenazopyridine (Pyridium), sulfonamides, and elevated nitrites.[26,32]

- False negatives can occur with prolonged sample exposure to light, stale urine specimen, high levels of nitrites, or formaldehyde.[26]

Protein

- Dipstick analysis for protein detects albumin and is most sensitive to high levels of albuminuria and will not detect other proteins or small amounts of albumin. Normally, protein amounts in urine should be negative to trace. When protein is present, it is referred to as proteinuria and can be reported as 1+ (30 mg/dL), 2+ (100 mg/dL), 3+ 300 mg/dL), or 4+ (2000 mg/dL or more).
- Urine dipstick does not accurately or consistently detect moderate albuminuria levels between 30 and 300 mg/day (formerly referred to as microalbuminuria).[28] Since moderate albuminuria is a sign of early kidney disease, glomerular injury, and risk of kidney disease progression, urine dipstick should not be used to monitor or screen for proteinuria.[26,28,32] Instead, urine samples can be sent for quantitative measurement of albuminuria (albumin: creatinine or protein: creatinine ratio).[28]
- Etiologies of proteinuria are many, with some that are transient and others that are persistent. Transient proteinuria is particularly common in children.[44] Examples of transient proteinuria causes include infection, fever, dehydration, and orthostatic (postural) proteinuria.
- Examples of persistent proteinuria include, but are not limited to, preeclampsia, congestive heart failure (CHF), renal dysfunction, acute tubular necrosis, heavy metal poisoning, chronic kidney disease, glomerular sclerosis, nephrotic syndrome, and malignancy.[22,26,28,32,44] A thorough history and physical examination (especially looking for the presence of edema) will help evaluate for more serious causes.
- Heavy proteinuria with minimal or absent hematuria is indicative of non-proliferative diseases including severe diabetic nephropathy and amyloidosis. Evaluation for these causes is indicated with persistent, high levels of proteinuria.
- False positives can occur in setting of concentrated urine, alkaline specimens, hematuria, phenazopyridine (Pyridium), quaternary ammonia compounds, or recent use of radiocontrast agents.[24,28,32,44,45]
- False negatives can occur in the setting of dilute specimen, acidic specimen, or in the presence of non-albumin protein.[24,28,32]
- Follow-up any proteinuria greater than 1+ by performing a urine protein/creatinine ratio on a random or 24-hour urine sample.[44] Other follow-up should be directed by differential diagnoses that are based on history and physical examination.

pH

- Normal urine pH is between 5.0 and 8.0 with the usual range being 4.5 to 6.5.
- Table 151.4 assists with interpretation of the urine pH.

Blood

- The urinalysis test pad for blood detects heme. Red blood cells (RBCs) in the urine (hematuria), free hemoglobin in the urine (hemoglobinuria), or myoglobin in the urine (myoglobinuria) can all cause a positive reading on urine dipstick for blood; therefore, urine dipstick alone cannot be used to

TABLE 151.4: pH VARIATIONS

URINE pH	ETIOLOGY
Alkaline (>6.5–8.0)	Hyperventilation
	Presence of urease-producing bacteria
	Renal tubular acidosis
	Stale specimen (common)
	Vegetarian diet
	Vomiting
Acidic (<4.5–5.0)	Cranberry juice
	Dehydration
	Diarrhea
	Emphysema
	High protein diet
	Potassium depletion
	Starvation

Sources: Data from Fogazzi GB, Verdesca S, Garigali G. Urinalysis: core curriculum 2008. *Am J Kidney Dis.* 2008;51(6):1052–1067. doi:10.1053/j.ajkd.2007.11.039; Simerville JA, Maxted WC, Pahira JJ. Urinalysis: a comprehensive review. *Am Fam Physician.* 2005;71(6):1153–1162; Queremel Milani DA, Jialal I. Urinalysis. In: *StatPearls.* StatPearls Publishing; 2021. http://www.ncbi.nlm.nih .gov/books/NBK557685/; Wad R. Urinalysis in the diagnosis of kidney disease. In: Carhan GC, ed. *UpToDate.* UpToDate; 2022. https://www.uptodate.com/contents/urinalysis-in-the-diagnosis-of-kidney-disease

diagnose hematuria. A normal result is negative. Positive results on urine dipstick are quantified as trace, small (+), moderate (2+), or large (3+).[22,26,28,32,37,46]

- A positive dipstick for blood should be followed-up with microscopic analysis to determine if hematuria is present. Hematuria confirmed on microscopic analysis is termed "asymptomatic microhematuria" (AMH), which should only be used to refer to the presence of RBC in the urine on microscopic analysis (and not by dipstick).[16,19] RBC on microscopic analysis is not seen in myoglobinuria and hemoglobinuria.[44]

- Common etiologies of hematuria include UTI, renal calculi, glomerulonephritis, malignancy, pyelonephritis, trauma, use of anticoagulants, strenuous exercise, recent sexual activity, and exposure to toxic chemicals.[22,26,28,32,43,44,46]

- Etiologies of hemoglobinuria include hemolytic anemia, strenuous exercise, severe burns, transfusion reaction, and infections, such as malaria.[22,26,28,32,46]

- Etiologies of myoglobinuria include rhabdomyolysis, seizures, extensive exertion, drug abuse, and alcohol overdose.[26,28,32]

- False-positive results (for dipstick testing) can result from semen or dehydration.[26,28,32,44] Menstruation can also cause a positive finding.

- False-negative results can occur in the presence of ascorbic acid (vitamin C), captopril, dilute urine, acidic urine specimens, or proteinuria.

- The presence of UTI is not always the only reason for AMH, and some patients could still have malignancy.[47] Therefore, for those patients with AMH in the setting of UTI, a repeat microscopic urinalysis should be completed 1 to 2 weeks after UTI therapy completion.[48] If hematuria persists, urology referral is indicated.[20,21,46]

- A negative urine dipstick test for blood along with the absence of LE and nitrites helps rule out the possibility of UTI.[43] Likewise, consider LE and nitrites when interpreting positive blood on urine dipstick. If LE and nitrites are absent and microscopic urinalysis shows AMH, consider non-infectious causes (especially malignancy) over cystitis.

Specific Gravity

- Specific gravity reflects the kidneys' ability to concentrate or dilute urine and is based on the number and size of dissolved particles within the urine.[22,26,28] The reference interval is 1.005 to 1.030 (greater than 1.030 reflects a more concentrated specimen; less than 1.005 reflects dilute urine).
- Dilute urine may be seen in diabetes insipidus, hyperaldosteronism, diuretic use, and impaired renal function.
- Concentrated urine may be seen in dehydration, nephrotic/nephritis syndrome, and syndrome of inappropriate diuretic hormone.
- Large particles in the urine, such as dextran solution, radiopaque contrast media, and protein, can result in a falsely elevated specific gravity.[28,32]
- Alkaline urine can lead to a falsely decreased specific gravity.[28,32]
- Specific gravity has not shown high sensitivity or specificity for any one condition and does not predict osmolality.[49]

Ketones

- Urine dipstick testing uses the nitroprusside reaction for detection of ketones. This reaction detects acetoacetate, which only accounts for 20% of ketones produced in ketoacidosis (β-hydroxybutyrate accounts for the majority of ketones).[50,51] Ketones are not normally found in urine.
- Presence of ketones in the urine is called "ketonuria." Ketonuria is reported as trace (5 mg/dL), small (15 mg/dL), moderate (40 mg/dL), or large (80 to 160 mg/dL).[52]
- Differential diagnoses of ketonuria include uncontrolled diabetes, ketoacidosis (alcohol or diabetic), low carbohydrate diet, starvation, pregnancy, and vomiting.[22,24,26,32,53]
- Urine ketone testing by dipstick is often used to evaluate for diabetic ketoacidosis (DKA) in those with a blood sugar greater than 250 mg/dL and has good sensitivity when used in this manner. However, it has poorer specificity than point-of-care β-hydroxybutyrate (β-OHB), which is often used in addition to urine ketone testing.[28,54,55] In a seminal study with emergency department patients, ketonuria had 95% sensitivity for DKA, but only 80% specificity.[56]
- False positives can occur in the presence of elevated specific gravity, acidic urine, and pharmacotherapy with mesna (Mesnex), levodopa, or captopril.[26,32] Additionally, ketonuria may persist during ketoacidosis recovery since β-OHB is converted to acetoacetate, before being completely cleared from the body.[51]
- False negatives can occur in a stale urine specimen or in acidotic states caused primarily by non-acetoacetate ketones.[26,32]

Bilirubin

- Heme from recycled RBCs is converted by the spleen to bilirubin and then released into circulation in an unconjugated form. After reaching the liver, bilirubin is combined, or conjugated, with glucuronic acid.[57,58] Bilirubin that is noted in the urine reflects this conjugated form of bilirubin, since only conjugated bilirubin is water soluble. Bilirubin is not normally found in urine.

■ Presence of bilirubin in the urine is called "bilirubinuria" and reported as small (+), moderate (2+), or large (3+) amounts. Differential diagnosis for bilirubinuria includes liver disease, biliary obstruction, acetaminophen overdose, or congenital forms of hyperbilirubinemia.[26,28,32]

■ False positives occur in the presence of phenazopyridine (Pyridium).

■ False negatives can occur in the presence of chlorpromazine, selenium, and in stale urine specimens.[26,32]

■ Follow-up of bilirubinuria should include evaluation of liver enzymes and serum bilirubin.

Glucose

■ Glucose is filtered by the glomerulus and reabsorbed by the distal tubule. When excess amounts of filtered glucose exceed the capacity of the distal tubule to reabsorb it (called the renal threshold) or the distal tubule absorptive capacity is dysfunctional, excess glucose is excreted in the urine. Although it is normal for scant amounts of glucose (25 mg/dL) to be excreted in the urine, these amounts are too small to be detected by urine dipstick methods.[59] Therefore, the normal result for glucose on urine dipstick is negative.

■ Presence of glucose in the urine is called "glycosuria." It generally occurs when plasma levels are higher than what the kidney is able to reabsorb (usually greater than 100 to 180 mg/dL) and it is reported as trace (100 mg/dL), 1+ (250 mg/dL), 2+ (500 mg/dL), 3+ (1,000 mg/dL), or 4+ (2,000 mg/dL or more).[22,24,26,28,32,52]

■ Differential diagnosis for glycosuria includes diabetes, pregnancy, Cushing's syndrome, Fanconi syndrome, use of sodium-glucose cotransporter-2 (*SGLT2*) inhibitors, and recent glucose administration.[26,28,32] Follow-up of positive results includes serum or plasma glucose and glycosylated hemoglobin (HgB A1C).

■ False positives can occur in the presence of levodopa or ketones.[26,28,32]

■ False negatives can occur with dilute urine, uric acid, and high doses of ascorbic acid (vitamin C).[26,28,32]

■ Urine dipstick testing for glucose lacks adequate sensitivity to screen for gestational diabetes mellitus (GDM).[60]

Microscopic Analysis

Cells

Red Blood Cells

■ The normal amount of RBC in the urine is 2 RBCs or fewer per high power field (HPF).[22,23,26,28]

■ Internationally, most guidelines agree that 3 or more RBCs per HPF on just one microscopic urinalysis defines asymptomatic microscopic hematuria (AMH) and warrants evaluation for urologic malignancy.[61,62] However, the American College of Obstetricians and Gynecologists and the American Urogynecologic Society contend that not all females with AMH need to be evaluated for urologic malignancy. Those who are never-smokers and 50 years old or younger may not need evaluation as long as microscopic analysis shows 25 or fewer RBC/HPF.[63]

- Causes of AMH include vigorous exercise, intercourse, UTI, urolithiasis, glomerular disease, kidney trauma, and urologic malignancy.[22,23,26,28,43,61] AMH is most suspicious for malignancy in males 35 or older to 40 years old, and when it is persistent, urologic malignancy has been noted even in patients with intermittent/transient AMH.[61] For this reason, clinical history/physical examination is paramount and care must be taken not to miss urologic malignancy.
- False negatives may occur if the specimen is not refrigerated. Lysis of RBCs can be seen as early as 90 minutes at room temperature.[64]
- False positives on microscopic evaluation for RBC are rare.
- Differential diagnosis of persistent AMH in children is usually accomplished by considering causes arising from the glomerulus versus other sites.[44]
  - **Glomerulus:** IgA nephropathy (will usually note gross hematuria with illness and AMH between illness), Henoch-Schönlein purpura (HSP), thin basement membrane disease, Alport syndrome, and postinfectious glomerulonephritis
  - **Nonglomerulus:** hypercalciuria, nephrolithiasis, nutcracker syndrome
- AMH associated with dysmorphic RBC, RBC casts, and proteinuria is suspicious for proliferative glomerular disease. If this is associated with rapidly declining kidney function, it constitutes a nephrologic emergency.[28]
- In patients with AMH, evaluate blood urea nitrogen, creatinine, estimated glomerular filtration rate, RBC count, and spot or 24-hour protein.[61]
- Male sex, smoking history, and age older than 50 all increase the risk for urologic malignancy. If these patients have AMH, follow-up should include urologic referral.[48]

White Blood Cells

- The normal amount of white blood cells (WBC) in the urine is 2 to 5 WBC per HPF or fewer. Eosinophils and neutrophils are the most common types of WBCs noted.[22]
- More than 5 WBC per HPF (pyuria) can indicate UTI, noninfectious cystitis, urine contaminant from genital secretions, interstitial nephritis, nephrolithiasis, malignancy, glomerulonephritis, acute renal failure, sexually transmitted infections, or noninfectious cystitis.[26–28,30–32] Highly concentrated urine may also result in more than 5 WBC in the absence of disease.[36]
- The presence of WBC on microscopic urinalysis in symptomatic patients has a sensitivity of 95% and specificity of 71% for UTI.[43]
- Consider specific gravity when interpreting severity of pyuria, especially in young children. Children with UTI and dilute urine samples may have as few as three WBC per HPF while those with concentrated urine will have more.[36–38]
- False negatives may occur if the specimen is not refrigerated or is dilute. Significant decrease in WBC concentrations can be seen as early as 90 minutes at room temperature.[33]

Epithelial Cells

- Three types of epithelial cells may be noted on microscopic examination.[22,26,28]

- Squamous cells are the most common and are considered normal as long as fewer than 15 to 20 per HPF are observed. They are usually found from the distal urethra and genitalia.[26,65] When seen in high numbers with leukocytes and bacteria, this may be associated with contamination from genital (vaginitis) secretions and may predict poorer performance of the urinalysis.[66]
- Transitional cells arise from the epithelium lining of the urinary tract (kidney to bladder in females and distal urethra in males). The cells can occur with UTI, but more often present concern for underlying urologic disease.[22,26,28]
- Renal cells arise from renal tubules and, if present, signify a more concerning kidney issue such as infection (pyelonephritis), ischemia, malignancy, acute tubular necrosis, or toxicity (heavy metal poisoning or drug toxicity).[22,26,28]

Bacteria

- Bacteria can be seen in UTI and in cases of contamination with normal flora.

Fungi, Parasites, or Semen

- Fungi and parasites are not normally seen, but if present they may be from contamination from vaginal yeast or trichomonas infections. They also may be seen in cases of trichomonal urethritis.
- Semen is occasionally encountered if there has been recent sexual activity. If it is encountered outside of sexual activity history, it may be an indication of sexual abuse.

Casts

- Urinary casts are cylindrical-like aggregations formed in the renal tubule and named for the primary cell or matrix composition. Casts should not be present in normal circumstances. When present, they reflect acute or chronic kidney injury/disease and should warrant consultation with nephrology.[22,26,28] Table 151.5 lists the differential diagnoses of urinary casts.
- In patients with acute kidney injury, the presence of granular or epithelial casts is strongly suggestive of acute tubular necrosis.[28]

TABLE 151.5: DIFFERENTIAL DIAGNOSIS OF URINARY CASTS	
RBC casts	Glomerulonephritis and acute tubular necrosis/injury
WBC casts	Pyelonephritis, interstitial nephritis, or glomerulonephritis
Hyaline casts	Chronic kidney disease, low perfusion of kidney (sluggish urine flow), concentrated urine, dehydration, exercise, fever, or diuretic use
Epithelial casts	Acute tubular necrosis, acute interstitial nephritis, and glomerulonephritis
Granular casts	Acute or chronic renal disease. Can also be seen after stress/exercise
Waxy casts	Renal insufficiency (acute or chronic) or advanced renal failure
Fatty casts	Marked proteinuria, severe crush injuries, and nephrotic syndrome
Renal tubular casts	Tubular necrosis

Sources: Data from Fogazzi GB, Verdesca S, Garigali G. Urinalysis: core curriculum 2008. *Am J Kidney Dis.* 2008;51(6):1052–1067. doi:10.1053/j.ajkd.2007.11.039; Queremel Milani DA, Jialal I. Urinalysis. In: *StatPearls.* StatPearls Publishing; 2021. http://www.ncbi.nlm.nih.gov/books/NBK557685/; Wad R. Urinalysis in the diagnosis of kidney disease. In Carhan GC, ed. *UpToDate.* UpToDate; 2022. https://www.uptodate.com/contents/urinalysis-in-the-diagnosis-of-kidney-disease

■ False negatives can occur if the specimen is not refrigerated. Significant decrease in cast concentrations can be seen as early as 90 minutes at room temperature.[64]

Crystals

■ Crystals are a byproduct of metabolism of certain substances or related to pharmaceutical use. Sulfonamides, ciprofloxacin, atazanavir, acyclovir, and methotrexate are known pharmaceuticals that cause crystal formation in urine.[22,26,28]

■ The concentration of substances as well as urine pH impacts formation. Specimen handling and timely evaluation are important as incidental crystals (e.g., uric acid crystals) can occur in the absence of disease if more than 2 hours have passed since urine collection.[22,26,28]

■ Crystals may be indicative of pathology or can be normal. More often than not, they are an incidental finding. In one report, up to 8% of urine samples had crystals present (uric acid, calcium oxalate, or calcium phosphate).[22,26,28]

■ Cystine crystals are seen only with cystinuria, a recessive inherited disease associated with nephrolithiasis. Other types of crystals are listed in Table 151.6.

PEARLS & PITFALLS

■ Multiple organizations recommend screening for asymptomatic bacteria in pregnancy by urine culture, but not by urinalysis since sensitivity is not high enough.[10–12,67,68]

TABLE 151.6: SUMMARY OF CRYSTALS (BESIDES CYSTINE) THAT MAY BE FOUND IN URINE

CALCIUM OXALATE	URIC ACID
• Most commonly seen crystal • Associated urine pH typically <5.8 (range <5.5-6.7) • Seen in normal patient as well as with pathology • Seen with ingestion of high oxalate foods (chocolate, rhubarb, almonds, spinach) • May be associated with urolithiasis • Can result from gastric bypass surgery or other causes of malabsorption of oxalate (orlistat, pancreatitis) as well as drugs breaking down into the calcium oxalate crystal (vitamin C, ethylene glycol)	• Occurs in acidic urine • Can be seen in specimens that have delayed processing or if refrigerated prior to evaluation • Seen in normal patient as well as with pathology • Pathology associated with uric acid crystals includes uric acid nephrolithiasis, rhabdomyolysis, and tumor lysis syndrome
AMORPHOUS PHOSPHATE (CALCIUM AND MAGNESIUM PHOSPHATE)	**TRIPLE PHOSPHATE**
• Occurs in alkaline urine • Seen in normal patient as well as with pathology • Associated with decreased urine volume, calcium-rich diet, prolonged immobilization, overactive parathyroids, bony metastases • Magnesium phosphate crystals may be seen in UTIs with urease-producing organisms (Proteus or Klebsiella)	• Found in alkaline urine • Not usually normal • Associated with infection from urease producing bacteria (Proteus, Klebsiella, Ureaplasma urealyticum, Corynebacterium urealyticum)

- Urine should be evaluated within 1 to 2 hours of collection. If this is not possible, refrigeration of specimen between 2 °C and 8 °C for up to 24 hours is acceptable.[22,26,28]
- Theoretically, a morning first void specimen is the ideal specimen for evaluation for UTI as it should have the least amount of genital or periurethral contaminant. However, there is no clinical data to support this theory.[27]
- When collecting urinalysis for urine culture in women, there is evidence that midstream urinalysis with or without cleansing has equal risk for sample contamination.[69]
- In a patient with UTI symptoms, a positive LE, but negative urine culture/sensitivity, consider the possibility of trichomonas, chlamydia, or *Ureaplasma urealyticum*.[23]
- Do not assume hematuria is from menstruation or sexual activity; use repeat urinalysis to confirm.
- In patients with a positive urine dipstick for blood, but negative RBC on urine microscopy, repeat microscopy three times before ruling out intermittent AMH, since it can be associated with malignancy.[46]
- For diagnosis of UTI, three small studies with adult females found urinalysis by dipstick performed as well as urinalysis by microscopy.[70–72] A metanalysis in the pediatric population showed that urinalysis by dipstick has similar accuracy to urine microscopy, but that urine cultures should still be performed on children with dysuria if there is suspicion of a false-negative urinalysis.[73] For children 24 months or younger, urine culture is always recommended by guidelines to confirm/refute UTI.[74]
- In adults, diagnosis of UTI can sometimes be done without laboratory testing. The symptom of dysuria in the absence of vaginal discharge has high accuracy for prediction of UTI.[75]

PATIENT EDUCATION

- https://www.healthlabtesting.com/-/media/health-lab/pdfs/patient -instructions/urine--urinalysis-or-culture-and-susceptibility-studies .pdf?la=en&hash=162A3CFA8BA78A2FAE5AA0FDB4BAB860

RELATED DIAGNOSES AND ICD-10 CODES

Dysuria	R30
Pyuria	B99.9
Asymptomatic microscopic hematuria	R31.21
Gross hematuria	R31.0
Other chromoabnormalities of urine (positive urine dipstick; negative RBC on microscopic analysis or no microscopic analysis done)	R82.91

REFERENCES

Full list of references can be accessed through Springer Publishing Company Connect™ at the following link: http://connect.springerpub.com/content/reference-book/ 978-0-8261-8843-4/part/part03/toc-part/ch151

152. URINE ALBUMIN

Debra Hain and Nancy C. Tkacs

PHYSIOLOGY REVIEW

Nephrons are the functional units of the kidney, with each kidney having about one million nephrons. Nephron functions consist of two major components. First, glomerular capillaries are the site of *glomerular filtration*, movement of water and small solutes (electrolytes, glucose, amino acids, urea, creatinine, and numerous other biomolecules and wastes) from the plasma to Bowman's space. Second, the nephron tubule that receives the fluid entering Bowman's space conducts *reabsorption from and secretion into* the filtered fluid, progressively retaining needed water and solutes while concentrating wastes for excretion in the urine. Glomerular filtration occurs through a three-layer barrier consisting of pores between capillary endothelial cells, a dense basement membrane rich in negative charges that repel proteins, and filtration slits between the processes of surrounding epithelial cells (podocytes).[1]

As a relatively low molecular weight plasma protein, small amounts of albumin can enter the urine space. In a healthy kidney, this albumin is reabsorbed by the tubules and should not be detectable in the urine. Systemic diseases such as diabetes, hypertension, systemic lupus erythematosus, and various other conditions induce progressive damage to the glomerular filtration barrier. This damage manifests initially as a small, but detectable rate of albumin excretion in the urine—microalbuminuria. Measurements of albumin excretion sometimes use timed urine collections, with albumin excretion expressed as mg/minute, mg/hour, or mg/24 hours. An alternative is to assay a single, early morning spot urine sample, followed by dividing the albumin concentration by the creatinine concentration (albumin/creatinine ratio).[2] Urine albumin measurements are made quantitatively by immunoassay and are specific to albumin.[3]

OVERVIEW OF LABORATORY TESTS

- Urine albumin concentration should be measured in patients with known chronic kidney disease (CKD) or those with risk factors for chronic kidney disease, including diabetes, hypertension, and lupus. Microalbumin (CPT code 82043) and creatinine (CPT code 82570) are needed to calculate the urine albumin to creatinine ratio (ACR). Microalbumin measurements alone can be performed on urine collected over an identified period of time, generating an estimate of albumin excretion over that period. Abnormal results should be followed up with an additional test, since urinary albumin excretion increases with variables such as exercise and postural changes. Testing for microalbumin can be done three ways[4]:
  - 24-hour urine collection with creatinine (CPT code 82570)
    - Able to measure creatinine clearance

■ Not done on regular basis because it is cumbersome and prone to inaccurate results due to over- and under-collection
■ Results are validated by quantifying the 24-hour urine creatinine excretion and comparing this to the expected urine creatinine
● Timed (4-hour or overnight) collection (CPT code 82043)
● Measurement of the ACR in a random spot urine sample (CPT codes 82570 and 84156) (preferred screening method)
■ This is easily obtained in the office.
■ Patients should not exercise within 24 hours of the test (vigorous exercise will cause a transient increase in microalbumin).
■ ACR can be elevated independent of kidney disease, so one should consider other causes (see the text that follows).

INDICATIONS

Screening

Microalbuminuria, as a marker of kidney damage, is an early sign of progressive cardiovascular disease and kidney disease in people with diabetes. Microalbuminuria is also a predictor of kidney disease progression and reflects the effect of diabetic kidney disease and other cardiovascular complications on the kidneys (Box 152.1).[5]

■ Universal screening is not recommended. At this time, the United States Preventive Services Task Force (USPSTF)[6] recommendations are inactive. Past recommendations opposed screening for CKD in asymptomatic adults without diagnosed CKD. The American College of Physcians[7] recommends against screening in those who are asymptomatic and without risk factors. However, the USPSTF suggest that there is minimal risk of screening people at risk for CKD. Individuals at risk of CKD (see Box 152.1) should be screened annually for CKD.[8]

Targeted screenings guidelines are as follows:

■ The 2020 International Society of Hypertension Global Hypertension Practice Guidelines[9] recommend screening for kidney disease in adults with hypertension by obtaining microalbumin and evaluating urinary ACR.

Box 152.1: Risk Factors for Chronic Kidney Disease

■ Diabetes mellitus*
■ Hypertension*
■ Cardiovascular disease
■ Family history of CKD
■ Hyperlipidemia
■ Obesity
■ Adults over age 70
■ Non-Hispanic Black adults

*Most common causes.

■ The International Society of Nephrology recommends screening those at highest risk, such as individuals with diabetes, hypertension, family history, and cardiovascular disease.[10]

■ The American Diabetes Association[11] and National Kidney Foundation KDOQI Clinical Practice Guidelines[12] recommend screening for proteinuria in all people with type 2 diabetes at the time of diagnosis and, if the urinalysis is negative for protein, to obtain microalbumin. For people with type 1 diabetes, screening should begin 5 years after the diagnosis. Individuals with diabetes should be screened annually for CKD that can be attributed to diabetic kidney disease.

■ The NIH Joint National Committee on Prevention, Detection, Evaluation, and Treatment of High Blood Pressure[13] recommends screening individuals with hypertension for kidney disease that includes ACR.

Diagnosis and Evaluation

■ The presence of persistent microalbuminuria is diagnostic for kidney damage. There is variability in urinary albumin excretion (varies throughout the day and from day to day), so two of three urine ACR results collected over a 3- to 6-month period of time must be abnormal in order to diagnosis microalbuminuria.[8]

■ Microalbuminuria has been proposed to be an acute phase reactant that increases with inflammation.[14]
  ● Ischemia
  ● Reperfusion
  ● Burns
  ● Sepsis
  ● Surgery

■ Other organic specific-inflammatory conditions[14–17]
  ● Peritonitis
  ● Obstructive respiratory disease
  ● Hepatitis
  ● Bowel diseases
  ● Pancreatitis
  ● Rheumatoid arthritis
  ● Psoriasis

■ In third-trimester pregnancies, the presence of microalbuminuria may indicate future sequelae of preeclampsia.[18]

Monitoring

■ When microalbuminuria is present, it is important to institute evidence-based measures to decrease the risks of cardio-metabolic complications and slow the progression of kidney disease.[5]

■ In people with diabetic kidney disease, it is essential to achieve glycemic control to slow the progression of CKD. Urinary ACR should be monitored on an annual basis.[8]

■ Patients with urinary albumin greater than 30 mg/g Cr and/or an eGFR less than 60 mL/min/1.73 m^2 should be monitored twice annually to guide therapy.[11]

INTERPRETATION

■ The normal albumin excretion rate (AER) is less than 30 mg/day, whereas persistent albumin secretion is between 30 and 300 mg/day (moderately increased albuminuria–microalbuminuria; Table 152.1).[4,14]

■ The immunoturbidimetric assay is reliable and has greater than 95% sensitivity and specificity to detect very low levels of albuminuria.[17]

■ Estimating a urine albumin with dipstick can result in false-positive and false-negative results because the urine albumin concentration is determined by the urine volume as well as albuminuria. This can be minimized by obtaining repeated measurements on early morning specimens.

● Obtaining a urinary ACR in an untimed urine specimen can reduce the risk of false-positive or false-negative results.

● There must be at least two of three specimens that are within the moderately increased or severely increased albuminuria range over a 3- to 6-month period of time to diagnosis with kidney disease.

● An elevated urinary ACR must be persistent for at least 3 months for diagnosis of moderate albuminuria (see Table 152.1).[15]

● Adults with hypertension and microalbuminuria at any time, baseline, and follow-up have a significant risk for cardiovascular events.[16]

FOLLOW-UP

■ Screening is affected by differences in laboratory methods, urine samples studied, and the definitions of microalbuminuria, which can lead to variable results, so it is important to follow-up with the same laboratory parameters each time.

■ If there is a positive test, it should be repeated twice within 3 to 6 months.

■ If two of the three tests are positive, then treatment should be started. Follow-up is not clear in those with nondiabetic kidney disease; recommendations for follow-up should be based on the patient's risk. For example, in someone with hypertension, testing could be done every 3 years depending on the risk for CKD and/or cardiovascular disease.[19]

PEARLS & PITFALLS

■ Micro- or macroalbuminuria should be distinguished from proteinuria, which is assessed by dipstick urine tests and semi-quantified as trace, 1+, 2+, 3+, or 4+.

TABLE 152.1: CATEGORIES OF PROGRESSIVE CHANGES IN ALBUMIN EXCRETION RATE AND ALBUMIN/CREATININE RATIO INDICATIVE OF KIDNEY DISEASE

MEASURE	NORMAL TO MILDLY INCREASED	MODERATELY INCREASED	SEVERELY INCREASED
AER mg/24 h	<30	30–300	>300
ACR mg/mmol m/g	<3	3–30	>30
	<30	30–300	>300

Source: Data from Levey AS, Inker LA, Coresh J. "Should the definition of CKD be changed to include age-adapted GFR criteria?" Con: the evaluation and management of CKD, not the definition, should be age-adapted. *Kidney Int.* 2020;97:37. doi:10.1016/j.kint .2019.08.032

- Urinary albumin excretion can be affected by hypertension or recent strenuous exercise, both of which increase its level.
- Adults who have abnormal levels of urinary albumin—for example, moderate microalbuminuria—have significant risk for all-cause mortality, cardiovascular disease, and long-term risk for CKD that can progress to end-stage kidney disease (ESKD).
- In adults with large muscle mass, in whom creatinine excretion may be higher than 1,000 mg/day, the urinary ACR will underestimate albuminuria.
- In an adult who is cachectic or has small muscle mass, in whom the creatinine excretion may be lower than 1,000 mg/day, the urinary ACR will overestimate albuminuria.
- One of the most important predictors of CKD progression, cardiovascular disease, and premature mortality is elevated albuminuria.[20]

PATIENT EDUCATION

- https://www.mayoclinic.org/tests-procedures/microalbumin/about/pac-20384640
- https://medlineplus.gov/lab-tests/microalbumin-creatinine-ratio/

RELATED DIAGNOSES AND ICD-10 CODES

Chronic kidney disease	N18
Chronic kidney disease, stage 1	N18.1
Chronic kidney disease, stage 2 (mild)	N18.2
Chronic kidney disease, stage 3 (moderate)	N18.3
Chronic kidney disease, stage 3 unspecified	N18.30
Chronic kidney disease, stage 3a	N18.31
Chronic kidney disease, stage 3b	N18.32
Chronic kidney disease, stage 4 (severe)	N18.4
Chronic kidney disease, stage 5	N18.5
End-stage renal disease	N18.6
Chronic kidney disease, unspecified	N18.9
Type 1 diabetes mellitus with diabetic chronic kidney disease	E10.22
Type 2 diabetes mellitus with diabetic chronic kidney disease	E11.22
Hypertensive chronic kidney disease with stage 1 through stage 4 chronic kidney disease	I12.9
Hypertensive heart and chronic kidney disease with stage 5 chronic kidney disease or end-stage renal disease	I12.0
Hypertensive heart and chronic kidney disease without heart failure, with stage 1 through stage 4 chronic kidney disease, or unspecified chronic kidney disease	I13.10

| Preexisting hypertensive chronic kidney disease complicating childbirth | O10.22 |
| Unspecified preeclampsia, unspecified trimester | O14.90 |

REFERENCES

Full list of references can be accessed through Springer Publishing Company Connect™ at the following link: http://connect.springerpub.com/content/reference-book/ 978-0-8261-8843-4/part/part03/toc-part/ch152

---

153. URINE CREATININE CLEARANCE

Joelle D. Hargraves and Kelly Small Casler

PHYSIOLOGY REVIEW

The prevalence of chronic kidney disease (CKD), defined as abnormalities of structure or function of the kidneys for 3 months or longer, is approximately 14% in the United States.[1-3] Criteria used to determine CKD are glomerular filtration rate (GFR) of less than 60 mL/min/1.73 m^2 and/or one or more markers of kidney damage such as albuminuria, structural/histologic abnormalities, urine sediment abnormalities, tubular disorders, or kidney transplantation.[1-6] Risk factors for CKD include diabetes, hypertension, and family history.[1] The National Institute of Diabetes and Digestive and Kidney Diseases reports that approximately 468,000 have end-stage kidney disease (ESKD) requiring dialysis.[1] Black individuals are at a 3.7 times higher risk for developing ESKD while Asian Americans and Native Americans are approximately 1.5 times more likely compared to Caucasians.[1]

OVERVIEW OF LABORATORY TESTS

The National Kidney Foundation affirms that the best overall measure of kidney function is GFR.[7-10] While the National Kidney Foundation has deemed measurement of an exogenous filtration marker (e.g., clearance of insulin following injection) as the gold standard for measuring GFR, it is generally not done due to complexity and expense.[2,9] Therefore, methods to estimate GFR have been developed. Measured creatinine clearance (CrCl) is one such method. Creatinine is a waste product excreted by the kidneys.[7-9] The CrCl by 24-hour timed urine collection (CPT code 003004) reflects the volume of blood plasma cleared of creatinine over time.[2,7-9] For the test, a urine creatinine level and serum creatinine (CPT code 82565) level are compared using the formula that follows. The result is reported in mL/minute for a standard adult body surface area (1.73 m^2).[10]

$$\text{Creatinine Clearance} = \frac{(\text{urine creatinine} \times \text{total urine volume})}{(\text{plasma creatinine} \times \text{time})}$$

CrCl can also be estimated (sometimes referred to as predicted) (eCrCl) using the Cockcroft-Gault (CG) calculation that follows.

$$\text{CrCl (male)} = ([140 - \text{age}] \times \text{weight in kg})/(\text{serum creatinine} \times 72)$$
$$\text{CrCl (female)} = \text{CrCl (male)} \times 0.85$$

Limitations of the calculation should be considered including that it was developed with limited sample diversity (Caucasian men) and prior to standardization of creatinine measurement by laboratories.[11] Additionally, the calculation can overestimate measured CrCl.[12] Therefore, the relevance of its use to clinical practice is controversial.[13] Additionally, multiple modifications to the original CG calculation result in confusion surrounding the best way to estimate CrCl. It can be calculated using ideal body weight, total body weight, adjusted body weight, or without body weight.[14,15] There is disagreement as to which is better, with a meta-analysis finding that calculation using no body weight more closely estimated CrCl[15] while some authorities suggest that any method is acceptable.[19] Finally, because eCrCl uses creatinine, it will be inaccurate in patients with physiologic variation in creatinine (extremes of muscle mass, vegetarian or high-protein diet, extremes of age, malnutrition or obesity, skeletal muscle disease, paraplegia, quadriplegia, limb amputation, and pregnancy).

INDICATIONS

Screening and Diagnosis and Evaluation

■ When eGFR based on serum creatinine is suspected to be inaccurate, measured CrCl is an alternative method to estimate GFR and screen for or diagnose impairment of kidney function.[3,5] It is also the preferred method to estimate GFR in special circumstances (evaluation for kidney organ donation or monitoring drugs with significant nephrotoxicity or narrow therapeutic indices).[2]

Monitoring

■ eCrCl or measured CrCl are used to monitor renal function or guide dosing decisions during pharmacotherapy with renally excreted medications.[16-19]

INTERPRETATION

■ The normal range for CrCl varies by gender.[10] Adjustment for BSA is needed for pediatric patients.[10]
Male: 85 to 125 mL/min
Female: 75 to 115 mL/min
■ Reduced CrCl is associated with kidney impairment and can be seen in a variety of conditions summarized in Box 153.1.[16] Increased CrCl (hyperfiltration) is seen in diabetes mellitus (early stage), pregnancy, high cardiac output, infection, large dietary protein intake, plasma volume expansion, and exercise.

FOLLOW-UP

■ Urine albumin levels and urine albumin-to-creatine ratios are necessary to fully evaluate a patient with reduced CrCl and determine the severity of kidney impairment.[3-6]

Box 153.1: Differential Diagnoses for Reduced Creatinine Clearance

■ Acute kidney injury
■ Chronic kidney disease
■ Diabetic nephropathy
■ Interstitial nephritis
■ Lupus nephritis
■ Multiple myeloma
■ Nephrolithiasis
■ Nephrotic syndrome
■ Polycystic kidney disease
■ Preeclampsia
■ Urinary obstruction

Sources: Data from Chen TK, Knicely DH, Grams ME. Chronic kidney disease diagnosis and management: a review. *JAMA.* 2019;322(13):1294–1304. doi:10.1001/jama.2019.14745; Inker LA, Astor BC, Fox CH, et al. KDOQI US commentary on the 2012 KDIGO clinical practice guideline for the evaluation and management of CKD. *Am J Kidney Dis.* 2014;63(5):713–735. doi:10.1053/j.ajkd.2014.01.416; Johns Hopkins Medicine. *24-Hour Urine Collection.* https://www.hopkinsmedicine.org/health/treatment-tests-and-therapies/24hour-urine-collection#:~:text=All%20urine%2C%20after%20the%20first,this%20time%2C%20it%20is%20OK; Kidney Disease Improving Global Outcomes (KDIGO) CKD Work Group. KDIGO 2012 clinical practice guideline for the evaluation and management of chronic kidney disease. *Kidney Int Suppl.* 2013;3:1–150. https://kdigo.org/wpcontent/uploads/2017/02/KDIGO_2012_CKD_GL.pdf; National Institute of Diabetes and Digestive and Kidney Diseases. *Frequently Asked Questions eGFR.* https://www.niddk.nih.gov/health-information/professionals/clinical-tools-patient-management/kidney-disease/laboratory-evaluation/frequently-asked-questions; National Kidney Foundation. *Frequently Asked Questions About GFR Estimates.* https://www.kidney.org/sites/default/files/12-10-4004_FAQ-ABE.pdf; Nicoll D, Mark Lu C, McPhee SJ. Lab tests, Creatinine Clearance. In: Nicoll D, Mark Lu C, McPhee SJ, eds. *Guide to Diagnostic Tests.* 7th ed. McGraw-Hill; 2017; Shahbaz H, Gupta M. Creatinine clearance. In: *StatPearls.* StatPearls Publishing; 2021. https://www.ncbi.nlm.nih.gov/books/NBK544228/; Vassalotti JA, Centor R, Turner BJ, Greer RC, Choi M, Sequist TD. Practical approach to detection and management of chronic kidney disease for the primary care clinician. *Am J Med.* 2016;129(2):153. doi:10.1016/j.amjmed.2015.08.025

■ Other follow-up tests will be based on both the differential diagnoses for kidney impairment etiology and any underlying chronic diseases that can further impair kidney function (diabetes).

PEARLS & PITFALLS

■ Medication dosing guidelines for renally excreted medications make recommendations based on measured or estimated CrCl, since these methods are used in pharmacokinetic research during medication development.[17–19]
■ eGFR can be used instead of CrCl to guide medication dosing. For patients with extremes of BSA or body weight, first determine eGFR and then convert to eCrCl by multiplying by the quotient of the patient's BSA (in m^2)/1.73 m^2.[12,18,19]
■ In patients with unstable kidney function (critical illness) or physiologic states that can make creatinine inaccurate, order a measured CrCl rather than estimated CrCl. This is especially important when using medications with narrow therapeutic indices or high risk of nephrotoxicity.[12,19]
■ CrCl overestimates measured GFR by 10% to 20% since total urinary creatinine includes not only creatinine that is filtered by the glomerulus but also creatinine that is secreted from the proximal/distal tubules (approximately 15%).[2,8–10,20,21]

Box 153.2: 24-Hour Urine Collection Instructions

1. Obtain plastic container(s) from the laboratory performing the study.
2. Void and flush the commode as the bladder must be empty prior to starting urine collection.
3. Document the start date and time the urine collection commenced (immediately after voiding).
4. Collect urine in a urinal toilet hat, urinal, or bedpan for specimen collection. Do not put toilet paper in the collection device.
5. Collect all urine including any mixed with stool over the next 24 hours.
6. Carefully transfer urine into the plastic container. Follow laboratory-specific directions regarding storage (e.g., room temperature versus placing the container in a basin or cooler filled with ice).
7. Note the d ate and time when urine collection finished.
8. Transport the plastic container(s) to the laboratory for processing.

- To determine safe pharmaceutical doses for transgender patients on gender-affirming hormone therapy for 6 months or longer, use CrCl reference intervals based on gender identity. Drug dosing for transgender patients not on gender-affirming hormone therapy or using it for less than 6 months should be based on sex at birth.[22,23]
- Because transgender patients have not been included in studies regarding the accuracy of calculations for eGFR or eCrCl, clinicians should consider the imprecisions of estimates in these patients. It may be beneficial to calculate estimates using the calculations for both males and females and determine a range that reflects the potential eCrCl for the patient. Alternatively, measuring CrCl will also provide clear information[22,23]
- Monitoring creatinine alone without using it to estimate GFR may result in over- or underestimation of kidney function.[2,3,7-9]
- Collection of urine for 24 hours is often inconvenient and associated with collection errors resulting in inaccurate results.[2,9] To improve accuracy of CrCl, the patient and caregivers must understand key concepts including that the bladder must be empty prior to starting urine collection (Box 153.2).[9,16,24]

PATIENT EDUCATION

- https://www.nationwidechildrens.org/family-resources-education/health
-wellness-and-safety-resources/helping-hands/24-hour-urine-specimen
-collection-guidelines

RELATED DIAGNOSES AND ICD-10 CODES

Abnormal results of kidney function studies	R94.4

REFERENCES

Full list of references can be accessed through Springer Publishing Company Connect™
at the following link: http://connect.springerpub.com/content/reference-book/
978-0-8261-8843-4/part/part03/toc-part/ch153

154. URINE CULTURE AND SENSITIVITY

Joan E. Zaccardi and Kelly Small Casler

PATHOPHYSIOLOGY REVIEW

Bacteriuria refers to the presence of bacteria in urine, which is normally sterile. Asymptomatic bacteriuria (ASB) is the presence of a bacteria colony count in the urine that would usually be consistent with infection, without presentation of local or systemic signs and symptoms. When bacteriuria causes symptoms, urinary tract infection (UTI) is diagnosed. UTIs that are localized to the bladder are termed "cystitis," while those that ascend to the kidneys are termed "pyelonephritis."[1,2]

UTIs are one of the most common bacterial infections encountered by clinicians. Frequency, urgency, dysuria, suprapubic pressure or pain, and hematuria are the most common signs and symptoms of UTI and diagnosis can often be made by history alone.[1-3] Uropathogenic *Escherichia coli* (UPEC, aka. *E. coli*) is a bacterium normally found in the bowel and is responsible for the majority (75%) of uncomplicated UTIs. Other common causative pathogens are identified in Box 154.1.[3] In complicated UTI, the prevalent bacteria is *E. coli* (65%), followed by *Enterococcus faecalis* (11%) *K. Pneumoniae* (8%), and *Candida* spp (7%).[4]

OVERVIEW OF LABORATORY TESTS

Urine culture (CPT code 87086) and sensitivity (CPT codes 87184 or 87186) (Urine C&S) is a laboratory test used to complement diagnosis of UTIs and guide antibiotic treatment plans.[1-8] They are usually completed after a history, physical examination, and urinalysis lead a clinician to suspect UTI.[1] Urine C&S is considered the gold standard in diagnosing UTIs but is costly, and waiting 3 to 5 days for results can delay treatment.[4-6] Therefore, many UTIs are treated after history and physical examination and urinalysis alone. However, urine culture is indicated if the diagnosis is unclear or if the patient is at risk for complicated UTI (Table 154.1).[9-11]

Box 154.1: Common Causative Pathogens of Uncomplicated Urinary Tract Infection

- *Escherichia coli (75%)*
- *Klebsiella (K.) pneumoniae (6%)*
- *Staphylococcus (S.) saprophyticus (6%)*
- *Enterococcus faecalis (5%)*
- *Group B Streptococcus (GBS) (3%)*
- *Proteus (P.) mirabilis (2%),*
- *Staphylococcus (S) aureus (1%),*
- *Candida* spp *(1%).*

TABLE 154.1: INTERPRETATION OF URINE CULTURE AND SENSITIVITY	
OBTAINED BY:	**COLONY COUNT THRESHOLD FOR POSITIVE***
Catheterization	≥50,000 CFUs/mL
Clean catch	≥100,000 (10⁵) CFUs/mL
Suprapubic aspiration	≥1,000 (10³) CFUs/mL

*Diagnosis of urinary tract infection (UTI) can still be made when counts are less than these thresholds if signs and symptoms are consistent with UTI and there is a single pathogen.

ASB, asymptomatic bacteria; CFUs/mL, colony-forming units per mililiter.

Sources: Data from Mattoo TK, Shaikh N, Nelson CP. Contemporary management of urinary tract infection in children. *Pediatrics.* 2021;147(2):e2020012138. doi:10.1542/peds.2020-012138; Nicolle LE, Gupta K, Bradley SF, et al. Clinical practice guideline for the management of asymptomatic bacteriuria: 2019 update by the infectious Diseases Society of America. *Clin Infect Dis.* 2019;68(10):e83–e110. doi:10.1093/cid/ciy1121; Roberts KB, Wald ER. The diagnosis of UTI: colony count criteria revisited. *Pediatrics.* 2018;141(2):e20173239. doi:10.1542/peds.2017-3239

If bacteria are identified in the culture sample, the amount of growth is quantified with a colony count. Sensitivity testing against a standard profile of antibiotics is also performed. Sensitivity of the bacteria to each antibiotic is rated as susceptible, intermediate, or resistant depending on the lowest concentration (in ug/ml) of an antibiotic that inhibits the growth of the bacteria.[1, 8-11]

Urine samples for C&S can be obtained at the same time a sample for urinalysis is collected. Collection techniques will vary depending on the patient situation. In noncatheterized patients, a midstream voided urine (voiding first in toilet and then in container) is the preferred way to collect the specimen and avoids contamination.[1-4,7] There is insufficient evidence to recommend for or against peri-urethral cleansing prior to midstream collection in adults, but it is recommended for children.[8] Children can sit backwards on the toilet to help separate the labia.[9] Sterile urine bags or diaper collection of urine is not recommended, and therefore non-toilet trained children may require catheterization or suprapubic bladder aspiration.[8,9] To obtain a urine sample aseptically from an indwelling catheter, clean the needless port and aspirate the urine from the port with a sterile syringe.[6]

INDICATIONS

Screening

- The United States Preventive Services Task Force (USPSTF) recommends screening for ASB using Urine C&S in pregnant people at 12 to 16 weeks' gestation.[12]
- The Infectious Diseases Society of America and American Society for Microbiology recommend screening for ASB with Urine C&S prior to undergoing urologic surgery.[10,13]
- The American College of Obstetricians and Gynecologists, Society for Post-Acute and Long-Term Care Medicine, and USPSTF recommend against screening for asymptomatic bacteria with Urine C&S in nonpregnant people of any age.[6,12,14]

The American Academy of Pediatrics recommends that febrile children ages 2 to 24 months without identified sources for infection should be screened for UTI using Urine C&S.[9]

Diagnosis and Evaluation

■ Urine C&S is used to complement the diagnosis of UTI in patients with dysuria, suprapubic pain/tenderness, urinary frequency, urgency, and/or gross hematuria. However, Urine C&S is not needed in all cases of suspected UTI. Diagnosis can be made with history, physical, and dipstick urinalysis alone; in some instances, a urinalysis may not even be required.[15]
Patients who should have Urine C&S as part of the diagnostic workup of UTI include pediatric patients[9] and those with risk factors for complicated UTI (Box 154.2).

Monitoring

■ Urine C&S is not used for monitoring in pediatric or adult conditions.[6,9]

INTERPRETATION

■ Urine C&S is considered positive depending on the number of colonies that grow (Table 154.1).
■ A culture showing multiple/mixed pathogens is suspicious for contamination.[4-8]

FOLLOW-UP

■ If symptoms persist for 3 or more days after treatment with antibiotics, follow-up testing with another clean, midstream Urine C&S is warranted.[4-6]
■ Diagnostic imaging studies may be needed for those with a complicated UTI, structural abnormalities of the urinary tract, history of trauma or surgery in the area, recurrent infections, or unresolved infection after

---

Box 154.2: Risk Factors for a Complicated Urinary Tract Infection

■ Anatomical/structural abnormalities of the urinary tract
■ Diabetes mellitus
■ Immunocompromise (HIV/AIDS, immunosuppressive medication use)
■ Older age
■ Patient with indwelling catheters or intermittent catheterization use
■ Pregnancy
■ Pre- or post-surgery/procedure of the urinary tract
■ Prior history of recurrent, resistant, or complicated UTI
■ Suspected sepsis
■ Symptoms suggestive of pyelonephritis (fever or flank pain)

Sources: Data from Hanno PM. Lower urinary tract infections in women and pyelonephritis. In: Hanno PM, Guzzo TJ, Malkowicz SB, Wein AJ, eds. *Penn Clinical Manual of Urology.* 2nd ed. Saunders/Elsevier; 2014:110–132.; Mayne S, Bowden A, Sundvall P-D, Gunnarsson R. The scientific evidence for a potential link between confusion and urinary tract infection in the elderly is still confusing—a systematic literature review. *BMC Geriatr.* 2019;19(1):32. doi:10.1186/s12877-019-1049-7; Yang B, Foley S. Presentation and diagnosis. In: Yang B, Foley S, eds. *Female Urinary Tract Infections in Clinical Practice.* Springer; 2020:11–16. doi:10.1007/978-3-030-27909-7

treatment with antibiotics.[1-3,7,16,17] Studies that may be performed include ultrasound, CT urography, MRI, urodynamic evaluation, or cystoscopy.
- Those with recurrent UTIs may need urology referral.

PEARLS & PITFALLS

- Recent antibiotic use may mask the presence of pathogens in a urine C&S.
- Other factors such as the use of diuretics or consumption of large amounts of fluid can interfere with results of a urine C&S by decreasing the number of bacteria present in the specimen.
- Results can also be affected by faulty collection techniques and/or handling errors, causing contamination of the specimen. Samples must be refrigerated after collection.[8,14,18]
- Some laboratories will automatically order a Urine C&S on urinalysis specimens that test positive for nitrites.
- In primary care patients without risk factors for complicated UTI, some studies have found that the method of urine sample collection does not matter. Midstream collections with and without cleansing and random urine samples all had similar contamination rates.[19,20]
- UTIs are seen more often in patients with a vagina compared to patients with a penis. Patients with a vagina have a short urethra that is conducive to invasion of ascending bacteria from the urogenital area.[1,2,7]
- Beware of false-negative risk with Urine C&S. Some laboratories will not report growth on cultures if there is less than 10^4 colony counts despite studies that document the occurrence of UTI even in the presence of 10^2 CFU/mL.[15]
- Patients with a prostate do not usually experience UTI until after age 50 when prostate enlargement and outlet obstruction become an issue.[3]
- Patients with spinal cord injury may have alternate symptoms of UTI: autonomic dysreflexia and uneasiness.[21]
- False negatives are commonly seen in urine cultures in patients with chronic prostatitis.[22-24]

PATIENT EDUCATION

- https://labtestsonline.org/tests/urine-culture

RELATED DIAGNOSES AND ICD-10 CODES

Urinary tract infection	N39.0 (site not specified)
Acute cystitis	N30.0
• With hematuria	N30.01
• Without hematuria	N30.00
Other chronic cystitis without hematuria	N30.20
Interstitial cystitis	N30.1
Recurrent UTI (other chronic cystitis without hematuria)	N30.20
Personal history of urinary tract infections	Z87.440

REFERENCES

Full list of references can be accessed through Springer Publishing Company Connect™ at the following link: http://connect.springerpub.com/content/reference-book/ 978-0-8261-8843-4/part/part03/toc-part/ch154

---

155. URINE CYTOLOGY

Rebecca Hunt

PATHOPHYSIOLOGY REVIEW

In the United States, bladder cancer is the fourth most common cancer diagnosis for men and tenth most common cancer diagnosis for women.[1] The development of bladder cancer can be due to genetic disorders, molecular changes, and environmental exposures, most notably smoking.[2] Bladder cancer is diagnosed most often after a person develops unexplained hematuria. Diagnosis is most commonly made through cystoscopy, CT imaging, and urine cytology.[3] Urine cytology not only aids in diagnosis but is useful in surveillance for bladder cancer recurrence.[4]

OVERVIEW OF LABORATORY TESTS

Urine cytology is the most well-established bladder cancer biomarker available (CPT core 88108). Urine cytology is not a laboratory test, but rather a microscopic evaluation of urine for exfoliated cells.[4] A positive test is determined to be positive by a cytopathologist (determining a positive test is not the job of the ordering provider). The test is completed by collecting a urine sample, which is then evaluated by cytopathology after the sample is smeared onto a slide. Many of the features that are present in cancer are subjective, which leads to a wide variety of interpretations and a lack of consistency. Consequently, the accuracy of cytology can vary among pathologists.[4] Cytology interpretation includes a variety of possible results including, but not limited to, atypical, atypical-suspicious, and nondiagnostic. The Paris System for Reporting Urine Cytology (PSRUC) was developed in recent years in an effort to standardize interpretations or urine cytology.

Urine cytology has a varying level of sensitivity. Despite this, it is a highly specific test. According to a 2016 systemic review, urine cytology sensitivity is on average 40% and the specificity is greater than 90%.[5] As a result, urine cytology has a role in aiding in the diagnosis of bladder cancer but is not recommended for primary screening or diagnosis.

INDICATIONS

Screening
- Urine cytology has not proven to provide the sensitivity and specificity necessary to be clinically beneficial for universal screening.[6]

Diagnosis and Evaluation

■ Urine cytology is used in the differential diagnosis of hematuria to detect neoplastic cells in the urine that might be a sign of nonmuscle-invasive bladder cancer or muscle-invasive bladder cancer. Urine cytology is used along with cystoscopy and CT urogram in the diagnostic process.[6]

Monitoring

■ Urine cytology is used with cystoscopy for surveillance after bladder cancer treatments every 6 months for 2 years. After 2 years, the recommendation is to complete cytology and cystoscopy annually thereafter.[6]

INTERPRETATION

■ Interpretation of the most common urine cytology findings are illustrated in Table 155.1.[8–10]
■ High grade urothelial carcinoma (HGUC) should be suspected when[7]:
  ● At least 5 to 10 abnormal cells
  ● Large nuclei (nucleus occupies more than 70% of the cytoplasm)
  ● Moderate to severe hyperchromatic nuclei
  ● Marked irregular nuclear membrane
  ● Coarse/clumped chromatin

FOLLOW-UP

■ Table 155.2 reviews the follow-up for abnormal results.[8–10]

PEARLS & PITFALLS

■ Urine cytology should not be used alone to evaluate for bladder cancer.

PATIENT EDUCATION

■ https://www.cancer.org/cancer/bladder-cancer.html

TABLE 155.1: INTERPRETATION OF URINE CYTOLOGY RESULTS

REPORTED FINDING	RISK OF MALIGNANCY %
Unsatisfactory/nondiagnostic	<5% to 10%
Negative for malignancy	5% to 10%
Atypical urothelial cells	8% to 35%
Suspicious for high grade urothelial neoplasm	50% to 90%
Low grade urothelial neoplasm	10%
High grade urothelial carcinoma	>90%

TABLE 155.2: FOLLOW-UP TESTING	
CYTOLOGY INTERPRETATION	**CLINICAL STEPS**
Unsatisfactory/nondiagnostic	Repeat cytology in 3 months. If high clinical suspicion, consider cytology and cystoscopy.
Negative for malignancy	Follow clinically as needed
Atypical urothelial cells	Follow clinically as needed. Consider use of ancillary testing based on suspicion level
Suspicious for high grade urothelial neoplasm	More aggressive follow-up, cystoscopy, biopsy
Low grade urothelial neoplasm	More aggressive follow-up, cystoscopy, biopsy
High grade urothelial carcinoma	More aggressive follow-up, cystoscopy, biopsy

RELATED DIAGNOSES AND ICD-10 CODES

Malignant neoplasm of trigone of bladder	C67.0
Malignant neoplasm of dome of bladder	C67.1
Malignant neoplasm of lateral wall of bladder	C67.2
Malignant neoplasm of anterior wall of bladder	C67.3
Malignant neoplasm of posterior wall of bladder	C67.4
Malignant neoplasm of bladder neck	C67.5

REFERENCES

Full list of references can be accessed through Springer Publishing Company Connect™ at the following link: http://connect.springerpub.com/content/reference-book/978-0-8261-8843-4/part/part03/toc-part/ch155

156. URINE DRUG SCREEN/TEST

Dayna Jaynstein

PATHOPHYSIOLOGY REVIEW

Many drugs are eliminated in urine through renal excretion. The speed and extent to which drugs are eliminated renally is influenced by several factors including water solubility and protein-binding properties of the drug, urine acidity, and kidney function.

OVERVIEW OF LABORATORY TESTS

Urine drug testing (UDT) is commonly utilized in multiple clinical scenarios including evaluation of altered mental status, identification of substance use disorders, confirmation of sobriety, and for medication adherence. UDTs may be offered as "panels" which indicate how many substances the test examines for. A five-panel UDT (frequently referred to as the "Federal Five" secondary to its use in government job screening) is the most commonly used UDT and tests for the presence of amphetamines, cannabinoids, cocaine, opiates, and phencyclidine (PCP).[1] Additional substances frequently tested for include benzodiazepines, barbiturates, and methadone.

UDTs are a screening tool. They do not quantify the amount of a substance present; rather, they tell you if a substance is present at all.[2] This inherently makes UDTs highly sensitive, but nonspecific. Further, individual patient metabolism and pharmacodynamics can significantly affect UDTs. While once considered a routine part of many patient evaluations, there continues to be significant professional and societal debate as to the utility of UDTs. Clinicians should have clear understanding as to when a UDT should be ordered and fully understand the limitations associated with UDT.

There are two main types of UDTs: immunoassay and gas chromatography-mass spectrometry (GC-MS).[3] Immunoassay testing, which uses antibodies to detect the presence of drugs or metabolites, is the most common form of testing and considered the initial test in clinical practice.[1,3] While immunoassay testing is relatively easy to obtain, cheap, and highly sensitive, immunoassay UDTs lack specificity and can result in frequent false positives and false negatives, which will then require secondary confirmation testing.[1] In clinical practice, the standard UDT order is for an immunoassay test. GC-MS is considered a confirmatory test rather than an initial screening test and is often ordered after a positive result has been obtained on immunoassay testing.

Drug testing can be obtained from urine, blood, hair, sweat, saliva, and nails, with urine being the most commonly used.[3] Blood samples tend to show substances much sooner after ingestion than urine testing.[3] UDT can be performed as a point-of-care test or done within the laboratory and takes less than an hour to result. Typically, a minimum of 30 mLs of urine is needed and many processes and evaluation procedures exist to verify normal urine characteristics and discourage tampered specimens.[1]

Standard reference ranges vary by test and further deviate based on what the UDT is being used to evaluate. For example, UDTs used by employers typically have lower cutoff values than tests used in clinical practice. Clinicians must understand that these reference ranges can vary significantly, and it is possible for patients to be positive on one test and negative on another. Further, many tests have high false-positive rates. In one of the most comprehensive analyses of the positive predictive value (PPV) of UDTs, PPV was 100% for cannabinoids, 100% for cocaine, 86.8% for opiates, 74.6% for benzodiazepines, and 9.3% for amphetamines.[4]

Amphetamines

Amphetamine assays are the most difficult to interpret. Most amphetamine assays are created to detect amphetamine, dextroamphetamine, methamphetamine, methylenedioxyethylamphetamine, methylenedioxyamphetamine, and methylenedioxymethylamphetamine (MDMA). However, there are numerous other substances, many commonly prescribed medications, that can lead to a false-positive, including amantadine, bupropion, labetalol, phentermine, phenylephrine, promethazine, pseudoephedrine, ranitidine, and trazodone.[3] Clinicians should make sure they assess all medications the patient is on when interpreting the results. Further, clinicians should be aware that methylphenidate is not detected by the amphetamine immunoassay and the assay has a low overall sensitivity (50%) in detecting MDMA.[3]

Benzodiazepines

Benzodiazepines are commonly prescribed medications and clinicians must consider normal pharmacologic use versus abuse when interpreting UDTs. Benzodiazepine assays will not differentiate between single-use and long-standing use, abuse, or dependence.[3] Overall, there are a few agents that produce false positives or false negatives on benzodiazepine screen. Sertraline and oxaprozin can cause false positives, while some benzodiazepine assays may not detect midazolam, chlordiazepoxide, flunitrazepam, alprazolam, lorazepam, and clonazepam.[3,5]

Cannabinoids

Secondary to being highly lipophilic, tetrahydrocannabinol (THC) and its metabolites are slowly released into the urine. Therefore, a UDT can be positive up to 1 week after a single use, and long-term use can produce a positive result more than 30 days after last use.[3] False positives are fairly rare but can be seen from efavirenz and proton-pump inhibitors. It is highly unlikely for a UDT to be positive from occasional passive inhalation of THC or ingestion of hemp-containing foods such as tea and oil.[3] Adding Visine to urine samples has led to false-negative results on immunoassay testing but does not interfere with GS-MS testing.[3]

Cocaine

UDTs have a high predictive value for cocaine ingestion. False positives are nearly non-existent on cocaine screening UDTs.[3] A few case studies have suggested that coca plant leaves (such as those used in teas) can produce a false positive, but this is debated. Children exposed to secondhand smoke from crack cocaine can have a positive screen as well.[3]

Opioids

UDTs used for opioid screening typically test for the metabolites of heroin and codeine (mainly morphine).[1,3] Clinicians must have a solid understanding of the limitations of opioid UDTs. Most opioid UDTs do not screen for fentanyl, oxycodone, or methadone.[3] Opioid immunoassays do not differentiate between opiates; therefore, GS-MS may be necessary to definitively screen for heroin. Ingestion of moderate amounts of poppy seeds, dextromethorphan, diphenhydramine, quinine, fluroquinolones, rifampin, and verapamil can lead to false-positive results.[3]

Phencyclidine

Phencyclidine, or PCP, was initially introduced as an anesthetic in the 1950s. While it has been discontinued for human use, PCP is still used within veterinary medicine and can be laced with other drugs.[3] Several medications can lead to a false-positive result including dextromethorphan, diphenhydramine, doxylamine, ibuprofen, ketamine, meperidine, tramadol, and venlafaxine.[3]

INDICATIONS

Screening

- Universal screening is not endorsed by any organization.
- Guidelines from the CDC and American Pain Society recommend periodic UDTs for adherence to treatment but leave the frequency of testing up to individual providers.[6,7]

Diagnosis and Evaluation

- UDT can be used in the evaluation of acutely altered patients or those suffering from coma, seizures, agitation, delirium, and psychosis.[2]
- UDT can be used to evaluate for medication compliance and sobriety.

Monitoring

- The 2018 CDC Guideline for Prescribing Opioids for Chronic Pain recommends clinicians can use UDTs prior to initiating opioid therapy and monitoring UDTs annually to assess that prescribed medications are being used and illicit drugs are not.[8]

INTERPRETATION

- Each test has a minimum threshold level. A sample must surpass that threshold level in order for the test to demonstrate a positive. UDTs used within clinical practice tend to have slightly higher threshold levels than those used in employment screening.[1]
- Clinicians should be familiar with the detection windows for each substance (Table 156.1).[1,3]

FOLLOW-UP

- Positive results on an immunoassay test may require confirmatory testing via GC-MS.
- Many drug-specific assays exist to further characterize a positive result. For example, it can be difficult to assess a patient who is being prescribed hydrocodone for concurrent heroin use; therefore, a specific heroin assay test exists.

PEARLS & PITFALLS

- A typical five-panel UDT only tests for amphetamines, cannabinoids, cocaine, opiates, and PCP.

TABLE 156.1: TIME URINE DRUG TESTING WILL STAY POSITIVE AFTER INGESTION OF SUBSTANCE	
SUBSTANCE	**TIME UDT WILL STAY POSITIVE AFTER INGESTION**
Amphetamines	48 hours
Barbiturates:	
Short-acting	24 hours
Long-acting	3 weeks
Benzodiazepines:	
Short-acting	48 hours
Long-acting	10 to 30 days
Cannabinoids:	
Single use	3 days
Moderate use	5 to 7 days
Daily use	10 to 14 days
Chronic, heavy use	Over 30 days
Cocaine	2 to 4 days
Opioids:	
Codeine	48 hours
Heroin (morphine)	48 hours
Hydrocodone	2 to 3 days
Hydromorphone	2 to 3 days
Methadone	3 to 5 days
Oxycodone	2 to 4 days
Phencyclidine	8 days

■ Typical opioid drug screens only test for nonsynthetic opioids which excludes buprenorphine, fentanyl, methadone, oxycodone, and oxymorphone.

■ High false-positive rates can be seen on many assays. Clinicians should review the patient's other medications for causes of false positives and obtain confirmatory testing if results are questionable.

■ A study conducted within 141 VA facilities evaluated outcomes after increasing UDT. They found that "higher levels of urine drug screening (UDS) implementation from 2010-2013 were associated with lower risk of suicide and drug overdose events."[9]

■ Results may differ based on the test's threshold levels. For example, a patient may test negative on one UDT and positive on a UDT that has lower threshold levels.

■ Occasional passive inhalation of THC does not surpass threshold levels to have a positive UDT.[1,3,5]

■ Poppy seed ingestion can lead to a positive opiate test. Casual ingestion does not appear to cause a positive, but moderate or regular ingestion does.[3,5]

- UTDs do not provide information on length of time from use, amount used, and current intoxication level.[3]
- The time for a UDT to become positive after screening can vary by tests or may not even be known. This is a significant limitation, especially in the evaluation of an acutely intoxicated patient. Clinicians may opt to order a serum level over a urine test in these situations.
  - PCP UDTs become positive 8 hours after ingestion.[3]
  - Highly lipophilic benzodiazepines, such as diazepam, cannot be detected in the urine until 36 hours after ingestion.[3]

PATIENT EDUCATION

- https://www.SAMHSA.gov
- https://www.CDC.gov

RELATED DIAGNOSES AND ICD-10 CODES

Substance abuse	F19.10
Opioid abuse, uncomplicated	F11.10
Other stimulant abuse, uncomplicated	F15.10

REFERENCES

Full list of references can be accessed through Springer Publishing Company Connect™ at the following link: http://connect.springerpub.com/content/reference-book/ 978-0-8261-8843-4/part/part03/toc-part/ch156

157. URINE OSMOLALITY

Meleana Burt

PHYSIOLOGY REVIEW

Osmolality is a key mechanism in fluid homeostasis since fluid normally moves from areas of low osmolality to high osmolality. Osmolality is monitored and adjusted by the endocrine and renal system. For example, in response to vasopressin (also called antidiuretic hormone), collecting ducts in the kidneys increase water reabsorption, leading to increased urine osmolality. Measurement of urine osmolality can assist in the diagnosis of certain conditions. For example, syndrome of inappropriate antidiuretic hormone (SIADH) results from excess vasopressin causing higher-than-normal levels of urine osmolality. Conversely, diabetes insipidus, where vasopressin production is hampered, can result in decreased urine osmolality.

OVERVIEW OF LABORATORY TESTS

Laboratory evaluation of urine osmolality (CPT code 83935) can be assessed by ordering a random clean catch urine sample. The amount of urine needed for the collection is 0.5 to 2 mL. Urine osmolality is a measurement of urine concentration or dissolved particles in the urine. It is a good indicator of the kidney's ability to dilute or concentrate the urine and maintain water balance of the extracellular fluid.[1] Urine osmolality is the main regulator of the antidiuretic hormone in the body, which helps to maintain water balance during fluctuations of fluid intake and loss.[2,3]

Osmolarity and osmolality are often used interchangeably since both reflect the amount of particles dissolved in a certain amount of water.[3] Osmolarity is a measurement of the number of moles of a solute in a liter of solution while osmolality is a measurement of the number of moles of a solute in a kilogram of solution.[3] Osmolality is the preferred term.

Older adult patients will have a lower maximum osmolality due to age-related reductions in the kidney's ability to concentrate the urine.[4] For each year beyond the age of 20, the upper range of osmolality decreases about 5 mOsm/kg.[1]

INDICATIONS

Screening
- Not used.

Diagnosis and Evaluation
- Used to evaluate those with increased urine output (more than 2,000 mL/day)
  - If the urine osmolality is decreased, differential diagnoses include renal tubular necrosis, diabetes insipidus, overhydration, kidney failure, hyponatremia, or severe pyelonephritis.[5–7]
- Used to evaluate those with decreased/low urine output (less than 500 mL/day)
  - If the urine osmolality is increased, differential diagnoses include Addison's disease, heart failure, hypernatremia, dehydration, renal artery stenosis, shock, diabetes (glucosuria), and SIADH secretion.[5–7]
- Used also in the evaluation of polyuria, polydipsia, hyponatremia, hypernatremia, and acute kidney injury (AKI).[8–10]

Monitoring
- Used to monitor response to therapy.

INTERPRETATION
- Reference interval: 500 to 800 mOsm/kg H_2O[11]

FOLLOW-UP
- Urine osmolality may be repeated when the underlying cause for elevated or decreased urine osmolality has been corrected or the patient's hydration level is at a steady state.

- Urine sodium, serum/plasma osmolality, and serum electrolytes are often needed in addition to urine osmolality to evaluate patients with polyuria or polydipsia.[9]

PEARLS & PITFALLS

- The best time of day to collect the urine sample for urine osmolality is in the late afternoon as a morning specimen will be the most concentrated and will alter results.[7,12]
- It is important to understand that plasma osmolality and urine osmolality reveal different things. Plasma osmolality reveals the body's ability to maintain total body water balance while the urine osmolality reveals the body's ability to balance water intake and loss through antidiuretic activity. Urine osmolality reveals whether the process of maintaining water balance is intact while serum osmolality reveals the outcome of maintaining water balance.[2]
- Urine osmolality is a superior test to urine-specific gravity in revealing an accurate urine concentration and dilution because the specific gravity considers the weight of particles in the urine. Abnormal particles with a higher weight such as glucose, protein, and radiocontrast can disproportionately increase the specific gravity of the urine but will not impact the osmolality since it measures the number of particles.[1,3,8]
- Urine osmolality can be used to calculate the urine osmolol gap (UOG), which is a qualitative way to measure the concentration of urine ammonium. The UOG helps to determine if a patient with chronic metabolic acidosis has impaired renal excretion of ammonium. The proper renal response to chronic metabolic acidosis is to increase the excretion of more hydrogen ions in the urine, in the form of ammonium. The UOG will be increased in patients with a normal renal response to chronic metabolic acidosis. The UOG will be decreased in patients with an impaired renal response to chronic metabolic acidosis.[13]
- Urine osmolality is measured as part of a water deprivation test. Restricting water intake should trigger release of antidiuretic hormone (ADH) resulting in increases in urine osmolality. Water deprivation with impaired secretion of endogenous ADH leads to a dilute urine and low urine osmolality.[9]
- According to a 2015 Cochrane review, urine osmolality lacks diagnostic accuracy for diagnosing water-loss dehydration.[14]
- Patients with low urine osmolality may be at risk for poorer outcomes in chronic kidney disease (CKD).[15]

PATIENT EDUCATION

- https://medlineplus.gov/ency/article/003609.htm?utm_source=email&utm_medium=share&utm_campaignmplus_share[6]

RELATED DIAGNOSES AND ICD-10 CODES

| Hypo-osmolality or hyponatremia | E87.1 | AKI (acute kidney injury) | N17.9 |
| Polyuria | R35 | Diabetes insipidus or primary polydipsia | E23.2 |

REFERENCES

Full list of references can be accessed through Springer Publishing Company Connect™ at the following link: http://connect.springerpub.com/content/reference-book/ 978-0-8261-8843-4/part/part03/toc-part/ch157

158. URINE PROTEIN

Jonathan D. Savant

PHYSIOLOGY REVIEW

A variety of proteins are found in the urine, primarily serum proteins that pass through the filtration barrier and those that originate in the renal tubules or urinary tract. Large (molecular weight greater than 20,000 Daltons) and/or strongly charged serum proteins generally do not pass through the filtration mechanism, while low molecular weight proteins may pass through but are largely reabsorbed. Hence, the urine of healthy individuals may contain a small amount of protein whereas urinary protein excretion greater than 150 mg/day is considered abnormal (proteinuria), and greater than 3.5 g/day is classified as nephrotic range proteinuria.[1-3]

Proteinuria can be classified as transient or persistent. Transient proteinuria is related to temporary changes in glomerular permeability and is generally benign (e.g., exercise, dehydration, stress) or self-limited [e.g., fever, seizures, urinary tract infection (UTI)]. Persistent proteinuria can be classified according to glomerular, tubular, or overflow etiologies.[4-6]

Of these, the most common type is glomerular proteinuria, which is related to increased permeability of the glomerular capillary walls and is a sensitive marker of glomerular disease. Tubular proteinuria results from deficient reabsorption of low molecular weight proteins and is related to tubulointerstitial and some glomerular diseases. Overflow proteinuria results from overproduction of particular proteins that overwhelm kidney filtration and reabsorption mechanisms, as seen in multiple myeloma or hemoglobinuria.

The most common cause of benign proteinuria is orthostatic proteinuria, which is related to prolonged standing. Orthostatic proteinuria is found in approximately 2% to 5% of post-pubertal adolescents and accounts for 90% of asymptomatic proteinuria in teenagers; it is less common in adults over the age of 30.[7] This benign etiology can be distinguished by an absence of proteinuria on a first morning urine sample (collected after 8 hours of lying down).

Albumin is the primary protein found in the urine of those with proteinuric kidney diseases. Healthy young adults typically excrete less than 10 g/day of albumin in the urine while older adults may excrete a larger amount. Amounts greater than 30 mg/day of albumin are considered "moderately increased" (formerly termed "microalbuminuria") and amounts of more than 300 mg/day are "severely increased" (formerly termed "macroalbuminuria").[2,8] There is some evidence that albuminuria is more common among Black, as compared to White, individuals.[9] This poorly understood and multifactorial racial disparity may be due to a higher prevalence in Black individuals of hypertension and diabetes, certain proteinuric kidney diseases (e.g., FSGS), genetic factors (e.g., *APOL1* variant), or institutional/societal factors, such as barriers to accessing healthcare and socioeconomic deprivation.[10-12]

OVERVIEW OF LABORATORY TESTS

Point-of-Care Urine Dipstick and Urinalysis

Proteinuria is assessed by chemical analysis of the urine. This analysis can be performed by point-of-care (POC) dipstick reagent strips or by sending to the laboratory for full urinalysis (which also includes microscopic and macroscopic analysis) (CPT code 8100X). POC dipstick is performed by inserting the reagent strip into the urine sample and comparing the color of the strip to the manufacturer-provided color interpretation guide. Estimates of the urine protein content on dipstick are reported as "negative," "trace," 1+ (30 mg/dL), 2+ (100 mg/dL), 3+ (300 mg/dL), or 4+ (1,000 mg/dL). Benefits of the POC dipstick include the relative speed of results, although it may be less accurate. Dipstick results can be manually read by the tester or by using an automated reader. The automated reader is the preferred method as it is less subject to human error (e.g., ambient lighting, tester inexperience, or visual impairment).[2] False-positive results can occur in urine that is alkaline (elevated pH), highly concentrated (elevated specific gravity), contains other constituents (e.g., blood, pus, semen, vaginal secretions), or with certain medications.[1,13] False-negative results can occur with dilute urine or failure to detect non-albumin or low molecular weight proteins (therefore, they are less sensitive to tubular as compared to glomerular proteinuria). Nevertheless, urine dipstick does perform well with detecting significant proteinuria (sensitivity 96%, specificity 87%), and a negative dipstick has a high negative predictive value for moderately (97.6%) and severely (100%) increased albuminuria.[13,14]

Urinalysis by laboratory evaluation includes chemical analysis as well as macroscopic/visual analysis (e.g., color, clarity) and microscopic analysis after centrifuge (e.g., cellular components, casts, sediment). As with the POC dipstick, urinalysis has a high sensitivity for the detection of heavy proteinuria, but it may not detect lower levels of clinically significant proteinuria.

Spot Total Urine Protein and Creatinine Ratio, Spot Urine Albumin Creatinine Ratio, and Timed, or 24-Hour, Urine Protein Creatinine Ratio

Given that the amount of urine protein can fluctuate throughout the day, the 24-hour urine protein creatinine ratio test (CPT codes 84156 and 82575) involves taking multiple samples of urine over a 24-hour period and sending each for analysis. This was formerly considered the gold standard. Collection of all urine throughout the day (a 24-hour urine specimen) may be more informative than a one-time or "spot" urine collection in some cases. However, 24-hour urine samples are cumbersome, inconvenient, and prone to collection error.

Spot measurements of total urine protein or urine albumin concentrations can vary due to a variety of factors, particularly hydration status. Simultaneous measurement of urine creatinine helps adjust for this variability, expressed as a urine protein-to-creatinine ratio (UPCR) (CPT codes 84155 and 82570) or urine albumin-to-creatinine ratio (UACR) (CPT codes 82043 and 82570). Both UPCR and UACR approximate 24-hour protein and albumin excretion, respectively (i.e., a UACR of 30 mg/g and 300 mg/g correspond to excretion of 30 mg/day and 300 mg/day of albumin). A 2005 systematic review showed a strong correlation between UPCR and 24-hour urine protein (correlation coefficient, r >0.9).[15] UACR may be preferred in conditions where albumin is the primary protein (e.g., glomerular diseases, diabetic nephropathy) as opposed to tubulointersitital diseases, for which UPCR is preferred. UACR is also thought to be more sensitive to lower levels of proteinuria.[16]

Urine Protein Electrophoresis
Urine protein electrophoresis (UPEP) (CPT code 84166) is used to identify specific light chain proteins in the urine, such as Bence Jones protein associated with multiple myeloma.

INDICATIONS

Screening
Along with estimates of glomerular filtration rate (eGFR), urine protein can be included as a component of screening for and staging of chronic kidney disease (CKD).

- The U.S. Preventive Services Task Force (USPSTF) has concluded that there is insufficient evidence to assess the risk versus benefit in routine CKD screening in asymptomatic adults ("I statement").[17]
- The American College of Physicians (ACP) and the American Academy of Family Physicians (AAFP) recommend against screening for CKD in adults with symptoms or risk factors.[18]
- The American Academy of Pediatrics and American Society of Pediatric Nephrology recommend against routine screening with a urinalysis in otherwise healthy pediatric patients.[19]
- A 2015 Cochrane systematic review found insufficient data to recommend screening the general population with urine dipstick.[20]
- Several professional organizations and multiple guidelines recommend annual screening for CKD in patients with risk factors, such as diabetes, hypertension, cardiovascular disease, and HIV.[2,8,16,21–25] Additionally, patients with older age, obesity, or a family history of CKD may be considered for screening.[18,26]
  - Per the Kidney Disease Improving Global Outcomes (KDGIO) guidelines, the preferred tests for screening of CKD (in decreasing order of preference) are UACR, UPCR, dipstick (automated), and dipstick (manual).[8] First morning urine samples are preferred. Positive dipstick tests should be confirmed with quantitative assessment.
- Baseline screening/monitoring for renal dysfunction can be performed when prescribing drug therapy with potential renal effects.
- USPSTF and American College of Obstetricians and Gynecologists (ACOG) recommend against screening for proteinuria in pregnant individuals without symptoms of or risk factors for preeclampsia.[27] If tests of proteinuria are

indicated clinically, 24-hour or spot UPCR should be used as opposed to POC dipsticks.

Diagnosis and Evaluation

■ Tests for proteinuria are helpful in the workup of various signs/symptoms, such as:
  ● Edema/anasarca (concern for nephrotic syndrome, CHF, cirrhosis)
  ● Arthralgias, mouth ulcers, characteristic rashes (concern for autoimmune/connective tissue diseases with renal involvement)
  ● Polyuria, polydipsia, blurry vision, parasthesia (concern for diabetes mellitus)
  ● Elevated BP, headache, visual changes (workup of symptomatic hypertension)

Monitoring

■ Orthostatic proteinuria typically resolves with age, but an annual assessment of proteinuria should be considered to monitor for progression.[5]
■ Transient causes of proteinuria generally do not need continued monitoring after resolution/removal of the inciting event.
■ Higher levels of proteinuria are associated with a quicker progression to end-stage renal disease (ESRD), more cardiovascular events, and increased mortality in patients with kidney disease.[6] As such, proteinuria should be assessed to monitor for disease progression and treatment efficacy (e.g., renin-angiotensin-aldosterone system [RAAS] blockade with angiotensin-converting enzyme/angiotensin receptor blocker [ACEi/ARB] therapy) at least annually in patients with CKD[8] and in patients with proteinuria associated with DM[21] and/or hypertension (HTN).[28]

INTERPRETATION

■ There are many causes of proteinuria. Assessment should include a detailed medical/family history and physical examination.[1,4,5] See Table 158.1 for a list of common causes by type of proteinuria.
■ Table 158.2 reviews interpretation of urine protein tests.

FOLLOW-UP

■ Determine if proteinuria is transient or persistent; consider benign causes (e.g., particularly orthostatic proteinuria in adolescents).
■ Confirm urine dipstick results by urinalysis, ratios (UPCR/ UACR), and/or 24-hour collection.
■ Urinalysis with microscopy can identify sediment suggestive of glomerular disease (e.g., dysmorphic red blood cell's (RBC's)/RBC casts and white blood cell's (WBC's)/WBC casts without evidence of infection)
■ Serum creatinine or cystatin C-based estimates of glomerular filtration rate help evaluate for stage of CKD.
■ As indicated, screen for HTN and DM, including blood pressure, metabolic panel for serum creatinine/glucose, and Hgb A1c.

TABLE 158.1: COMMON CAUSES OF PROTEINURIA

PROTEINURIA TYPE	COMMON CAUSES
Transient	Fever, emotional stress, heavy exercise, seizures, UTI, CHF
Orthostatic	Benign postural proteinuria
Persistent:	
• Glomerular	Primary glomerular (e.g., FSGS, minimal change disease, IgA nephropathy)
	Secondary glomerular (e.g., SLE, Alport's)
	Diabetic nephropathy
• Tubular	Drugs/ heavy metals, interstitial nephritis, Fanconi syndrome
• Overflow	Hemoglobinuria, myoglobinuria, multiple myeloma

CHF, congestive heart failure; FSGS, focal segmental glomerulosclerosis; IgA, immunoglobulin A; SLE, systemic lupus erythematosus; UTI, urinary tract infection.

Sources: Data from Rovin BH. Assessment of urinary protein excretion and evaluation of isolated non-nephrotic proteinuria in adults. In: Glassock RJ, Curhan GC, Lam AQ, eds. *UpToDate.* UpToDate; 2021. https://www.uptodate.com/contents/assessment-of-urinary -protein-excretion-and-evaluation-of-isolated-non-nephrotic-proteinuria-in-adults; Simerville JA, Maxted WC, Pahira JJ. Urinalysis: a comprehensive review. *Am Fam Physician.* 2005;71:1153–1162. https://www.aafp.org/afp/2005/0315/p1153.html

TABLE 158.2: INTERPRETATION OF PROTEINURIA MEASUREMENTS

ALBUMINURIA GRADING PER KDIGO	DIPSTICK	SPOT URINE PROTEIN	UPCR	UACR	24 HR PROTEIN	24 HR ALBUMIN
Normal to mildly increased (A1)	Neg to 1+	<30 mg/dL	<200 mg/g (<0.2 g/g)	<30 mg/g	<150 mg/ day	<30 mg/day
Moderately increased (A2)	-	-	-	30 to 300 mg/g	-	30 to 300 mg/day
Severely increased (A3)	1+ to 3+	>30 mg/dL	>200 mg/g (>0.2 g/g)	>300 mg/g	>500 mg/ day	>300 mg/day
Nephrotic range	3+ to 4+	-	-	>2.2 g/g	>3.5 g/day	>3 g/day

24 hr, 24-hour urine specimen; KDIGO, Kidney Disease Improving Global Outcomes; UACR, urine albumin creatinine ratio; UPCR, urine protein creatinine ratio.

Sources: Data from KDIGO and NICE Guidelines; Cassia MA, Pozzi FE, Bascapè S, et al. Proteinuria and albuminuria at point of care. *Nephrology @ Point of Care.* 2016. doi:10.5301/pocj.5000194; Eknoyan G, Lameire N, Eckardt K, et al. KDIGO 2012 clinical practice guideline for the evaluation and management of chronic kidney disease. *Kidney Int.* 2013;3:5–14. https://kdigo.org/wp-content/ uploads/2017/02/KDIGO_2012_CKD_GL.pdf; National Institute for Health and Care Excellence. Chronic kidney disease in adults: assessment and management [*NICE Guideline CG182*]. Published July 23, 2014. https://www.nice.org.uk/guidance/cg182

■ Assess lipid levels, serum albumin, and for evidence of edema/anasarca with nephrotic range proteinuria.
■ Send a urine culture for complicated UTI(s).
■ Obtain a kidney ultrasound to assess for structural causes (e.g., reflux nephropathy).
■ Refer to a nephrologist and consider a kidney biopsy to assess glomeruli histologically, particularly with persistent nephrotic range proteinuria.

- Obtain an UPEP if there is suspicion for significant non-albumin proteinuria (e.g., suspicion of multiple myeloma with hypercalcemia, anemia, and bone pain).

PEARLS & PITFALLS

- While evidence-based practice does not support universal screening of proteinuria, clinical practice may vary. The benefits (potential identification of early disease resulting in reduction of morbidity/mortality and future treatment costs) should be weighed against the risk (benign proteinuria/false positives leading to inappropriate workup/invasive testing, patient anxiety, etc.).
- Consider environmental/patient-related factors contributing to unreliable dipstick testing and measured protein assessment.
- For confirmatory testing, patients should be educated to avoid strenuous activity and to stay well-hydrated.
- Urine creatinine is impacted by muscle mass, so ratios (UACR and UPCR) may be falsely elevated in patients with large muscle mass and falsely decreased in cachectic patients.
- UACR is more sensitive to lower levels of clinically significant proteinuria as compared to UPCR and dipstick.

PATIENT EDUCATION

- https://www.kidney.org/atoz/content/know-your-kidney-numbers-two-simple-tests

RELATED DIAGNOSES AND ICD-10 CODES

Proteinuria	R80	Chronic kidney disease	N18
Isolated proteinuria	R80.0	Nephrotic syndrome	N04
Persistent proteinuria, unspecified	R80.1	Glomerulonephritis	N05.9
Orthostatic proteinuria, unspecified	R80.2	Type 2 diabetes mellitus with diabetic nephropathy	E11.21
Bence Jones proteinuria	R80.3	Hypertensive chronic kidney disease	I12.9
Other proteinuria	R80.8	Kidney transplant status	Z94.0
Proteinuria, unspecified	R80.9		

REFERENCES

Full list of references can be accessed through Springer Publishing Company Connect™ at the following link: http://connect.springerpub.com/content/reference-book/978-0-8261-8843-4/part/part03/toc-part/ch158

159. URINE STONE ANALYSIS

Joan E. Zaccardi and Kelly Small Casler

PATHOPHYSIOLOGY REVIEW

Urolithiasis occurs when minerals or crystals precipitate into calculi (stones) in the urinary system. Calculi most often form unilaterally and within the renal pelvis, calyces, and bladder. They remain small (2 to 3 mm) within the pelvis but may become larger as they travel toward the bladder.[1] Calcium calculi are the most common, occurring either as calcium oxalate or calcium phosphate stones. Calculi composed of struvite and uric acid stones are also possible. Several genetic and environmental factors influence and contribute to the formation of urolithiasis (Table 159.1).[2]

OVERVIEW OF LABORATORY TESTS

Urine stone analysis(CPT code 82365) and 24-hour urine composition (sometimes called renal stone risk panel or kidney stone urine test) are two tests available to guide management of urolithiasis. For urine stone analysis, the urine is strained and the stone sent for analysis by infrared spectroscopy, x-ray diffraction, or chemical analysis.[1-4] The 24-hour urine composition will have multiple CPT codes depending on the components analyzed. A typical 24-hour urine composition measures total urine volume and pH in addition to calcium, oxalate, uric acid, citrate, sodium, potassium, magnesium, and creatinine levels. Excess levels are clues to contributing factors or underlying conditions for calculi and guide preventative efforts for future events.[2]

INDICATIONS

Screening
■ Neither urine stone analysis nor 24-hour urine analysis composition are used for screening purposes.

TABLE 159.1: GENETIC AND ENVIRONMENTAL FACTORS IN URINARY CALCULI	
GENETICS	**ENVIRONMENTAL**
Idiopathic hypercalciuria	Dietary factors
Primary hyperoxaluria types 1, 2, 3	Obesity
Distal renal tubular acidosis (RTA)	Diabetes
Cystinuria	Geographic location: Southeast United States
Lesch-Nyhan syndrome	

Source: Data from Pearle MS, Goldfarb DS, Assimos DG, et al. Medical management of kidney stones: AUA guideline. *J Urol.* 2014;192(2):316–324. doi:10.1016/j.juro.2014.05.006

Diagnosis and Evaluation

- Urine stone analysis is recommended at least once for patients with urolithiasis. It is used to diagnose the type of calculi so that underlying causes can be corrected and future recurrences prevented.[2]
- 24-hour urine composition can be offered to all patients with urolithiasis, but strongest recommendations for its use are made for patients with anatomic or genetic conditions predisposing to future urolithiasis, patients with one kidney, or patients with recurrent stone disease.[5] Two collections on two different days are completed as soon as 6 weeks after stone passage as long as the patient is free from pain, infection, and obstruction and is able to resume usual physical activity, fluid intake, and diet.[2,6] Note that recommendations for this test mainly rely on expert opinion, though there is some evidence that the information obtained accurately guides prevention efforts (diet change, medications) and minimizes stone reoccurrence.[7-9] However, in one study, 24-hour urine composition analysis only predicted stone type 64% of the time.[10] Part of the reason for these findings may be that patients can develop multiple stone types.

Monitoring

- Repeat stone analysis can be completed to monitor patients with repeat episodes of urolithiasis.[2]
- Repeat 24-hour urine composition is recommended 6 months after initiation of future stone preventative measures and annually (to monitor effectiveness of diet changes or medications). The test may be ordered more frequently if patients have recurrent disease or do not respond to prevention efforts.[2,3]

INTERPRETATION

- Interpretation of stone analysis is reviewed in Table 159.2.[11,12]
- Table 159.3[13-17] summarizes interpretation of the 24-hour urine composition test.

TABLE 159.2: INTERPRETATION OF STONE ANALYSIS

TYPE OF STONE	POSSIBLE UNDERLYING CONDITIONS OR CONCERNS
Uric acid	Gout; high purine diet
Cystine	Cystinuria
Struvite	Recurrent UTI risk with urea-splitting organisms (Proteus)
Calcium phosphate	RTA Type 1, primary hyperparathyroidism, medullary sponge kidney
Calcium oxalate	Primary hyperoxaluria or overabsorption of oxalate (inflammatory bowel disease; cystic fibrosis)

RTA, renal tubular acidosis; UTI, urinary tract infection.

Sources: Data from Hulton S-A. The primary hyperoxalurias: a practical approach to diagnosis and treatment. *Int J Surg.* 2016;36: 649–654. doi:10.1016/j.ijsu.2016.10.039; Rumsby G. Genetic defects underlying renal stone disease. *Int J Surg.* 2016;36:590–595. doi:10.1016/j.ijsu.2016.11.015

▪ Use urine pH (on 24-hour urine composition) to evaluate what crystals are most likely to precipitate and form stones.[18]
  ● Calcium oxalate stones are more likely with acidic pH (less than 6.0) and uric acid stones are more likely with a very acidic pH (less than 5.5).
  ● Calcium phosphate and struvite stones are more likely with an alkaline pH (>7.2).

FOLLOW-UP

▪ If signs of concurrent UTI on microscopy or history/physical, urine culture and sensitivity is indicated.[2,19,20]
▪ If stone analysis reveals uric acid stone, serum uric acid can be assessed.[2–4]
▪ If concerns for sepsis or severe infection, a complete blood count may be warranted.
▪ If hypercalciuria or calcium phosphate stone, a serum calcium level and parathyroid hormone are warranted to check for hyperparathyroidism.[2]
▪ If renal tubular acidosis (RTA) is suspected, an ammonium chloride load test can be considered.
▪ For undetermined stone types, a nitroprusside test can help evaluate for cystinuria.[5]

TABLE 159.3: INTERPRETATION OF 24-HOUR URINE COMPOSITION		
ANALYTE	**ABNORMAL IF:**	**IF ABNORMAL, UNDERLYING CONDITION TO TARGET WITH PREVENTION EFFORTS**
Urinary creatinine excretion	<15–18 mg/kg or > 20–24 mg/kg	n/a*
Urinary calcium excretion	>200–300 mg/24 hours	Hypercalciuria
Urine citrate excretion	<400 mg/24 hours	Hypocitraturia
Urine uric acid excretion	>800 mg/24 hours	Hyperuricemia
Urine magnesium	<60 mg/24 hours	Hypomagnesuria
Oxalate	>40 mg/24 hours	Hyperoxaluria
Sodium	>200 mEq/24 hours	Excess sodium^
Potassium	<25 mEq/24 hours	Too little potassium^

*Use creatinine excretion to determine the adequacy of urine collected. Adequate collection of volume should be determined before proceeding with interpretation.

^Calcium is more likely to precipitate under these conditions.

Note: Exact cutoffs may vary; clinicians should use local laboratory reference limits.

Sources: Data from Curhan GC, Taylor EN. 24-h uric acid excretion and the risk of kidney stones. *Kidney Int.* 2008;73(4):489–496. doi:10.1038/sj.ki.5002708; Ennis JL, Asplin JR. The role of the 24-h urine collection in the management of nephrolithiasis. *Int J Surg.* 2016;36:633–637. doi:10.1016/j.ijsu.2016.11.020; Leslie SW, Sajjad H, Bashir K. 24-hour urine testing for nephrolithiasis interpretation. In: *StatPearls.* StatPearls Publishing; 2021. http://www.ncbi.nlm.nih.gov/books/NBK482448; Rao LV, Snyder LM, eds. *Wallach's Interpretation of Diagnostic Tests: Pathways to Arriving at a Clinical Diagnosis.* 11th ed. Wolters Kluwer; 2021; Song S, Thomas I-C, Ganesan C, et al. Twenty-four hour urine testing and prescriptions for urinary stone disease–related medications in veterans. *CJASN.* 2019;14(12):1773–1780. doi:10.2215/CJN.03580319

- Diagnostic imaging can be used to assess for new stone formation or to follow stones that still may be in the urinary system. Noncontrast CT is the usual first choice with renal/bladder ultrasound used in pregnant patients and children.[2,21]

PEARLS & PITFALLS

- Patients may experience more than one stone composition type in their lifetime.
- For patients with symptomatic urolithiasis, urinalysis and microscopy may show hematuria, leukocytes, and bacteria. If crystals are noted during microscopy, it may be a clue to stone type.
- A 24-hour urine composition can reduce the risk of recurrence; however, many patients do not complete testing so clinician education and follow-up with patients is important.[22,23]
- Diabetes is a high-risk factor for developing kidney stones.[4]
- RTA is suspected in consistently high alkaline pH (greater than 6.0) especially if combined with hypercitraturia and calcium phosphate stones.[14]
- If ordering a 24-hour urine composition, make sure to use the results. One analysis showed less than half of patients who had this test were prescribed appropriate medication and diet therapy.[17]

PATIENT EDUCATION

- https://uroweb.org/guideline/urolithiasis

RELATED DIAGNOSES AND ICD-10 CODES

Calculus of the kidney	N20.0	Other lower urinary tract calculus	N21.8
Calculus of the ureter	N20.1	Calculus of lower urinary tract, unspecified	N21.9
Calculus in the urethra	N21.1	Calculus of kidney with calculus of ureter	N20.2
Calculus in the bladder	N21.0		
Urinary calculus, unspecified	N20.9		

REFERENCES

Full list of references can be accessed through Springer Publishing Company Connect™ at the following link: http://connect.springerpub.com/content/reference-book/ 978-0-8261-8843-4/part/part03/toc-part/ch159

160. VAGINITIS TESTING—BACTERIAL VAGINOSIS

Deanna Hunt

PHYSIOLOGY REVIEW

Bacterial vaginosis (BV) is caused by an imbalance of the vaginal flora, with a decrease in *Lactobacillus* genus and an increase in BV-related bacterium. BV is not caused by one organism but is instead the result of an increase in multiple anaerobic and facultative bacteria.[1] Thirty-five bacterial species have been identified to date to cause BV and are listed in Box 160.1.[2] Symptoms of BV include a vaginal discharge with a fishy odor; however, some women are asymptomatic.[2,3]

OVERVIEW OF LABORATORY TESTS

BV can be diagnosed through a variety of tests which are described in the text that follows. Cost of testing may be a factor to consider in the selection, and the cost of testing depends on the test ordered. DNA testing ranges from $27 to $49, compared to $5 to $10 with microscopy.[4] Microscopy and Gram stain methods are the preferred testing options according to current clinical guidelines from the American College of Obstetricians and Gynecologists (ACOG), Centers for Disease Control and Prevention (CDC), and Infectious Diseases Society of America (IDSA).[5-7]

Gram Stain
The Gram stain is considered the gold standard test for the diagnosis of BV but is not often ordered. The Gram stain looks for three primary morphotypes: large Gram-positive rods (*Lactobacillus*), small Gram-positive or Gram-variable rods

---

Box 160.1: Bacteria Known to Contribute to Bacterial Vaginosis

- Aerococcus
- Anaerococcus
- Atopobium vaginae*
- Gardnerella vaginalis*
- Gemella
- Leptotrichia amnionii*
- Megasphaera types*
- Peptostreptococcus spp
- Porphyromonas asaccharolytica*
- Prevotella species*
- Sneathia sanguinegens*
- Veillonella genera

*More common causes

(*Gardnerella* and *Bacteroides*), and lastly, curved Gram-negative or Gram-variable rods (*Mobiluncus*). The Gram stain is examined according to the Nugent score, a standardized scoring system used for the diagnosis of BV. A slide is examined for the number of normal flora compared with the three bacterial morphotypes described previously. Results range from 0 to 3 (normal flora), 4 to 6 (mixed flora), and 7 to 10 (diagnosis of BV). A drawback to the Nugent score is that results are not available at the time of an office visit due to the expertise needed to read and interpret the slides. Other disadvantages of the Nugent score are the subjectivity of the test, and the inability to identify newer morphotypes.[2]

Microscopy

Microscopy is beneficial in some settings where a quick diagnosis is needed or in settings where other laboratory testing is not available. Microscopy is easy to perform but does require a trained clinician. When using saline microscopy (also called wet mount) (CPT code 87210), Amsel's criteria guide BV diagnosis (Box 160.2). Amsel's criteria requires the presence of at least three of the following criteria to diagnose BV: vaginal discharge, vaginal pH greater than 4.5, 20% of epithelial cells appearing as clue cells, and a positive amine, or "whiff" test (fishy odor after addition of 10% potassium hydroxide to vaginal sample). The sensitivity for Amsel's criteria ranges from 37% to 70% and specificity ranges from 94% and 99%.[1]

Point-of-Care Tests

Another option for testing BV is with point-of-care (POC) tests. One POC method measures sialidase levels in vaginal secretions (CPT code 87905). Sialidases are produced by bacteria including *Gardnerella* and *Bacteroides* species. The test is a quick dipstick with a relatively high sensitivity and specificity (sensitivity 88% to 91%; specificity 91% to 98%).[2] Another POC test available detects metabolic products of *G. vaginalis* and concurrently measures vaginal pH. Sensitivity for this test is 91% and the specificity is 61%.[1]

Molecular Test

Two molecular diagnostic assays available for the diagnosis of BV are direct probe assays and nucleic acid amplification tests (NAATs). Direct probe assays are placed into vaginal fluid at which point the DNA probe binds to sequences from a bacterium, ultimately detecting the presence of bacteria. More commonly used are the NAATs, with sensitivities of 95.9% and specificities of 93.7%.

Box 160.2: Amsel Criteria for Bacterial Vaginosis

Three out of the four criteria must be met:

- Thin, homogenous vaginal discharge
- Positive whiff test (fishy odor is produced when vaginal secretions are mixed with 10% potassium hydroxide)
- At least 20% of epithelial cells appear as clue cells
- Vaginal pH greater than 4.5

Several NAATs products are available. The different NAATs available differ slightly in the bacterial causative agents they test for and are often referred to as vaginitis or vaginitis-plus panels. Usually, the vaginitis panel includes testing for *G. vaginalis* only; however, the vaginitis-plus panels detect additional bacterial species seen in BV including *A. vaginae*, BVAB2, *Lactobacilli crispatus*, and *Megasphaera* type 1. Clinicians should review the test panels available at their practice site to confirm that they are achieving the extent of testing desired. Some vaginitis-plus panels do not include *G. vaginalis* to avoid misinterpretation of results, as *G. vaginalis* is also normal vaginal flora, and detection does not necessarily mean BV is present.[2]

Vaginal discharge samples can be clinician or patient collected. In a well-designed cross-sectional study evaluating the efficacy of clinician swabs and self-collected swabs in the diagnosis of vaginitis, the accuracy of testing with the two collection methods were similar, indicating self-collected samples are a valid alternative.[8,9]

INDICATIONS

Screening

- Routine screening for BV is not recommended.
- The United States Preventive Services Task Force (USPSTF) recommends against screening for BV in pregnant patients who are not at increased risk for preterm delivery (Grade D).[7]
  - High levels of evidence (meta-analysis) revealed that antibiotic therapy was shown to be effective at eliminating BV during pregnancy but did not reduce the risk of premature birth before 37 weeks.[4]

Diagnosis and Evaluation

- Patients with signs/symptoms of BV (Table 160.1) warrant diagnostic testing with one of the previously discussed methods.

Monitoring

- Routine testing in asymptomatic women and retesting (test of cure) are not recommended because these bacteria can be part of normal flora.[6]

INTERPRETATION

- Molecular testing and point-of-care tests: positive or negative.[1]
- Microscopy: see Table 160.1 and Figure 160.1

FOLLOW-UP

- If sexually transmitted infections (STI) cannot be ruled out as the cause of symptoms, STI testing will be needed.

PEARLS & PITFALLS

- Many microbial tests test for the detection of several different causes of vaginal discharge at once: *Candida albicans*, *Trichomonas vaginalis*, and *Gardnerella vaginalis*.[10]

TABLE 160.1: COMPARISON OF THREE MOST COMMON REASONS FOR SYMPTOM OF VAGINAL DISCHARGE

	VULVOVAGINAL CANDIDIASIS (VVC)	TRICHOMONIASIS	BACTERIAL VAGINOSIS (BV)
Signs/Symptoms	Itching Soreness Painful intercourse Vulvar erythema White, clumpy vaginal discharge	Thin, green vaginal discharge Vulvar/vaginal erythema Malodorous discharge Vaginal burning Painful intercourse Dysuria	Malodorous vaginal discharge Gray, thin vaginal discharge
Amine test (whiff test) findings	Negative	Positive	Positive
Wet mount (saline microscopy) findings	Rod shape lactobacilli present White blood cells	Motile trichomonads White blood cells	Loss of rod-shaped lactobacilli Increased coccobacilli 20% of epithelial cells appear as clue cells
10% Potassium hydroxide microscopy findings	Hyphae or pseudohyphae	No findings	No findings
pH	<4.5	>4.5	>4.5

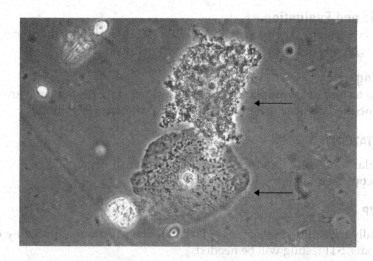

FIGURE 160.1. Clue cells on microscopy. Description: This photomicrograph of a vaginal smear specimen depicts two epithelial cells, a normal epithelial cell (bottom arrow) and an epithelial "clue cell" (top arrow) with its exterior covered by bacteria, giving the cell a roughened, stippled appearance. The presence of clue cells is a sign that the patient has bacterial vaginosis. *Source:* Courtesy of Centers for Disease Control and Prevention/M. Rein. https://phil.cdc.gov/Details.aspx?pid=14574

- Vaginal discharge should be collected from the posterior fornix and side walls of the vagina.[10]
- Although patient-collected swabs are an appropriate option for testing, do not underestimate the utility of clinician examinations that can be concurrently done at the time of clinician-collected specimens.[11,12]

PATIENT EDUCATION

- https://medlineplus.gov/lab-tests/bacterial-vaginosis-test

RELATED DIAGNOSES AND ICD-10 CODES

Bacterial vaginosis	N76.0
Vaginal discharge	N89.8

REFERENCES

Full list of references can be accessed through Springer Publishing Company Connect™ at the following link: http://connect.springerpub.com/content/reference-book/978-0-8261-8843-4/part/part03/toc-part/ch160

---

161. VAGINITIS TESTING—CANDIDA

Deanna Hunt and Kelly Small Casler

PHYSIOLOGY REVIEW

Vulvovaginal candidiasis (VVC) is one of three common conditions, along with trichomoniasis and bacterial vaginosis (BV) (compared in Table 161.1), that cause vaginal discharge and inflammation.[1] These conditions are commonly referred to as vaginitis. VVC is caused by yeast species, most often by *Candida albicans*, but other species of candida including *glabrata, parapsilosis,* and *tropicalis* are also possible etiologies.[2,3] Risk factors for VVC include antibiotic use, pregnancy, immunosuppression, use of hormonal contraceptives, sexual activity, and diabetes mellitus.[4] The signs and symptoms of VVC include vaginal itching and soreness, dyspareunia, dysuria, vaginal edema, and thick, white, cottage-cheese-like discharge.[4,5] Oftentimes, diagnosis of VVC is made on self-reported symptoms; however, the sensitivity and specificity of diagnosis based on symptoms alone is very low.[6] It is therefore important to consider the clinical examination, laboratory testing, and symptoms experienced by the patient. On clinical examination, signs of VVC include vulvar edema, fissures, excoriations, and a thick, curdy, and white vaginal discharge.[4]

OVERVIEW OF LABORATORY TESTS

A patient presenting with vaginal or vulvar complaints should be evaluated for vaginitis. Testing can include co-testing for other causes of vaginitis or vaginal discharge. Individual laboratory testing for candida alone is not common. The types of testing available are reviewed in this section and samples may be collected either by the clinician or the patient.[7,8] All testing options, except rapid testing, are considered appropriate options based on current clinical guidelines from the American College of Obstetricians and Gynecologists (ACOG), Centers for Disease Control and Prevention (CDC), and Infectious Diseases Society of America (IDSA).[4,9,10]

Culture

The gold standard for diagnosing VVC is through a culture (CPT code 87102). A culture is especially important in the diagnosis of complicated and recurrent VVC infections, but is not often used outside of these situations, due to the long turnaround time for results and labor intensive process.[4,9,10]

Microscopy

Saline microscopy, or wet mount, and potassium hydroxide (KOH) preparation are commonly used when VVC is suspected. Preparation of slides for this test is reviewed in Box 161.1 and Figure 161.1. Both saline and KOH preparations may demonstrate budding yeasts, hyphae, or pseudo hyphae, but use of 10% KOH improves the visualization of yeast, and should be used with wet mount to evaluate for VVC.[4] Even with 10% KOH preparations, accuracy of microscopy can be poor. Compared to fungal culture, 10% KOH microscopy has a sensitivity of 39.6% to 57.5%, a specificity of 89.4% to 90.4%, negative predictive value of 81.4%, and a positive predictive value of 72.2%.[11,12] For these reasons, other laboratory tests have been developed to improve accuracy of diagnostic confirmation.

Molecular Test

Microbial molecular tests use polymerase chain reaction (PCR) and DNA probe hybridization testing methodology to test for the most common candida species

---

Box 161.1: How to Prepare a Wet Mount

1. Collect vaginal secretions sample using a cotton swab.
2. Place in small test tube or like container that contains a few drops of normal saline.*
3. Smear sample on laboratory slide in circular motion.^
4. Place cover slip over sample.
5. Examine under microscope.
6. Add potassium hydroxide to the sample after completion and hold the slide near your nose, smelling for a fishy odor. A fishy odor is a positive "whiff" test (this is useful in the diagnosis of bacterial vaginosis).

*It is usually best to perform pH testing between step 1 and 2.

^If also performing a potassium hydroxide (KOH) prep for suspected yeast/candida: to the right of the first sample, prepare a second sample in a like manner, adding KOH to the second sample only prior to step 4.

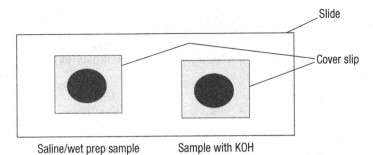

FIGURE 161.1. Preparation of a wet mount and potassium hydroxide slide.

involved in VVC.[13–15] Sensitivity of these methods ranges from 84.7% to 91.7% and specificity ranges from 94.9% to 99% (highest accuracy is seen for *Candida albicans* and lowest seen for *Candida glabrata*).[16] It is important that the clinician reviews the species of candida that various molecular testing products assess for, as not all possible VVC causing yeast species may be included on panel testing.

Rapid Testing
Lateral flow assay for rapid testing at the point of care is another option to evaluate for VVC. This test can provide results within 10 minutes and provides up to 77.4% sensitivity.[12]

INDICATIONS
Screening
- Routine screening for VVC is not recommended.

Diagnosis and Evaluation
- Laboratory testing for VVC is appropriate when signs and symptoms appear as described in Table 161.1.

Monitoring
- Candida species and anaerobes can be normal flora in asymptomatic women, so retesting (test of cure) is not recommended as long as the patient no longer has symptoms.[4]

INTERPRETATION

- **Molecular and rapid testing**: positive or negative[1]
- **Microscopy**: positive if hyphae, pseudo hyphae, or yeast buds are identified. See Figure 161.2.

FOLLOW-UP

- pH testing may help confirm the diagnosis of VVC.
- If patients are having recurring bouts of candida, be sure to consider testing for possible diabetes mellitus, impaired fasting glucose, or other conditions associated with immunosuppression.[6]

TABLE 161.1: COMPARISON OF VAGINITIS

	VULVOVAGINAL CANDIDIASIS (VVC)	TRICHOMONIASIS	BACTERIAL VAGINOSIS (BV)
Signs/Symptoms	• Itching • Soreness • Painful intercourse • Vulvar erythema • White, clumpy vaginal discharge	• Thin, green vaginal discharge • Vulvar/vaginal erythema • Malodorous discharge • Vaginal burning • Painful intercourse • Dysuria	• Malodorous vaginal discharge • Gray, thin vaginal discharge
Amine test (whiff test) findings	Negative	Positive	Positive
Wet mount (saline microscopy) findings	Rod shape lactobacilli present White blood cells	Motile trichomonads White blood cells	Loss of rod-shaped lactobaccili Presence of clue cells Increased coccobaccili
10% Potassium hydroxide microscopy findings	Hyphae or psuedohyphae	No findings	No findings
pH	<4.5	>4.5	>4.5

PEARLS & PITFALLS

■ Vaginal discharge should be collected from the posterior fornix and side walls of the vagina.[14]

■ When a patient presents with vaginal complaints, consider a comprehensive approach to rule out sexually transmitted infections

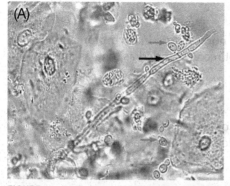 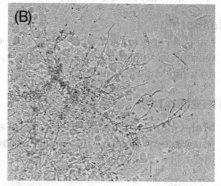

FIGURE 161.2A/B. Microscopy findings for vulvovaginal candidiasis. (A) Saline vaginal wet mount at 40× magnification showing hyphae at the black arrow and budding yeast on the gray arrow. **(B)** 10% potassium hydroxide mount at 10× magnification showing multiple hyphae visible. In the background, the outline of the dissolving epithelial cells (due to the potassium hydroxide) is seen. *Source:* Spach DH, Muzny CA. Vaginitis. *National STD Curriculum.* Updated October 12, 2021. https://www.std.uw.edu/go/comprehensive-study/vaginitis/core-concept/all#vulvovaginal-candidiasis

- The diagnosis of VVC requires physical examination and testing. The combination of thick white discharge and vulvar pruritis is neither sensitive nor specific on its own for diagnosis.[3]
- A drawback to multiplex panels is that they may discover yeast or bacteria that are not causing a pathologic problem. In the absence of signs or symptoms of VVC, treatment would be considered inappropriate because 10% to 20% of women harbor *Candida* species within the vagina.[4]

PATIENT EDUCATION

- https://www.cdc.gov/fungal/diseases/candidiasis/genital/index.html
- https://www.cdc.gov/std/tg2015/candidiasis.htm

RELATED DIAGNOSES AND ICD-10 CODES

Vaginal candidiasis	B37.3
Vaginal discharge	N89.8
Vaginal itching	N89.8

REFERENCES

Full list of references can be accessed through Springer Publishing Company Connect™ at the following link: http://connect.springerpub.com/content/reference-book/ 978-0-8261-8843-4/part/part03/toc-part/ch161

---

162. VITAMIN B12

Debra Hain

PHYSIOLOGY REVIEW

Vitamin B12 is a water-soluble vitamin required for formation of the hematopoietic cells (red blood cells, white blood cells, and platelets), as well as the development, myelination, and function of the central nervous system and for DNA synthesis. Methylcobalamin and 5-deoxyadenosylcobalamin are the metabolically active forms; hydroxocobalamin and cyanocobalamin become biologically active after they are converted to methylcobalamin and 5-deoxyadenosylcobalamin. Vitamin B12 is naturally present in some foods but added to others; it is bound to protein in the food and must be released before it is absorbed. This process begins in the mouth when food is mixed with saliva. The freed vitamin B12 then binds with haptocorrin, a cobalamin-binding protein in the saliva. Vitamin B12 continues to be released from the food matrix by the activity of hydrochloric acid and gastric protease in the stomach. It is there that it binds to haptocorrin.

In the duodenum, digestive enzymes free the vitamin B12 from the haptocorrin and then it binds with the intrinsic factor (IF). IF is a transport and delivery binding protein secreted by the stomach's parietal cells. This becomes a complex that is absorbed by the distal ileum by receptor-mediated endocytosis. If vitamin B12 is added to fortified foods and with dietary supplements, it is already in a free form and does not have to undergo the separation as previously described. B12 deficiency causes reversible megaloblastic anemia, demyelinating neurologic disease, or both.[1] Methylmalonic acid (MMA) is a vitamin B12-associated metabolite that is a very sensitive marker of vitamin B12 deficiency.[2]

OVERVIEW OF LABORATORY TESTS

Vitamin B12 (CPT code 82607) is measured using a competitive chemiluminescence assay that has an estimated sensitivity of about 95% and specificity of about 80% or less in symptomatic patients. The assay binds to the IF following dissociation from binding proteins with a readout based on the amount of unbound IF remaining.

INDICATIONS

Screening

Universal screening is not recommended. Targeted screening for individuals at risk for B12 deficiency may be warranted if one or more risk factors are present. Those at risk should be screened with a complete blood count and vitamin B12 level.[2] Targeted screenings should be considered in patients with the following conditions and considerations[2-4]:

- Difficulty absorbing vitamin B12 from food, lack of IF (e.g., pernicious anemia), post-gastrectomy syndrome (includes Roux-en-Y gastric bypass)
- Use of metformin for more than 4 months, proton-pump inhibitors, or histamine H_2 blockers for more than 12 months
- Alcohol abuse
- Older adults (75 and older) who are at risk for deficiency, especially those with atrophic gastritis and those with *Helicobacter pylori* infection
- Individuals with gastrointestinal disorders (e.g., celiac disease, inflammatory bowel disease such as Crohn's disease)
- Vegetarians who don't consume animal products or rare animal products (e.g., eggs, dairy, meat)
- Malabsorption syndrome
- Individuals with neurologic symptoms such as paresthesia, fatigue, numbness, poor motor concentration, memory problems
- Individuals with diabetes

Diagnosis and Evaluation

- Individuals with macrocytic anemia or macrocytosis with oval or hypersegmented neutrophils or pancytopenia
- Individuals exhibiting signs and symptoms of vitamin B12 deficiency including gait and balance disturbance, depression, confusion, memory impairment, mouth and tongue soreness, easily fatigued with exertion, palpitations, and skin pallor.

■ Diagnosis may require obtaining a MMA level. See MMA chapter (Chapter 115) for more information and Figure 162.1.

Monitoring
■ Varies depending on the cause and treatment. If there is a known cause, re-evaluate with a complete blood count (CBC), vitamin B12 and folate level(s) 3 to 12 months after discontinuing therapy.
  ● Reticulocyte count increases in the first 1 to 2 days.

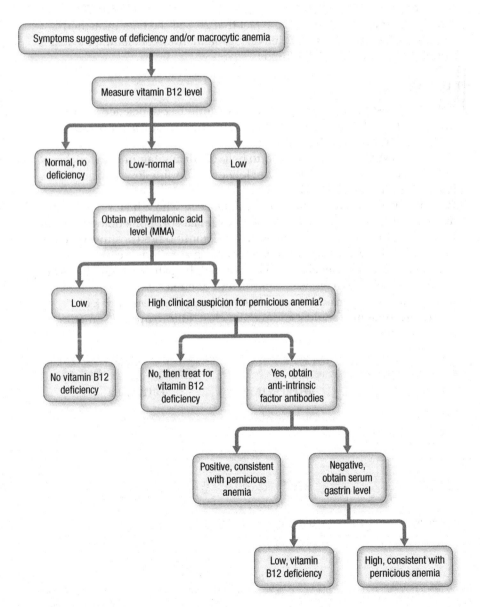

FIGURE 162.1. Algorithm for evaluating B12 deficiency.

- Anemia starts to improve in 1 to 2 weeks and normalizes within 4 to 8 weeks.
- Hypersegmented neutrophils disappear within approximately 2 weeks.
- Vitamin B12 levels increase to normal range.
■ Monitoring should continue until a complete response has been achieved.

INTERPRETATION

■ False-negative and false-positive values are common with the use of a laboratory- reported lower limit of the normal range as the cutoff for deficiency; this may be due to the fact that 20% of the total measured vitamin B12 is on the cellular delivery protein, transcobalamin; the rest is bound to haptocorrin (Table 162.1).[5,6]

FOLLOW-UP

■ Follow-up testing for individuals with vitamin B12 deficiency is based on the cause, if known. For patients where the etiology is not known, additional testing may be required.
■ A serum MMA level may be used to help confirm vitamin B12 deficiency. When serum vitamin B12 levels are low or borderline-low, plasma MMA concentrations are elevated.
■ Patients diagnosed with vitamin B12 deficiency whose history and physical assessment is not suggestive of dietary or malabsorption etiology should be tested for pernicious anemia with anti-IF antibodies (positive predictive value = 95%) especially when a patient has an autoimmune disorder.[2] If this is negative, a gastrin level should be ordered. If gastrin is high, this is also consistent with the diagnosis of pernicious anemia.
■ Individuals with pernicious anemia may have an increased risk of gastrointestinal malignancy and require close follow-up and sometimes additional testing.

TABLE 162.1: B12 REFERENCE LEVELS

B12 LEVEL	INTERPRETATION	FOLLOW-UP
Above 300 pg/mL The sensitivity is lower in individuals with anti-intrinsic factor antibodies	Normal; deficiency is unlikely	None needed
200–300 pg/mL (150–399 pg/mL is low-normal)	Borderline; deficiency possible	Additional testing may be needed; consider MMA level
Below 200 pg/mL	Low; consistent with deficiency	Additional testing may be appropriate to determine the diagnosis

*Sensitivity of about 90%.

Sources: Data from Anthony AC. Megaloblastic anemias. In: Hoffman R, Benz EJ, Shattil SJ, et al., eds. *Hematology: Basic Principles and Practice.* 4th ed. Churchill Livingstone; 2005:519; Matchar DB, McGrory DC, Millington DS, Feussner JR. Performance of the serum cobalamin assay for diagnosis of cobalamin deficiency. *Am J Med Sci.* 1994;308:276. doi:10.1097/00000441-199411000-00004

■ Additional testing should be done if anemia is present to assess for other causes of anemia (e.g., iron levels, copper deficiency, infection, hypothyroidism, myelodysplastic syndrome).

PEARLS & PITFALLS

■ The first step in prevention of vitamin B12 deficiency is identifying patients at risk.[2]

■ If anti-IF results are negative but you still think the patient may have pernicious anemia you may consider obtaining a serum gastrin level; an elevation is consistent with the diagnosis of pernicious anemia.

■ Patients with pernicious anemia may have other hematologic findings that are consistent with normocytic anemia.[2]

■ The Schilling test, once used to diagnosis pernicious anemia, is no longer available.

■ Ingestion of vitamin C can increase serum vitamin B12.

■ Switch from oral to parenteral therapy if there are concerns about absorption or if there is a suboptimal response to treatment; however, ensure the patient is taking the oral form before switching to the parenteral form.

■ There is low toxicity for vitamin B12 because even at large doses, vitamin B12 is considered to be safe because the body does not absorb excess amounts.[7]

■ Holotranscobalamin (biologically active form of vitamin B12) can be used to help diagnose vitamin B12 deficiency but may not be superior to serum B12 for detection of vitamin B12 deficiency. Considering the cost of the test and the limited diagnostic advantage, it is not the best choice.[8]

■ Homocysteine is elevated in both vitamin B12 and folate deficiencies. MMA is only elevated in vitamin B12 deficiency.

■ A systematic review and metanalysis was conducted to evaluate the association between serum and plasma vitamin B12 levels in pregnant women and birth weight and length of gestation. The researchers reported that having a lower maternal vitamin B12 level was linked to preterm birth.[9] Lower vitamin B12 levels have also been associated with preeclampsia.[10] Vitamin B12 deficiency (concentration less than 200 pg/mL) in pregnancy is associated with a higher risk of gestational diabetes.[11] Although there are no current guidelines recommending vitamin B12 screening and monitoring in this population, these research studies clearly indicate the importance of monitoring B12 levels in pregnant women. All women should be screened for anemia; if macrocytic anemia is present, the cause is most likely vitamin B12 deficiency.

■ Certain conditions (e.g., multiple myeloma, HIV infection, pregnancy, oral contraceptive use, and diphenylhydantoin administration) may be associated with low serum vitamin B12 levels, giving the appearance of vitamin B12 deficiency. Other conditions may erroneously make vitamin B12 appear normal but are actually low; these include occult malignancy, myeloproliferative neoplasm, alcoholic liver disease, kidney disease, nitrous oxide exposure, and certain inborn errors of metabolism.

■ Symptoms and any associated anemias may take several months to improve.

PATIENT EDUCATION

- https://ods.od.nih.gov/pdf/factsheets/VitaminB12-Consumer.pdf
- https://www.health.harvard.edu/a_to_z/vitamin-b12-deficiency-a-to-z

RELATED DIAGNOSES AND ICD-10 CODES

Pernicious anemia	281.0
Vitamin B12 deficiency	281.1
Megaloblastic anemia	D53

REFERENCES

Full list of references can be accessed through Springer Publishing Company Connect™ at the following link: http://connect.springerpub.com/content/reference-book/978-0-8261-8843-4/part/part03/toc-part/ch162

---

163. VITAMIN D

Kelly Small Casler

PHYSIOLOGY REVIEW

Vitamin D is a fat-soluble vitamin needed for normal mineralization of bone and normal absorption of calcium. It also has a role in cell function, immune system homeostasis, and neuromuscular physiology. The two main forms of vitamin D are vitamin D2 (ergocalciferol) and vitamin D3 (cholecalciferol) and they can be obtained from sun exposure or from the diet (fish, eggs, and vitamin D fortified milk).[1] Vitamin D must undergo conversion in the body to become physiologically active. First, vitamin D is converted to 25-hydroxyvitamin D [25(OH)D_3], also called calcidiol, by the liver and then the kidney converts 25 (OH)D to 1,25-dihydroxyvitamin D [1,25(OH)$_2D_3$], called calcitriol (Figure 163.1). Calcitriol acts on the gastrointestinal system to influence calcium absorption from the diet.

OVERVIEW OF LABORATORY TESTS

Laboratory evaluation of vitamin D status can be assessed by 25(OH)D (CPT code 82306) or 1, 25(OH)D (CPT code 82652). In the majority of cases, 25 (OH)D should be ordered over 1,25 (OH)D because 25 (OH) D accurately reflects the stores of vitamin D in the body and is not influenced by parathyroid hormone (PTH) or other hormones, in contrast to 1,25(OH)D.[2] In rare cases, such as hyperkalemia or end stage renal disease, 1,25 (OH) D is indicated, but it will be unlikely to be abnormal unless there is severe vitamin D deficiency.

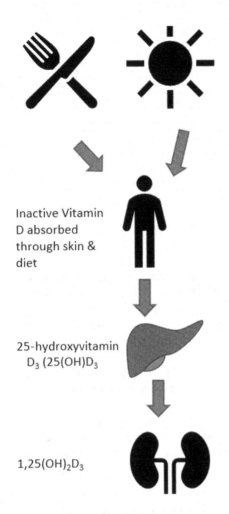

Inactive Vitamin D absorbed through skin & diet

25-hydroxyvitamin D_3 ($25(OH)D_3$)

$1,25(OH)_2D_3$

FIGURE 163.1. Vitamin D physiology.

INDICATIONS

Screening

- Universal screening is overused and discouraged by several groups due to lack of evidence to support.[3–5]
  - The United States Preventive Services Task Force determined there is insufficient evidence to universally screen adults for vitamin D deficiency.[6]
  - The United States Endocrine Society and American Society for Clinical Pathology recommend against screening individuals for vitamin D deficiency.
  - The American College of Obstetricians and Gynecologists recommends against screening pregnant individuals.[7]
  - Pediatric endocrine guidelines recommend against universal screening.[8]
- Consider targeted screening in those with vitamin D deficiency risk factors as listed in Box 163.1[8–13]
- Kidney Disease Improving Global Outcomes (KDIGO) and the National Kidney Association both recommend screening with 25 (OH)D in chronic kidney disease, but don't make frequency suggestions.[14]

Box 163.1: Risk Factors for Vitamin D Deficiency

- Antiseizure mediations
- Chronic kidney disease
- Hepatic failure
- Hyperparathyroidism
- Malabsorption (cystic fibrosis, inflammatory bowel disease, or bariatric surgery)
- Obesity (BMI >30 kg/m^2)
- Osteomalacia
- Osteoporosis
- Recurrent fractures
- Rickets

Diagnosis and Evaluation

- 25 (OH)D is used to assist in diagnosis of osteomalacia and rickets and to evaluate the cause of abnormal parathyroid hormone, phosphorus, and/or calcium values.[15–17]
- 25 (OH)D is used to evaluate for vitamin D deficiency as a contributing factor to statin-induced myalgia, although the data on this association are conflicting.[18,19]
- The evidence is conflicting regarding the association of fatigue as a symptom of vitamin D deficiency, but most research argues against evaluating 25(OH)D due to fatigue only.[20–24]
- Hypercalcemia, hyperkalemia, hypoparathyroidism, suspicion of sarcoidosis or granulomatous disease, and end-stage renal disease are the few indications for testing 1, 25 (OH) D instead of or in addition to 25 (OH) D.[2]

Monitoring

- Low levels of evidence (expert opinion) recommend monitoring vitamin D status every 3 to 4 months after initiation of vitamin D supplementation.[8,15–17]

INTERPRETATION

- Presently, there is a lack of agreement on definitions for vitamin D insufficiency/deficiency and if the category of insufficiency is really needed.[25] Table 163.1 summarizes current clinical practice interpretation

TABLE 163.1: INTERPRETATION OF 25(OH)D

	ADEQUATE LEVELS	VITAMIN D INSUFFICIENCY	VITAMIN D DEFICIENCY
The Endocrine Society[16]	≥30 ng/mL	21–29 ng/mL	≤ 20 ng/mL
Institute of Medicine and Global Consensus Group[10,11]	≥20 ng/mL	12–20 ng/mL	<12 ng/mL

guidelines although two of the three recommendations are a decade old. More recent evidence analysis supports a level less than 20 ng/mL as the cutoff for vitamin D deficiency.[3,26]

■ There is little consensus on a safe upper reference limit for 25 (OH)D. Suggestions seem to be between 50 and 80 ng/mL, but vitamin D toxicity has not been documented with levels less than 88 ng/mL.[27]

FOLLOW-UP

■ If vitamin D deficiency is diagnosed, follow-up laboratory work should include parathyroid hormone to evaluate for hyperparathyroidism, hypoparathyroidism, or osteomalacia.[8,17] PTH will be decreased in osteomalacia and hypoparathyroidism and elevated in hyperparathyroidism.

■ With severe levels of vitamin D deficiency (less than 10 to 12 ng/mL), clinicians should check PTH to evaluate for osteomalacia.[9,15] PTH will be low with osteomalacia.

■ Vitamin D levels should improve within 3 to 4 months of vitamin D replacement; if they don't, patients should be evaluated for malabsorption problems. For example, order tissue transglutaminase antibodies to evaluate for celiac disease.[28]

■ Evaluate for hypercalcemia and hypercalciuria if vitamin D toxicity is identified.

■ Since vitamin D levels influence calcium absorption, evaluation for hypocalcemia is warranted and vitamin D deficiency is noted.

PEARLS & PITFALLS

■ The Black population has lower baseline levels of 25 (OH) D compared to other populations, but this has not been shown to correlate to an increased risk of fractures.[28]

■ Between 2000 and 2019, there was an 83-fold increase in vitamin D testing, much of it unnecessary screening.[29]

■ 25 (OH)D reflects vitamin D status and the amount of vitamin D obtained from food and sunlight, but does not reflect vitamin D stores.[1]

■ The National Institute of Standards and Technology released vitamin D laboratory testing standards in 2009; prior to that, there was significant variability in testing practices and reported values between laboratories.[9,21]

■ There is little risk for osteomalacia and rickets unless 25(OH)D is less than 12 ng/mL.[10]

■ Older adult patients have trouble absorbing vitamin D.[24]

■ Testing to separate out the levels of vitamin D2 and D3 are not necessary or evidence-based.[28]

■ Several studies have attempted to develop valid risk factor scoring systems to guide when it is necessary to screen for vitamin D insufficiency. More study is needed before these scoring systems are ready for practice.[30]

■ Some evidence argues it may be more cost effective to provide vitamin D supplementation in obese pediatric patients with insufficient vitamin D intake, rather than screening for deficiency.[31]

PATIENT EDUCATION

- http://www.choosingwisely.org/patient-resources/vitamin-d-tests/

RELATED DIAGNOSES AND ICD-10 CODES

Vitamin D deficiency, unspecified	E55.9
Adult osteomalacia, unspecified	M83. 9
Active rickets	E55.0

REFERENCES

Full list of references can be accessed through Springer Publishing Company Connect™ at the following link: http://connect.springerpub.com/content/reference-book/ 978-0-8261-8843-4/part/part03/toc-part/ch163

---

164. VON WILLEBRAND DISEASE PANELS

Samara Linnell and Kate Sustersic Gawlik

PHYSIOLOGY REVIEW

Blood components are essential for oxygen and nutrient transport. There are various proteins and cell fragments found in the blood that react with one another to form a clot to stop bleeding, and to achieve a balance between clotting and bleeding, known as homeostasis.[1] Sometimes there are congenital genetic mutations that can occur, where individuals do not have enough of the needed clotting components and are at increased risk for bleeding disorders.[2] One of the proteins that blood needs in order to clot is von Willebrand factor (VWF). VWF helps a clot form by increasing platelet aggregation and by serving as a carrier protein for coagulation factor VIII, stabilizing its procoagulant activity. The major function of VWF is serving as adhesive glycoprotein for platelet–platelet and platelet to vessel hemostatic interactions. VWF protein originates in the endothelium and megakaryocytes and is stored in the alpha platelet granules.[1] When people have either a deficiency in VWF or the VWF protein does not properly function, they have von Willebrand disease (VWD).

There are three main types and several subtypes of VWD. Type 1 is the most common type (85% of VWD) and is an autosomal inherited disorder that occurs in roughly one in 100 individuals. Both men and women are equally affected.[2-5] This is the mildest form of VWD and is due to low levels of VWF. These individuals may also have a deficiency of factor VIII. Type 2 has four subtypes (2A, 2B, 2C, and 2D) and occurs when VWF does not properly function. Type 3 is the least common type (3% of VWD) and is where the person has little to no

VWF and low levels of factor VIII. This is the most severe form of VWD.[2] There is also a rare occurrence of acquired von Willebrand syndrome (or acquired VWD) where it develops alongside other conditions, such as lymphoproliferative, autoimmune, myeloproliferative, or cardiovascular disorders.[6] The acquired form may be related to a medication or even nonhematologic malignancies. It is believed to happen when a presence of antibodies lessens VWF.[4] When there is not enough of VWF, it can lessen the amount of factor VIII available and contribute further to bleeding risk in individuals. Individuals with VWD usually bleed with trauma rather than having spontaneous bleeding. However, the disease presents with varying degrees of severity.[3,4] VWF is also an acute phase reactant so it can be elevated during times of inflammation and/or stress.

OVERVIEW OF LABORATORY TESTS

Initial laboratory evaluation of VWD should be completed using the following laboratory tests[4,7,8]:

- vWF antigen (vWF:Ag) (CPT code 85246) is a latex immunoassay that measures the quantity of VWF protein.
- Ristocetin cofactor (RCoF) (also known as von Willebrand factor activity) helps test the functioning of the VWF protein activity (CPT code 85245).
- Factor VIII (FVIII) is an activity-clotting factor in the cascade that is important in joining factor IX and X to help form a clot (CPT code 85335).

These laboratory tests in combination are useful for the diagnosis of VWD, differentiation of VWD subtype, and differentiation of VWD from hemophilia A.

INDICATIONS

Screening

The evidence does not support universal or routine use of screening for VWD. Consider targeted screening for VWD when there is:

- Positive family history of VWD, bleeding disorder, or bleeding including any extended family members[4]

Diagnosis and Evaluation

Consider screening with an initial VWD evaluation with the following patients:[3-5,8]

- Presenting with unknown bleeding disorder or bleeding problem
- Any individual with menorrhagia history that is consistent off oral contraceptives
- Any individual with International Society of Thrombosis and Haemostasis (ISTH)/ Scientific Standardization Committee (SSC) bleeding assessment tool score of 6 or greater
- Following any postpartum hemorrhage
- Reported personal history of VWD but without supporting documentation
- Abnormal laboratory result(s) (e.g., prolonged activated partial thromboplastin time [aPTT] that corrects on 1:1 mixing study, high/low platelet count)
- Liver or kidney disease

■ Blood or bone marrow disorder
■ With two or more of the following reported signs/symptoms: easy bruising, bruises with lumps, bleeding gums, unexplained blood in the stool, spontaneous nose bleeds, prolonged bleeding, heavy menses, excessive postoperative bleeding, heavy bleeding following dental extractions, joint bleeds, iron deficiency or unexplained anemia, or history of blood transfusions or postpartum hemorrhage

Monitoring

■ Monitoring of VWD levels should be considered in the following circumstances:
  ● In known VWD patient during third trimester pregnancy to formulate a delivery plan
  ● Following major surgery and when treating with factor
  ● During stimate or desmopressin (DDAVP) challenge to determine how significantly levels respond to treatment
  ● Prior to surgery/procedures to form a pre/post-surgery plan
  ● Postoperatively to determine treatment needs, especially major surgery
  ● To formulate a neuro-axial anesthesia plan
  ● To determine therapeutic efficacy of treatment with DDAVP or VWF concentrates in patients with VWD

INTERPRETATION

Establishing the diagnosis of VWD in individuals who have type 2 and type 3 subtypes can typically be determined based on the initial VWD tests.[4] Type 1 diagnosis is often more difficult due to a variety of contributing factors but is typically defined as individuals who have VWF levels below 30 IU/dL.[4] As previously noted a combination of vWF:Ag, RCoF, and factor VIII can be used to assist in both diagnosis and differentiation of type of VWD. Reference values can be found at https://www.nhlbi.nih.gov/health-topics/diagnosis-evaluation-and-management-of-von-willebrand-disease/von-willebrand-disease-full-report.

■ If VWD does not seem to be the accurate diagnosis based on the VWF initial panel, consider a different clotting factor deficiency or possible delta storage pool platelet deficiency disorder.[1]
■ Individuals of blood group "O" may have lower plasma von Willebrand factor (VWF) antigen than those of other ABO blood groups. Normal individuals of blood group "O" may have plasma VWF antigen as low as 40% to 50%.[4]
■ Aging increases VWF levels, which can move into the normal reference range the older a person gets. This does not mean they no longer have VWD; therefore, they should always be reevaluated for any surgeries and similar situations.
■ DDAVP will increase VWF levels.
■ Refer to https://www.nhlbi.nih.gov/health-topics/diagnosis-evaluation-and-management-of-von-willebrand-disease/von-willebrand-disease-full-report for a laboratory assessment algorithm.

FOLLOW-UP

- Since VWF is an acute phase reactant, it can be falsely elevated due to stress or inflammation and may require repeat testing to identify low levels. Refer to Table 164.1 for causes of elevated VWF.
- Reevaluate previous and current bleeding issues to ensure treatment is tailored to the individual. Not everyone, for example, will respond well to DDAVP and/or antifibrinolytics such as tranexamic acid (Lysteda).[7] Gathering details about an individual's bleeding, such as menstrual cycles and nose bleeds, will help to guide ongoing treatment. Past surgery bleeding information will help guide upcoming treatments for future procedures and surgeries. If they are experiencing ongoing bleeding issues, they should be screened for and followed for any iron deficiency anemia (IDA) with a CBC and iron studies.
- When one or more of the initial VWF tests come back abnormal, the patient should be referred to a hematology specialist for specialized VWD studies including VWF:RCo to VWF:Ag ratio, multimer distribution, collagen binding, RIPA or platelet binding, FVIII binding, platelet VWF studies, and DNA sequencing of the VWF gene.

PEARLS & PITFALLS

- Laboratory testing should be guided by the patient history and physical examination findings.[4]
- Perform a bleeding assessment tool (BAT) at the office visit to better define the individual bleeding disorder.[8]
- If a person has a very severe bleeding history and only borderline VWF levels, consider additional testing to better define their type of VWD/genetic testing. Treatment should be considered based on severity of bleeding history and borderline levels. Women are affected by their VWD more due to having menstrual cycles and heavy bleeding issues.
- When taking a menstrual history, consider "heavy cycles" as being subjective and obtain detailed objective data: Is there any flooding? How often do pads and/or tampons need to be changed; duration of cycle;

TABLE 164.1: CAUSES OF INCREASED AND DECREASED LEVELS OF VON WILLEBRAND FACTOR

DECREASED LEVELS OF VWF	INCREASED LEVELS OF VWF
Congenital von Willebrand disease	• Estrogen/oral contraceptive use
• Types 1, 2, and 3	• Exercise
Acquired von Willebrand disease (AVWD)	• Excessive crying in a child
• Autoimmune disorders	• Inflammation (acute-phase reactant)
• Hypothyroidism	• Liver disease
• Lymphoproliferative disorders	• Pregnancy
• Monoclonal gammopathies	• Stress/Anxiety
	• Surgery
	• Thrombotic thrombocytopenic purpura/hemolytic uremic syndrome
	• Vasculitis

VWF, von Willebrand factor.

regular or irregular; always been this pattern? Occasionally a woman will say she does not have heavy cycles, but when asked these details, it is considered heavy.
■ Consider referral to hematologist after screening for consultation.

PATIENT EDUCATION

■ https://www.cdc.gov/ncbddd/vwd/facts.html
■ https://www.mayoclinic.org/diseases-conditions/von-willebrand
  -disease/symptoms-causes/syc-20354978

RELATED DIAGNOSES AND ICD-10 CODES

Von Willebrand disease	D68.0
Menorrhagia	N92.0
Epistaxsis	R04.0
Coagulation defect, unspecified	D68.9

REFERENCES

Full list of references can be accessed through Springer Publishing Company Connect™ at the following link: http://connect.springerpub.com/content/reference-book/
978-0-8261-8843-4/part/part03/toc-part/ch164

165. WHITE BLOOD CELLS AND THE DIFFERENTIAL COUNT

Kelly Small Casler

PATHOPHYSIOLOGY REVIEW

White blood cells (WBCs), or leukocytes, are responsible for the immune response of the human body. There are five types of WBCs. Two types (monocytes and lymphocytes) are categorized as agranulocytes, due to a lack of granules in their cytoplasm. The other three types (neutrophils, basophils, and eosinophils) are categorized as granulocytes, and play a large role in acute infection response. Neutrophils have the largest role, being initially recruited to the site of infection. If too many neutrophils are consumed during the infection response, the bone marrow increases production and releases them into circulation at a more immature stage.[1] This results in what is often termed a "left shift" where more bands (immature neutrophils), metamyelocytes, and/or myelocytes are seen in circulation than usual. A left shift is usually only seen in more severe bacterial infections since normally, the body should have enough circulating mature neutrophils to target infection.[1] With bacterial infection, WBC count initially decreases and then eventually becomes elevated. If infection is severe enough for a left shift to occur, it will usually be seen in the first 12 to 24 hours while the WBC is decreased and before the WBC recovers/elevates. Resolution of infection is signaled by movement of the WBC back to normal reference intervals and disappearance of the left shift.[1,2]

OVERVIEW OF LABORATORY TESTS

The numbers of WBCs are most often measured as a component of the complete blood count (CBC). A total WBC number can also be provided through point-of-care testing; this method is popular in clinics where frequent monitoring is needed (e.g., oncology).[3] When a CBC is ordered with a differential, a count and percentage of the five different subtypes of WBCs is provided. Differentials can be performed automatically (by laboratory machine) or manually (by laboratory staff), the latter being more expensive.[4] Automated differentials are generally more accurate than manual, but there are a handful of conditions that require a manual differential, such as when leukemia or platelet clumping is suspected.[5] Laboratory analyzers will also flag specimen reports for a manual differential if certain abnormalities are detected, although this process is not perfect.[5-7]

INDICATIONS

Screening
■ Used to screen newborns at risk for neonatal sepsis.[8]

Diagnosis and Evaluation
■ Used to assist in the differential diagnosis when infection is suspected.
■ Used to evaluate a variety of signs and symptoms including fatigue, hepatosplenomegaly, recurrent infections, and fever (especially if source undetermined).
■ A differential count is rarely needed when ordering an initial evaluation of a CBC or WBC, but it is helpful in the differential diagnosis if leukocytosis/leukopenia is detected.[9]

Monitoring
■ Used in monitoring for side effects of certain medications such as disease-modifying anti-rheumatic drugs (DMARDS).[10,11]
■ Used in monitoring of absolute neutrophil count (ANC) to detect the rare complication of agranulocytosis during clozapine administration. Monitor weekly for the first 6 months of clozapine administration, then every 2 weeks for the next 6 months and then monthly.[12]
■ Used along with platelets and red blood cell counts to monitor for side effects of chemotherapy. Exact intervals of monitoring vary with agent.[13]
■ A CBC with WBC differential is monitored every 4 to 12 weeks in patients on hydroxyurea therapy for sickle cell disease.[14]
■ Monitor for resolution of abnormalities after resolution of underlying event.

INTERPRETATION

- See Tables 165.1, 165.2,[15] and 165.3 for one set of reference intervals and possible causes of abnormal results. It is recommended to use reference intervals provided by the clinician's laboratory.
- Leukemoid reaction (leukocytosis of 50 to 100 × 10³ cells/μL) can be seen in the first few hours to days of certain severe infections.
- Hyperleukocytosis (leukocytosis greater than 100 × 10³ cells/μL) is a clinical emergency due to the risk of leukostasis. The problem is only usually seen in leukemias and myeloproliferative disorders.[16]
- Elevations of WBCs or ANC are sometimes used to evaluate for bacterial infection. However, the sensitivity and specificity are not strong.
  - For a WBC greater than 15 × 10³ cells/μL, there is a 64% to 82% sensitivity and 67% to 75% specificity for bacterial infection. The positive likelihood ratio (LR) is 1.9 to 2.7.[17]
  - For a ANC greater than 10 × 10³ cells/μL, there is a sensitivity of 64% to 76% and specificity of 76% to 81% with positive LR of 3 to 3.3.[17]
- Neutropenia is graded by severity of ANC reductions on the WBC differential and helps determine susceptibility to severe infection
  - **Mild:** ANC 1,000 to 2,000 cells (1 to 2 × 10³ cells/μL)
  - **Moderate:** 500 to 1,000 cells (0.5 to 1.0 × 10³ cells/μL)
  - **Severe (agranulocytosis):** less than 500 cells (less than 0.5 × 10³ cells/μL)

FOLLOW-UP

- When infection is severe enough to cause a left shift, it may be beneficial to evaluate for C-reactive protein elevations as a sign of bacterial infection.[1]
- Unexplained, persistent elevations or decreases should warrant consideration for hematology referral.

PEARLS & PITFALLS

- In one study for CBC evaluation upon admission to neonatal intensive care, cord blood provided equivalent accuracy compared to venous blood.[18]
- Pseudoleukopenia is possible with conditions that cause cryoglobulin agglutination while pseudoleukocytosis can be seen in platelet clumping.[19]

TABLE 165.1: INTERPRETATION OF WHITE BLOOD CELL ABNORMALITIES	
LEUKOPENIA[13,28]	**LEUKOCYTOSIS***[,15,28]
Deficiencies of vitamin B12, copper, or folate	Chronic inflammatory conditions
Immune deficiencies and autoimmune conditions	Chronic smokers
Infections	Early viral response
Leukemia	Medications (most common: corticosteroids, lithium, beta agonists)
Medications	Stress (causes neutrophilia)

*Most commonly due either to neutrophilia or lymphocytosis.

TABLE 165.2: INTERPRETATION OF WHITE BLOOD CELL DIFFERENTIAL ABNORMALITIES—GRANULOCYTES (ALSO CALLED POLYMORPHONUCLEAR CELLS)

GRANULOCYTE (PHYSIOLOGY)	REFERENCE INTERVALS[20] (×10³ CELLS/μL)	TERM USED IF LOW; POSSIBLE CAUSES	TERM USED IF HIGH; POSSIBLE CAUSES
Neutrophils (Phagocytosis/ "First responders")	Total: 1.8–7.7 Bands: 0–0.7	**Neutrophilia** • Bone marrow stimulation, infection (viral or bacterial) • Inflammation • Asplenia (decreased removal of cells) • Medications (steroids) • Stress • Autoimmune disease • Leukemia • Smoking	**Neutrophilia** • Bone marrow stimulation, infection (viral or bacterial) • Inflammation • Asplenia (decreased removal of cells) • Medications (steroids) • Stress • Autoimmune disease • Leukemia • Smoking
Eosinophils (Binds with IgE to target parasites)	0.0–0.45	**Eosinopenia*** • Bacterial infections (co-occurring leukocytosis) • Stress reactions • Medications (steroid) • Nutrition deficiency	**Eosinophilia** • Menstruation • Eosinophilic esophagitis • **C**: connective tissue disease • **H**: helinthic (parasites) • **I**: idiopathic • **N**: neoplasia (leukemia) • **A**: allergies/asthma medications
Basophils (Histamine/ prostaglandin release)	0.01–0.2	**Basopenia*** • Ovulation • Nutrition • Glucocorticoids	**Basophilia** • CML • Parasites • Allergic conditions • Oral contraceptive pills • Hodgkin's disease

*Can be difficult to define since 0 is considered normal range.

CML, chronic myelogenous leukemia; WBC, white blood cell.

Source: Data from Vajpayee N, Graham SS, Bern S. Basic examination of blood and bone marrow. In: McPherson RA, Pincus MR, eds. *Henry's Clinical Diagnosis and Management by Laboratory Methods.* 23rd ed. Elsevier; 2017:510–539.

- ▪ WBC normal ranges do differ by age and race, but are not influenced by gender as with red blood cells (RBC).[20] Research is ongoing on developing more accurate reference ranges by decades of age.[21]
- ▪ Elevations in the ANC, WBC count, and band count, when used as combined findings, may predict bacterial infection.[22] The following have been proposed for cutoffs for prediction: WBC greater than 15 to 20 × 10³ cells/μL, bands greater than 1,500 cells (1.5 × 10³ cells/μL), and band:neutrophil ratio greater than 0.2.[17]

TABLE 165.3: DIAGNOSIS OF WHITE BLOOD CELL DIFFERENTIAL ABNORMALITIES—AGRANULOCYTES

AGRANULOCYTE (PHYSIOLOGY)	REFERENCE INTERVALS[20] (×10³ CELLS/µL)	TERM USED IF LOW; POSSIBLE CAUSES	TERM USED IF HIGH; POSSIBLE CAUSES
Lymphocytes (B cells, antibodies; T/NK cells, humoral immunity)	1.0–4.8	**Lymphocytopenia** • Steroids; recent infection • HIV/AIDs (T cells); humoral immune deficiency (B cells) • Autoimmune • Aplastic anemia	**Lymphocytosis** • Leukemia • Adrenal problems • Infection (esp. viral), hypersensitivity reactions • Splenomegaly can sequest granulocyte causing a relative lymphocytosis • Atypical lymphocytes • Smoking
Monocytes/ Macrophages (Phagocytosis, cytokine production, antigen presentation)	0.0–0.8	**Monocytopenia** • Steroids • Infections • Aplastic anemia, AML • Menstruation	**Monocytosis** • Asplenia • Infection recovery • Cushing syndrome • Stress response • Viral syndrome • Smoking • Autommune conditions • Infection with EBV, protozoa, rickettsia, or TB • CML (with levels >1 or 10%)

AIDS, acquired immunodeficiency syndrome; CML, chronic myelogenous leukemia; EBV, Epstein-Barr virus; HIV, human immunodeficiency virus; NK, natural killer cells; TB, tuberculosis.

Sources: Data from McPherson RA, Pincus MR, eds. *Henry's Clinical Diagnosis and Management by Laboratory Methods.* 23rd ed. Elsevier; 2017; Rao LV, Snyder LM, eds. *Wallach's Interpretation of Diagnostic Tests: Pathways to Arriving at a Clinical Diagnosis.* 11th ed. Wolters Kluwer; 2021.

- Leukocytosis can be seen in post-splenectomy for several months (post-splenectomy results in more leukocytes in circulation since they are not being stored in the spleen, as usual).[16]
- Band count can be normal even in serious bacterial infections such as infective endocarditis and meningitis.[23,24]
- Band count can rise postoperatively or after parenteral nutrition.[23,24]
- When considering differential diagnoses related to abnormalities in WBCs, make sure to consider whether it is an acute or chronic change and the clinical findings of the patient.[16]
- In studies, Black populations have been found to have a lower baseline neutrophil count than White populations.[25]
- The expense of monitoring for clozapine-induced agranulocytosis often leads to alternative medicines being chosen.[26]

- Automated differentials can underestimate band counts.[4]
- Noninvasive monitoring of WBC that doesn't require blood draw is a focus of current research.[27]

PATIENT EDUCATION

- https://www.redcrossblood.org/donate-blood/dlp/white-cells-and -granulocytes.html

RELATED DIAGNOSES AND ICD-10 CODES

Fever	R50.9
Fatigue	R53.83
Leukocytosis	D72.829
Leukopenia	D72.819

REFERENCES

Full list of references can be accessed through Springer Publishing Company Connect™ at the following link: http://connect.springerpub.com/content/reference-book/ 978-0-8261-8843-4/part/part03/toc-part/ch165

166. WEST NILE VIRUS

Catherine A. Stubin

PATHOPHYSIOLOGY REVIEW

West Nile virus (WNV) is an RNA virus belonging to the family *Flaviviridae* of viruses, and is the leading cause of arthropod-borne viral illness in the continental United States.[1-3] WNV is primarily transmitted to humans by mosquitoes that have bitten infected birds or infected other diseased humans.[3] The virus is not passed through handling or consumption of infected birds or directly from person-to-person; however, there have been cases of WNV being transmitted to others through blood donations, organ transplants, and from a mother to child during pregnancy, delivery, or through breast milk.[1,4]

An estimated 70% to 80% of human WNV infections are asymptomatic.[1,2,5] Symptomatic patients usually develop mild manifestations which include fever, headache, myalgia, arthralgia, skin rash, and lymphadenopathy that can last a few days to several weeks and usually subside on their own.[5] Sensorineural hearing loss has occasionally been reported in association with WNV infection.[6] The incubation period for WNV disease is typically 2 to 6 days but ranges from 2 to 14 days and can be several weeks in immunocompromised patients.[5]

Less than 1% of WNV-infected patients develop West Nile neuroinvasive disease, which typically presents as encephalitis, meningitis, or acute flaccid paralysis.[1,2] Common symptoms of West Nile neuroinvasive disease may include those symptoms generally seen in WNV with the addition of confusion, weakness, numbness, and tremors.[2,4] Less common symptoms include imbalance, paresthesias, focal sensory loss, and ataxia, while uncommon symptoms include seizures, coma, para- or tetraplegia, and parkinsonism.[5,7] Risk factors for developing West Nile neuroinvasive disease from WNV infection include older age, history of solid organ transplantation, and other immunosuppressive conditions.[5,8] WNV disease in organ transplant recipients has been associated with a high incidence (70%) of West Nile neuroinvasive disease, an incidence much greater than the 1% reported in the general population.[8]

West Nile neuroinvasive disease occurs in all age groups and both sexes but more often impacts older persons and males, particularly older men.[1,5] The association between increasing age and increasing West Nile neuroinvasive disease incidence is likely the result of differences in immunity that occur with aging.[1,2] The reason for the higher incidence of this neuroinvasive disease among males is unknown.[1,2] The prognosis for patients with severe West Nile neuroinvasive disease is generally poor. Hospitalization rates for patients with this neuroinvasive disease are high (greater than 85%) in all age groups, but mortality rates escalate significantly with increasing age.[1,2] There is no effective therapy for West Nile neuroinvasive disease,[2,9] and only 37% of individuals with this disease will experience full recovery of cognitive, physical, and functional domains.[7,10]

There are no licensed human vaccines to prevent WNV and no specific treatments for WNV.[1,4,5,10] The patient is generally treated with only supportive care. WNV disease is a nationally notifiable condition, and cases are reported to the Centers for Disease Control and Prevention (CDC) by local public health authorities.[1,5,10]

OVERVIEW OF LABORATORY TESTS

Antibody Testing

Antibody testing is primarily used to help diagnose a current or recent infection. WNV IgM antibody testing (CPT code 86789) is the primary test performed on the serum or cerebrospinal fluid (CSF) of symptomatic patients.[5,11] IgM antibodies, the first to be produced by the immune system in response to a WNV infection, are usually detectable 3 to 8 days after onset of illness and persist for 30 to 90 days.[5,11] The level of antibody continues to rise for a short time period and will then taper off and fall below detectable levels.

The presence of WNV-specific IgM in blood or CSF provides good evidence of recent infection but may also be positive after infection with any related arboviruses (such as the St. Louis Encephalitis virus and Japanese Encephalitis virus), or from nonspecific reactivity.[5,12] For this reason, whenever possible, positive WNV IgM tests should be confirmed by another method before a diagnosis is established and officially reported to the CDC. The confirmatory neutralization antibody test, plaque-reduction neutralization testing (PRNT), is performed at state public health or CDC laboratories.[12] PRNT can help determine the specific infecting flavivirus by confirming whether the detected antibodies are capable of binding and inactivating the WNV.[5,12] It is not possible to know with certainty if WNV IgM positives reflect true WNV positives without performing PRNTs.[12]

WNV IgG antibodies (CPT code 86788) generally are detected shortly after IgM antibodies and persist for many years following a symptomatic or asymptomatic infection.[11] Testing for WNV IgG antibodies can sometimes be used in conjunction with IgM testing to help detect the presence of a recent or previous WNV infection. The IgG WNV test may be ordered once with the IgM test or ordered initially and then again 2 to 4 weeks later to determine if titers are rising or falling.[5] When a blood or organ recipient becomes infected with WNV, both IgM and IgG antibodies may be ordered on the donor, who is frequently asymptomatic, to help determine whether that person was the source of the infection.[11]

NUCLEIC ACID AMPLIFICATION

Reverse Transcriptase-Polymerase Chain Reaction

A nucleic acid amplification test (NAAT) (CPT code 87798) amplifies and measures the WNV's genetic material (RNA) to detect the presence of the virus.[11,12] Nucleic acid testing can use many different methods to amplify nucleic acids and detect the virus, including reverse transcription polymerase chain reaction (RT-PCR). RT-PCR can be performed on serum, CSF, and tissue specimens that are collected early in the course of illness and, if results are positive, can confirm an infection with the virus often before antibodies to the virus are detectable.[5] Within the first few days of illness, WNV RNA may be detected in CSF or serum using RT-PCR; however, the likelihood of detection using this method is relatively low as there must be a certain amount of virus present in the sample in order to detect it and viral RNA is often absent by the time of symptom onset.[5,12,13] Since humans are secondary hosts of WNV (birds are the primary hosts), virus levels in humans are usually relatively low and do not persist for very long.[13]

RT-PCR is most useful as a screen for WNV in donated units of blood, tissue, or organs; for detecting WNV in the blood of living tissue and organ donors; and for testing birds and mosquito pools to detect the presence and spread of WNV in the community.[13] Driven by a continuous high number of WNV infection cases, an all-year universal donor screening has been implemented nationwide in the United States.[4,11] Donors suspected of having WNV in their blood are notified and referred for counseling.[11] As an additional tool in reducing WNV in the blood supply, blood collection centers have recently started asking potential donors during WNV season if they have had symptoms of a WNV infection, such as a recent fever or headache.[11] RT-PCR may also be used to test the blood or tissues of a patient postmortem to determine whether WNV may have caused or contributed to their death.[13]

Other Testing for West Nile Virus Disease

Viral cultures and immunohistochemistry can also be used to detect WNV, although they are not used in routine testing. Viral cultures can be performed on serum, CSF, and tissue specimens that are collected early in the course of illness and, if results are positive, can confirm an infection. Immunohistochemistry (IHC) can detect WNV antigen in formalin-fixed tissue.[5]

INDICATIONS

Screening

■ There is no indication for universal, targeted, or asymptomatic screening.

Diagnosis and Evaluation

WNV illness should be examined in any person with a febrile or acute neurologic illness who has had recent exposure to mosquitoes, blood transfusion, or organ transplantation, especially during the summer months in areas where virus activity has been reported.[5]

■ WNV should also be considered in any infant born to a mother infected with WNV during pregnancy or while breastfeeding.
■ Other arboviruses, such as the St. Louis Encephalitis virus and Japanese Encephalitis virus, should also be contemplated in the differential etiology of suspected WNV disease.
■ Routine clinical laboratory studies are nonspecific for the diagnosis of WNV illness.[5]
■ In patients with West Nile neuroinvasive disease, CSF examination also shows lymphocytic pleocytosis, but neutrophils may predominate early in the course of illness.[12]
■ Brain magnetic resonance imaging is frequently normal, but signal abnormalities in the basal ganglia, thalamus, and brainstem may be seen in patients with encephalitis, and in the anterior spinal cord in patients with poliomyelitis.[5]

Monitoring

■ Once diagnosed, no further monitoring is needed.

INTERPRETATION

■ For laboratory case confirmation, at least one of the following four criteria must be met[1,2]:
  ● Isolation of the virus from blood or CSF
  ● Detection of WNV nucleic acid in blood or CSF
  ● Detection of WNV specific IgM antibodies in CSF
  ● Detection of anti-WNV IgM antibodies in high titer and detection of anti-WNV IgG antibodies, and confirmation by neutralization
■ Probable cases have virus-specific IgM antibodies in CSF or serum, but with no further testing performed.[1,2]

Refer to Table 166.1[14,15] for reference ranges and interpretation criteria.

FOLLOW-UP

There is no recommendation for follow-up testing.

PEARLS & PITFALLS

■ WNV epidemics are a substantial economic burden on healthcare resources.[16]

TABLE 166.1: TEST TYPES, REFERENCE INTERVALS, AND INTERPRETIVE CRITERIA

TEST TYPE	RANGE	INTERPRETIVE CRITERIA
West Nile Virus Antibodies (IgM) Serum and CSF	West Nile Virus Ab (IgM) <0.90	**<0.90:** Antibody not detected **0.90–1.10:** Equivocal **>1.10:** Antibody detected
West Nile Virus Antibodies (IgG) Serum and CSF	West Nile Virus Ab (IgG) <1.30	**<1.30:** Antibody not detected **1.30–1.49:** Equivocal **>1.49:** Antibody detected
Reverse Transcriptase-Polymerase Chain Reaction (RT-PCR)		**Mean detection:** 7.43 copies/mL 95%; detection cutoff: 28.16 copies/mL

Source: Quest Diagnostics. *West Nile Virus.* https://testdirectory.questdiagnostics.com

- Clinicians should remain attentive for the possible transmission of WNV through blood transfusion or organ transplantation, and promptly report these cases to the appropriate state and local health departments.[5]
- Clinicians should consider arboviral infections in patients with aseptic meningitis or encephalitis, perform appropriate diagnostic testing, and report cases to state and local health departments.[17]
- WNV neuroinvasive disease might be undiagnosed due to either lack of testing or inappropriate testing.[9,17]
- WNV prevention depends on community efforts to reduce mosquito populations and blood donation screening to minimize alternative routes of transmission.[1]

PATIENT EDUCATION

- https://www.cdc.gov/westnile/resourcepages/communication-resources.html
- https://www.cdc.gov/westnile/resources/pdfs/wnvfactsheet_508.pdf
- https://www.doh.wa.gov/YouandYourFamily/IllnessandDisease/WestNileVirus/EducationandMediaMaterials

RELATED DIAGNOSES AND ICD-10 CODES

West Nile virus infection, unspecified	A92.30[18]
West Nile virus infection with encephalitis	A92.31[18]
West Nile virus infection with other neurologic manifestation	A92.32[18]
West Nile virus infection with other complications	A92.39[18]
Mosquito-borne viral fever, unspecified	A92.9[18]

REFERENCES

Full list of references can be accessed through Springer Publishing Company Connect™ at the following link: http://connect.springerpub.com/content/reference-book/978-0-8261-8843-4/part/part03/toc-part/ch166

167. ZIKA VIRUS

Lindsay Jamison Wolf

PATHOPHYSIOLOGY REVIEW

Zika virus is a virus in the genus Flavivirus and in the family Flaviviridae.[1] In 1947, Zika virus was isolated from a nonhuman primate for the very first time. The following year, in 1948, in the continent of Africa, Zika virus was isolated from mosquitos.[1] Zika virus is primarily spread through the bite of an infected Aedes species mosquito (Ae. *Aegypti* and Ae. *Albopictus*).[1] Zika virus can be sexually transmitted from an infected individual to their sexual partner, even if this individual remains asymptomatic from infection.[2] Additionally, Zika virus can be passed perinatally from an infected woman to their fetus. Infection during pregnancy can cause birth defects and/or fetal demise.[2] Other modes of transmission include through blood and/or blood products, organ transplant, and laboratory exposure.[3]

Zika RNA persists nearly three times longer in a pregnant woman's serum than a nonpregnant individual. Because of this, and the severity of risks to the unborn fetus, the diagnostic approach for the pregnant woman differs from that of nonpregnant individuals.[4,5] The clinical presentation of Zika virus includes fever, rash, headache, arthralgia, conjunctivitis, and muscle pain.[6-8]

Similar to the clinical manifestations of the Zika virus, Dengue virus has been shown to co-circulate with the Zika and present similar physical symptoms including high fever, severe muscle pain, and headache. Unlike Zika virus, Dengue virus has been known to be associated with hemorrhage; however, it is not typically associated with conjunctivitis like the Zika virus.[9] For the similar clinical presentation and strong co-circulation potential, it is recommended to concurrently test for Dengue virus and Zika virus in some cases.

OVERVIEW OF LABORATORY TESTS

There are several different tests that can be used to determine the diagnosis of Zika virus: the real time reverse-transcription polymerase chain reaction (rRT-PCR) for Zika RNA (CPT code 87662), Zika serology by Zika immunoglobulin M (IgM) (CPT code 86794), and the plaque reduction neutralization test (PRNT).[6,10-16] Zika RNA's can be detected in urine after viremia has waned to an undetectable level.[6] Nucleic acid amplification test (NAAT) is a general term used to describe all molecular tests that detect viral genomic material. NAAT is the preferred method of diagnosis because it can confirm evidence of infection. Zika virus testing should not be performed on patient populations outside of the recommendations.[12] Different tests should be ordered based on risk factors, exposures, length of time since symptoms started, and travel history (Table 167.1).

The World Health Organization (WHO) has established the sensitivity of laboratory tests, but limited information on the diagnostic accuracy of laboratory tests for congenital Zika virus in fetuses and neonates exists. The WHO has made this a research priority, but there are currently no systematic reviews that address this accuracy.[3] The text that follows provides guidance on neonatal testing:

Laboratory testing for Zika virus infection in the neonate includes the following[17]:

- Serum and urine for Zika virus RNA via real-time rRT-PCR
- Serum Zika virus immunoglobulin M (IgM) enzyme-linked immunosorbent assay (ELISA)
- Cerebrospinal fluid (CSF) RNA (via rRT-PCR) as well as Zika virus IgM

TABLE 167.1: ZIKA TESTING BASED ON RISK FACTORS, EXPOSURES, AND TRAVEL HISTORY

CASE	IGM	RRT-PCR	NAAT
Asymptomatic pregnant persons living in or with recent travel to United States and its territories	Not recommended	Not recommended	Not recommended
Asymptomatic pregnant persons with recent travel to an area with Zika risk	Not recommended	Not recommended	Not recommended
Symptomatic pregnant women who had recent travel to areas with active Dengue transmission and risk of Zika	Zika not recommended Dengue only*	Not recommended	Dengue – blood** Zika – urine**
Symptomatic pregnant women who have had sexual intercourse with someone who lives in or recent travel to Zika risk area	Not recommended	Not recommended	Zika only***
Pregnant women who have a fetus with prenatal ultrasound consistent with congenital Zika virus infection who live in or traveled to area of Zika risk	Zika blood	Not recommended	Zika**** Blood and urine

*If positive, provides enough evidence of Dengue infection and no further testing is needed.

**Specimen should be collected ASAP after onset of symptoms and up to 12 weeks after symptom onset.

***If positive, repeat on newly extracted RNA from same specimen to rule out false positive.

****If Zika NAAT is negative and IgM positive, confirmatory PRNTs (plaque reduction neutralizing test) should be ordered.

IGM, immunoglobulin M; NAAT, nucleic acid amplification test; RRT-PCR, reverse-transcription polymerase chain reaction.

Source: Adapted from Centers for Disease Control and Prevention. Emergency preparedness and response: recognizing, managing, and reporting Zika virus infections in travelers returning from Central America, South America, the Caribbean, and Mexico. http://emergency.cdc.gov/han/han00385.asp.

■ The initial samples should be collected from the infant within the first few days after birth to distinguish between congenital, perinatal, and postnatal infection[2]

INDICATIONS

Screening

■ Zika virus testing should not be performed as part of routine preconception testing except in an epidemic region. During an epidemic, Zika virus screening should be performed at each prenatal visit.[2,10-12]

■ At prenatal visits, clinicians should verbally screen pregnant women for possible exposure to Zika.[2,10-12]

■ If travel-associated Zika virus exposure has occurred, and/or the patient lives in an endemic region, the patient should be screened for Zika virus symptoms.[2,10-12]

Diagnosis and Evaluation

■ Clinical suspicion of Zika virus based on clinical presentation, places and dates of travel, and activities.

● Symptoms of Zika virus are similar to other viruses and include an acute onset of fever, a maculopapular rash, headache, arthralgias, conjunctivitis, and/or myalgias. Symptoms last for several days to a week and are typically mild in nature. The differential diagnoses list is broad due to this common clinical presentation. Differential diagnoses should include Dengue, leptospirosis, malaria, rickettsia, measles, group A streptococcus, rubella, chikungunya virus, parvovirus, adenovirus, and enterovirus.

■ All pregnant women with symptoms of Zika virus and a positive history of sexual intercourse without a condom with a person who tested positive for the Zika virus should be screened.[10-12]

■ All patients, pregnant or not pregnant with positive symptoms and history of sexual exposure to a person who lives in or has traveled to areas of Zika virus risk, even if the person was never symptomatic, should be screened.[10-12]

■ All newborns born to mothers with positive Zika virus infection during pregnancy should be screened (see Table 167.1).[17]

■ Newborns who have clinical or neuroimaging findings indicating congenial Zika virus with a maternal epidemiologic link suggesting possible transmission (which includes paternal exposure) should be screened, regardless of maternal Zika virus test results.[18]

Monitoring

Once diagnosis has been established, no further monitoring of laboratory level(s)are needed.[1]

INTERPRETATION

■ Tables 167.2 and 167.3 provide information about infant and maternal testing results for the Zika virus.[2]

TABLE 167.2: INFANTILE ZIKA VIRUS TESTING

INFANT TEST RESULT		INTERPRETATION
NAAT	**IgM**	
Positive	Any result	Confirmed CZV
Negative	Non-negative	Probable CZV
Negative	Negative	Unlikely CZV

CZV, congenital Zika virus; IgM, immunoglobulin M; NAAT, nucleic acid amplification test.

TABLE 167.3: MATERNAL AND FETAL TISSUE TESTING FOR COMPLETED PREGNANCIES

PREGNANCY OUTCOME	IF MATERNAL ZIKA VIRUS TEST RESULT SHOW:		
	Acute Zika virus infection	Zika virus timing of infection unknown	>12 weeks after symptom onset or exposure, with either negative maternal Zika virus IgM, or no maternal testing conducted
Live birth, possible Zika virus-associated birth defects	**Placental testing**		
	Not indicated	Consider for the aid of maternal diagnosis	Not indicated
Live birth, no obvious Zika virus-associated birth defects at birth	**Placental testing**		
	Not indicated	May be considered on a case-by-case basis	Not indicated
Pregnancy loss, possible Zika virus-associated birth defects	**Placental and fetal tissue testing:**		
	Consider aiding in fetal diagnosis	Consider aiding in fetal and maternal diagnosis	Not indicated
Pregnancy loss, no obvious Zika virus-associated birth defects	**Placental and fetal tissue testing:**		
	Consider aiding in fetal diagnosis	Consider aiding in fetal and maternal diagnosis	Not indicated

(*Continued*)

TABLE 167.3: MATERNAL AND FETAL TISSUE TESTING FOR COMPLETED PREGNANCIES (*CONTINUED*)

PREGNANCY OUTCOME	IF MATERNAL ZIKA VIRUS TEST RESULT SHOW:		
Infant death following live birth	Placental and fetal autopsy tissue:		
	Consider aiding in infant diagnosis	Consider aiding in infant and maternal diagnosis	Not indicated

Source: Adapted from Ciapponi A, Matthews S, Cafferata ML, et al. Laboratory tests for diagnosis of congenital Zika virus in fetuses and neonates. *Cochrane Database of Syst Rev.* 2020;(7):CD013676. doi:10.1002/14651858.CD013676.

FOLLOW-UP

- Maternal antibodies will wane in neonatal serum after approximately 18 months. If neonatal PRNT is positive at birth, repeating the test after 18 months can confirm or rule out infection.[15]
- For the similar clinical presentation and strong co-circulation potential, it is recommended to concurrently test for Dengue virus and Zika virus in some cases. See Table 167.1 for guidance on when to run this test.

PEARLS & PITFALLS

- Clinicians should encourage pregnant patients and their partners to check the CDC website for information regarding the Zika virus prior to traveling if there is concern there may be Zika in the region in which they are traveling. The CDC website has up-to-date traveler information as well as current regional Zika virus distributions and outbreaks.
  - https://wwwnc.cdc.gov/travel/page/zika-travel-information
  - https://www.cdc.gov/zika/geo/index.html
- The CDC Zika virus tool kit can be found at https://www.cdc.gov/zika/hc-providers/index.html.
- There is no evidence of Zika virus transferring to a child from the mother through breast milk intake or breastfeeding. At the certainty of the present, evidence is low.[19]

PATIENT EDUCATION

- www.cdc.gov/zika/pdfs/fs-zika-basics.pdf
- https://www.mayoclinic.org/diseases-conditions/zika-virus/symptoms-causes/syc-20353639

RELATED DIAGNOSES AND ICD-10 CODES

Zika virus disease, Zika virus fever, Zika virus infection, Zika NOS	A92.5
Contact with and (suspected) exposure to Zika virus	Z20.821

Other specified mosquito-borne viral fever	A92.8
Other viral diseases complicating pregnancy, first trimester	O98.511
Congenital Zika virus disease	P35.4
Encounter for other suspected maternal and fetal conditions ruled out	Z03.79

REFERENCES

Full list of references can be accessed through Springer Publishing Company Connect™ at the following link: http://connect.springerpub.com/content/reference-book/978-0-8261-8843-4/part/part03/toc-part/ch167

168. ZINC

Stephanie C. Evans and Kate Sustersic Gawlik

PHYSIOLOGY REVIEW

Zinc is an essential trace element, a mineral, which is most abundant intracellularly in the body. Zinc is a critical mineral for many regulatory functions of the body. The mineral is required for the activity of over 300 enzymes in the body, and is important in immune function, protein synthesis, wound healing, and other cellular activities. Zinc supports normal growth and development beginning with pregnancy and on through adolescence. The body requires daily intake of zinc as there is no specialized storage of zinc in the body systems.[1]

The mineral is taken up through intestinal absorption if the diet is appropriate in foods with zinc. Zinc deficiency related to diet may occur when the dietary intake is not sufficient or if absorption is blocked due to high levels of copper or iron in the diet. Zinc depletion may occur in patients with large surface area burns, open wounds, or in gastrointestinal loss in diseases such as ulcerative colitis and Crohn's disease.[2] The Recommended Dietary Allowance (RDA) for adults 19+ years is 11 mg a day for men and 8 mg for women. Pregnant and lactating women require slightly more at 11 mg and 12 mg, respectively.[3,4]

OVERVIEW OF LABORATORY TESTS

Laboratory evaluation of zinc (CPT code 84630) is assessed and completed using a nonhemolyzed serum sample, using the laboratory methodology of inductively coupled plasma/mass spectrometry (ICP/MS). Hemolysis of the blood may provide false elevated zinc levels. Serum testing of zinc has limitations. It cannot detect marginal deficiency and is affected by daily fluctuations and inflammation.[5] Urine zinc is also available but is an insensitive biomarker. It is somethings used as an indicator of acute toxicity.[5]

INDICATIONS

Screening

Universal screening of zinc levels is not recommended. Consider targeted screening for zinc deficiency in individuals who are exhibiting signs of zinc deficiency and have the following risk factors[4,6-12]:

- Gastrointestinal absorption disorders or chronic diarrhea (e.g., ulcerative colitis, Crohn's disease, short bowel syndrome, malabsorption syndrome)
- Vegetarians
- Sickle cell disease
- Cystic fibrosis
- Individuals with alcohol addiction
- Burn patients with acrodermatitis
- Macular degeneration
- Pregnant and lactating individuals
- Bariatric surgery
- Older infants who are exclusively breast fed
- Individuals with sickle cell disease
- Growth retardation (infants)

Diagnosis and Evaluation

Consider diagnostic testing in individuals with signs or symptoms of either zinc deficiency or overload. Both severe zinc deficiency and zinc toxicity are rare. Signs/symptoms of zinc deficiency include[4,13,14]:

- Growth retardation
- Loss of appetite
- Impaired immune function
- Weight loss
- Delayed healing of wounds
- Smell/taste abnormalities
- Mental lethargy

More severe cases cause hair loss, diarrhea, delayed sexual maturation, impotence, hypogonadism in males, and eye and skin lesions. Zinc deficiency can still be present in the absence of clinically relevant serum zinc levels. Signs/symptoms of zinc overload include[4,13,14]:

- Nausea
- Vomiting
- Anorexia
- Abdominal cramps
- Altered iron function
- Low copper status
- Low high-density lipoproteins (HDL)
- Diarrhea
- Headaches

Monitoring

■ Zinc should be monitored at least annually in patients following bariatric surgery.[15]

INTERPRETATION

Normal Zinc Levels:

■ Age of patient 0 to 10 years: 0.60 to 1.20 mcg/mL
■ Age of patient 11 years or older: 0.66 to 1.10 mcg/mL
■ A low plasma zinc concentration is typically defined as a value less than 0.60 to 0.65 mcg/mL, but this level can vary by laboratory.
■ Zinc can be elevated or decreased due to a variety of external conditions (see Table 168.1).

FOLLOW-UP

There is no follow-up testing needed unless the deficiency is due to an underlying condition.

PEARLS & PITFALLS

■ Zinc is essential for normal smell and taste.[1]
■ Poor zinc levels will impair wound healing.[11]
■ Zinc excess is not often a clinical concern as it is excreted in feces.[3]
■ Foods rich in zinc: shellfish, oysters, crab, lobster, beef, poultry, pork, legumes, nuts, seeds, whole grains, and fortified breakfast cereals.[2,3]
■ Fortification of foods with zinc may improve the serum zinc status of populations if zinc is the only micronutrient used for fortification.
■ The findings of this review suggest that routine zinc supplementation probably made little or no difference in reducing the risk of preterm births in women of probable low zinc status.[16]

TABLE 168.1: FACTORS THAT INCREASE AND DECREASE ZINC LEVELS	
DECREASED ZINC LEVELS	**INCREASED ZINC LEVELS**
Decreased albumin	Fasting
Infection	Zinc supplementation
Inflammation	
Malnutrition	
Oral contraceptives	
Pregnancy	
Stress	

- There is not enough evidence to show that routine zinc supplementation in women results in an effect on other clinically relevant outcomes, including mortality (perinatal and neonatal), birthweight, small-for-gestational-age, or low birthweight.[8]
- There is no convincing evidence that zinc supplementation to infants or children results in improved motor, mental development, or asthma control.[17,18]
- The benefits of preventive zinc supplementation in infants outweigh the harms in areas where the risk of zinc deficiency is relatively high in infants and children especially in low resource countries.[9,10,14]

PATIENT EDUCATION

- https://ods.od.nih.gov/pdf/factsheets/Zinc-Consumer.pdf

RELATED DIAGNOSES AND ICD-10 CODES

- Endocrine, nutritional, and metabolic diseases

Malnutrition	E40-E46
Dietary zinc deficiency	E60

REFERENCES

Full list of references can be accessed through Springer Publishing Company Connect™ at the following link: http://connect.springerpub.com/content/reference-book/978-0-8261-8843-4/part/part03/toc-part/ch168

INDEX

Note: Page numbers in *italics* denote figures and tables.

- NIPS is considered a screening test only, not a diagnostic test. A positive result should be followed up by discussion with the pregnant female regarding the importance of definitive invasive testing by CVS (appropriate for gestational weeks 10 to 13) or amniocentesis (usually between gestational weeks 15 to 22).[7]
- Follow-up testing is guided by the differential diagnosis. The differential diagnosis for a positive result on cfDNA includes trisomy 21, trisomy 18, trisomy 13, sex chromosome abnormalities (Turner syndrome, Klinefelter syndrome), vanishing twin, fetal mosaicism, maternal mosaicism, and maternal cancer.[8]
- The Society for Maternal-Fetal Medicine recommends that NIPS NOT be followed by second trimester serum screening tests for aneuploidy.[9]

PEARLS & PITFALLS

- Prenatal genetic screening by a variety of approaches is appropriate to offer to all patients, regardless of maternal age.[3]
- cfDNA testing sensitivity and specificity are somewhat lower in twin pregnancies; however, data are still being collected and the test will still be informative for trisomy 21.[10]
- Laboratories reporting cfDNA results should always include data about the fetal fraction in the sample. The test can be repeated if the fetal fraction is 4% or less; however, the mother should be told that low fetal fraction can be an indication of aneuploidy.[11]
- Clinicians must be sensitive to parental beliefs and wishes regarding response to findings. cfDNA screening that shows a high likelihood of fetal aneuploidy should be followed up by genetic counseling. Additional definitive testing can further inform parental decision-making.
- Unusual results on cfDNA screening can be caused by maternal malignancy. Although this is a rare finding, it warrants additional follow-up and referral.

PATIENT EDUCATION

- https://medlineplus.gov/genetics/understanding/testing/nipt/#:~:text=Noninvasive%20prenatal%20testing%20(NIPT)%2C,in%20a%20pregnant%20woman's%20blood.

RELATED DIAGNOSES AND ICD-10 CODES

Maternal care for chromosomal abnormality in fetus, unspecified	Q35.1XX0	Trisomy 18, mosaicism	Q91.1
		Trisomy 18, translocation	Q91.2
Trisomy 21, nonmosaicism	Q90.0	Trisomy 18, unspecified	Q91.3
Trisomy 21, masoicism	Q90.1	Trisomy 13, nonmosaicism	Q91.4
Trisomy 21, translocation	Q90.2	Trisomy 13, mosaicism	Q91.5
Trisomy 18, nonmosaicism	Q91.0	Trisomy 13, translocation	Q91.6

chromosome number. Detection rate by cell-free DNA is highest for trisomy 21, ahead of trisomy 18. Trisomy 13 is rare and detection rate is limited due to low case numbers.[3]

INDICATIONS

Screening

- American College of Obstetrics and Gynecology recommends offering screening to all pregnant females after 9 to 10 weeks gestation, with appropriate patient education.[3]
- cfDNA screening can be recommended as a follow-up to an abnormal first trimester screen that includes tests of nuchal translucency by ultrasound, serum human chorionic gonadotropin (hCG), pregnancy-associated plasma protein A (PAPP-A), and alpha-fetoprotein (AFP).[3]
- cfDNA screening may be offered to those who have higher risk of a fetus with aneuploidy based on advanced maternal age, previous pregnancy losses, or history of prior pregnancy resulting in fetus with aneuploidy.

Diagnosis and Evaluation

- This is not used as a diagnostic test.

Monitoring

- This is not used for monitoring.

INTERPRETATION

- The detection rate (DR) of cfDNA for trisomy 21 in a 2017 meta-analysis (studies of singleton pregnancies) was 99.7% and the false-positive rate (FPR) was 0.04%. For trisomy 18 the DR was 97.9% and the FPR was 0.04%. For trisomy 13 the DR was 99.0% and FPR was 0.04%; for monosomy X the DR was 95.8% and the FPR was 0.14%[4]
- Sensitivity of cfDNA to detect trisomy 21, 18, and 13 was reported in an additional meta-analysis using data from the general population as well as a data set on high-risk pregnancies. For the general population, sensitivity of cfDNA to detect trisomy 21 was 99.3% while specificity was 99.9%, while sensitivity and specificity for trisomies 18 and 13 could not be determined due to low case numbers. In a high-risk population, sensitivity for trisomy 21 was 99.8%, with specificity of 99.9%; sensitivity for trisomy 18 was 97.7% and sensitivity for trisomy 13 was 97.5%. Pooled specificity for all three trisomies was 99.9%[5]
- The positive predictive value of cfDNA screening increases as maternal age increases (and as rates of aneuploidy increase). For maternal age 20, the positive predictive value for trisomy 21 is 38% to 80%; for maternal age 40, the positive predictive value rises to 91% to 99%.[3,6]

FOLLOW-UP

- If a "no-call" result is reported, usually due to low fetal fraction, the test may be repeated.